Difficult Decisions in Surgery: An Evidence-Based Approach 1

Series Editor
Mark K. Ferguson

For further volumes:
http://www.springer.com/series/13361

Mark K. Ferguson

Editor

Difficult Decisions in Thoracic Surgery

An Evidence-Based Approach

Third Edition

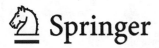 Springer

Editor
Mark K. Ferguson
Department of Surgery
The University of Chicago
Chicago, IL
USA

ISBN 978-1-4471-6403-6   ISBN 978-1-4471-6404-3   (eBook)
DOI 10.1007/978-1-4471-6404-3
Springer London Heidelberg New York Dordrecht

Library of Congress Control Number: 2014941452

Printed on acid-free paper

Springer is part of Springer Science+Business Media (www.springer.com)

To Phyllis – I could not have hoped for a better partner on this journey.

Preface

I am pleased to offer readers Edition 3 of *Difficult Decisions in Thoracic Surgery*. The series was planned to include new editions every 3–4 years, and this volume follows on the heels of two successful prior editions. I am grateful for the positive feedback from many readers who use the information in these books to help guide their clinical practices and for the compliments from educators who found the data and discussions valuable for their trainees.

The format of this volume is similar to that of the past two editions. A table of contents was developed that focused on current areas of controversy in general thoracic surgery, and authors with recognized expertise were invited to examine evidence relevant to the controversies. Their charge was to develop best practice recommendations based on published evidence, and to also provide a statement as to their personal approaches to these challenging clinical topics. One change for this edition was that authors were asked to construct their reviews based on PICO (patient population, intervention, comparator group, and outcomes measured) formatting, helping to clarify the question for the author/reader and to direct the appropriate literature search and analysis.

The authors were asked to work within a very tight timetable to ensure that the content was as up-to-date as possible. In fact, the author list and table of contents were developed less than a year before the publication date of this volume. Creating a print publication that involves so many moving parts in such a short time frame speaks to the dedication of the authors and the publisher to the concept of evidence-based medicine. They recognize the need for timely and accurate information to inform practicing physicians. I am grateful for their invaluable contributions.

Overall, 35 of the 55 clinical chapters in this volume are new compared to Edition 2, and all of the remaining 20 chapters were written by new authors. When viewed collectively, the three editions comprise over 100 unique clinical topics authored by over 140 senior authors, which makes the series a great resource for surgeons and trainees.

The success of these editions has engendered a plan to publish similar volumes in a newly developed series titled "Difficult Decisions in Surgery". The current volume is the first of the series. We hope to publish 3–4 volumes annually, ultimately covering a dozen subspecialty areas in great general surgery. The volumes will be edited by recognized authorities in their fields and new editions of each volume will be published every 3–4 years with updated information and new clinical topics. This will result in an entire library of up-to-date information of immediate use to specialty surgeons around the world. I envision that the series will serve as a teaching aid, an invaluable clinical tool, and as a source of inspiration for clinical research.

As always, I am grateful to my colleagues nationally and internationally for their friendship and cooperation. I am indebted to our trainees, who continue to ask important questions that illustrate the wide gaps that exist in our clinical knowledge. The ongoing pursuit by these esteemed professionals of evidence fostering excellence is the inspiration for this work.

Chicago, IL, USA   Mark K. Ferguson, MD
May, 2014

Contents

Contributors

Udo Abah, MBChB, MRCS Department of Cardiothoracic Surgery, Papworth Hospital, Cambridge, UK

Marco E. Allaix, MD Department of Surgery, Center for Esophageal Diseases, University of Chicago Pritzker School of Medicine, Chicago, IL, USA

Nasser K. Altorki, MB, BCh Department of Surgery, Division of Cardiothoracic Surgery, Weill Cornell Medical College-New York Presbyterian Hospital, New York, NY, USA

Rafael S. Andrade, MD Section of Thoracic and Foregut Surgery, Division of Cardiothoracic Surgery, University of Minnesota, Minneapolis, MN, USA

Marco Anile, MD, PhD Department of Thoracic Surgery, University of Rome Sapienza, Rome, Italy

Mara B. Antonoff, MD Division of Cardiothoracic Surgery, Washington University School of Medicine, St. Louis, MO, USA

Peter Baik, DO Lung Cancer Program, Swedish Medical Center, First Hill, Seattle, WA, USA

Richard G. Berrisford Peninsula Oesophagogastric Unit, Derriford Hospital, Plymouth, Devon, UK

Thomas Birdas, MD Division of Cardiothoracic Surgery, Indiana University School of Medicine, Indianapolis, IN, USA

Shanda H. Blackmon, MD, MPH Division of Thoracic Surgery, Departments of Thoracic Surgery and General Surgery, Houston Methodist Hospital, Texas, Weill Cornell Medical College, Houston, TX, USA

Alessandro Brunelli, MD Department of Thoracic Surgery, Ospedali Riuniti Ancona, Ancona, Italy

Christopher Cao, MBBS, BSc (Med) The Systematic Reviews Unit, The Collaborative Research (CORE) Group, Sydney, Australia

The Baird Institute for Applied Heart and Lung Surgical Research, Sydney, Australia

Shamus R. Carr, MD Division of Cardiothoracic Surgery, University of Utah and Huntsman Cancer Institute, Salt Lake City, UT, USA

Apoorva Krishna Chandar, MBBS, MA, MPH Division of Gastroenterology, Louis Stokes Cleveland VA Medical Center, Case Western Reserve University, Cleveland, OH, USA

Andrew C. Chang, MD Section of Thoracic Surgery, University of Michigan Health System, Ann Arbor, MI, USA

Kezhong Chen, MD Department of Thoracic Surgery, Peking University People's Hospital, Beijing, People's Republic of China

Benedict D.T. Daly, MD Department of Surgery, Boston Medical Center, Boston University School of Medicine, Boston, MA, USA

R. Duane Davis, MD, MBA Division of Cardiothoracic Surgery, Department of Surgery, Duke University Medical Center, Durham, NC, USA

Alberto de Hoyos, MD, FACS, FCCP Division of Thoracic Surgery, Northwestern Memorial Hospital, Northwestern University Feinberg School of Medicine, Chicago, IL, USA

Malcolm DeCamp, MD, FACS, FCCP Division of Thoracic Surgery, Northwestern Memorial Hospital, Northwestern University Feinberg School of Medicine, Chicago, IL, USA

Todd L. Demmy, MD Department of Thoracic Surgery, Roswell Park Cancer Institute, Buffalo, NY, USA

Daniele Diso, MD, PhD Department of Thoracic Surgery, University of Rome Sapienza, Rome, Italy

Peter Downey, MD Department of Surgery, Columbia University Medical Center, New York-Presbyterian Hospital, New York, NY, USA

Janet P. Edwards, MD, MPH Division of Thoracic Surgery, Foothills Medical Centre, Calgary, AB, Canada

Yngve Falck-Ytter, MD, AGAF Division of Gastroenterology, Louis Stokes Cleveland VA Medical Center, Case Western Reserve University, Cleveland, OH, USA

Richard H. Feins, MD Division of Cardiothoracic Surgery, Department of Surgery, University of North Carolina, Chapel Hill, NC, USA

Mark K. Ferguson, MD Department of Surgery, The University of Chicago, Chicago, IL, USA

Department of Thoracic Surgery, Peking University People's Hospital, Beijing, China

Alfonso Fiorelli, MD, PhD Chirurgia Toracica, Seconda Università di Napoli, Piazza Miraglia, Napoli, Italy

Samuel J. Ford, MB, ChB, PhD, FRCS Peninsula Oesophagogastric Unit, Derriford Hospital, Plymouth, Devon, UK

Clara S. Fowler, MSLS Research Medical Library, The University of Texas MD Anderson Cancer Center, Houston, TX, USA

Joseph S. Friedberg, MD Department of Surgery, University of Pennsylvania, Philadelphia, PA, USA

PENN Presbyterian Medical Center, Philadelphia, PA, USA

Henning A. Gaissert, MD Department of Thoracic Surgery, Massachusetts General Hospital, Boston, MA, USA

Sabha Ganai, MD, PhD Department of Surgery, Simmons Cancer Institute, Southern Illinois University School of Medicine, Springfield, IL, USA

Laurissa Gann, MSLS Research Medical Library, The University of Texas MD Anderson Cancer Center, Houston, TX, USA

Puja Gaur, MD Division of Thoracic Surgery, Brigham and Women's Hospital, Boston, MA, USA

Zaninotto Giovanni, MD, FACS General Surgery Unit, "SS. Giovanni e Paolo" Hospital, University of Padova, Venice, Italy

Felice Granato, MD, PhD Department of Thoracic Surgery, Papworth Hospital, Cambridge, UK

Tyler R. Grenda, MD Section of Thoracic Surgery, University of Michigan, Ann Arbor, MI, USA

Sean C. Grondin, MD, MPH Division of Thoracic Surgery, Foothills Medical Centre, Calgary, AB, Canada

Brian C. Gulack, MD Department of Surgery, Duke University Medical Center, Durham, NC, USA

Benjamin E. Haithcock, MD Division of Cardiothoracic Surgery, University of North Carolina at Chapel Hill, Chapel Hill, NC, USA

Zane Hammoud, MD, FACS Department of Thoracic Surgery, Henry Ford Hospital, Detroit, MI, USA

Karen Harrison-Phipps, FRCS (CTh) Thoracic Surgery Department, Guy's Hospital, London, UK

Matthew G. Hartwig, MD Department of Surgery, Duke University Medical Center, Durham, NC, USA

Axel Haverich, MD Department of Thoracic, Transplant and Cardiovascular Surgery, Hannover Medical School, Hannover, Germany

Joshua A. Hemmerich, PhD Department of Medicine, The University of Chicago, Chicago, IL, USA

Casey P. Hertzenberg, MD Department of Cardiothoracic Surgery, University of Kansas Hospital, Kansas City, KS, USA

Arielle Hodari, MD Department of Thoracic Surgery, Henry Ford Hospital, Detroit, MI, USA

David H. Ilson, MD, PhD Gastrointestinal Oncology Service, Department of Medicine, Memorial Sloan Kettering Cancer Center, New York, NY, USA

Philipp Jungebluth, MD Division of Ear, Nose, and Throat (CLINTEC), Advanced Center for Translational Regenerative Medicine (ACTREM), Karolinska Institutet, Stockholm, Sweden

Hirofumi Kawakubo, MD, PhD Department of Surgery, Keio University School of Medicine, Tokyo, Japan

Yuko Kitagawa, MD, PhD Department of Surgery, Keio University School of Medicine, Tokyo, Japan

Vani J.A. Konda, MD Section of Gastroenterology, Department of Medicine, University of Chicago Medical Center, Chicago, IL, USA

Christian Kuehn, MD Department of Thoracic, Transplant and Cardiovascular Surgery, Hannover Medical School, Hannover, Germany

Gabriel D. Lang, MD Department of Gastroenterology, Hepatology, and Nutrition, University of Chicago, Chicago, IL, USA

Michael Lanuti, MD Division of Thoracic Surgery, Massachusetts General Hospital, Harvard Medical School, Boston, MA, USA

Françoise Le Pimpec-Barthes, MD Department of Thoracic Surgery and Lung Transplantation, Pompidou European Hospital, Paris-Descartes University, Paris, France

Xiao Li, MD Department of Thoracic Surgery, Peking University People's Hospital, Beijing, China

Yun Li, MD Department of Thoracic Surgery, Peking University People's Hospital, Beijing, People's Republic of China

Moishe Liberman, MD, PhD Division of Thoracic Surgery, CHUM Endoscopic Tracheobronchial and Oesophageal Center (C.E.T.O.C.), University of Montreal, Montreal, QC, Canada

Donald E. Low, MD, FACS, FRCS(c) Digestive Disease Institute, Esophageal Center of Excellence, Virginia Mason Medical Center, Seattle, WA, USA

Marco Lucchi, MD Division of Thoracic Surgery, Cardiac Thoracic and Vascular Department, Azienda Ospedaliero-Universitaria Pisana, Pisa, Italy

Paolo Macchiarini, MD, PhD Division of Ear, Nose, and Throat (CLINTEC), Advanced Center for Translational Regenerative Medicine (ACTREM), Karolinska Institutet, Stockholm, Sweden

Giuseppe Marulli, MD, PhD Thoracic Surgery Division, Department of Cardiac, Thoracic and Vascular Sciences, University of Padova, Padova, Italy

David J. McCormack, BSc (Hons) MRCS Cardiothoracic Surgery Department, King's College Hospital, London, UK

Anna L. McGuire, MD Department of Thoracic Surgery, The Ottawa Hospital, Ottawa, ON, Canada

Rudy Mercelis, MD Department of Neurology, Antwerp University Hospital, Edegem (Antwerp), Belgium

Robert E. Merritt, MD Department of Surgery, Ohio State University – Wexner Medical Center, Columbus, CA, USA

Bryan F. Meyers, MD MPH Division of Cardiothoracic Surgery, Washington University School of Medicine, Columbus, OH, USA

Timothy M. Millington, MD Department of Thoracic Surgery, Massachusetts General Hospital, Boston, MA, USA

DuyKhanh P. Mimi Ceppa, MD Division of Cardiothoracic Surgery, Department of Surgery, Indiana University School of Medicine, Indianapolis, IN, USA

Nathan M. Mollberg, DO Department of Cardiothoracic Surgery, University of Washington Medical Center, Seattle, WA, USA

Tamas F. Molnar, MD, DSci Department of Operational Medicine, Faculty of Medicine, University of Pécs, Pécs, Hungary

Jacob R. Moremen, MD Division of Cardiothoracic Surgery, Department of Surgery, Indiana University School of Medicine, Indianapolis, IN, USA

Septimiu Murgu, MD Department of Medicine, The University of Chicago, Chicago, IL, USA

Basil S. Nasir, MBBCh Division of Thoracic Surgery, CHUM Endoscopic Tracheobronchial and Oesophageal Center (C.E.T.O.C.), University of Montreal, Montreal, QC, Canada

Katie S. Nason, MD, MPH Department of Cardiothoracic Surgery, University of Pittsburgh, Pittsburgh, PA, USA

Brant K. Oelschlager, MD Department of Surgery, Center for Videoendoscopic Surgery, Center for Esophageal and Gastric Surgery, University of Washington, Seattle, WA, USA

Department of Surgery, Center for Esophageal and Gastric Surgery, University of Washington, Seattle, WA, USA

Parise Paolo, MD General Surgery Unit, "SS. Giovanni e Paolo" Hospital, University of Padova, Venice, Italy

Marco G. Patti, MD Department of Surgery, Center for Esophageal Diseases, University of Chicago Pritzker School of Medicine, Chicago, IL, USA

Eitan Podgaetz, MD Section of Thoracic and Foregut Surgery, Division of Cardiothoracic Surgery, University of Minnesota, Minneapolis, MN, USA

Varun Puri, MD Division of Cardiothoracic Surgery, Washington University School of Medicine, St. Louis, MO, USA

Federico Rea, MD Thoracic Surgery Division, Department of Cardiac, Thoracic and Vascular Sciences, University of Padova, Padova, Italy

Szilard Rendeki, MD Department of Operational Medicine, Faculty of Medicine, University of Pécs, Pécs, Hungary

Erino Angelo Rendina, MD Department of Thoracic Surgery, Sant'Andrea Hospital, University of Rome Sapienza, Rome, Italy

Eleonora Lorillard Spencer Cenci Foundation

David Rice, MB, BCh Department of Thoracic and Cardiovascular Surgery, University of Texas MD Anderson Cancer Center, Houston, TX, USA

Gaetano Rocco, MD, FRCSEd Division of Thoracic Surgery, Department of Thoracic Surgery and Oncology, National Cancer Institute, Pascale Foundation, Naples, Italy

Michele Salati, MD Department of Thoracic Surgery, Ospedali Riuniti Ancona, Ancona, Italy

Mario Santini, MD Chirurgia Toracica, Seconda Università di Napoli, Napoli, Italy

Marco Scarci, MD, PGCTS, FRCS Department of Thoracic Surgery, Papworth Hospital NHS Foundation Trust, Cambridge, UK

Henner M. Schmidt, MD Digestive Disease Institute, Esophageal Center of Excellence, Virginia Mason Medical Center, Seattle, WA, USA

Joshua Sonett, MD Division of Thoracic Surgery, Columbia University Medical Center, New York-Presbyterian Hospital, New York, NY, USA

Sadeesh Srinathan, MD, MSc, FRCS (C), FRCS (C/TH) Section of Thoracic Surgery, Winnipeg Health Sciences Centre, Winnipeg, MB, Canada

Brendon M. Stiles, MD Department of Surgery, Division of Cardiothoracic Surgery, Weill Cornell Medical College-New York Presbyterian Hospital, New York, NY, USA

R. Sudhir Sundaresan, MD Department of Surgery,, The Ottawa Hospital, University of Ottawa, Ottawa, ON, Canada

Scott James Swanson, MD Division of Thoracic Surgery, Brigham and Women's Hospital, Boston, MA, USA

Hiryoya Takeuchi, MD Department of Surgery, Keio University School of Medicine, Tokyo, Japan

Eric Vallières, MD, FRCSC Lung Cancer Program, Swedish Cancer Institute, Seattle, WA, USA

Paul E. Van Schil, MD, PhD Department of Thoracic and Vascular Surgery, Antwerp University Hospital, Edegem (Antwerp), Belgium

Kellie Van Voorhis, BS Department of Medicine, The University of Chicago, Chicago, IL, USA

Panos Vardas, MD Division of Cardiothoracic Surgery, Indiana University School of Medicine, Indianapolis, IN, USA

Gonzalo Varela, MD, PhD Thoracic Surgery Service, Department of Thoracic Surgery, Salamanca University Hospital and Medical School, Salamanca, Spain

Thomas K. Varghese Jr., MD, MS, FACS Department of Surgery, Harborview Medical Center, University of Washington, Seattle, WA, USA

Nirmal K. Veeramachaneni, MD Department of Cardiothoracic Surgery, University of Kansas Hospital, Kansas City, KS, USA

Federico Venuta, MD Department of Thoracic Surgery, University of Rome Sapienza, Rome, Italy
Eleonora Lorillard Spencer Cenci Foundation

Jun Wang, MD Department of Thoracic Surgery, Peking University People's Hospital, Beijing, People's Republic of China

Christopher Wigfield, MD, MD, FRCS (C/TH) Department of Surgery, Section of Cardiac and Thoracic Surgery, University of Chicago Medical Center, Chicago, IL, USA

Trevor Williams, MD, MPH Department of Surgery, Section of Cardiac and Thoracic Surgery, University of Chicago, Chicago, IL, USA

Elizabeth Won, MD Gastrointestinal Oncology Service, Department of Medicine, Memorial Sloan Kettering Cancer Center, New York, NY, USA

Robert B. Yates, MD Department of Surgery, Center for Videoendoscopic Surgery, University of Washington, Seattle, WA, USA

Sai Yendamuri, MD Department of Thoracic Surgery, Roswell Park Cancer Institute, Buffalo, NY, USA

Chapter 1
Introduction

Introduction

Dorothy Smith, an elderly and somewhat portly woman, presented to her local emergency room with chest pain and shortness of breath. An extensive evaluation revealed no evidence for coronary artery disease, congestive heart failure, or pneumonia. A chest radiograph demonstrated a large air-fluid level posterior to her heart shadow, a finding that all thoracic surgeons recognize as being consistent with a large paraesophageal hiatal hernia. The patient had not had similar symptoms previously. Her discomfort was relieved after a large eructation, and she was discharged from the emergency room a few hours later. When seen several weeks later in an outpatient setting by an experienced surgeon, who reviewed her history and the data from her emergency room visit, she was told that surgery is sometimes necessary to repair such hernias. Her surgeon indicated that the objectives of such an intervention would include relief of symptoms such as chest pain, shortness of breath, and postprandial fullness, and prevention of catastrophic complications of giant paraesophageal hernia, including incarceration, strangulation, and perforation. Ms. Smith, having recovered completely from her episode of a few weeks earlier, declined intervention, despite her surgeon's strenuous encouragement.

She presented to her local emergency room several months later with symptoms of an incarcerated hernia and underwent emergency surgery to correct the problem. The surgeon found a somewhat ischemic stomach and had to decide whether to resect the stomach or just repair the hernia. If resection was to be performed, an additional decision was whether to reconstruct immediately or at the time of a subsequent operation. If resection was not performed, the surgeon needed to consider a

M.K. Ferguson, MD
Department of Surgery, The University of Chicago,
5841 S. Maryland Avenue, MC5040, Chicago, IL 60637, USA
e-mail: mferguso@surgery.bsd.uchicago.edu

M.K. Ferguson (ed.), *Difficult Decisions in Thoracic Surgery*,
Difficult Decisions in Surgery: An Evidence-Based Approach 1,
DOI 10.1007/978-1-4471-6404-3_1, © Springer-Verlag London 2014

variety of options as part of any planned hernia repair: whether to perform a gastric lengthening procedure; whether a fundoplication should be constructed; and whether to reinforce the hiatal closure with non-autologous materials. Each of these intraoperative decisions could importantly affect the need for a subsequent reoperation, the patient's immediate survival, and her long-term quality of life. Given the dire circumstances that the surgeon was presented with during the emergency operation, it would have been optimal if the emergent nature of the operation could have been avoided entirely. In retrospect, which was more correct in this hypothetical situation, the recommendation of the surgeon or the decision of the patient?

Decisions are the stuff of everyday life for all physicians; for surgeons, life-altering decisions often must be made on the spot, frequently without what many might consider to be necessary data. The ability to make such decisions confidently is the hallmark of the surgeon. However, decisions made under such circumstances are often not correct or even well reasoned. All surgeons (and many of their spouses) are familiar with the saying "…often wrong, but never in doubt." As early as the fourteenth century physicians were cautioned never to admit uncertainty. Arnauld of Villanova wrote that, even when in doubt, physicians should look and act authoritative and confident [1]. In fact, useful data do exist that could have an impact on many of the individual decisions regarding elective and emergent management of the giant paraesophageal hernia scenario outlined above. Despite the existence of these data, surgeons tend to make decisions based on their own personal experience, anecdotal tales of good or bad outcomes, and unquestioned adherence to dictums from their mentors or other respected leaders in the field, often to the exclusion of objective data. It is believed that only 15 % of medical decisions are scientifically based [2], and it is possible that an even lower percentage of thoracic surgical decisions are so founded. With all of our modern technological, data processing, and communication skills, why do we still find ourselves in this situation?

Early Surgical Decision Making

Physicians' diagnostic capabilities, not to mention their therapeutic armamentarium, were quite limited until the middle to late nineteenth century. Drainage of empyema, cutting for stone, amputation for open fractures of the extremities, and mastectomy for cancer were relatively common procedures, but few such conditions were diagnostic dilemmas. Surgery, when it was performed, was generally indicated for clearly identified problems that could not be otherwise remedied. Some surgeons were all too mindful of the warnings of Hippocrates: "…physicians, when they treat men who have no serious illness, … may commit great mistakes without producing any formidable mischief … under these circumstances, when they commit mistakes, they do not expose themselves to ordinary men; but when they fall in with a great, a strong, and a dangerous disease, then their mistakes and want of skill are made apparent to all. Their punishment is not far off, but is swift in overtaking both the one and the other [3]." Others took a less considered approach to their craft, leading Hunter to liken a surgeon to "an armed savage who attempts to get that by force which a civilized man would get by stratagem [4]."

Based on small numbers of procedures, lack of a true understanding of pathophysiology, frequently mistaken diagnoses, and the absence of technology to communicate information quickly, surgical therapy until the middle of the nineteenth century was largely empiric. For example, by that time fewer than 90 diaphragmatic hernias had been reported in the literature, most of them having been diagnosed postmortem as a result of gastric or bowel strangulation and perforation [5]. Decisions were based on dogma promulgated by word of mouth. This has been termed the "ancient era" of evidence-based medicine [6].

An exception to the empiric nature of surgery was the approach espoused by Hunter in the mid-eighteenth century, who suggested to Jenner, his favorite pupil, "I think your solution is just, but why think? Why not try the experiment?" [4]. Hunter challenged the established practices of bleeding, purging, and mercury administration, believing them to be useless and often harmful. These views were so heretical that, 50 years later, editors added footnotes to his collected works insisting that these were still valuable treatments. Hunter and others were the progenitors of the "renaissance era" of evidence-based medicine, in which personal journals, textbooks, and some medical journal publications were becoming prominent [6].

The discovery of x-rays in 1895 and the subsequent rapid development of radiology in the following years made the diagnosis and surgical therapy of a large paraesophageal hernia such as that described at the beginning of this chapter commonplace. By 1908 x-ray was accepted as a reliable means for diagnosing diaphragmatic hernia, and by the late 1920s surgery had been performed for this condition on almost 400 patients in one large medical center [7, 8]. Thus, the ability to diagnose a condition was becoming a prerequisite to instituting proper therapy.

This enormous leap in physicians' abilities to render appropriate ministrations to their patients was based on substantial new and valuable objective data. In contrast, however, the memorable anecdotal case presented by a master (or at least an influential) surgeon continued to dominate the surgical landscape. Prior to World War II, it was common for surgeons throughout the world with high career aspirations to travel to Europe for a year or two, visiting renowned surgical centers to gain insight into surgical techniques, indications, and outcomes. In the early twentieth century Murphy attracted a similar group of surgeons to his busy clinic at Mercy Hospital in Chicago. His publication of case reports and other observations evolved into the Surgical Clinics of North America. Seeing individual cases and drawing conclusions based upon such limited exposure no doubt reinforced the concept of empiricism in decision making in these visitors. True, compared to the strict empiricism of the nineteenth century there were more data available upon which to base surgical decisions in the early twentieth century, but information regarding objective short-term and long-term outcomes still was not readily available in the surgical literature or at surgical meetings.

Reinforcing the imperative of empiricism in decision making, surgeons often disregarded valuable techniques that might have greatly improved their efforts. It took many years for anesthetic methods to be accepted. The slow adoption of endotracheal intubation combined with positive pressure ventilation prevented safe thoracotomy for decades after their introduction into animal research. Wholesale denial of germ theory by US physicians for decades resulted in continued unacceptable infection rates for years after preventive measures were identified. These are just a few examples of how ignorance and its bedfellow, recalcitrance, delayed progress in thoracic surgery in the late nineteenth and early twentieth centuries.

Evidence-Based Surgical Decisions

There were important exceptions in the late nineteenth and early twentieth centuries to the empiric nature of surgical decision making. Among the first were the demonstration of antiseptic methods in surgery and the optimal therapy for pleural empyema. Similar evidence-based approaches to managing global health problems were developing in non-surgical fields. Reed's important work in the prevention of yellow fever led to the virtual elimination of this historically endemic problem in Central America, an accomplishment that permitted construction of the Panama Canal. The connection between the pancreas and diabetes that had been identified decades earlier was formalized by the discovery and subsequent clinical application of insulin in 1922, leading to the awarding of a Nobel prize to Banting and Macleod in 1923. Fleming's rediscovery of the antibacterial properties of penicillin in 1928 led to its development as an antibiotic for humans in 1939, and it received widespread use during World War II. The emergency use of penicillin, as well as new techniques for fluid resuscitation, were said to account for the unexpectedly high rate of survival among burn victims of the Coconut Grove nightclub fire in Boston in 1942. Similar stories can be told for the development of evidence in the management of polio and tuberculosis in the mid-twentieth century. As a result, the first half of the twentieth century has been referred to as the "transitional era" of evidence-based medicine, in which information was shared easily through textbooks and peer-reviewed journals [6].

Among the first important examples of the used of evidence-based medicine is the work of Semmelweiss, who in 1861 demonstrated that careful attention to antiseptic principles could reduce mortality associated with puerperal fever from over 18 % to just over 1 %. The effective use of such principles in surgery was investigated during that same decade by Lister, who noted a decrease in mortality on his trauma ward from 45 to 15 % with the use of carbolic acid as an antiseptic agent during operations. However, both the germ theory of infection and the ability of an antiseptic such as carbolic acid to decrease the risk of infection were not generally accepted, particularly in the United States, for another decade. In 1877 Lister performed an elective wiring of a patellar fracture using aseptic techniques, essentially converting a closed fracture to an open one in the process. Under practice patterns of the day, such an operation would almost certainly lead to infection and possible death, but the success of Lister's approach secured his place in history. It is interesting to note that a single case such as this, rather than prior reports of his extensive experience with the use of antiseptic agents, helped Lister turn the tide towards universal use of antiseptic techniques in surgery thereafter.

The second example developed over 40 years after the landmark demonstration of antiseptic techniques and also involved surgical infectious problems. Hippocrates described open drainage for empyema in 229 BC, indicating that "when empyema are opened by the cautery or by the knife, and the pus flows pale and white, the patient survives, but if it is mixed with blood and is muddy and foul smelling, he will die [3]." There was little change in the management of this problem until the introduction of thoracentesis by Trusseau in 1843. The mortality rate for empyema remained at 50–75 % well into the twentieth century [9]. The confluence of two important events, the flu pandemic of 1918 and the Great War, stimulated the formation of the US Army Empyema Commission in 1918. Led by Graham and Bell, this commission's recommendations for management included three basic principles: drainage, with avoidance of open pneumothorax; obliteration of the empyema cavity; and nutritional maintenance for the patient. Employing these simple principles led to a decrease in mortality rates associated with empyema to 10–15 %.

The Age of Information

These surgical efforts in the late nineteenth and early twentieth centuries ushered in the beginning of an era of scientific investigation of surgical problems. This was a period of true surgical research characterized by both laboratory and clinical efforts. It paralleled similar efforts in non-surgical medical disciplines. Such research led to the publication of hundreds of thousands of papers on surgical management. This growth of medical information is not a new phenomenon, however. The increase in published manuscripts, and the increase in medical journals, has been exponential over a period of more than two centuries, with a compound annual growth rate of almost 4 % per year (Fig. 1.1) [10]. In addition, the quality and utility of currently published information is substantially better than that of publications in centuries past.

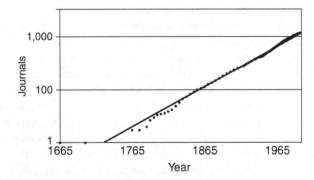

Fig. 1.1 The total number of active refereed journals published annually (Data from Mabe [10])

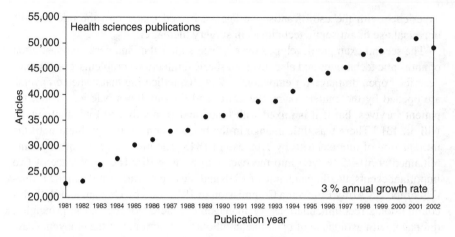

Fig. 1.2 Growth in the number of published health science articles published annually (Data from Mabe [10])

Currently there are more than 2,000 publishers producing works in the general field of science, technology, and medicine. The field comprises more than 1,800 journals containing 1.4 million peer-reviewed articles annually. The annual growth rate of health science articles during the past two decades is about 3 %, continuing the trend of the past two centuries and adding to the difficulty of identifying useful information (Fig. 1.2) [10]. There is also a trend towards decentralization of publication of biomedical data, which offers challenges to identifying useful information that is published outside of what are considered traditional journals [11]. For example, publication rates of clinical trials relevant to certain specialties vary from one to seven trials *per day* [12]. When confronting this large amount of published information, separating the wheat from the chaff is a daunting task. The work of assessing such information has been assumed to some extent by experts in the field who perform structured reviews of information on important issues and meta-analyses of high quality, controlled, randomized trials. These techniques have the potential to summarize results from multiple studies and, in some instances, crystallize findings into a simple, coherent statement.

An early proponent of such processes was Cochrane, who in the 1970s and 1980s suggested that increasingly limited medical resources should be equitably distributed and consist of interventions that have been shown in properly designed evaluations to be effective. He stressed the importance of using evidence from randomized controlled trials, which were likely to provide much more reliable information than other sources of evidence [13]. These efforts ushered in an era of high quality medical and surgical research. Cochrane was posthumously honored with the development of the Cochrane Collaboration in 1993, encompassing multiple centers in North America and Europe, with the purpose of "helping healthcare providers, policy makers, patients, their advocates and carers, make well-informed decisions about human health care by preparing, updating and promoting the accessibility of Cochrane Reviews [14]."

Methods originally espoused by Cochrane and others have been codified into techniques for rating the quality of evidence in a publication and for grading the strength of a recommendation based on the preponderance of available evidence. In accord with this, the clinical problems addressed in this book have been assessed using a modification of a single rating system (GRADE) that is outlined and updated in Chap. 2 [15].

Techniques such as those described above for synthesizing large amounts of quality information were introduced for the development guidelines for clinical activity in thoracic surgery, most commonly for the management of lung cancer, beginning in the mid-1990s. An example of these is a set of guidelines based on what were then current standards of care sponsored by the Society of Surgical Oncology for managing lung cancer. It was written by experts in the field without a formal process of evidence collection [16]. A better technique for arriving at guidelines is the consensus statement, usually derived during a consensus process in which guidelines based on published medical evidence are revised until members of the conference agree by a substantial majority in the final statement. An example of this iterative structure is the Delphi process [17]. The problem with this technique is that the strength of recommendations, at times, is sometimes diluted until there is little content to them. Some organizations that appear to have avoided this pitfall in the general of guidelines of interest to thoracic surgeons include The American College of Chest Physicians, the Society of Thoracic Surgeons, the European Society of Thoracic Surgeons, the European Respiratory Society, the American Thoracic Society, the National Comprehensive Cancer Network, the Society of Clinical Oncology, the British Thoracic Society, and the Society of Surgical Oncology, to name but a few.

Despite the enormous efforts expended by professional societies in providing evidence-based algorithms for appropriate management of patients, adherence to these published guidelines, based on practice pattern reports, is disappointing. Focusing again on surgical management of lung cancer, there is strong evidence that standard procedures incorporated into surgical guidelines for lung cancer are widely ignored. For example, fewer than 50 % of patients undergoing mediastinoscopy for nodal staging have lymph node biopsies performed. In patients undergoing major resection for lung cancer, fewer than 60 % have mediastinal lymph nodes biopsied or dissected [18]. Only one-third of physicians routinely assess diffusing capacity in lung cancer patients who are candidates for lung resection in Europe, and in the United States fewer than 60 % of patients who undergo major lung resection for cancer have diffusing capacity measured [19, 20]. Even at centers with expertise in preoperative evaluation adherence to evaluation algorithms can be challenging, especially for higher risk patients [21]. There are also important regional variations in the use of standard staging techniques and in the use of surgery for stage I lung cancer patients, patterns of activity that are also related to race and socioeconomic status [22, 23]. Failure to adhere to accepted standards of care for surgical lung cancer patients results in higher postoperative mortality rates [24, 25], and the selection of super specialists for one's lung cancer surgery confers an overall long-term survival advantage [26].

The importance of adherence to accepted standards of care, particular those espoused by major professional societies, such as the American College of Surgeons, The Society of Surgical Oncology, the American Society of Clinical Oncology, the American Cancer Society, the National Comprehensive Cancer Network, is becoming clear as the United States Centers for Medicare and Medicaid Services develops processes for rewarding adherence to standards of clinical care. This underscores the need for surgeons to become familiar with evidence-based practices and to adopt them as part of their daily routines. What is not known is whether surgeons should be rewarded for their efforts in following recommended standards of care, or for the outcomes of such care? Do we measure the process, the immediate success, or the long-term outcomes? If outcomes are to be the determining factor, what outcomes are important? Is operative mortality an adequate surrogate for quality of care and good results? Whose perspective is most important in determining success, that of the patient, or that of the medical establishment?

The Age of Data

We have now entered into an era in which the amount of data available for studying problems and outcomes in surgery is truly overwhelming. Large clinical trials involving thousands of subjects render databases measured in megabytes. As an example, for the National Emphysema Treatment Trial (NETT), which entered over 1,200 patients, initial data collection prior to randomization consisted of over 50 pages of data for each patient [27]. Patients were subsequently followed for up to 5 years after randomization, creating an enormous research database. The size of the NETT database is dwarfed by other databases in which surgical information is stored, including the National Medicare Database, the Surveillance Epidemiology and End Results (SEER), Nationwide Inpatient Sample (NIS), the American College of Surgeons National Surgical Quality Improvement Program (NSQIP), and the Society of Thoracic Surgeons (STS) database. Other foreign national and international databases contain similar large amounts of information.

Medical databases are of two basic types: those that contain information that is primarily clinical in nature, especially those that are developed specifically for a particular research project such as the NETT, and administrative databases that are maintained for other than clinical purposes but that can be used in some instances to assess clinical information and outcomes, an example of which is the National Medicare Database. Information is organized in databases in a hierarchical structure. An individual unit of data is a field; a patient's name, address, and age are each individual fields. Fields are grouped into records, such that all of one patient's fields constitute a record. Data in a record have a one-to-one relationship with each other. Records are compiled in relations, or files. Relations can be as simple as a spreadsheet, or flat file, in which there is a one-to-one relationship between each field.

More complex relations contain many-to-one, or one-to-many, relationships among fields, relationships that must be accessed through queries rather than through simple inspection. An example is multiple diagnoses for a single patient, or multiple patients with a single diagnosis. Ultimately, databases become four-dimensional complex clinical and research resources as time emerges as an important factor in assessing outcomes and the changing molecular signatures of cancers, as examples [28].

In addition to collection of data such as those above that are routinely generated in the process of standard patient care, new technological advances are providing an exponential increase in the amount of data generated by standard studies. An example is the new 640 slice computed tomography scanner, which has vastly expanded the amount of information collected in each of the x-y-z axes as well as providing temporal information and routine 3-D reconstruction capabilities during a routine CT scan. The additional information provided by this technology has created a revolutionary, rather than evolutionary, change in diagnostic radiology. Using this technology, virtual angiograms can be performed, three dimensional reconstruction of isolated anatomic entities is possible, and radiologists are discovering more abnormalities than clinicians know what to do with.

A case in point is the use of CT as a screening test for lung cancer. Rapid low-dose CT scans were introduced in the late 1990s and were quickly adopted as a means for screening high risk patients for lung cancer. The results of this screening were mixed. Several reports suggested that the number of radiographic abnormalities identified was high compared to the number of clinically important findings. For example, in the early experience at the Mayo clinic over 1,500 patients were enrolled in an annual CT screening trial, and in the 4 years of the trial, over 3,100 indeterminate nodules were identified, only 45 of which were found to be malignant [29]. Similar results were reported by others during screening or surveillance activities [30]. Many additional radiographic abnormalities other than lung nodules were also identified. In addition, the increase in radiation exposure owing to more complex exams and more frequent exams led to concerns about radiation-induced neoplasms, an unintended consequence of the good intentions of those performing lung cancer screening [31, 32]. However, recent reports of improved lung cancer survival resulting from screening appropriately selected individuals for screening has led to formal recommendations for screening such populations [33, 34]. This is changing the practice of medicine, even though cost-effectiveness of such interventions has not been demonstrated.

What Lies in the Future?

What do we now do with the plethora of information that is being collected on patients? How do we make sense of these gigabytes or terabytes of data? It may be that we now have more information than we can use or that we even want. Regardless, the trend is clearly in the direction of collecting more, rather than less, data, and it behooves us to make some sense of the situation. In the case of additional radiographic findings resulting from improved technology, new algorithms have already been refined for evaluating nodules and for managing their follow-up over time, and have yielded impressive results in the ability of these approaches to identify which patients should be observed and which patients should undergo biopsy or surgery [35, 36]. What, though, of the reams of numerical and other data than pour in daily and populate large databases? When confronting this dilemma, it useful to remember that we are dealing with an evolutionary problem, the extent of which has been recognized for decades. Eliot aptly described this predicament in *The Rock* (1934), lamenting:

> Where is the wisdom we have lost in knowledge?
> Where is the knowledge we have lost in information?

To those lines one might add:

> *Where is the information we have lost in data?*

One might ask, in the presence of all this information, are we collecting the correct data? Evidence-based guidelines regarding indications for surgery, surgical techniques, and postoperative management are often lacking. We successfully track surgical outcomes of a limited sort, and often only in retrospect: complications, operative mortality, and survival. We don't successfully track patient's satisfaction with their experience, the quality of life they are left with as a result of surgery, and whether they would make the same decision regarding surgery if they had to do things over again. Perhaps these are important questions upon which physicians should focus. In addition to migrating towards patient-focused rather than institutionally-focused data, are we prepared to take the greater leap of addressing more important issues requiring data from a societal perspective, including cost-effectiveness and appropriate resource distribution (human and otherwise) and utilization? This would likely result in redeployment of resources towards health prevention and maintenance rather than intervention. Such efforts are already underway, sponsored not by medical societies and other professional organizations, but by those paying the increasingly unaffordable costs of medical care.

Insurance companies have long been involved, through their actuarial functions, in identifying populations who are at high risk for medical problems, and it is likely that they will extend this actuarial methodology into evaluating the success of surgical care on an institutional and individual surgeon basis as more relevant data become available. The Leapfrog Group, representing a consortium of large commercial enterprises that covers insurance costs for millions of workers, was founded to differentiate levels of quality of outcomes for common or very expensive diseases, thereby potentially limiting costs of care by directing patients to better outcome centers. These efforts have three potential drawbacks from the perspective of the surgeon. First, decisions made in this way are primarily fiscally based, and are not patient focused. Second, policies put in place by payors will undoubtedly lead to regionalization of health care, effectively resulting in de facto restraint of trade affecting those surgeons with low individual case volumes or comparatively poor outcomes for a procedure, or who work in low volume centers. Finally, decisions about point of care will be taken from the hands of the patients and their physicians. The next phase of this process will be requirements on the part of payors regarding practice patterns, in which penalties are incurred if proscribed patterns are not followed, and rewards are provided for following such patterns, even if they lead to worse outcomes in an individual patient.

Physicians can retain control of the care of their patients in a variety of ways. First, they must make decisions based on evidence and in accordance with accepted guidelines and recommendations. This text serves to provide an outline for only a fraction of the decisions that are made in a thoracic surgical practice. For many of the topics in this book there are preciously few data that can be used to formulate a rational basis for a recommendation. Practicing physicians must therefore become actively involved in the process of developing useful evidence upon which decisions can be made. There are a variety of means for doing this, including participation in randomized clinical trials, entry of their patient data (appropriately anonymized) into large databases for study, and participation in consensus conferences aimed at providing useful management guidelines for problems in which they have a special interest. Critical evaluation of new technology and procedures, rather than merely adopting what is new to appear to the public and referring physicians that one's practice is cutting edge, may help reduce the wholesale adoption of what is new into patterns of practice before its value is proven.

Conclusion

Decisions are the life blood of surgeons. How we make decisions affects the immediate and long-term outcomes of care of our patients. Such decisions will also, in the near future, affect our reimbursement, our referral patterns, and possibly our privileges to perform certain operations. Most of the decisions that we currently make in our surgical practices are insufficiently grounded in adequate evidence. In addition, we tend to ignore published evidence and guidelines, preferring to base our decisions on prior training, anecdotal experience, and intuition as to what is best for an individual patient.

Improving the process of decision making is vital to our patients' welfare, to the health of our specialty, and to our own careers. To do this we must thoughtfully embrace the culture of evidence-based medicine. This requires critical appraisal of reported evidence, interpretation of the evidence with regards to the surgeon's target population, and integration of appropriate information and guidelines into daily practice. Constant review of practice patterns, updating management algorithms, and critical assessment of results is necessary to maintain optimal quality care. Documentation of these processes must become second nature. Unless individual surgeons adopt leadership roles in this process and thoracic surgeons as a group buy into this concept, we will find ourselves marginalized by outside forces that will distance us from our patients and discount our expertise in making vital decisions.

References

1. Kelly J. The great mortality. An intimate history of the black death, the most devastating plague of all time. New York: Harper Collins; 2006.
2. Eddy DM. Decisions without information. The intellectual crisis in medicine. HMO Pract. 1991;5:58–60.
3. Hippocrates. The genuine works of Hippocrates. Charles Darwin Adams (Ed, Trans). New York: Dover. 1868.
4. Moore W. The knife man: the extraordinary life and times of John Hunter, father of modern surgery. New York: Broadway Books; 2005.
5. Bowditch HI. A treatise on diaphragmatic hernia. Buffalo Med J Mon Rev. 1853;9:65–94.
6. Claridge JA, Fabian TC. History and development of evidence-based medicine. World J Surg. 2005;29:547–53.
7. Hedblom C. Diaphragmatic hernia. A study of three hundred and seventy-eight cases in which operation was performed. JAMA. 1925;85:947–53.
8. Harrington SW. Diaphragmatic hernia. Arch Surg. 1928;16:386–415.
9. Miller Jr JI. The history of surgery of empyema, thoracoplasty, Eloesser flap, and muscle flap transposition. Chest Surg Clin N Am. 2000;10:45–53.
10. Mabe MA. The growth and number of journals. Serials. 2003;16:191–7.
11. Druss BG, Marcus SC. Growth and decentralization of the medical literature: implications for evidence-based medicine. J Med Libr Assoc. 2005;93(4):499–501.
12. Hoffman T, Erueti C, Thorning S, Glasziou P. The scatter of research: cross sectional comparison of randomised trials and systematic reviews across specialties. BMJ. 2012;344:e3223.
13. Cochrane AL. Effectiveness and efficiency. Random reflections on health services. London: Nuffield Provincial Hospitals Trust; 1972.
14. Cochrane Collaboration Website. Available at http://www.cochrane.org/. Accessed Jun 2014.
15. Guyatt G, Gutterman D, Baumann MH, Addrizzo-Harris D, Hylek EH, Phillips B, Raskob G, Zelman Lewis S, Schunemann H. Grading strength of recommendations and quality of evidence in clinical guidelines: report from an American College of Chest Physicians Task Force. Chest. 2006;129:174–81.
16. Ginsberg R, Roth J, Ferguson MK. Lung cancer surgical practice guidelines. Society of Surgical Oncology practice guidelines: lung cancer. Oncology. 1997;11:889–92. 895.
17. Linstone HA, Turoff M, editors. The Delphi method: techniques and applications. A comprehensive book on Delphi method. http://www.is.njit.edu/pubs/delphibook/ Accessed 6 Jan 2014.
18. Little AG, Rusch VW, Bonner JA, Gaspar LE, Green MR, Webb WR, Stewart AK. Patterns of surgical care of lung cancer patients. Ann Thorac Surg. 2005;80:2051–6.
19. Charloux A, Brunelli A, Bolliger CT, Rocco G, Sculier JP, Varela G, Licker M, Ferguson MK, Faivre-Finn C, Huber RM, Clini EM, Win T, De Ruysscher D, Goldman L, European Respiratory Society and European Society of Thoracic Surgeons Joint Task Force on Fitness for Radical Therapy. Lung function evaluation before surgery in lung cancer patients: how are recent advances put into practice? A survey among members of the European Society of Thoracic Surgeons (ESTS) and of the Thoracic Oncology Section of the European Respiratory Society (ERS). Interact Cardiovasc Thorac Surg. 2009;9:925–31.
20. Ferguson MK, Gaissert HA, Grab JD, Sheng S. Pulmonary complications after lung resection in the absence of chronic obstructive pulmonary disease: the predictive role of diffusing capacity. J Thorac Cardiovasc Surg. 2009;138:1297–302.
21. Novoa NM, Ramos J, Jiménez MF, González-Ruiz JM, Varela G. The initial phase for validating the European algorithm for functional assessment prior to lung resection: quantifying compliance with the recommendations in actual clinical practice. Arch Bronconeumol. 2012;48(7):229–33.
22. Shugarman LR, Mack K, Sorbero ME, Tian H, Jain AK, Ashwood JS, Asch SM. Race and sex differences in the receipt of timely and appropriate lung cancer treatment. Med Care. 2009;47:774–81.

23. Coburn N, Przybysz R, Barbera L, Hodgson D, Sharir S, Laupacis A, Law C. CT, MRI and ultrasound scanning rates: evaluation of cancer diagnosis, staging and surveillance in Ontario. J Surg Oncol. 2008;98:490–9.
24. Birkmeyer NJ, Goodney PP, Stukel TA, Hillner BE, Birkmeyer JD. Do cancer centers designated by the National Cancer Institute have better surgical outcomes? Cancer. 2005;103:435–41.
25. Tieu B, Schipper P. Specialty matters in the treatment of lung cancer. Semin Thorac Cardiovasc Surg. 2012;24(2):99–105.
26. Freeman RK, Dilts JR, Ascioti AJ, Giannini T, Mahidhara RJ. A comparison of quality and cost indicators by surgical specialty for lobectomy of the lung. J Thorac Cardiovasc Surg. 2013;145(1):68–74.
27. Naunheim KS, Wood DE, Krasna MJ, DeCamp Jr MM, Ginsburg ME, McKenna Jr RJ, Criner GJ, Hoffman EA, Sternberg AL, Deschamps C, National Emphysema Treatment Trial Research Group. Predictors of operative mortality and cardiopulmonary morbidity in the National Emphysema Treatment Trial. J Thorac Cardiovasc Surg. 2006;131:43–53.
28. Surati M, Robinson M, Nandi S, Faoro L, Demchuk C, Rolle CE, Kanteti R, Ferguson BD, Hasina R, Gangadhar TC, Salama AK, Arif Q, Kirchner C, Mendonca E, Campbell N, Limvorasak S, Villaflor V, Hensing TA, Krausz T, Vokes EE, Husain AN, Ferguson MK, Karrison TG, Salgia R. Proteomic characterization of non-small cell lung cancer in a comprehensive translational thoracic oncology database. J Clin Bioinform. 2011;1(8):1–11.
29. Crestanello JA, Allen MS, Jett JR, Cassivi SD, Nichols 3rd FC, Swensen SJ, Deschamps C, Pairolero PC. Thoracic surgical operations in patients enrolled in a computed tomographic screening trial. J Thorac Cardiovasc Surg. 2004;128:254–9.
30. van Klaveren RJ, Oudkerk M, Prokop M, Scholten ET, Nackaerts K, Vernhout R, van Iersel CA, van den Bergh KA, van 't Westeinde S, van der Aalst C, Thunnissen E, Xu DM, Wang Y, Zhao Y, Gietema HA, de Hoop BJ, Groen HJ, de Bock GH, van Ooijen P, Weenink C, Verschakelen J, Lammers JW, Timens W, Willebrand D, Vink A, Mali W, de Koning HJ. Management of lung nodules detected by volume CT scanning. N Engl J Med. 2009;361:2221–9.
31. Smith-Bindman R, Lipson J, Marcus R, Kim KP, Mahesh M, Gould R, Berrington de González A, Miglioretti DL. Radiation dose associated with common computed tomography examinations and the associated lifetime attributable risk of cancer. Arch Intern Med. 2009;169:2078–86.
32. Berrington de González A, Mahesh M, Kim KP, Bhargavan M, Lewis R, Mettler F, Land C. Projected cancer risks from computed tomographic scans performed in the United States in 2007. Arch Intern Med. 2009;169:2071–7.
33. Jaklitsch MT, Jacobson FL, Austin JH, Field JK, Jett JR, Keshavjee S, MacMahon H, Mulshine JL, Munden RF, Salgia R, Strauss GM, Swanson SJ, Travis WD, Sugarbaker DJ. The American Association for Thoracic Surgery guidelines for lung cancer screening using low-dose computed tomography scans for lung cancer survivors and other high-risk groups. J Thorac Cardiovasc Surg. 2012;144(1):33–8.
34. Moyer VA on behalf of the U.S. Preventive Services Task Force. Screening for lung cancer: U.S. Preventive Services Task Force recommendation statement. Ann Intern Med. 2013. doi:10.7326/M13-2771. Published online 31 Dec 2013.
35. MacMahon H, Austin JH, Gamsu G, Herold CJ, Jett JR, Naidich DP, Patz Jr EF, Swensen SJ, Fleischner Society. Guidelines for management of small pulmonary nodules detected on CT scans: a statement from the Fleischner Society. Radiology. 2005;237:395–400.
36. Naidich DP, Bankier AA, MacMahon H, Schaefer-Prokop CM, Pistolesi M, Goo JM, Macchiarini P, Crapo JD, Herold CJ, Austin JH, Travis WD. Recommendations for the management of subsolid pulmonary nodules detected at CT: a statement from the Fleischner Society. Radiology. 2013;266(1):304–17.

Part I
Evaluations and Decisions

Chapter 2
Evidence Based Medicine: Quality of Evidence and Evaluation Systems

Apoorva Krishna Chandar and Yngve Falck-Ytter

Abstract Clinical care is increasingly informed by clinical practice guidelines. Well-formulated guidelines are transparent and actionable, and provide guidance through quality-rated evidence resulting into graded recommendations. In this chapter, we discuss a methodologically rigorous, yet simple rating system. Prior rating systems consisted of rigid, study type driven hierarchies. In contrast, the GRADE framework is outcomes-centric and explicit in its evidence rating criteria. GRADE also emphasizes that final guideline recommendations should not solely rely on the quality of evidence, but also on the balance between benefits and downsides, and consider patient values and preferences and resource use.

Keywords Rating systems • Clinical practice guidelines • GRADE • PICO • Quality of evidence • Strength of recommendations • Values and preferences • Resource utilization • Evidence based medicine

Introduction

Evidence based medicine is defined as "a systematic approach to clinical problem solving which allows the integration of the best available research evidence with clinical expertise and patient values" [1]. Arguably, the most important application of evidence based medicine is the development of clinical practice guidelines. Commenting on clinical practice guidelines, the Institute of Medicine [2] says:

Clinical Practice Guidelines are statements that include recommendations intended to optimize patient care. They are informed by a systematic review of evidence and an assessment

A.K. Chandar, MBBS, MA, MPH • Y. Falck-Ytter, MD, AGAF (✉)
Division of Gastroenterology, Louis Stokes Cleveland VA Medical Center,
Case Western Reserve University, 10701 East Blvd., Cleveland, OH 44106, USA
e-mail: apoorva.chandar@case.edu; yngve.falck-ytter@case.edu

M.K. Ferguson (ed.), *Difficult Decisions in Thoracic Surgery*,
Difficult Decisions in Surgery: An Evidence-Based Approach 1,
DOI 10.1007/978-1-4471-6404-3_2, © Springer-Verlag London 2014

of the benefits and harms of alternative care options. To be trustworthy, guidelines should be based on a systematic review of the existing evidence; be developed by a knowledgeable, multidisciplinary panel of experts and representatives from key affected groups; consider important patient subgroups and patient preferences, as appropriate; be based on an explicit and transparent process that minimizes distortions, biases, and conflicts of interest; provide a clear explanation of the logical relationships between alternative care options and health outcomes, and provide ratings of both the quality of evidence and the strength of recommendations; and be reconsidered and revised as appropriate when important new evidence warrants modifications of recommendations.

As knowledge grows exponentially, clinicians' treatment decisions increasingly depend on well done clinical practice guidelines [3]. However, a major impediment to the implementation and adoption of such guidelines is that they are often confusing and not actionable. The lack of clarity in guidelines creates confusion for not only the healthcare provider, but for patients as well. On the other hand, good clinical practice guidelines are actionable and easy to understand. In order to formulate clinical practice guidelines that can effectively guide clinicians and consumers, guidelines need to be derived from the best available evidence from which information can be obtained to support clinical recommendations.

Systematically developed guidelines have the potential to improve patient care and health outcomes, reduce inappropriate variations in practice, promote efficient use of limited healthcare resources and help define and inform public policy [4]. Despite an explosion in the field of guideline development in recent years, guidelines often lack transparency and useful information.

In the past, guideline developers usually relied solely on evidence hierarchies to determine the "level of evidence" with randomized controlled trials (RCTs) always being considered high level evidence and observational studies to be of lower quality. Such hierarchies suffer from oversimplification as RCTs can be flawed and well done observational studies may be the basis of higher quality evidence. Although the past 30 years have shown an enormous increase in evidence rating systems, almost all relied on a variation of those simple hierarchies. In addition, strong recommendations were routinely attached to high levels of evidence without regard to potentially closely balanced benefits and harms trade-offs which usually does require eliciting patient values and preferences and instead should result in conditional recommendations.

GRADE began as an initiative to offer a universally acceptable, sensible and transparent approach for grading the quality of evidence and strength of recommendations (http://www.gradeworkinggroup.org/). With the overarching goal of having a single system that avoids confusion and is methodologically rigorous, yet avoids the shortcomings of other systems, the GRADE framework helps to formulate clear, precise and concise recommendations. The uses of the GRADE framework are twofold:

1. Defines the strength recommendations in the development of clinical practice guidelines
2. Assist in rating the quality of evidence in systematic reviews and other evidence summaries on which those recommendations are based

   The GRADE framework has been widely adopted (>80 societies and organizations) including the WHO, the COCHRANE collaboration, the American Thoracic Society, and the European Society of Thoracic Surgeons [5]. In this chapter, we elaborate the GRADE approach to rating the quality of evidence and implications for strong and weak guideline recommendations and how patient values and preferences as well as resource use considerations can change those recommendations.

The GRADE Approach

Defining the Clinical Question

In GRADE, the starting point is the formulation of a relevant and answerable clinical question. It is essential to formulate a well-defined clinical question for more than one reason: On the one hand, it helps to bring emphasis on the focus and scope of the guideline and, and on the other, it helps to define the search strategy which will be used to identify the body of evidence. The PICO strategy that assists in defining a clinical question is detailed in Table 2.1.

What Outcomes Should We Consider for Clinical Decision Making?

Not all outcomes are equally important. Clinical questions in practice guidelines often contain several outcomes, some of which may or may not be useful for decision making. GRADE categorizes outcomes in a hierarchical fashion by listing outcomes that are critical to decision making (such as mortality), outcomes that are important but not critical for decision making (post-thoracotomy pain syndrome) and outcomes that are less important (hypertrophic scar resulting from thoracotomy incision). Such a step-wise rating is important because in GRADE, unlike other guideline systems that rate individual studies, quality of the available evidence is rated for individual outcomes across studies (Fig. 2.1). The reasoning behind this is that quality frequently differs across outcomes, even within a single study.

Table 2.1 The PICO approach to define a clinical question

P	Patient population	Describes the patient population being targeted by the intervention (e.g., patients with Barrett's esophagus)
I	Intervention	Describes the intervention that is being studied (e.g., minimally invasive esophagectomy for Barrett's esophagus with high grade dysplasia)
C	Comparator	Describes the intervention to which the study intervention is being compared to (e.g., radio frequency ablation)
O	Outcomes	Describes the outcomes which includes benefits and downsides (e.g., all-cause mortality, progression to esophageal adenocarcinoma, quality of life)

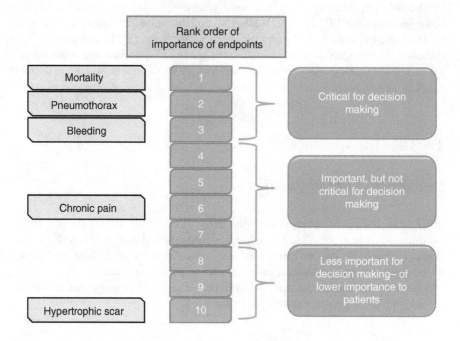

Fig. 2.1 Illustration of ranking outcomes according to importance to patients for assessing benefits and risks of open thoracotomy

Guideline panels should specify the comparator explicitly. In particular, when multiple treatment options are involved (such as surgical vs. nonsurgical treatments for symptomatic giant bullae in COPD), it should be specified whether the recommendation is suggesting that all treatments are equally recommended or that some interventions are recommended over others. In the same context, the choice of setting (such as resource poor vs. adequate resources or high volume vs. low volume centers) needs to be taken into consideration. Guideline panels should be aware of the audience and the setting they are targeting when formulating guidelines. We will elaborate further on resource use later in this chapter.

Grading the Quality of Evidence

The quality of evidence is the extent to which our confidence in a comparative estimate of an intervention effect is adequate to support a particular recommendation. For the rest of the chapter we will therefore use the terms "confidence in the evidence" and "quality of evidence" interchangeably.

Table 2.2 Quality of evidence

High quality	We are very confident that the true effect lies close to that of the estimate of the effect
Moderate quality	We are moderately confident in the estimate of effect: The true effect is likely to be close to the estimate of effect, but possibility to be substantially different
Low quality	Our confidence in the effect is limited: The true effect may be substantially different from the estimate of the effect
Very low quality	We have very little confidence in the effect estimate: The true effect is likely to be substantially different from the estimate of effect

Following the formulation of a PICO based clinical question is the crucial process of reviewing and grading the quality of evidence associated with the clinical question. For instance, a question like 'surgical management of non-small cell lung cancer' might give us a large number of studies, which might include randomized clinical trials (RCTs), observational studies and case series conducted in different settings, involve various kinds of surgeries and target different patient populations. Indeed, this becomes a challenge for review authors and guideline developers alike as they are presented with an enormous body of evidence. GRADE offers a formal way of rating the quality of this large body of evidence by providing detailed guidance for authors of systematic reviews and guidelines. GRADE defines the quality of evidence as the confidence we have in the estimate of effect (benefit or risk) to support a particular decision [6]. Although confidence in the evidence is continuous, GRADE uses four distinct categories to conceptualize evidence quality (Table 2.2).

Rating the Quality of Evidence from Randomized Controlled Trials

In GRADE, outcomes that are informed from RCTs start as high quality evidence. However, RCTs vary widely in quality. Methodological limitations (risk of bias), particularly related to the design and execution of RCTs can often lower the quality of evidence for a particular outcome. GRADE uses five different, well defined criteria to rate down the quality of evidence from RCTs (Table 2.3).

Limitations in Study Design

Proper randomization and adequate allocation concealment, which prevents clinicians and participants becoming aware of upcoming assignments are important strategies to protect from bias. Inadequate allocation concealment leads to exaggerated estimates of treatment effect [9]. Major limitations in study design may lead to rating down the quality of evidence for an outcome. However, assessment of whether

Table 2.3 Rating the quality of evidence for each important outcome

For outcomes informed by RCTs, start as high confidence, then rate down to moderate, low or very low confidence in the evidence

For outcomes informed by observational studies, start as low confidence, then either rate down or, on rare occasions, rate up to moderate or high confidence in the evidence

Checklist	Things to look out for
Risk of bias	RCTs: major limitations, such as lack of allocation concealment, lack of blinding, large losses of follow-up, failure of intention-to-treat analysis, and a study terminated early for benefit. Consider using the Cochrane risk of bias tool [7]
	Observational studies: assess risk of confounding by examining the selection of exposed and non-exposed cohort, comparability of the cohort and issues with assessment and adequacy of follow-up of the outcomes of interest. Consider using the Newcastle-Ottawa quality assessment tool [8]
Inconsistency	Widely differing estimates of the treatment effect (variability in results or heterogeneity)
Indirectness	Population: e.g., differences in age, gender, comorbidities
	Intervention: e.g., similar but not identical intervention
	Comparator: e.g., difference in comparator intervention
	Outcomes: e.g., use of surrogate outcomes, short-term vs. long-term
	No head-to-head comparison of two interventions
Imprecision	Wide confidence intervals/small sample size/few events that make the result uninformative
Publication bias	High probability of failure to report studies (likely because no effect was observed)
Magnitude of effect	Large magnitude of association: RR >2.0 or RR <0.5
	Very large magnitude of association: RR >5.0 or RR <0.2
	Two or more observational studies, direct evidence, no plausible confounders, no threats to validity, sufficiently precise estimate
Dose-response	Presence of a dose-response gradient
Plausible confounders	Unaccounted, plausible biases from observational evidence that moves the result in the direction of underestimating the apparent treatment effect (all plausible confounding would reduce a demonstrated effect; all plausible confounding would suggest a spurious effect when results show no effect)

or not a methodological shortcoming, such as lack of blinding, may have had a substantial impact on an estimate of effect is important as there are situations where lack of blinding may not materially impact a particular outcome. Another issue that is commonly encountered with RCTs is losses to follow up. Again, losses to follow up may not always require rating down if there are few and proportionate losses to follow up in both treatment and control groups. However, disproportionate losses to follow up can either increase (due to greater losses in the control group) or decrease (due to greater losses in the treatment group) the treatment effect [10]. The way in which RCTs are analyzed is another important criterion to consider in study design. Intention-to-treat (ITT) analysis is the preferred method of analysis of RCTs.

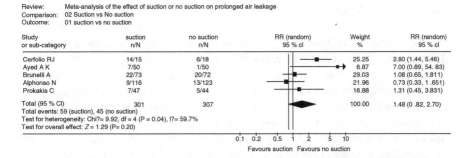

Fig. 2.2 Effect of suction vs. non-suction on prolonged air leakage showing widely varying estimate of effects and substantial heterogeneity among studies (I-squared of ~60 %) (Reprinted from Deng et al. [12], with permission)

However, it is documented that the intention-to-treat approach is often inadequately described and inadequately applied in RCT and deviations from ITT analysis are common [11]. RCTs should be carefully reviewed to determine if they adopted the ITT approach for a particular outcome. Lastly, authors of systematic reviews and guideline developers should exercise caution when they encounter trials that are stopped early for benefit, particularly when such trials contribute considerable weight to a meta-analysis as they might produce a spurious improvement in the treatment effect [12, 13].

Inconsistency of Study Results

Confidence in the estimate of effect may require rating down for inconsistency, if the magnitude and direction of effects across different studies varies widely (heterogeneity of study results). Variability in treatment effects across studies usually is the result of varying populations or interventions. However, when the reasons for inconsistency across studies cannot be identified, the confidence in the evidence may be lower. Consider for example the effect of suction vs. non-suction on prolonged air leakage to the underwater seal drains following pulmonary surgery. A meta-analysis of available RCTs showed varying effect estimates and direction of effect resulting in an I-squared of residual heterogeneity of close to 60 %, which could be considered substantial and it would not be unreasonable to rate down for inconsistency (Fig. 2.2) [14].

It is particularly important to remember that in GRADE, the quality of evidence is not rated up for consistency, it is only rated down for inconsistency. Several criteria may help decide whether heterogeneity exists: the point estimates vary widely across studies; minimally or non-overlapping confidence intervals; statistical test for heterogeneity shows a low p-value; I-squared value (percentage of variability due to heterogeneity rather than chance) is large [15].

Indirectness of Evidence

GRADE defines several sources of indirectness. For example, differences in patient characteristics (age, gender and race), differences in interventions or comparators (similar but not the same intervention or comparators), indirectness of outcomes (direct outcome measures vs. surrogate outcome measures) and indirect comparisons (e.g., lack of head-to-head trials of competing surgical approaches). All sources of indirectness can result in lowering our confidence in the estimate of effects. However, it is necessary to remember that when direct evidence is limited in quantity or quality, indirect evidence from other populations may be considered and the quality need not necessarily be rated down with proper justification for not doing so. For example, although direct evidence about the safety and effectiveness of prophylaxis of VTE prevention in patients undergoing thoracic surgery is limited, the ACCP anti-thrombotic guidelines did not rate down for indirectness as they felt that the evidence about relative risks from studies of patients undergoing general or abdominal-pelvic surgery could be applied with little or no indirectness to thoracic surgery [16]. Another domain of indirectness is duration of follow-up for certain outcomes. GRADE recommends that guideline developers should always indicate the length of follow up to which the estimate of absolute effect refers. This length of follow up is a time frame judged appropriate to balance the risk-benefit consequences of alternative treatment strategies. Longer follow up periods are associated with higher risk differences between intervention and control. This could potentially lead to important differences in readers' perception of the apparent magnitude of effect. Often, extending the time frame involves the assumption that event rates will stay constant over time [17].

Of particular importance is the categorization of outcome measures into direct and surrogate outcomes. In the absence of data on patient-important outcomes, surrogates could contribute to the estimation of the effect of an intervention on the outcomes that are important. Post-surgical asymptomatic deep vein thrombosis detected by screening venography or ultrasound surveillance is an example of a surrogate outcome [18]. It is to be noted that despite the relative importance of direct outcomes, both direct and surrogate outcomes should be reported in studies because the audience for guideline developers and systematic reviews might want to see both before making appropriate decisions.

Imprecision

Imprecision is usually determined by examining the confidence intervals. Usually, studies with few enrolled patients and/or few events have wider confidence intervals. Additionally, our confidence in the evidence is lowered when the 95 % confidence interval fails to exclude important benefit or important harm. Consider for example the long-term outcome of dilation requirements when using 180-degree laparoscopic anterior fundoplication (180-degree LAF) versus laparoscopic Nissen fundoplication (LNF) for GERD [19]. Although the partial fundoplication showed

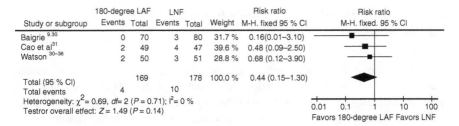

Fig. 2.3 Five-year dilatation rate of 180-degree laparoscopic anterior fundoplication vs. laparoscopic Nissen fundoplication for GERD (Reprinted from Broeders et al. [17], with permission)

less than half the rate of dilatations, few events in the studies and generally low sample sizes did not allow for a precise estimate even after pooling the results, and the 95 % confidence interval crosses one (Fig. 2.3).

Publication Bias

When there is sufficient evidence that trials have not been reported (especially when treatment effects are negligibly small or absent), this may lead to an overestimation of effect and decrease our confidence in the evidence. Such trials, more commonly than not, are industry funded and small. Authors of systematic reviews and clinical guidelines should show due diligence in checking for any unreported trial results by verifying with clinicaltrials.gov for registered, but potentially unpublished, trials. Systematic reviews provide a way of detecting publication bias by examining the funnel plot, for example, to help detect potential publication bias.

Rating Up the Quality of Evidence from Observational Studies

Outcomes deriving their evidence from observational studies usually start as low confidence in the evidence (low quality evidence). The reason for this is that observational studies are unable to fully control for unknown confounders. However, there are situations where evidence from observational studies should be considered to provide higher quality evidence. GRADE recommends rating up the quality of evidence in several instances. Evidence from well-done observational studies without known residual confounding, large magnitude of effect will usually increase our confidence that an effect exists and it would be reasonable to rate up the quality of evidence. For example, surgical resection with curative intent of esophageal cancer shows a very large relative magnitude of effect in reduction of mortality compared to best supportive care [20]. Another reason for rating up the evidence quality is the presence of a dose response gradient. Table 2.3 gives an overview of when to rate up or rate down the quality of evidence obtained from observational studies.

Moving from Quality of Evidence to Formulating Recommendations

Strength of a recommendation reflects the extent to which we can be confident that the beneficial effects of an intervention clearly outweigh its undesirable effects [21]. Even though GRADE suggests rating the quality of evidence for each outcome in an ordinal fashion to assist systematic review authors and guideline developers to arrive at an outcome-specific rating of confidence, the final rating of confidence in the evidence (overall quality of evidence for a particular PICO question) will need to be determined before making recommendations. GRADE specifies that the over-all quality of evidence is driven by the lowest quality of evidence of an outcome that is critical for decision making [22]. For instance, we might be confident about an intervention's benefit, but as long as there is a harm associated with this intervention that is considered critical for decision making (and, for example, rated as moderate quality of evidence), the overall quality of evidence across all critical outcomes in regards to the PICO question should remain at moderate despite the high quality of evidence for benefit.

While acknowledging that the strength of recommendations is, in fact, a contin-uum, GRADE offers a binary classification for strength of recommendations: strong and weak (conditional). Such a dichotomous system provides clear, simple, easily understandable, and readily implementable directions with clear implications for patients, clinicians and policy-makers. Table 2.4 provides an overview of this classification.

The strength of recommendation is guided not merely by the quality of the evi-dence—high quality evidence doesn't necessarily always indicate strong recom-mendations, and strong recommendations can sometimes arise from lower quality evidence [23]. Though the quality of evidence is the primary starting point in guid-ing the strength of a recommendation, additional, but separate factors such as bal-ance between desirable and undesirable effects, patients' values and preferences, and uncertainty regarding wise use of resources arising from a recommendation are equally important in the GRADE system and may change the strength or even the direction of a recommendation [6]. When guideline panels strongly recommend an intervention, they are confident that the desirable effects clearly outweigh the unde-sirable effects and that almost all fully informed patients, with reasonable certainty will opt for the intervention. GRADE identifies 4 important factors that can impact the overall quality of evidence and thereby influence the strength of recommenda-tions (Table 2.5).

Resource Use

Resource use varies widely over time and across geographical settings. While an intervention with higher costs is unlikely to be strongly recommended over an equally effective lower cost alternative, it is essential to consider the context of

Table 2.4 Health care implications of GRADE defined strengths of recommendations

Strength of recommendation	Implications for patients	Implications for clinicians	Implications for policy makers
Strong	Most individuals in this situation would want the recommended course of action and only a small proportion would not	Most individuals should receive the intervention	The recommendation can be adopted as a performance indicator in most situations
	Formal decision aids are not likely to be needed to help individuals make decisions consistent with their values and preferences, but could help with the implementation	Adherence to this recommendation according to the guidelines could be used as a quality criterion or a performance indicator	
Weak (conditional)	The majority of individuals in this situation would want the suggested course of action, but many would not	Be prepared to help people to make a decision that is consistent with their own values and preferences	Policy-making will require substantial debates and involvement of many stakeholders
	Decision aids may be useful in helping individuals make decisions consistent with their values and preferences	Use decision aids and implement shared decision making approaches	

recommendation and hence, guideline panels must be specific about the setting to which a recommendation applies [21].

Resource use studies might be conducted concurrently within the framework of an empirical study such as clinical trial or using a decision model that typically uses secondary data collected from several sources. Cost utilization and resource utilization might be particularly important in surgical treatments.

GRADE recommends assessing resource implications in two steps [24]. First, consider whether resource use is important (or critical) for making the recommendation. Second, consider specific items of resource use and their potential impact on different strategies. For a detailed explanation of application of GRADE to resource use, we refer the readers to other relevant GRADE publications [24, 25].

Presenting Summary of Findings

GRADE offers a way of displaying a comprehensive, but condensed summary of key outcomes and their importance in a summary of findings (SoFs) table. A SoFs table usually contains all important outcomes necessary for clinical decision

Table 2.5 GRADE determinants of the strength of recommendation

GRADE category	Example of a **strong** recommendation	Example of a **weak** (conditional) recommendation
Quality of evidence	A large number of high quality RCTs has shown that plain chest X-ray screening does not reduce lung cancer mortality	Only case series have examined the effectiveness of diaphragmatic repair for the treatment of hepatic hydrothorax in patients who are not eligible for TIPS
Balance of benefits versus harms and burdens	The success of an initial pleural aspiration attempt in stable patients with large spontaneous pneumothorax is sufficiently high with acceptable risks and low costs compared to VATS	180 ° laparoscopic anterior fundoplication compared to Nissen fundoplication reduces the incidence of procedure related dysphagia and need for dilatation, but at a cost of increased rate of re-operation and residual reflux symptoms
Values and preferences	Younger patients with early stage non-small cell lung cancer will invariably place a higher value on the life prolonging effects of post-surgical adjuvant chemotherapy over treatment toxicity	Older patients with early stage non-small cell lung cancer may not place a higher value on the life prolonging effects of post-surgical adjuvant chemotherapy over treatment toxicity
Resource use (e.g., cost)	The relative low cost of chest catheter insertion for the treatment of large primary spontaneous pneumothorax	The high cost of adding bevacizumab to initial chemotherapy regimens in patients with advanced non-small cell lung cancer

making, shows the quality of evidence across studies for a particular outcome and the associated relative and absolute effects [22]. When meta-analyses are accompanied by such SoFs tables, they can prove useful for guideline developers while developing recommendations. GRADE recommends limiting the number of outcomes to approximately 7 for each SoFs table, as it is unlikely that more outcomes will lead to better overview of the data and judgments made [17]. If there are more than seven outcomes, combining certain similar outcomes might become necessary (such as symptomatic deep vein thrombosis and pulmonary embolism into one category of "venous thrombotic events"). It is not uncommon to find systematic reviews that address more than one comparison, evaluate an intervention in two disparate populations or examine the effects of a number of interventions for the same clinical problem. Such systematic reviews are also likely to be accompanied by more than one SoFs table [26]. A GRADE summary of findings table showing five important outcomes for using heparin compared to no heparin in lung and other cancers with no other indication for anticoagulation [27] is shown in Fig. 2.4.

heparin compared to no heparin for patients with cancer who have no other therapeutic or prophylactic indication for anticoagulation

Patient or population: patients with cancer who have no other therapeutic or prophylactic indication for anticoagulation
Settings: outpatient
Intervention: heparin
Comparison: no heparin

Outcomes	Illustrative comparative risks* (95% CI)		Relative effect (95% CI)	No of Participants (studies)	Quality of the evidence (GRADE)	Comments
	Assumed risk	Corresponding risk				
	no heparin	heparin				
Mortality Follow-up: 12 months	Medium risk population		RR 0.93 (0.85 to 1.02)	2531 (8 studies)	⊕⊕⊕◯ moderate[1,2,3]	
	649 per 1000	604 per 1000 (552 to 662)				
Symptomatic VTE Follow-up: 12 months	Medium risk population		RR 0.55 (0.85 to 1.02)	2264 (7 studies)	⊕⊕⊕⊕ high	
	29 per 1000	16 per 1000 (11 to 24)				
Major bleeding Follow-up: 12 months	Medium risk population		RR 1.3 (0.59 to 2.88)	2843 (9 studies)	⊕⊕⊕◯ moderate[1,4]	
	7 per 1000	9 per 1000 (4 to 20)				
Minor bleeding Follow-up: 12 weeks	Medium risk population		RR 1.05 (0. 75 to 1.46)	2345 (7 studies)	⊕⊕⊕◯ moderate[1,4]	
	27 per 1000	28 per 1000 (20 to 39)				
Health related quality of life the Uniscale and the Symptom Distress Scale (SDS) ; Better indicated by lower values Follow-up: 12 months	See comment	See comment	Not estimable[5]	0 (1 study)	⊕⊕◯◯ low[6]	

*The basis for the assumed risk (e.g. the median control group risk across studies) is provided in footnotes. The corresponding risk (and its 95% confidence interval) is based on the assumed risk in the comparison group and the relative effect of the intervention (and its 95% CI).
CI: Confidence interval ; RR: Risk ratio;

GRADE Working Group grades of evidence
High quality: Further research is very unlikely to change our confidence in the estimate of effect.
Moderate quality: Further research is likely to have an important impact on our confidence in the estimate of effect and may change the estimate.
Low quality: Further research is very likely to have an important impact on our confidence in the estimate of effect and is likely to change the estimate.
Very low quality: We are very uncertain about the estimate.

1 Vast majority of studies had allocation concealment , and used blinded outcome and adjudication. We did not downgrade although there was some concern about lack of blinding in some studies; the overall risk of bias was felt to be very low.
2 There is moderate heterogeneity among studies included in the analysis of death at 12 months (12 =41 %). The subgroup analysis for mortality at 12 months was statistically significant and suggested survival benefit in patients with SCLC but not in patients with advanced cancer. Overall we decided to downgrade by one level when considering these issues along with imprecision.
3 CI interval includes effects suggesting benefit as well as no benefit.
4 CI includes possibility of both harms or benefits.
5 The scores for the 2 scales were similar for the 2 study groups, both at baseline and at follow-up
6 High risk of bias and only 138 patients enrolled.

Fig. 2.4 Summary of findings table showing five relevant pooled outcomes for heparin therapy compared to no heparin in lung and other cancers where there is no therapeutic or prophylactic indication for anticoagulation (Reprinted from Akl et al. [27], with permission)

How Should Clinical Guidance Be Worded?

Guideline authors should choose appropriate phrasing to disseminate their findings. GRADE advises the use of standardized language to express strong and weak recommendations for or against an intervention. Such standardized wording would be: "We recommend to use…" or "We recommend against the use of …" for strong recommendations and "We suggest to use…" or "We suggest against the use of…"

for weak recommendations [22]. For example, a weak recommendation would be worded like this: "For thoracic surgery patients who are at high risk for major bleeding, we suggest the use of mechanical prophylaxis, preferably with optimally applied intermittent pneumatic compression, over no prophylaxis" [16].

Applying GRADE

Figure 2.5 illustrates a high level overview of the GRADE system. With its clarity, simplicity and methodological rigor, GRADE lends itself for application to grading the quality of evidence for a wide range of evidence summaries, from systematic reviews of interventions, diagnostic tests and strategies to formal health technology assessments or presentations that can be more easily utilized by health care providers by including actionable recommendations, such as clinical practice guidelines, care paths, or decision support systems (top half illustrating the supporting systematic review; lower half the moving-to-recommendations process).

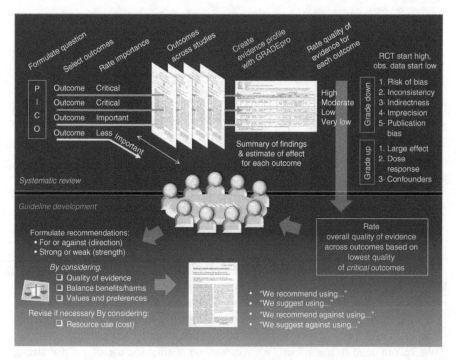

Fig. 2.5 An overview of the GRADE system (Reprinted from Falck-Ytter and Guyatt [28] with permission)

Conclusion

A common, simple, yet rigorous rating system can reduce confusion and increase the transparency when formulating recommendations in guidelines, textbooks and other evidence summaries. It allows surgeons to engage the patient in a shared decision-making process when recommending care based on varying levels of confidence in the evidence and different trade-offs between benefits and downsides as well as uncertainty of patient's values and preferences [29].

Although evidence quality ratings within the GRADE approach have shown to be reproducible, [30] the main goal is to provide transparent and explicit judgments. GRADE is the only system to recognize that quality may differ across outcomes and specifically addresses this issue by being outcomes-centric. GRADE provides explicit, detailed and comprehensive criteria for rating the quality of evidence. Finally, not only does GRADE define quality of evidence and strength of recommendations as two related but separate concepts, but also makes the transition from rating the quality of evidence to formulating clinically sensible recommendations a transparent process by including additional domains important for decision making: patient's values and preferences, balance between harms and burdens, and resource use.

References

 1. Sackett D, Strauss S, Richardson W, et al. Evidence-based medicine: how to practice and teach EBM. 2nd ed. Edinburgh: Churchill Livingstone; 2000.
 2. IOM (Institute of Medicine). Clinical practice guidelines we can trust. Washington, DC: The National Academies Press; 2011.
 3. Mendelson D, Carino TV. Evidence-based medicine in the United States – de rigueur or dream deferred? Health Aff Millwood. 2005;24(1):133–6.
 4. Sultan S, Falck-Ytter Y, Inadomi JM. The AGA institute process for developing clinical practice guidelines part one: grading the evidence. Clin Gastroenterol Hepatol. 2013;11(4):329–32.
 5. Organizations that have endorsed or that are using GRADE: GRADE Working Group. 2013. Available from: http://www.gradeworkinggroup.org/society/. Cited Oct 30 2013.
 6. Falck-Ytter Y, Kunz R, Guyatt GH, Schunemann HJ. How strong is the evidence? Am J Gastroenterol. 2008;103(6):1334–8.
 7. Schulz KF, Grimes DA. Allocation concealment in randomised trials: defending against deciphering. Lancet. 2002;359(9306):614–8.
 8. Guyatt GH, Oxman AD, Vist G, Kunz R, Brozek J, Alonso-Coello P, et al. GRADE guidelines: 4. Rating the quality of evidence – study limitations (risk of bias). J Clin Epidemiol. 2011;64(4):407–15.
 9. Hollis S, Campbell F. What is meant by intention to treat analysis? Survey of published randomised controlled trials. BMJ. 1999;319(7211):670–4.
10. Bassler D, Briel M, Montori VM, Lane M, Glasziou P, Zhou Q, et al. Stopping randomized trials early for benefit and estimation of treatment effects: systematic review and meta-regression analysis. JAMA. 2010;303(12):1180–7.

11. Guyatt GH, Briel M, Glasziou P, Bassler D, Montori VM. Problems of stopping trials early. BMJ. 2012;344:e3863.
12. Deng B, Tan QY, Zhao YP, Wang RW, Jiang YG. Suction or non-suction to the underwater seal drains following pulmonary operation: meta-analysis of randomised controlled trials. Eur J Cardiothorac Surg. 2010;38(2):210–5.
13. Guyatt GH, Oxman AD, Kunz R, Woodcock J, Brozek J, Helfand M, et al. GRADE guidelines: 7. Rating the quality of evidence – inconsistency. J Clin Epidemiol. 2011; 64(12):1294–302.
14. Gould MK, Garcia DA, Wren SM, Karanicolas PJ, Arcelus JI, Heit JA, et al. Prevention of VTE in nonorthopedic surgical patients: antithrombotic therapy and prevention of thrombosis, 9th ed: American College of Chest Physicians evidence-based clinical practice guidelines. Chest. 2012;141(2 Suppl):e227S–77.
15. Guyatt GH, Oxman AD, Santesso N, Helfand M, Vist G, Kunz R, et al. GRADE guidelines: 12. Preparing summary of findings tables-binary outcomes. J Clin Epidemiol. 2013;66(2):158–72.
16. Guyatt GH, Norris SL, Schulman S, Hirsh J, Eckman MH, Akl EA, et al. Methodology for the development of antithrombotic therapy and prevention of thrombosis guidelines: antithrombotic therapy and prevention of thrombosis, 9th ed: American College of Chest Physicians evidence-based clinical practice guidelines. Chest. 2012;141(2 Suppl):53S–70.
17. Broeders JA, Roks DJ, Ahmed Ali U, Watson DI, Baigrie RJ, Cao Z, et al. Laparoscopic anterior 180-degree versus Nissen fundoplication for gastroesophageal reflux disease: systematic review and meta-analysis of randomized clinical trials. Ann Surg. 2013;257(5): 850–9.
18. Lee JS, Urschel DM, Urschel JD. Is general thoracic surgical practice evidence based? Ann Thorac Surg. 2000;70(2):429–31.
19. Higgins JP, Altman DG, Gotzsche PC, Juni P, Moher D, Oxman AD, et al. The Cochrane collaboration's tool for assessing risk of bias in randomised trials. BMJ. 2011;343:d5928.
20. Wells GA, Shea B, O'Connell D, Peterson J, Welch V, Losos M, et al. The Newcastle-Ottawa Scale (NOS) for assessing the quality of nonrandomised studies in meta-analyses. 2000. http://www.ohri.ca/programs/clinical_epidemiology/oxford.asp, accessed 4 May 2014.
21. Guyatt GH, Oxman AD, Kunz R, Falck-Ytter Y, Vist GE, Liberati A, et al. Going from evidence to recommendations. BMJ. 2008;336(7652):1049–51.
22. Falck-Ytter Y, Guyatt GH. Guidelines: rating the quality of evidence and grading the strength of recommendations. In: Burneo JG, Demaerschalk BM, Jenkins ME, editors. Neurology: an evidence-based approach. New York: Springer; 2012. p. 25–41.
23. Guyatt GH, Oxman AD, Vist GE, Kunz R, Falck-Ytter Y, Alonso-Coello P, et al. GRADE: an emerging consensus on rating quality of evidence and strength of recommendations. BMJ. 2008;336(7650):924–6.
24. Brunetti M, Shemilt I, Pregno S, Vale L, Oxman AD, Lord J, et al. GRADE guidelines: 10. Considering resource use and rating the quality of economic evidence. J Clin Epidemiol. 2013;66(2):140–50.
25. Guyatt GH, Oxman AD, Kunz R, Jaeschke R, Helfand M, Liberati A, et al. Incorporating considerations of resources use into grading recommendations. BMJ. 2008;336(7654): 1170–3.
26. Guyatt G, Oxman AD, Akl EA, Kunz R, Vist G, Brozek J, et al. GRADE guidelines: 1. Introduction-GRADE evidence profiles and summary of findings tables. J Clin Epidemiol. 2011;64(4):383–94.
27. Akl EA, Gunukula S, Barba M, Yosuico VE, van Doormaal FF, Kuipers S, et al. Parenteral anticoagulation in patients with cancer who have no therapeutic or prophylactic indication for anticoagulation. Cochrane Database Syst Rev. 2011;4:CD006652. doi:10.1002/14651858. CD006652.pub3.

28. Falck-Ytter Y, Guyatt G. Guidelines: rating the quality of evidence and grading the strength of recommendations. In: Burneo J, Demaerschalk B, Jenkins M, editors. Neurology – an evidence based approach. New York: Springer; 2011.
29. Feuerstein JD, Gifford AE, Akbari M, Goldman J, Leffler DA, Sheth SG, et al. Systematic analysis underlying the quality of the scientific evidence and conflicts of interest in gastroenterology practice guidelines. Am J Gastroenterol. 2013;108(11):1686–93.
30. Mustafa RA, Santesso N, Brozek J, Akl EA, Walter SD, Norman G, et al. The GRADE approach is reproducible in assessing the quality of evidence of quantitative evidence syntheses. J Clin Epidemiol. 2013;66(7):736–42.

Chapter 3
Decision Analytic Techniques and Other Decision Processes

Varun Puri and Bryan F. Meyers

Abstract Clinical decision making is complex and guided by a number of factors including medical evidence, personal experience and intuition. "Decision analysis" is a process that provides a framework for examining the clinical scenario, synthesizing the available evidence, and providing a recommendation for action. Decision analysis techniques are increasingly used in clinical medicine to develop health policy, clinical algorithms, and for cost-effectiveness analysis. An overview of the techniques, interpretation, and application of decision analysis is presented here.

Keywords Decision analysis • Cost-effectiveness analysis • Markov modeling

Introduction

Nearly all clinical care results from some sort of decision process. Decisions that influence patient care can range from bedside choices concerning routine laboratory testing to health policy decisions about permitting and paying for new and expensive treatment options for specific illnesses. Similarly, the consequences of healthcare decisions can be seen in the outcomes of individual patients as well as generational shifts in the management of disease processes.

Decision making in healthcare is inherently complex and often influenced by a multitude of factors. These include the availability of competing alternatives; information about the risks, costs and downstream effects of these individual options; and the point of view or perspective from which one must make the decision. The process of formally and simultaneously considering the available evidence and

V. Puri, MD (⊠) • B.F. Meyers, MD MPH
Division of Cardiothoracic Surgery, Washington University School of Medicine,
St. Louis, MO, USA
e-mail: puriv@wustl.edu; meyersb@wustl.edu

M.K. Ferguson (ed.), *Difficult Decisions in Thoracic Surgery*,
Difficult Decisions in Surgery: An Evidence-Based Approach 1,
DOI 10.1007/978-1-4471-6404-3_3, © Springer-Verlag London 2014

comparing options with the objective of maximizing desirable outcomes is called
decision analysis. Though decision analysis has its roots in engineering and economic systems, it has been increasingly utilized in the field of medicine to clarify
thinking and guide management decisions [1, 2]. Several authors have also applied
this methodology to common thoracic surgical problems [3–9].

Application of Decision Analytic Techniques

Common scenarios in clinical medicine where decision analysis might be most useful fall into one of three categories which are described below with relevant
examples.

Action Versus Inaction

Certain clinical situations require an active choice between an intervention and
watchful waiting. A common scenario in thoracic surgery is an incidentally detected
solitary pulmonary nodule [5]. The framework for decision analysis here begins
with a consideration of all the available options. These include watchful waiting
with a further CT scan in 3–6 months (relative inaction) or immediate action alternatives which include CT-PET scan, percutaneous or bronchoscopic biopsy, or proceeding directly with surgery. Proper consideration of the risk of malignancy prior
to any of these interventions is of paramount importance. As an example, the risk of
a nodule being malignant is higher in a 65 year old smoker than in a 45 year old
non-smoker. Similarly, the likelihood of cancer in a 2 cm spiculated lesion is much
higher than that in a 9 mm ground glass opacity. These defining characteristics
greatly influence the positive and negative predictive values of the tests (also called
post-test probabilities) and must be considered and defined in the decision analysis.
The careful formulation of the question is paramount in the construction of a worthwhile decision analysis. In the examples above, one would expect a different answer
for the two extreme examples, so it would be unlikely that those two patients would
be evaluated with the same decision analysis. The question must be very specific,
and the results of the subsequent decision analysis would only generalize to situations consistent with the specific parameters defined in advance.

Next, one looks at each of the possible options for action and considers the consequences of each of these choices. For this, it is important to consider the sensitivity,
specificity, and accuracy of each of these tests, in the setting in which they will be
employed. A false positive test will lead to an unnecessary operation while a false
negative test might result in a missed or delayed cancer diagnosis and the potential
for progression and increased long term risk of mortality. The consequences of inaction (watchful waiting) may be the appropriate avoidance of an unnecessary operation in the event that the lesion is actually benign, or an inappropriate delay in
treatment for what turns out to be a lung cancer. Finally the advantages of treatment,

such as an early diagnosis and an increased chance of avoiding cancer-related mortality, and the disadvantages, such as perioperative costs and adverse outcomes, are factored into the decision analysis. The end-points in analysis can vary and range from minimizing costs, to minimizing cancer deaths, to minimizing intervention-related adverse effects, or to maximizing overall length of life. Though, superficially these objectives appear similar, the analysis is usually performed with a specific end-point in mind. Rarely, the decision analysis will evaluate two options that result in the same qualitative outcome and they are compared on measures of cost or time efficiency. More commonly, the measured end-points are more complex like a simultaneous assessment of costs, length of life and quality of life. The more complex the endpoint, the more likely that decision analysis techniques will be helpful in elucidating and clarifying the differences between the choices studied.

Choice Among Various Actions That Seem Plausible

Another common application of decision analytic techniques is a comparison of viable alternatives when one option is not known to be clearly superior. As an example, unsuspected mediastinal lymph node metastases may be encountered at the time of proposed resection for lung cancer [3]. The two principal alternatives are: (a) Proceed with the planned resection; or, (b) Stop the operation without a resection in order to administer neoadjuvant chemotherapy or chemoradiotherapy, and then attempt resection at a later date in the absence of progression or clinical decline. In this cited example, the authors considered an array of possible events after the primary resection option including operative mortality, survival with adjuvant treatment, and survival with no adjuvant treatment. Similarly, for the scenario where resection is postponed until after induction therapy, they considered the probabilities of various consequences; mortality related to the exploration, the receipt of chemoradiation without a subsequent resection, and successful progression from induction therapy to resection. Investigators may estimate the likelihood of each of these scenarios from previously published literature, utilize their own clinical data, or employ a combined approach. In this particular study, the authors chose to perform a cost-effectiveness analysis. The enquiry shed light on that clinical decision by estimating the overall costs of treatment and the expected survival and quality-adjusted survival for the two competing treatment options to facilitate a decision and subsequent research.

Optimizing Timing or Interval of Action

Decision analysis can also be employed to propose the appropriate timing of interventions. As an example, the optimal follow-up strategy after resection for esophageal cancer is a matter of debate. Various groups advocate frequency of follow-up ranging from 3 to 12 month intervals. An appropriate use of decision analysis could be to compare two alternatives; intensive follow-up with axial imaging, clinic visits, and lab tests every 3 months, versus a less intensive approach with imaging performed at annual clinic visits only. For both strategies, one would consider the probabilities of detection of recurrence and the likelihood of survival with and without treatment for recurrence. Subsequently a model could be created to with a view towards optimizing resource utilization and avoiding unnecessary interventions.

Technical Aspects

The decision analysis process is best conducted using a standard approach. Briefly, one must first define the problem and clarify the objectives in the problem-solving process. Next, one must enumerate the alternatives and how these choices affect downstream events with their probabilities and values. Finally, we consider the balance of benefits and adverse outcomes of each option. Hunink et al. [10] have described this **PROACTIVE** approach to decision analysis.

P – Problem(s) – Define Problem Explicitly

The details of the problem must be described as precisely as possible because the performance characteristics of the intervention and many of the subsequent probabilities and outcomes will be highly associated to those defining details. This step also involves a consideration of the natural history of the problem and likely consequences of inaction. It is often useful to create a "consequence table" enumerating outcomes for the watchful waiting approach.

R – Reframe

Consider the problem from multiple perspectives including those of the patient, family members, society, and the clinician. This is useful as it is common for a disease process to pose different challenges to these stakeholders. For example: a screening question might pose minimal health impact on the vast majority of patient stakeholders who do not have the screened condition, but a huge impact on the small minority who are found to have the disease being sought. The answer in such a decision analysis will often hinge on the costs of screening and the costs of care prevented or required as a result of a positive screen. Certainly, the net benefit of such a program might vary if you consider from various perspectives: patient, society, or payor.

O – Objective – Focus on the Objective(s)

Is the goal to save lives, or save money or to strike a balance between the two? There may be more than one objective and it is important to understand any trade-offs between objectives. A "means" objective is an intermediate step (e.g. performing surgery for lung cancer) and is not considered to be intrinsically valuable while a "fundamental" objective (e.g. long-term survival after surgery for lung cancer) has intrinsic value. Means objectives might be useful for surrogate endpoints when the downstream events from that point are predictable and the fundamental objective is either distant in time or expensive to measure.

A – Alternatives

Consider all relevant alternatives. It is useful to broadly consider alternatives in three categories; inaction, intervention, and information (e.g. ordering more tests before making a decision).

C – Consequences/Chances

Model the consequences and estimate the chances, or probability, of these consequences. The consequences (positive and negative) of each alternative can be tabulated into a balance sheet. The likelihood of each of these consequences needs to be estimated and the search for these probabilities can be an important part of the entire decision analysis. The sum of all outcome probabilities for an individual action always adds up to 1.

T – Trade-offs

Identify and estimate the value trade-offs. Valuation of consequences requires assessing the importance of each potential consequence. Here, patient reported outcomes are often a key. As an example, if one is interested in survival after treatment for cancer, quality of life estimates further refine the valuation. A more meaningful assessment of utility of an intervention is quality-adjusted survival. The Quality Adjusted Life Year (QALY) is a measure that integrates the length of life and the quality of life. The basic idea underlying the QALY assumes that a year of life lived in perfect health is worth 1 QALY (1 Year of Life × 1 Utility value = 1 QALY) and that a year of life lived in a state of less than perfect health is worth less than 1 QALY. A variety of techniques are available to assess the utility of each disease state and thus calculate QALYs.

I – Integrate

To integrate the evidence and values, one formally calculates the expected value of each option. In some analyses, this is referred to as "rolling up" the decision tree to come up with a preferred alternative and some numerical estimates that justify the preference. Sophisticated computer programs are available to perform this step.

V – Value

Optimize the expected value. The underlying principle of decision analysis is to maximize the expected utility. The probability of reaching each outcome (e.g. survival free of disease, survival with burden of disease, death) is multiplied by the calculated value of that outcome, and for each choice in the decision tree, the sums of these products are added to create the expected average value for that choice. The choice of the expected value to measure may stem from an aim to maximize desirable outcomes (QALYs) or to minimize cost or harm. Alternatively, a more complex end-point may be chosen like in a cost-effectiveness analysis.

E –Explore/Evaluate

Explore the assumptions and evaluate uncertainty. Decision analysis uses locally observed or researched values as estimates of both probabilities and value of outcomes. If there is uncertainty about these numbers, it may change the recommendation. Hence it is imperative to determine if the recommendation is "sensitive" to plausible changes in probabilities and utility values. Such an analysis is called a "sensitivity analysis" and may be conducted by varying one (1-way sensitivity analysis) or more than one (n-way sensitivity analysis) variable simultaneously across the range of clinically meaningful values and reassessing the model. In some cases, the outcome will change very little in response to large swings in a data point (insensitive) while in other cases, a particular data input will be very influential and thus more important to the analysis.

Creating a Decision Tree

Now let us examine how these principles can be applied in creating a decision tree. A decision tree (Fig. 3.1) reads from left to right and begins with a decision node (square) that frames the question being evaluated. At this point in the analysis, an intervention is selected, in this case a choice between two competing treatment

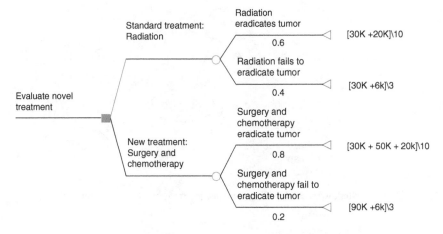

Fig. 3.1 A generic decision tree for cost-effectiveness analysis for treatment of cancer

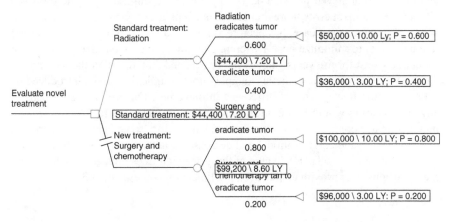

Fig. 3.2 Rolled back decision tree depicting the overall costs and the utilities associated with either treatment option

options for lung cancer. From there, a series of probability nodes (circles) reflects the likelihood of downstream events for patients subjected to any of the interventions. In this overly simplistic model, the possible outcomes with either treatment arm are limited to success and failure. The probabilities of these outcomes (a number between 0 and 1) are indicated. The probabilities of outcomes for each intervention add up to 1. Finally, the terminal nodes (triangles) represent final states for the analysis and are labeled with the costs expended to reach that state (for cost effectiveness analyses) as well as the estimated utilities for patients reaching that terminal state. In this case, the costs are provided in dollars and beneficial outcomes are described in QALYs. Figure 3.2 shows a decision tree after rolling it back. "Rolling back" a decision tree refers to an analysis that starts at the terminal nodes of the tree

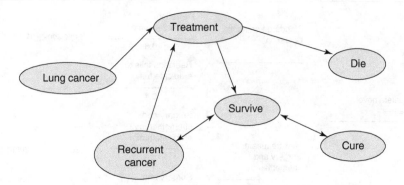

Fig. 3.3 A simple Markov model depicting the transition from one state of health to another

and works backward to the initial decision node, determining the costs expended and the values achieved for each decision pathway. In this example, the proposed alternative treatment costs more, but provides a longer expected survival. The standard treatment, or base case, has been recommended in this model as the decision tree here aims to minimize cost. Different end points (e.g. maximizing survival or minimizing cost for life years gained) can be selected that may alter the recommendation. While this is a very simple example, more complexity can be introduced by acknowledging finer grades of difference in outcomes. For instance, cure without any complication would be the ideal outcome in any decision tree, but cure with minor or major complications might lead to similar life expectancy with increased cost (to manage the complications) and decreased quality of life (as a consequence of the complications). The real value of these decision trees increases as their complexity begins to approximate that seen in clinical outcomes (Fig. 3.3).

Special Situations

Cost-Effectiveness Analysis (CEA)

CEA refers to a unique situation in decision analysis whereby the objective is to maximize population health benefits for any given level of resources. The same approach may be used given a preset health benefit goal, with the objective of minimizing the cost of attaining it. Such an analysis is often performed from a payer's perspective. In this perspective the costs of therapy are those experienced by the payer of treatment. Alternate approaches are to consider the societal perspective or a combined approach. In a combined perspective analysis, the costs of treatment are those experienced by the payer, minus the monetary gains to society from an individual who lives longer due to a more effective treatment. The costs of therapy may include direct medical costs, non healthcare costs (transportation, dietary changes, exercise programs etc.), caregiver time costs, loss of productivity, and costs of future healthcare interventions with longevity gained by treatment. Effectiveness of therapy is typically measured in QALYs. In a typical CEA, the incremental cost-effectiveness ratio (ICER) is estimated as the cost per life year (or quality-adjusted life year) gained over the patient's remaining lifetime by using a decision model and is a measure of cost-effectiveness. If one treatment modality is less costly and more effective than the other, it is labeled as dominant.

Markov Modeling

Thus far we have considered a linear model in the decision tree where a cohort moves forward in time. A state-transition model, also called a Markov model, is also commonly utilized in decision analyses. Markov models allow patients or groups of patients to transition from one state of health/disease to another as they move through the model. The specific strength of Markov models is this ability to reflect disease progression over time by using different health states or events. Therefore, these models are usually well understood by clinicians and can make direct use of traditional epidemiological survival data (e.g. annual rates, Kaplan-Maier curves, time-to-event distributions). A Markov model can be used to simulate both short-term processes (e.g. recovery after an operation), and long-term processes (e.g. an individual's life span).

Markov models can be analyzed in several ways. One of the most common is known as cohort simulation. A cohort of patients begins the model in any of the disease states and the cohort is then tracked for the duration of the model. The proportion of the cohort in any of the states at any point in time, and the mean duration in each state can be calculated. Alternatively, the Monte Carlo simulation (micro-simulation) approach operates at the level of the individual patient. Many hypothetical patients are passed individually through the model and their disease pathways recorded, replicating as closely as possible the process of interest. This allows investigators to simulate variability in outcome on both the individual and population level.

Other Clinical Applications of Decision Analysis

Healthcare Policy

Decision analysis techniques are implicitly and explicitly employed in the development of health policy. These applications range from recommendations from national and international working groups about management of specific disease processes, to cost-effectiveness analyses that inform whether or not certain treatment options are viable.

Clinical Protocols

Clinical protocols can be developed using the "PROACTIVE" approach and by eliminating the nonoptimal alternatives in a decision tree. This approach is relatively rigid and is most suitable when patient preference is less likely to alter the decision.

Patient Decision Aids

These are tools designed to inform patients about the alternatives where patient preference is critical in the decision making process. Decision analysis methodology is at the core of developing these instruments. These decision aids provide detailed information to patients but generally avoid making a specific recommendation and leave the final decision up to the patient-clinician team.

Benefits of Decision Analysis

Though decision analysis is not suitable for all clinical questions, it is clearly a useful technique for assisting complex and uncertain decisions, where the best option is not immediately apparent. Studying and performing DA clarifies the thinking of clinicians by forcing them to explicitly consider the known and the unknown elements of the decision process. Additionally, since decision analyses include the results of the most relevant research studies in the field, they promote evidence-based decisions. Also, it is likely that formal DA studies incorporate a more specific yet a comprehensive range of evidence than would be used in a more unstructured approach to decision making. Decision analysis provides a framework whereby clinicians can objectively communicate with colleagues and patients about the decision making process [1, 2]. By incorporating patient-centered outcomes like quality adjusted survival as measures of utility in decision processes, it encourages patients to be more involved in the decision process [1]. Decision analysis can be a catalyst for encouraging focused research in an area. This is particularly true when sensitivity testing leads to a change in the recommendation and thus generates both active discussion and testable hypotheses.

Drawbacks and Limitations of Decision Analysis

Since decision analysis is conducted with a specific end-point and a base case analysis which mirrors a clinical scenario, clinicians may have some difficulty applying the recommendations or thinking in the same framework when either the end-point or the clinical situation is altered. The methodology for decision analysis inherently requires making assumptions about the probabilities of events and values and these are supported by literature that may be of varying quality. Clinicians who are trained to interpret measurable individual data points and make decisions based upon them may be skeptical of recommendations generated by utilizing assumptions even though they may be based upon sound evidence.

Conclusion

Clinical decision making is complex and guided by a number of factors including medical evidence, personal experience and intuition. "Decision analysis" provides a framework for examining the clinical scenario, synthesizing the available evidence, and providing a recommendation for action. Decision analysis techniques are valuable tools in clinical medicine to develop health policy, clinical algorithms, and for cost-effectiveness analysis.

References

1. Elwyn G, Edwards A, Eccles M, Rovner D. Decision analysis in patient care. Lancet. 2001;358:571–4.
2. Richardson WS, Detsky AS. Users' guides to the medical literature. VII. How to use a clinical decision analysis. B. What are the results and will they help me in caring for my patients? Evidence Based Medicine Working Group. JAMA. 1995;273:1610–3.
3. Ferguson MK. Optimal management when unsuspected N2 nodal disease is identified during thoracotomy for lung cancer: cost-effectiveness analysis. J Thorac Cardiovasc Surg. 2003;126:1935–42.
4. Ferguson MK, Lehman AG. Sleeve lobectomy or pneumonectomy: optimal management strategy using decision analysis techniques. Ann Thorac Surg. 2003;76:1782–8.
5. Tsushima Y, Endo K. Analysis models to assess cost effectiveness of the four strategies for the work-up of solitary pulmonary nodules. Med Sci Monit. 2004;10:MT65–72.
6. Puri V, Crabtree TD, Kymes S, et al. A comparison of surgical intervention and stereotactic body radiation therapy for stage I lung cancer in high-risk patients: a decision analysis. J Thorac Cardiovasc Surg. 2012;143:428–36.
7. Puri V, Pyrdeck TL, Crabtree TD, et al. Treatment of malignant pleural effusion: a cost-effectiveness analysis. Ann Thorac Surg. 2012;94:374.
8. Shah A, Hahn SM, Stetson RL, et al. Cost-effectiveness of stereotactic body radiation therapy versus surgical resection for stage I non-small cell lung cancer. Cancer. 2013;119:3123–32.
9. Meyers BF, Haddad F, Siegel BA, et al. Cost-effectiveness of routine mediastinoscopy in computed tomography- and positron emission tomography-screened patients with stage I lung cancer. J Thorac Cardiovasc Surg. 2006;131:822–9; discussion 822–9.
10. Hunink MGM, Glasziou PP, et al. Elements of decision making in health care. In: Decision making in health and medicine. 1st ed. Cambridge/New York : Cambridge University Press; 2001. p. 1–33.

Chapter 4
Decision Making: The Surgeon's Perspective

Thomas K. Varghese Jr.

Abstract Delivery of medical advice is characterized by a process of weighing, prioritizing and structuring information given to a patient into a decision. In the ideal world, this is evidence-based. However, non-clinical factors can influence the decision-making process. The current chapter will briefly review models of the surgeon-patient relationship, and focus on those factors that influence the decision-making process from the surgeon's perspective. A subsequent chapter will focus on issues from the patient perspective.

Keywords Decision-making • Decision models • Evidence-based medicine • Non-clinical factors • Health care environment

Introduction

The history of lung volume reduction surgery (LVRS) in the United States exemplifies the influence of nonclinical determinants of care. LVRS was first used to treat emphysema in the 1950s. However, the procedure didn't catch favor until the early 1990s when reported successes from small case series led to a dramatic increase in its use nationwide despite variability in results, incomplete follow-up, and lack of data on patient selection criteria [1]. Factors that contributed to this included favorable media reports, patient advocacy group testimonials that influenced patient and surgeon attitudes about LVRS, the relative inexpensive nature of the procedure and generous reimbursement [2]. A National Heart, Lung, and Blood Institute (NHLBI)

T.K. Varghese Jr., MD, MS, FACS
Department of Surgery, Harborview Medical Center, University of Washington,
Box 359796, 325 Ninth Ave., Seattle, WA 98104, USA
e-mail: tkv@uw.edu

M.K. Ferguson (ed.), *Difficult Decisions in Thoracic Surgery*,
Difficult Decisions in Surgery: An Evidence-Based Approach 1,
DOI 10.1007/978-1-4471-6404-3_4, © Springer-Verlag London 2014

workshop of medical experts in September 1995 as well as critical analysis commissioned by the Centers for Medicare and Medicaid Services (CMS) concluded that the data on risks and benefits of the procedure were too inconclusive to warrant unrestricted Medicare reimbursement. However, as the analysis showed some patients appeared to benefit from the procedure, a clinical trial demonstrating the effectiveness of surgery was recommended [3].

The announcement of the National Emphysema Treatment Trial (NETT) was met with resistance from some in the surgical community who felt that there was enough evidence to warrant reimbursement in all cases [4]. The suspension of Medicare reimbursement in December 1995 until NETT was completed led to a dramatic decrease in the number of LVRS procedures [5]. As many third-party payers base their coverage plans on CMS guidelines, the policy likely influenced Non-Medicare patients and providers. Whether surgeons stopped performing the procedure because of lack of reimbursement or as an acknowledgement of scientific uncertainty is unknown. But the sharp decline in LVRS temporally related to CMS intervention is clear. NETT determined that a subgroup of patients with localized apical emphysema and poor exercise tolerance after exercise training were the most likely to benefit from LVRS [6], and subsequent CMS policy partly limited surgical decision-making as reimbursement was limited to eligible patients and surgeons.

Delivery of medical advice is characterized by a process of weighing, prioritizing and structuring information given to a patient into a decision. In the ideal world, this is evidence-based. However, non-clinical factors can influence the surgical decision-making process. There is a growing expectation for patient participation in their care, and passage of the Affordable Care Act (ACA) encourages greater use of shared decision-making [7]. Government policy is an example of how non-clinical factors can influence the surgical decision-making process.

Models of the Surgeon-Patient Relationship

The surgeon-patient relationship can be described based on the degree of decisional authority assumed by patients as the surgeon as agent, shared decision-making and informed decision-making models. The surgeon as agent is one where the physician is the expert adviser who incorporates the values of the patient when making a treatment recommendation. The surgeon elicits or assumes these values from the patient, and has total command over the decision-making process. As patient participation is limited, they may be subjected to biased treatment if the surgeon only gives limited treatment options or in the delivery of the same. On the other end of the spectrum is informed decision-making. Although the surgeon is recognized as the one who has technical expertise, in this model patients are the ones who elicit and understand information about their treatment choices. The surgeon in this instance doesn't give his/her opinion, but rather presents the patient with various options, allowing patients to arrive at their own conclusions (Fig. 4.1).

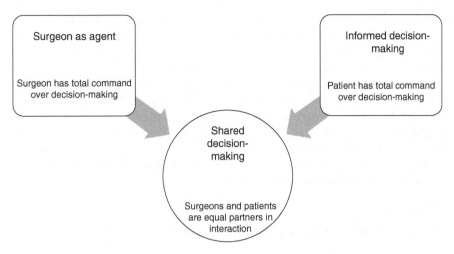

Fig. 4.1   Surgeon-patient relationship models

In between these two models is shared decision-making. Surgeons and patients are equal partners in this interaction, where each freely exchanges information and preferences about treatment options so that a mutually acceptable decision can be made. For situations where there isn't only one clearly superior course of treatment, shared decision-making can help to better align medical care with patients' preferences and values.

In surgery, the decision-making process is often situational. Patient autonomy and participation can be influenced by medical condition, surgeon factors, patient educational level, and availability of evidence-based information on the particular condition. We'll continue to explore the factors that influence the decision-making process from the surgeon's perspective, while a subsequent chapter will focus on issues from the patient's perspective.

Methodology for Evaluating Decision-Making Factors

Studies of nonclinical factors influencing clinical decision-making use qualitative or semi-quantitative research methodologies (surveys, case vignettes, decision-analysis modeling) that have methodological limitations [8]. Qualitative research (focus groups and key informant interviews) helps develop hypotheses that can then be evaluated using semi-quantitative methods. Surveys are at times difficult to interpret because limited generalizability to those who respond to the questionnaire, the degree of understanding of the questions by the responders, and the extent of socially normative responses by physicians. Socially normative responses occur when members of a group provide "acceptable" answers to questions when the "real" answer would generate negative social judgment. Socially normative answers are more common where responding individuals are identified. Subsequent quantitative evaluations of these issues may become difficult to do if the number of variables of interest and potential for confounding become overwhelming. Methods less familiar to surgeons, such as the factorial experimental design, may overcome these obstacles. Factorial design allows comparison of different groupings of categorical variables. For example, five dichotomized variables have 32 [2^5] unique groupings that can be analyzed using hierarchical logistic regression. The complexity of the calculations rises with the number of variables and combinations of variables, and thus even this study design has limitations. It is thus imperative that surgeons involved in these type of studies work with behavioralists and biostatisticians who are well-versed in alternative research designs.

Surgeon Factors Related to Clinical Decision-Making

The clinical decision-making process is often influenced by non-clinical factors from the surgeons' perspective. These factors include the surgeons' tolerance of uncertainty, risk-taking attitude, demographic characteristics, and their level of training.

Impact of Risk-Taking Attitude on Clinical Decision-Making

Reactions to uncertainty and attitudes towards risk intuitively have implications on clinical decision-making. However, there is a limit in our understanding of the degree to which this issue influences surgical care [10]. Instruments have been developed in an attempt to assess risk-taking in general among physicians. Nightingale [11] developed a two-question test that has been frequently used to assess the degree to which physicians view themselves as risk seeking or risk averse (Table 4.1). These questions assess respondents' willingness to gamble for their patients in both the face of gain and in the face of loss. Those who refuse to gamble for their patients in the face of loss are considered risk averse. In three studies that

Table 4.1 Questions used to assess relative risk preferences of surgeons

1. In a choice between two therapies for an otherwise healthy person
    (a) Treatment A: 100 % chance of increase in survival by 5 years as compared to the average person, 0 % chance of no increase in survival
    (b) Treatment B: 50 % chance of increase in survival by 10 years as compared to the average person, 50 % chance of no increase in survival
2. In a choice between two therapies for a sick person
    (a) Treatment A: 100 % chance of decrease in survival by 5 years as compared to the average person, 0 % chance of decrease in survival by 10 years as compared to the average person
    (b) Treatment B: 50 % chance of decrease in survival by 5 years as compared to the average person, 50 % chance of decrease in survival by 10 years as compared to the average person

Nightingale conducted [11–13], a significant correlation was found between resource utilization and risk preference in the face of loss. The more often physicians chose the risk averse gamble, the more likely they were to utilize additional resources to rule out uncertain outcomes. Most physicians in the setting of certain loss would rather minimize loss and fail in half of these attempts, than accept a certain loss. This fear of risk taking has been found to be less consistent in other studies [14], and varies based on mode of testing and across different cultures [15].

Impact of Surgeon Age

There is little data looking specifically at the impact of surgeon age and clinical decisions. Anecdotes have suggested many surgeons lack insight into the gradual degradation of their own skills. Age causes deterioration in physical and cognitive performance. Greenfield and Proctor identified cognitive factors that declined with age in surgeons including the ability to focus attention, the ability to process and correlate information and native intelligence [16]. Trunkey and Botney developed a series of tests, the "MicroCog", that were designed to detect impaired competence occurring late in a physician's career [17]. The tests measure reactivity, attention, numeric recall, verbal memory, visiospatial facility, reasoning and mental calculation. The authors found that in all physicians (including non-surgeons) that though they perform better than non-physicians, by age 75 they lose 25 % of their starting score. In a meta-analysis looking at all types of physicians, Choudhry and colleagues found that half of the 59 articles included for study reported declining measures of quality of care with increasing physician years in practice [18]. Other studies have shown that older physicians were less likely to adopt newly proven therapies, and may be less receptive to new standards of care [19–21]. In a study of 93 surgeons and anesthesiologists in Japan by Nakata and colleagues, the relationship between risk attitudes and demographic characteristics were explored in case vignettes assessing whether respondents were risk averse, risk neutral and risk seeking [22]. The only positive finding was with regards to age – the older the physician, the more risk averse they were. The study concluded that older physicians might shy away from risk, while younger physicians may be more willing to gamble.

However, it is unknown what influence emergence of the evidence-based care movement and maintenance of certification programs will have on any interaction of surgeon age and decision-making.

Impact of Surgeon Gender

There has been a dramatic change in the number of women entering the physician workforce over the past three decades [23]. Women make up close to half of all US residents and fellows – increasing from 21.5 % in 1980 to 45.4 % in 2010. Change however is coming more slowly in many of the surgical specialties, where women are still a distinctly small minority. As fewer than 5 % of cardiothoracic surgeons are women [24], the impact of surgeon gender and decision-making have not been assessed. There have been small studies comparing communication styles between male and female physicians [9]. Female doctors were found to actively facilitate patient participation on medical decisions by enacting methods such as partnership building, positive talk, question asking, and information giving [9, 25, 26]. Female doctors were less dominant verbally during clinic visits as compared to males and engaged in active discussions with patients.

Impact of Specialty Training

Surgeon specialty has been shown to be associated with better post-operative outcomes among high-risk operations [27]. Goodney and colleagues [28] demonstrated that board-certified thoracic surgeons have lower rates of operative mortality with lung resections compared to general surgeons, although they noted that other factors such as hospital volume also influenced a patient's operative risk of mortality. In a lung cancer resection study conducted by our group in the SEER-Medicare population [29], we found that board-certified general thoracic surgeons had greater long-term survival rates than those treated by general surgeons. General thoracic surgeons performed preoperative and intraoperative staging more often than general surgeons or cardiothoracic surgeons (those who performed both cardiac and thoracic procedures as part of their practice). In esophageal cancer surgery, Dimick and colleagues [30] found that specialty board certification in thoracic surgery was independently associated with lower operative mortality rates. Common themes in these studies were influence of provider volume on the overall effect, as well as more consistent process-of-care measures by specialty surgeons. As there is a trend towards increasing specialization amongst surgeons, other factors that may have influenced decision-making include training in the modern era, with inclusion of evidence-based protocols, and multi-disciplinary participation in tumor boards amongst specialists. It is unknown if subspecialty-trained surgeons are more risk seeking in their treatment options in light of additional training experience.

Healthcare System Factors Related to Clinical Decision Making

Impact of Practice Environment

The Patient Protection and Affordable Care Act (ACA) signed into law in March 2010 seeks to improve health care delivery in several ways, from access to quality to cost. ACA's goal was to create a movement of payment reforms, in which private insurance companies would follow the lead of successful government payment reforms, such as bundled payments, and ultimately create system-wide changes for reimbursement [31]. Changing the reimbursement structure for providers will inevitably create new issues for surgeons who are making decisions for their patients. Most of the payment reforms began in 2011 and 2012, and will continue through 2016. Two programs designed to restructure the way health care is delivered have been proposed under ACA, namely Patient-Centered Medical Homes (PCMHs) and Accountable Care Organizations (ACOs). These programs are designed to improve care coordination by encouraging use of electronic medical records, changing providers' financial incentives by including quality measures in reimbursement, and ultimately moving away from a fee-for-service to one where quality of care is valued [32].

The ACO movement has led to increased consolidation and integration in the medical marketplace. Hospitals are buying practices, which means that physicians are ceding autonomy to belong to the organizations to keep their market share intact and to have access to electronic record systems and other infrastructure that are expensive to capitalize. Awareness emerges for surgeons that their medical decisions can potentially negatively influence their income. This is not necessarily unethical, as cost containment has been recognized as an important circumstance in good decision-making [33]. There will be penalties, which could affect physician reimbursement. Adoption of rigid guidelines for the treatment of patients may limit individual surgeon decision-making, as well as expansion of treatment pathways and care plans. All of these are attempts at decreasing variation in care, decreasing length of stay, and reducing use of resources.

Surgeons in the Veterans Administration hospital system have participated for more than a decade in a systematic data-gathering and feedback system of outcomes for major surgery [34]. The National Surgical Quality Improvement Project (NSQIP) works to decrease variation in clinical outcomes by demonstrating to surgeons when their center is an "outlier" in performance. This system allows hospitals to target QI activities that may influence components of care, and subsequently decision-making.

Impact of Political Environment

Professional organizations can play a role in decision-making by effectively regulating surgeon-directed clinical practice. One example is the guidelines for laparoscopic resection of curable colon and rectal cancer [35] written by the Society of American Gastrointestinal and Endoscopic Surgeons (SAGES) and endorsed by the American Society of Colon and Rectal Surgeons (ASCRS). These guidelines give recommendations on tumor localization, diagnostic evaluation for metastases, preparation for operation, surgical technique, as well as minimum number of cases to gain proficiency. The society also noted that while robotic surgery appears feasible, that in the absence of long-term oncologic outcome studies, no clear recommendations were made. Guidelines such as these influence members, and are in stark contrast to the situation of non evidence-based decision-making that existed for LVRS prior to NETT.

The reporting of surgeon-specific outcome data is another example of the influence of the political environment. Outcome data were rarely reported prior to the mid-1980s [36]. The first release of hospital open heart surgery risk-adjusted mortality rates in December 1990 [37] and the first formal public report in December 1992 [38] marked the start of a new era. These performance reports, or physician report cards, have increased in frequency in recent years [39]. Advocates of this form of reporting believe they provide information about quality of care that consumers, employers, and health plans can use to improve their decision-making and to stimulate quality improvement among providers [40]. They may also appropriately promote regionalization of medical centers and consolidation of resources. However, physicians are concerned that risk adjustment strategies in these reports are not adequate. Without this confidence, publication of procedural mortality rates may result in physicians withholding procedures in high-risk patients. In a study by Narins and colleagues [39], the attitudes and experiences of cardiologists were surveyed about the influence of the New York Percutaneous Coronary Intervention (PCI) report card on their decision-making process. Eighty-nine percent agreed or strongly agreed that patients who might benefit from PCI may not receive the procedure as a result of public reporting of physician-specific mortality rates. Seventy percent agreed or strongly agreed that the presence of a scorecard influences whether they treat a critically ill patient with an expected high mortality rate. The authors concluded that unintended consequence of scorecards might be to adversely affect healthcare decisions for especially high-risk patients. Scorecards may also impair the development of new treatments because of the more restrictive clinical practice environment [40].

In light of these drawbacks, many have proposed revamping the current system to facilitate rapid and accurate access to outcome data in the local practice environment. Adoption of these efforts is often embraced as this occurs on a voluntary basis rather than in response to punitive restrictions. Examples of such grass-roots initiatives on a state level that are surgeon-led include those in the states of Michigan [41] and Washington [42, 43]. On a national level, the Society of Thoracic Surgeons (STS) is a leader in the development of a society-based, publicly reported, volunteer registry database that has made a tremendous impact on risk-stratification and outcomes in cardiothoracic surgery [44, 45]. Surgeons who participate in such database initiatives can utilize risk-stratified models to better inform their decision-making process.

The Choosing Wisely® initiative helps physicians and patients have important conversations necessary to ensure that timely and optimal care is delivered. Launched by the American Board of Internal Medicine (ABIM) Foundation, Choosing Wisely® enables physicians and patients to engage in conversation about the overuse of tests and procedures, and helps patients make smart and effective care choices [46]. The original campaign has evolved into a multi-year initiative where the ABIM Foundation has reached out to specialty societies to identify a list of five tests or procedures that may be overused or misused. Criteria for developing

Table 4.2 Society of thoracic surgeons Choosing Wisely® list

1. Patients who have no cardiac history and good functional status do not require preoperative stress testing before non-cardiac thoracic surgery
2. Do not initiate routing evaluation of carotid artery disease before cardiac surgery in the absence of symptoms or other high-risk criteria
3. Do not perform routine predischarge echocardiogram after cardiac valve replacement surgery
4. Patients with suspected or biopsy proven stage I non-small cell lung cancer do not require brain imaging before definitive care in the absence of neurologic symptoms
5. Before cardiac surgery there is no need for pulmonary function testing in the absence of respiratory symptoms

these lists include limiting to items that fall within the specialty; supported by evidence; documented and publicly available upon request; frequently ordered/costly; easy for a lay person to understand; and measurable/accountable. The STS participated in the February 2013 phase II release [47] (Table 4.2). These specialty generated lists help to empower physician-patient conversations and to avoid unnecessary procedures that may harm patients while driving up health care costs. Sixty-three specialty societies have joined the campaign, with additional lists targeted for early 2014.

Impact of the Medico-Legal Environment

Fear of lawsuits has had a dramatic effect on many specialties. Surgeons may be influenced by medico-legal risks in terms of their decision-making with certain operations in high-risk populations. The exact extent of this influence is unclear in the field of thoracic surgery. However, as a specialty that deals with a significant proportion of high-risk patients, it is certain that the cardiothoracic surgeon will face such a challenge in their career [48].

Summary

Although the ideal is to practice evidence-based medicine at all times, there are many non-clinical factors that influence the care that we provide. For every procedure there is sadly variability in operative and periprocedural care, with associated variations in outcomes between centers. Lapses in quality are a main driver in this variation. Further investigation into non-clinical factors may not only help to explain variation, but also serve as targets for change to improve outcomes. Areas of non-clinical influences include surgeon factors (such as risk-taking attitudes, age, gender, specialty training), and healthcare system factors (practice, political and medico-legal environment). Better assessment and control of these factors can lead to rational, consistent and appropriate care for our patients.

References

1. Cooper JD, Trulock EP, Triantafillou AN, et al. Bilateral pneumectomy (volume reduction) for chronic obstructive pulmonary disease. J Thorac Cardiovasc Surg. 1995;109:106–19.
2. Ramsey SD, Sullivan SD. Evidence, economics and emphysema: Medicare's long journey with lung volume reduction surgery. Health Aff (Millwood). 2005;24:55–66.
3. The National Emphysema Treatment Trial Research Group. Rationale and design of the National Emphysema Treatment Trial (NETT): a prospective randomized trial of lung volume reduction surgery. J Thorac Cardiovasc Surg. 1999;118:518–28.
4. Cooper JD. Paying the piper: the NETT strikes a sour note. National Emphysema Treatment Trial. Ann Thorac Surg. 2001;72:330–3.
5. Huizenga HF, Ramsey SD, Albert RK. Estimated growth of lung volume reduction surgery among Medicare enrollees: 1994 to 1996. Chest. 1998;114:1583–7.
6. National Emphysema Treatment Trial Research Group. A randomized trial comparing lung volume-reduction surgery with medical therapy for severe emphysema. N Engl J Med. 2003;348:2059–73.
7. Lee EO, Emanuel EJ. Shared decision making to improve care and reduce costs. Engl J Med. 2005;1:6–8.
8. Clark JA, Potter DA, McKinlay JB. Bringing social structure back into clinical decision making. Soc Sci Med. 1991;32:853–66.
9. Tubbs EP, Broekel Elrod JA, Flum DR. Risk taking and tolerance for uncertainty: implications for surgeons. J Surg Res. 2006;131:1–6.
10. Nightingale SD. Risk preference and laboratory use. Med Decis Making. 1987;7:168–72.
11. Nightingale SD. Risk preference and admitting rates of emergency room physicians. Med Care. 1988;26:84–7.
12. Nightingale SD. Risk preference and decision making in critical care situations. Chest. 1988;93:684–7.
13. Holtgrave DR, Lawler F, Spann SJ. Physicians' risk attitudes, laboratory usage, and referral decisions: the case of an academic family practice center. Med Decis Making. 1991;11:125–30.
14. Zaat JOM. General practitioners' uncertainty, risk preference and use of laboratory tests. Med Care. 1992;30:846–54.
15. Greenfield LJ, Proctor MC. When should a surgeon retire? Adv Surg. 1999;32:385–93.
16. Trunkey DD, Botney R. Assessing competency: a tale of two professions. J Am Coll Surg. 2001;192:385–95.
17. Choudhry NK, Fletcher RH, Soumerai SB. Systematic review: the relationship between clinical experience and quality of health care. Ann Intern Med. 2005;142:260–73.
18. Freiman MP. The rate of adoption of new procedures among physicians. The impact of specialty and practice characteristics. Med Care. 1985;23:939–45.
19. Hlatky MA, Cotugno H, O'Connor C, Mark DB, Pryor DB, Califf RM. Adoption of thrombolytic therapy in the management of acute myocardial infarction. Am J Cardiol. 1988;61:510–4.
20. Young MJ, Fried LS, Eisenberg J, Hershey J, Williams S. Do cardiologists have higher thresholds for recommending coronary arteriography than family physicians? Health Serv Res. 1987;22:623–35.
21. Nakata Y, Okuno-Fujiwara M, Goto T, Morita S. Risk attitudes of anesthesiologists and surgeons in clinical decision making with expected years of life. J Clin Anesth. 2000;12:146–50.
22. American College of Surgeons Health Policy Research Institute. The surgical workforce in the United States: profile and recent trends. Apr 2010. Accessed at http://www.acshpri.org/documents/ACSHPRI_Surgical_Workforce_in_US_apr2010.pdf.
23. Darves B. Women physicians in the specialties: making gains. N Eng J Med Career Center. 19 Sept 2012. Accessed at http://www.nejmcareercenter.org/article/women-physicians-in-the-specialties-making-gains/.
24. Roter DL, Hall JA. Why physician gender matters in shaping the physician-patient relationship. J Womens Health. 1998;7:1093–7.

25. Roter D, Lipkin Jr M, Korsgarrd A. Sex differences in patients' and physicians' communications during primary care medical visits. Med Care. 1991;29:1083–93.
26. Van den Bronk-Muinen A, Bensing JM, Kerssens JJ. Gender and communication style in general practice. Differences between women's health care and regular health care. Med Care. 1998;36:100–6.
27. Cowan Jr JA, Dimick JB, Thompson BG, et al. Surgeon volume as an indicator of outcomes after carotid endarterectomy: an effect independent of specialty practice and hospital volume. J Am Coll Surg. 2022;195:814–21.
28. Goodney PP, Lucas FL, Stukel TAA, Birkmeyer JD. Surgeon specialty and operative mortality with lung resection. Ann Surg. 2005;241:179–84.
29. Farjah F, Flum DR, Varghese Jr TK, et al. Surgeon specialty and long-term survival after pulmonary resection for lung cancer. Ann Thorac Surg. 2009;87:995–1006.
30. Dimick JB, Goodney PP, Orringer MB, Birkmeyer JD. Specialty training and mortality after esophageal cancer resection. Ann Thorac Surg. 2005;80:282–6.
31. Lee PV, Berenson RA, Tooker J. Payment reform – the need to harmonize approaches in Medicare and the private sector. N Engl J Med. 2010;362:3–5.
32. Ein D, Jefferson A. The patient protection and affordable care act: causes and effects. Ann Allergy Asthma Immunol. 2014;112:6–8.
33. Devettere RJ. Making health care decisions. In: Devettere RJ, editor. Practical decision making in health care ethics. Washington, DC: Georgetown University Press; 2000. p. 94.
34. Itani KM. Fifteen years of the National Surgical Quality Improvement Program in review. Am J Surg. 2009;198(5 Suppl):S9–18.
35. SAGES guidelines for laparoscopic resection of curable colon and rectal cancer. Feb 2012. Accessed at http://www.sages.org/publications/guidelines/guidelines-for-laparoscopic-resection-of-curable-colon-and-rectal-cancer/.
36. Topol EJ, Califf RM. Scorecard cardiovascular medicine. Its impact and future directions. Ann Intern Med. 1994;120:65–70.
37. Hannan EL, Kilburn Jr H, O'Donnell JF, et al. Adult open heart surgery in New York State. An analysis of risk factors and hospital mortality rate. JAMA. 1990;264:2768–74.
38. Epstein A. Performance reports on quality – prototypes, problems and prospects. N Engl J Med. 1995;333:57–61.
39. Narins CR, Dozier AM, Ling FS, Zareba W. The influence of public reporting of outcome data on medical decision making by physicians. Arch Intern Med. 2005;165:83–7.
40. Schneider EC, Epstein AM. Use of public performance reports: a survey of patients undergoing cardiac surgery. JAMA. 1998;279:1638–42.
41. Prager RL, Armenti FR, Bassett JS, et al. Cardiac surgeons and the quality movement: the Michigan experience. Semin Thorac Cardiovasc Surg. 2009;21:20–7.
42. Flum DR, Fisher N, Thompson J, et al. Washington State's approach to variability in surgical processes/outcomes: Surgical Clinical Outcomes Assessment Program (SCOAP). Surgery. 2005;138:821–8.
43. Aldea GS, Mokadam NA, Melford R, et al. Changing volumes, risk profiles, and outcomes of coronary artery bypass grafting and percutaneous coronary interventions. Ann Thorac Surg. 2009;87:1828–38.
44. Clark RE. The STS Cardiac Surgery National Database: an update. Ann Thorac Surg. 1995;59:1376–81.
45. Wright CD, Gaissert HA, Grab JD, et al. Predictors of prolonged length of stay after lobectomy for lung cancer: a Society of Thoracic Surgeons General Thoracic Database risk-adjustment model. Ann Thorac Surg. 2008;85:1857–65.
46. Cassel CK, Guest JA. Choosing Wisely: helping physicians and patients make smart decisions about their care. JAMA. 2012;307:1801–2.
47. Wood DE, Mitchell JD, Schmitz DS, et al. Choosing Wisely: cardiothoracic surgeons partnering with patients to make good health care decisions. Ann Thorac Surg. 2013;95(3):1130–5.
48. Mayer Jr JR. Ethical, legal and health policy challenges in contemporary cardiothoracic surgery: introduction. Semin Thorac Cardiovasc Surg. 2009;21:1–2.

Chapter 5
Decision Making: The Patient's Perspective

Joshua A. Hemmerich and Kellie Van Voorhis

Abstract Healthcare is moving towards a practice model involving patient participation for difficult decisions, such as whether or not to have surgery. For proper Shared Decision Making (SDM), the patients must be informed about their treatment options and the risks and benefits that go along with each so that they can apply their preferences in making the decision. SDM can be problematic in surgical clinics where time with patients is limited. Helping surgeons educate patients for SDM and incorporate the patient's preferences into the choice is a major challenge that requires research and guidance for those who see older sicker patients.

Keywords Shared decision making • Non-small cell lung cancer • Geriatric patients Patient knowledge

Introduction

Traditionally, healthcare has been delivered such that expert physicians have paternalistically guided patients towards the treatment they determined was best to address the patient's diagnosis. However, multiple forces are pushing healthcare and decision making about treatments towards a practice referred to as Shared Decision Making (SDM) for medical problems for which there is no standard of

J.A. Hemmerich, PhD (✉) • K. Van Voorhis, BS
Department of Medicine, The University of Chicago,
5841 S Maryland Ave, MC 6098, W700, Chicago, IL 60637, USA
e-mail: jhemmeri@medicine.bsd.uchicago.edu

M.K. Ferguson (ed.), *Difficult Decisions in Thoracic Surgery*,
Difficult Decisions in Surgery: An Evidence-Based Approach 1,
DOI 10.1007/978-1-4471-6404-3_5, © Springer-Verlag London 2014

care [1]. SDM involves the participation of both the physician and the informed patient. This paradigm shift extends beyond the primary care setting, where patients and physicians often have a well-established relationship, to specialty clinics, such as surgery, where the surgeon is charged with relatively limited, short-term care of the patient [2]. However, with more and more patients wishing not only for information, but also an active role in SDM for difficult decisions, such as whether or not to undergo a risky but potentially curative surgery, there is a premium put on ensuring patients are sufficiently equipped with the necessary knowledge. Failing to ensure patients are sufficiently informed when taking part in SDM is likely to have negative, dramatic, and irreversible consequences in surgical care.

A growing population of older people will continue fueling the proliferation of a diverse cancer patient population for which there exist limited data to guide treatment choices. Medical problems experienced by older and more clinically complex patients will require difficult decisions about higher risk surgical procedures, like resection of non-small cell lung cancer (NSCLC). In such decisions, where relevant evidence is limited and patient values and goals can be diverse, informed patients' preferences should be incorporated when making the choice. Consequently, this requires the sharing of information with the patient so that they are equipped with a good understanding of their situation and options. If the growing demand for SDM is to be met and executed appropriately, surgical care professionals must be prepared to inform patients and foster healthy SDM.

What Is Shared Decision Making?

SDM is a clinical approach in which informed patients actively share in making choices about their own care with their physicians. SDM is specifically required when, due to limitations of relevant medical evidence, none of the options are considered a true standard of care. For some health problems requiring SDM, there are trade-offs between options. Options are linked to various probabilistic outcomes that make the right decision reliant on patients' preferences [3]. The SDM process is a compound and ordered one that typically takes place in a face-to-face consultation between the patient and physician. The goal is to first deliver the important information and ensure its comprehension, and then deliberate over the options to settle on the preferred course of action.

Driving this transition from traditional paternalism towards SDM is the evolution of the physician-patient relationship towards a more collaborative model. It likely reflects changes in population demography as more paternalistic pre-baby boomers pass away and are replaced by later generation autonomous healthcare consumers, but SDM also receives pro-active international advocacy from many medical care providers, researchers, and ethicists as a moral imperative and strategy for improving care.

Call for Shared Decision Making

The practice of SDM has gained proponents, critics, and researchers from all around the world over the past two decades. An international panel of medical experts convening in 2010 came to a consensus and released the Salzburg Statement on Shared Decision Making, declaring that the implementation of effective SDM would make the single most profound improvement to healthcare quality [4]. The statement included instructions for health policy makers, as well as physicians and patients. It asserted that physicians have an ethical imperative to practice SDM with patients, engage in two way communication, field and answer patients' questions, and solicit patients' values and personal preferences. Physicians should also provide accurate and individually tailored information about treatment options and the uncertainties, benefits, and harms inherent in them. They must allow patients sufficient time to consider their options and recognize that most decisions need not be made immediately. The Salzburg Statement implored patients to recognize their right to participate, to voice their concerns, questions, and values, and seek out and utilize the highest quality information available [4].

Survey data indicate that the cancer patient population expresses desire for SDM, but that significant variance still exists in patient preferences for decisional control, as some patients still desire the physician to take a guiding role [5]. A qualitative interview study from 2010 indicated that older, frail patients expressed a desire for information but not necessarily to have input into the treatment choice [6]. Cancer patients often desire to have important information even when they indicated that they don't prefer a very active role in settling on the treatment choice. Though there will continue to be an overall increasing desire for information and continuing movement towards more patients wanting to be active participants in SDM, multiple decision making styles will persist.

Meeting the Requirement of Informed Patients in SDM

SDM is said to be performed effectively when patients accurately comprehend all of the necessary information regarding their options, identify their values and preferences, and determine which treatment choice gives them the best odds of realizing their goal [7]. Having a more equal informational footing, the patient and physician can often come to an agreement about what treatment best fits an individual patient's health state preferences and tolerance for risks, but if an agreement is not struck the patient's preferences should ultimately prevail [4].

In much of the SDM literature, the "important information" is only vaguely if ever defined, but it is, to some degree, specific to the diagnosis and available treatment options. When considering surgery for cancer, it is important that the patient know the essential information at the critical time because this treatment cannot be discontinued and is irreversible. This is a serious concern with older patients who are observed to take different strategies in decision making and bias their attention in ways that younger patients do not [8].

Unfortunately, nationally representative survey data suggest that patients do not know the relevant information about a disease, prognosis and available options at multiple important points in care [9]. As a result, an entire decision support aid movement has started with the mission of developing and verifying the quality of tools intended to improve patient knowledge, including tools relevant to cancer care and surgery [10, 11]. Many of these tools are intended to avoid ineffective SDM participation by uninformed or confused patients that could lead to treatment choices that do not match the patient's preferences and goals.

Several barriers to patient participation in SDM, which all could jeopardize patient education, have been identified and include dealing with multiple professionals unfamiliar with their preferences, diverse treatment strategies among physicians, fast patient turnover in hospitals, stressed medical personnel, and communication barriers [6]. All of these factors are risks that hinder the communication between patients and surgeons and contribute to patients having poor comprehension when a decision is to be made.

Impact of SDM on Clinical Outcomes

Currently, the downstream consequences for succeeding or failing to practice good SDM are not well-documented or understood. The rationale is that if a patient is to express their values, goals, and preferences and work with the physician to choose the treatment option that best fits, they must have an accurate understanding of the problem in their mind. There is some evidence that suggests that the quality of SDM is predictive of patient-centered, clinical and care-cost outcomes. Decision conflict is a construct that largely reflects how satisfied a patient is about their treatment decision shortly after making it and usually prior to fully realizing the treatment outcome. There is debate about the tenability and value of lowering patients' decision conflict [12]. But it seems that helping patients feel secure and confident in their treatment choice will benefit overall satisfaction with care.

Although, the ethics of SDM should make it immune to cost considerations, the potential to lower or raise costs is on many people's minds. Good SDM could improve satisfaction and functional outcomes, but poorly executed SDM could disproportionately increase costs and worsen clinical outcomes, satisfaction with care, and quality of life. Patients are unlikely to be as influenced by financial incentives as much as physicians sometimes are, but it is not a certainty how SDM will influence the cost of care until more appropriate and longitudinal data are available. However, some theories have been proposed as to how SDM might lower costs, and one in particular, costs of litigation, is highly relevant to surgery. Some data indicate that it is health care professionals' style as much as the content of their communication that predicts litigation. There is evidence that failures of SDM such as devaluing patient or family views, delivering information poorly, and failing to understand the patient's perspective of the problem were predictive of litigation [13–15]. It is clear that improving patient comprehension and participation in SDM could lower the high rate of litigation in surgery, and potentially decrease health care costs.

The Need for SDM in Surgical Care—The Example of Lung Cancer

The decision about whether or not to undergo lung resection for NSCLC is one example of the many difficult decisions in surgery, and one that will face more and more people. The global population is growing older because there are more people who are living to an older age. The U.S. population over age 65 is estimated to increase from 40 million in 2010 to 88 million in 2050 [16]. Sixty percent of early stage NSCLC patients are aged 65–84 [17]. With ever improving imaging techniques detecting more suspicious lung nodules, surgeons will continue to see an exponential growth of older early-stage NSCLC, patients with shorter remaining life expectancies, more comorbid conditions, and more extensive informational and decision support needs.

Surgeons deliberate over details. They take into account the characteristics of the patient, their diagnosis, and the risks associated with surgery, and then formulate a recommendation about whether or not having surgery is the best course of action. Although there are professional and financial biases pushing surgeons to recommend surgery, they recognize when a patient is not an ideal surgical candidate and that it might be advisable to consider other options.

When NSCLC is diagnosed, or suspected, the mass is evaluated for stage and location. Most early stage NSCLC tumors are operable and surgeons strive to remove the minimum necessary amount of lung tissue to remove all of the cancer. Treatment choices for NSCLC patients who are older, have significant co-morbid disease, or are otherwise not perfect surgical candidates, represents a problem that calls for SDM. When it is justifiable to either go to surgery or opt against going to the OR and instead consider radiation, the patient should be informed of the options and involved in SDM.

Early Stage NSCLC Treatment Options

When presenting to a thoracic surgery clinic for probable or confirmed NSCLC, patients are regularly evaluated on their surgical candidacy. Although surgical lung resection has been the most popular treatment choice for early stage (I or II) NSCLC for decades, the decision about having surgery is not obvious when the patient is at higher risk for complications or less likely to benefit from the operation. Without additional concerns, surgery is preferred because removing cancer from the patient's body provides the highest probability of 5 year survival. However, the immediate and long-term risks associated with surgery provide reason for pause, and more thorough pre-surgical assessment reveals that not all patients prove to be good surgical candidates.

Surgery

Depending on the stage and location of the tumor, several different types of procedures are possible ranging from pneumonectomy to a wedge resection which resects a minimum of healthy tissue. For highly fit surgical candidates with adequate pulmonary reserve [18], stage, and anatomy, the current standard of care is lobectomy to maximize the odds of cure.

Although scoring above pulmonary function thresholds predicts good surgical outcomes, lower scores are not prohibitive and the clinical complexity and the clinical diversity of patients has made it intractable to identify a criterion value of preoperative FEV_1 below which the surgical risk level should be considered excessive for all patients. There are insufficient data to provide guidelines for a diverse older patient population that presents a complex array of variables.

All of the aforementioned evaluation includes data from studies that did not include random assignment and that under-represents older patients and issues associated with a geriatric population. Consequently, there is no clear picture of actual surgical risk statistics for a diverse population of older patients with a wide array of co-morbid conditions, making the decision about surgery subject in part to individual patient preferences.

Radiation

Radiation therapy is the most common alternative to lung cancer surgery and doesn't have the immediate risks associated with surgical resection, but offers a 10–15 % lower cure rate relative to surgery [19]. For older or frailer patients who are at high risk for complications or don't anticipate a large survival-time benefit, it can be a preferable course that preserves healthy lung tissue and avoids the heightened perioperative risks to such a patient.

Problems with SDM and Surgery

The claim that patients are to be informed participants in SDM brings new challenges for both patients and their physicians because appropriate training and infrastructure for good SDM has largely not been put into place. As well, patients are usually not adequately prepared to get the most out of their face-to-face time with the surgeon.

Unfortunately, older patients are likely to have greater difficulty participating in SDM for multiple reasons. Older people represent a more diverse population than their younger counterparts because of their prevalence of a wide variety of medical conditions and physical functioning. Some older patients have a combination of medical conditions to be managed and an array of medications carrying various risks and side-effects. As the large influx of older patients floods into surgical clinics, these surgeons will be faced with tremendous challenges of delivering appropriate treatment to a diverse patient population, for which there are few data to guide treatment choices.

Patient Clinical Complexity

Many factors can make a patient a higher surgical risk and the decision about whether or not to have surgery more difficult. When the patient is not otherwise healthy, but instead has significant co-morbid health conditions or significantly diminished cardio-pulmonary function, they are less likely to benefit and are at higher risk for adverse outcomes. Outcomes can be expected to be worse in patients with more co-morbid burden [18]. Advanced age itself has become a difficult issue in surgical decisions as people are living longer and the population of advanced age adults is one of diverse health states. Some patients of advanced age are robust and highly functional, while others have difficulty with day to day endeavors and are vulnerable to further degradations of function and looming mortality.

There is a potentially important impact on surgical outcomes of the widely-recognized but poorly understood geriatric syndrome of physiological frailty [20–22]. Surgical clinics are currently not adept at assessing patient frailty, which could be a major determinant in perioperative experience and treatment outcomes. Some data show that patients' levels of physical exhaustion are predictive of major surgical complications in gastro-intestinal cancer resection, further suggesting that there is useful predictive information that is not captured in the traditional pre-operative evaluation [23].

Surgeons put the patient to the "eyeball test" regarding their fitness for surgery, supplementing what is captured in traditional pre-surgical evaluations, but much remains to be learned about the impact of frailty on surgical outcomes and how to predict it. Formal frailty testing is feasible and likely to out-perform the surgeon's intuitive judgment alone.

There is no clear criterion cutoff for any pre-surgical or physical evaluation that prohibits sending a patient to surgery and the available published data are not of sufficient quality or detail to set sound practice guidelines for a clinically diverse patient population. The process of assessing risk and probable outcomes for imperfect surgical candidates is somewhat fuzzy and speculative and, even with information on frailty, there remains a high amount of uncertainty regarding any individual patient's outcome. Consequently, without strict guidelines, SDM is called for so that patients know that their options lead to uncertain outcomes, but that there is information about their own surgical fitness worth knowing when deciding on treatment.

Difficulties in Patient Comprehension

Patients are never standing on the same ground as surgeons regarding foundational knowledge about disease and surgery. A substantial barrier to implementing effective SDM is helping patients understand the important facts about their disease and treatment options so that they are accurately informed at the time that they are participating in the decision making process. The devil is in the details because patients must know how their own clinical characteristics might impact the perioperative risks and probabilities of different outcomes. A verbatim comprehension of highly specific risk statistics appears to be neither necessary nor sufficient to guide decisions of physicians or patients if they do not derive the proper meaning [24, 25]. What is important is that patients understand what can be expected to happen if the disease goes untreated, what options are available to them to combat the disease, the goals of each treatment, the advantages and disadvantages of those options, and the uncertainty inherent in all. This is not always feasible for surgeons to convey or patients to comprehend, as current practice goes.

Non-demented older patients process information differently and sometimes implement strategies that are unlike those used by their younger counterparts. As cognitive abilities change over the life-span, there is sometimes a shift towards emotion-based information that can impact risk perception and decision making [8, 26]. Research shows that older adults in particular often use religious coping for health related stressors, and that coping can come in positive or negative forms, such that they can either alleviate or bring on psychological morbidity [27]. However, little is known about the impact religious thinking has on the treatment decisions of patients considering a risky, but potentially curable, cancer treatment options with varying risk and promise.

Lung cancer patients deciding about surgery sometimes hold beliefs that contradict evidence-based medicine and can potentially misguide their decisions. In thoracic oncology, some patients believe that cancer will spread during the surgery if the cancer, "hits the air" [28]. This belief is found to be predictive of the decision to forego surgery [29] and it was found to be widespread among a national sample of healthy survey respondents [30].

It is clear that patients' abilities to process information and the mental representations that they ultimately construct can make a big difference in which choice they make about treatment.

Surgical Practice

The traditional practice of surgery might also provide barriers to effectively satisfying the requirement of an informed patient in SDM. Ultimately, the goal of all surgeons is to do the best that they can for their patients. However, this requires separating out the often influential institutional and financially-driven goals to more clearly determine what is preferred by the patient. It is likely that the professional culture of surgery has worked against the adoption of SDM as common practice.

Surgeons focus on creating a feeling of confidence and optimism in their patients, which is somewhat at odds with delivering the "cold hard facts" and sometimes troubling risk information [2].

Surgeons strive to maintain an optimistic stance regarding the treatment that they provide and they often refer to an operation that removes all of the known cancer cells as a "cure" [31, 32]. This is thought to be integral part to the surgeon-patient relationship because putting patients into a positive state of mind is important to maximize hopes of a good outcome. The surgeon addresses the pre-surgical goal of comforting and convincing the patient that she or he is in good hands in the operating room and works to cultivate an optimistic attitude in the patient about surgery [32]. The operation is typically performed only in cases in which the surgeon believes that it is justifiable, given the patients level of surgical risk, and the patient agrees to do what the surgeon believes is best. However, eliciting optimism in patients is difficult to balance with delivering important information about risk, uncertainty, or trade-offs that might be viewed as unfavorable in order to allow them to be fully informed participants.

Additionally, surgeons have other incentives to make specific choices. There is little gain accrued when a patient is referred to radiation oncology, but surgeons receive financial incentives for patients going to the OR [31]. Many factors cast doubt that popular current practices in surgical clinics effectively help patients to be informed and to share in difficult decisions about whether or not to undergo surgery. Many of these motivations make assisting the patient in SDM a secondary concern, and even at odds with some of the surgeon's goals.

What Needs to Be Done

It will become increasingly important for surgical clinic staff to be able to effectively educate patients on the important information and engage in SDM with patients, as it becomes the prevailing practice of healthcare. With a growing population of older, more clinically complex patients presenting to surgery clinics, some changes to surgical care practices will be necessary. These changes include a premium put on identification of patients' informational needs and desire for participation, well-designed external patient education resources, and decision support that is integrated into the individual patient's surgical consultation.

Surgeons should ascertain what level of involvement each of their patients want in the decision making process. Even when an older, sicker or frailer patient desires a passive role in SDM, the surgeon should take account of the patient's preferences and risk tolerances for different outcomes. For patients wishing to provide input into the choice, participation in SDM involves first education, confirming that they comprehend the essential information about their cancer diagnosis and treatment options, then inviting them to express their desires. Participation by an uninformed patient can be counterproductive and lead to choices that are a poor fit for patients' goals or leave them poorly prepared and in the dark about what lies ahead.

As difficult as it is to share such information, a patient should know the progno-sis of their disease and the approximate time-frame in which it can be expected to advance and take their life. They should be told that there are options other than surgery (which is almost always the case), and that these might be worth exploring before making a choice, especially when they are not ideal surgical candidates. They should also know what treatment side-effects and health states are possible results from different treatments. A patient who wishes to eradicate their cancer in hopes of living as long as possible must be knowingly willing to accept a compara-tively higher risk of treatment related mortality and lasting morbidity. Such patients might choose to have surgery even if they are at a somewhat higher-risk for compli-cations or adverse outcomes because they desire what gives them the best hope of long-term survival. Conversely, a patient who believes that their remaining life-expectancy is too short to benefit from a high risk treatment offering a potential cure (5-year survival), should understand that they need not accept the risk of surgically-associated mortality and morbidities to do something to combat the malignancy, and instead could pursue radiation therapy, which could slow the cancer's advancement and better preserve healthy lung tissue.

Further research is needed to understand SDM in surgery and how to improve and support it. The current theories of SDM and the instrumentation used to mea-sure this process have been developed and used largely in primary care and, to a lesser degree, shown to be appropriate in oncology [33]. These instruments might not be well-tuned to measure and assess SDM or patient comprehension in surgical contexts and thus might have limited value in understanding the challenge that sur-gical professionals face when educating and sharing with their patients.

More research is needed to fully understand how to more reliably and consis-tently meet the unique decision support needs of older, clinically complex patients faced with a decision about curative surgery as they are likely to differ from those of patients in a primary care or medical oncology setting. The relatively short-term doctor patient relationship in surgical clinics, the trust required for effectively deliv-ering surgical consultation, the high-risk/high-reward prospects of surgery, and the relative urgency with which surgical patients must be informed, all make SDM a more difficult endeavor for surgical specialists than primary care physicians or even oncologists.

The specifics of each kind of surgery are important to SDM. There is limited support available for higher surgical risk early-stage NSCLC patients, and for patients facing decisions about many different surgical treatments. The majority of the decision research that has examined SDM in surgery has focused on breast can-cer patients. A formal review of 25 empirical articles published between 1986 and 2006 on breast cancer patients making surgical decisions report that patients' infor-mation needs were consistent and ranked (in order): chances for a cure, stage of disease, and treatment options [34]. Patient age and education predicted information needs and source use [34]. However, some research has examined patient-centered factors that predict the choice to have lung resection and show negative perceptions of the patient-physician interaction on a communication scale [29]. More research and development of sound SDM support aids and patient education is required to meet the needs for the swelling population of older and clinically diverse patients deciding about surgery.

For the time being, surgeons should strive to inform the patients presenting to their clinic, to the best of their ability, that there is no standard of care and that multiple courses of action are justifiable. They should also ascertain the degree to which each patient wishes to actively weigh options and participate in making the choice. And, as in all areas of health care, express an eager willingness to answer any questions the patient has and allow time to think over the surgery option, and all others, and explore information in greater detail before making a decision.

Summary

Patients' desired role in difficult decisions, like whether or not to undergo curative lung resection when deemed less than ideal surgical candidates, continues to shift towards active and informed participation in SDM with the physician. This change brings profound challenges to a specialty already overtaxed on time and resources because good SDM requires that patients are in a state of being accurately informed at the time of sharing in the decision. They must understand options, uncertainties, risks and potential tradeoffs. Currently, there appears to be a substantial number of patients presenting to surgical clinics who are not accurately informed and even have misconceptions that might steer them away from a treatment that suits their goals and preferences. Further research can help to illuminate the problems in SDM for surgery and how to solve them. It is likely that the burden of preparing patients for effective SDM in surgical clinics will have to be shared with professionals other than the surgeons because the surgical clinics are too limited, but for now surgeons should be aware of the importance of striving to maximize patients' understanding about their disease and treatment options so that the patients' values and preferences guide a treatment choice that is right for them.

References

1. Elwyn G, Edwards A, Kinnersley P, Grol R. Shared decision making and the concept of equipoise: the competences of involving patients in healthcare choices. Br J Gen Pract. 2000;50(460): 892–9.
2. Hollingham R. Blood and guts: a history of surgery. 1 U.S. edth ed. New York: Thomas Dunne Books/St. Martin's Press; 2009. 319 pp.
3. No Authorship i. Taking shared decision making more seriously. Lancet. 2011; 377(9768):784.
4. Seminar SG. Salzburg statement on shared decision making. Brit Med J. 2011;342:d1745.
5. Singh JA, Sloan JA, Atherton PJ, Smith T, Hack TF, Huschka MM, et al. Preferred roles in treatment decision making among patients with cancer: a pooled analysis of studies using the Control Preferences Scale. Am J Manag Care. 2010;16(9):688–96.
6. Ekdahl AW, Andersson L, Friedrichsen M. They do what they think is the best for me. Frail elderly patients' preferences for participation in their care during hospitalization. Patient Educ Couns. 2010;80(2):233–40.

7. Elwyn G, Miron-Shatz T. Deliberation before determination: the definition and evaluation of good decision making. Health Expect. 2010;13(2):139–47.

8. Peters E, Hess TM, Västfjäll D, Auman C. Adult age differences in dual information processes: implications for the role of affective and deliberative processes in older adults' decision making. Perspect Psychol Sci. 2007;2(1):1–23.

9. Fagerlin A, Sepucha KR, Couper MP, Levin CA, Singer E, Zikmund-Fisher BJ. Patients' knowledge about 9 common health conditions: the DECISIONS survey. Med Decis Making. 2010;30(5 Suppl):35S–52.

10. Fagerlin A, Lakhani I, Lantz PM, Janz NK, Morrow M, Schwartz K, et al. An informed decision? Breast cancer patients and their knowledge about treatment. Patient Educ Couns. 2006;64(1–3):303–12.

11. Whelan T, Levine M, Willan A, et al. Effect of a decision aid on knowledge and treatment decision making for breast cancer surgery: a randomized trial. JAMA. 2004;292(4):435–41.

12. Nelson WL, Han PKJ, Fagerlin A, Stefanek M, Ubel PA. Rethinking the objectives of decision aids: a call for conceptual clarity. Med Decis Making. 2007;27(5):609–18.

13. Ambady N, LaPlante D, Nguyen T, Rosenthal R, Chaumeton N, Levinson W. Surgeons' tone of voice: a clue to malpractice history. Surgery. 2002;132(1):5–9.

14. Levinson W, Roter DL, Mullooly JP, Dull VT, et al. Physician-patient communication: the relationship with malpractice claims among primary care physicians and surgeons. JAMA. 1997;277(7):553–9.

15. Beckman HB, Markakis KM, Suchman AL, Frankel RM. The doctor-patient relationship and malpractice. Lessons from plaintiff depositions. Arch Intern Med. 1994;154(12):1365–70.

16. Projections of the population by age and sex for the United States: 2010 to 2050 (NP2008-T12). In: Division P, editor. U.S. Cencus Bureau. August 14 2008.

17. Howlader NNA, Krapcho M, Garshell J, Neyman N, Altekruse SF, Kosary CL, Yu M, Ruhl J, Tatalovich Z, Cho H, Mariotto A, Lewis DR, Chen HS, Feuer EJ, Cronin KA. SEER cancer statistics review, 1975–2010. Bethesda: Institute NC. 2013.

18. Battafarano RJ, Piccirillo JF, Meyers BF, Hsu H-S, Guthrie TJ, Cooper JD, et al. Impact of comorbidity on survival after surgical resection in patients with stage I non–small cell lung cancer. J Thorac Cardiovasc Surg. 2002;123(2):280–7.

19. Brunelli A, Kim AW, Berger KI, Addrizzo-Harris DJ. Physiologic evaluation of the patient with lung cancer being considered for resectional surgery: diagnosis and management of lung cancer, 3rd ed: American College of Chest Physicians evidence-based clinical practice guidelines. Chest J. 2013;143(5_suppl):e166S–90.

20. Cicerchia M, Ceci M, Locatelli C, Gianni W, Repetto L. Geriatric syndromes in peri-operative elderly cancer patients. Surg Oncol. 2010;19(3):131–9.

21. Fried LP, Tangen CM, Walston J, Newman AB, Hirsch C, Gottdiener J, et al. Frailty in older adults: evidence for a phenotype. J Gerontol A Biol Sci Med Sci. 2001;56(3):M146–57.

22. Makary MA, Segev DL, Pronovost PJ, Syin D, Bandeen-Roche K, Patel P, et al. Frailty as a predictor of surgical outcomes in older patients. J Am Coll Surg. 2010;210(6):901–8.

23. Dale W, Hemmerich J, Kamm A, Posner MC, Matthews JB, Rothman R, et al. Geriatric assessment improves prediction of surgical outcomes in older adults undergoing pancreaticoduodenectomy: a prospective cohort study. Ann Surg. 2013; Publish Ahead of Print:10.1097/SLA.0000000000000226.

24. Reyna VF, Lloyd FJ. Physician decision making and cardiac risk: effects of knowledge, risk perception, risk tolerance, and fuzzy processing. J Exp Psychol Appl. 2006;12(3):179–95.

25. Reyna VF. A theory of medical decision making and health: fuzzy trace theory. Med Decis Making. 2008;28(6):850–65.

26. Finucane ML. Emotion, affect, and risk communication with older adults: challenges and opportunities. J Risk Res. 2008;11(8):983–97.

27. Pargament KI, Smith BW, Koenig HG, Perez L. Patterns of positive and negative religious coping with major life stressors. J Sci Study Relig. 1998;37(4):710–24.

28. DeLisser HM, Keirns CC, Clinton EA, Margolis ML. "The air got to it:" exploring a belief about surgery for lung cancer. J Natl Med Assoc. 2009;101(8):765–71.

29. Cykert S, Dilworth-Anderson P, Monroe MH, Walker P, McGuire FR, Corbie-Smith G, et al. Factors associated with decisions to undergo surgery among patients with newly diagnosed early-stage lung cancer. JAMA. 2010;303(23):2368–76.

30. Margolis M, Kaiser L, Christie J. Patient decisions to undergo surgery for early-stage lung cancer. JAMA. 2010;304(11):1165.

31. Katz P. The scalpel's edge: the culture of surgeons. Needham Heights: Allyn and Bacon; 1999.

32. Axelrod DA, Goold S. Maintaining trust in the surgeon-patient relationship: challenges for the new millennium. Arch Surg. 2000;135(1):55–61.

33. Butow P, Juraskova I, Chang S, Lopez A-L, Brown R, Bernhard J. Shared decision making coding systems: how do they compare in the oncology context? Patient Educ Couns. 2010;78(2):261–8.

34. O'Leary KA, Estabrooks CA, Olson K, Cumming C. Information acquisition for women facing surgical treatment for breast cancer: influencing factors and selected outcomes. Patient Educ Couns. 2007;69(1–3):5–19.

Part II
Lung

Chapter 6
Indications for Pretreatment Pathologic Mediastinal Staging in Non-small Cell Lung Cancer

Sai Yendamuri and Todd L. Demmy

Abstract The last decade has witnessed the evolution of several new methods of assessing the mediastinum of patients with non-small cell lung cancer. These include advances in radiologic imaging as well as advances in techniques enabling the pathological examination of lymph nodes before a multi-disciplinary discussion of the treatment plan. This chapter summarizes the available evidence for these modalities and provides a framework for decision making that the practicing clinician can use for the deployment of these techniques.

Keywords Lung cancer • Staging • Mediastinoscopy • Lymphadenectomy • VATS • VAMLA • TEMLA • EBUS • EUS

Introduction

Accurate staging is necessary for appropriate cancer therapy and is a hallmark of a good cancer program. Given that distant metastatic disease in non-small cell lung cancer (NSCLC) is often straightforward to diagnose, the main staging challenge in NSCLC is the determination of N stage. From a prognostic point of view, the most important decrement in survival is from N-null to N-positive patients. However, from a treatment planning point of view, the most important decision point is the presence or absence of N2 and N3 disease, i.e., mediastinal nodal disease. Several imaging

S. Yendamuri, MD
Department of Thoracic Surgery, Roswell Park Cancer Institute,
Elm & Carlton Streets, Buffalo, NY 14263, USA
e-mail: sai.yendamuri@roswellpark.org

T.L. Demmy, MD (✉)
Department of Thoracic Surgery, Roswell Park Cancer Institute,
Buffalo, NY 14263, USA
e-mail: todd.demmy@roswellpark.org

M.K. Ferguson (ed.), *Difficult Decisions in Thoracic Surgery*,
Difficult Decisions in Surgery: An Evidence-Based Approach 1,
DOI 10.1007/978-1-4471-6404-3_6, © Springer-Verlag London 2014

techniques such as computerized tomography (CT) and positron emission tomography with computerized tomography (PET-CT) can be used for this determination. Despite such imaging advances, a histological determination of mediastinal disease is often necessary. The focus of this chapter is to help the practicing clinician develop a framework to make the decision of *when* pathological staging of the mediastinum is required, rather than focusing on techniques that describe *how* to stage the mediastinum.

Search Strategy

A series of searches were performed in October 2013 in PUBMED (http://www.ncbi.nlm.nih.gov/pubmed/) using the logical argument "Lung Cancer AND X" with "X" changed to "mediastinal staging", "CT", "PET-CT", "mediastinoscopy", "EBUS", "EUS" and "VATS". The time interval was limited from 2007 to present. Some important earlier manuscripts were also cited. Information obtained was graded according to published GRADE guidelines [1]. In general, the strength of evidence for these studies is moderate to low, as it is has been difficult to execute large randomized controlled trials to evaluate such rapidly evolving technology.

Tools for Pathological Mediastinal Staging

In order of increasing invasiveness, tools for pathological mediastinal staging include endobronchial ultrasound guided fine needle aspiration (EBUS-FNA), endoscopic ultrasound guided fine needle aspiration (EUS-FNA), bronchoscopy with blind FNA, mediastinoscopy, transcervical extended mediastinal lymphadenectomy (TEMLA), video assisted mediastinal lymphadenectomy (VAMLA) and VATS. The performances of each of these modalities are summarized in Table 6.1.

Table 6.1 Accuracy of various mediastinal staging procedures

Modality	Sensitivity %	Specificity %	FP %/FN %	Morbidity
EBUS-FNA	93	100	1/28	Minimal
EUS-FNA	84	99.5	0.7/19	Minimal
Mediastinoscopy	78	100	0/11	Bleeding
				Recurrent laryngeal nerve injury (1 %)
TEMLA	94	100	0/2.8	Recurrent laryngeal nerve injury (2.3 %)
VAMLA	94	100	0/0.9	Recurrent laryngeal nerve injury (4.6 %)
VATS	75	100	0/7	Bleeding

EBUS-FNA endobronchial ultrasound guided fine needle aspiration, *EUS-FNA* endoscopic ultrasound guided fine needle aspiration, *TEMLA* transcervical extended mediastinal lymphadenectomy, *VAMLA* video assisted mediastinal lymphadenectomy, *VATS* video assisted thoracoscopic surgery, *FP* false positive rate, *FN* false negative rate

EBUS-FNA

EBUS–FNA has revolutionized the approach to surgical staging of the mediastinum over the last decade. Increasing familiarity with and adoption of this technique have yielded data showing reliability rivaling mediastinoscopy (considered the gold standard of pathologic pretreatment mediastinal assessment). EBUS has the advantage of being able to access most relevant mediastinal lymph nodes with minimal morbidity. EBUS is also attractive because it can be performed repeatedly without interfering with other staging techniques like mediastinoscopy. Staging EBUS should include, at the very least, examination of right and left paratracheal lymph node zones and the subcarinal lymph node station in addition to any other suspicious areas near the airway on imaging. At least three passes of each lymph node should be obtained [2, 3] and obtaining material for cell block is recommended to enhance diagnostic accuracy [4, 5].

EUS-FNA

EUS-FNA has been demonstrated to be useful to detect malignancy in select mediastinal lymph node stations such as levels 3, 7 and 8, but has limited advantage over EBUS. Some practitioners have combined EBUS and EUS ("medical mediastinoscopy") to obtain superior results [6]. However, EUS is not used widely as a standalone modality for staging the mediastinum.

Mediastinoscopy

Mediastinoscopy was the gold standard for staging the mediastinum before the advent of EBUS. During mediastinoscopy, at the very least bilateral paratracheal zones and the subcarinal lymph node station (levels 2, 4 and 7) should be sampled [7]. An extended mediastinoscopy technique can be used to access level 5,6 lymph nodes as well. Mediastinoscopy can be used to access most mediastinal lymph node stations and is safe and accurate in experienced hands. The primary problem with mediastinoscopy has been its variable effectiveness outside expert hands. In one study, a lymph node was biopsied in only 50 % of procedures [8]. Integrating video into the mediastinoscope probably improves node acquisition and safety [9]. In addition, the procedure necessitates a general anesthetic and has the potential for serious morbidity such as bleeding catastrophes and recurrent laryngeal nerve injury (1 %). While redo mediastinoscopy has been reported to be safe in expert hands [10], in general, it is not attempted by most surgeons. Therefore, restaging after neoadjuvant therapy is problematic if this modality is used to evaluate N2 disease before therapy is initiated.

TEMLA/VAMLA

Transcervical mediastinal lymphadenectomy is an extension of mediastinoscopy in which access to the mediastinum is obtained by a larger cervical incision and a sternal lift. Of all preresectional procedures, this approaches the results of transthoracic mediastinal lymphadenectomy most closely. While proven safe in a large single center series, it has not been widely adopted [11]. Therefore, data on its reproducibility is awaited. In addition, the rate of recurrent laryngeal nerve injury is somewhat higher (2.3 %). VAMLA uses a video-mediastinoscope to perform a systematic lymph node dissection instead of a sampling as done by standard mediastinoscopy. Similar to TEMLA, the lymph node dissection approaches that done by thoracotomy or VATS, but is associated with a higher incidence of recurrent laryngeal nerve injury (4–6 %) [12]. Arguably, the accuracy of TEMLA/VAMLA exceeds open or VATS dissections because the contralateral lymph node stations are accessible through the mid-line approach. Because TEMLA and VAMLA have not been widely adopted by surgeons, their availabilities are limited. Therefore, these techniques will not be discussed further in decision making for the rest of this chapter.

VATS

Video assisted thoracic surgery has become very popular and experienced surgeons can perform the same level of lymph node dissections that were previously performed by thoracotomy. However, this approach is invasive and can only access the ipsilateral mediastinum. Therefore, its use for mediastinal staging is reserved for special situations.

Decision Making and Recommendations—Balancing Risk, Benefit and Probability

In making a decision, the clinician has to balance the risk and benefit of an action and the probability of each arm of the decision. The benefit of attempting pretreatment pathological staging is twofold. The first is the avoidance of unnecessary surgery with its attendant mortality and morbidity in cases of occult multi-station N2 disease. The second is the potential for using neoadjuvant therapeutic strategies for single station N2 disease. This potential benefit is based on the accuracy of the various staging modalities discussed previously. Whereas accuracy of these modalities is dependent on the capabilities of local practitioners, for the purposes of this chapter, best published data will be used to make recommendations. The potential risk of pathologic staging depends on the procedure. While EBUS and EUS are very safe, mediastinoscopy and VATS carry some morbidity and even mortality. However, another "risk" is a false negative test, which is dependent on both the user and anatomic location of target nodes.

An important variable in this decision making is the probability of mediastinal disease. The most common imaging modalities used for this estimation are CT and PET-CT. CT scanning has a sensitivity and specificity of 51 and 86 % [13]. PET-CT scanning generally performs better – sensitivity and specificity of 77 and 86 %, respectively [14]. However, it is important to remember that the specificity and accuracy are based heavily on the patient population and the prevalence of inflammatory disease. In countries where this inflammatory incidence is low, performance characteristics are excellent. In other regions, specificity is lower due to other confounding mediastinal pathologies such as histoplasmosis, sarcoidosis, and tuberculosis [15].

Generally, a negative PET-CT indicates no N2 disease. This has been demonstrated in several retrospective analyses. Meyers et al. demonstrated that in clinical stage I lung cancer, the incidence of mediastinal metastasis is about 5 % [16]. A similar result was demonstrated by DeFranchi et al. from the Mayo clinic [17]. Both these studies, however, were based on clinical early stage lesions. If all lung cancer patients not having distant metastatic disease are included, the prevalence of occult (not detected by CT or PET-CT) is much higher, on the order of 10–15 % [18]. Several investigators have attempted to formulate and validate prediction systems for N2 disease with clinical criteria [19–21]. While these have the theoretical possibility of estimating the risk of mediastinal disease in an individual patient, they are based on small datasets and need significant refinement and validation before they can be recommended.

At this time broader categorizations of increased pre-test probability provide reasonable frameworks for clinical decision making. The presence of occult N2 disease is associated with the following clinical characteristics: large size (>3 cm), central tumors, adenocarcinoma or large cell carcinoma, high standardized value uptake (SUVmax) on PET-CT scan or clinical N1 disease [18, 19]. Based on the pre-test probability of mediastinal disease, the clinical situation can be classified into three categories in descending order of pre-test probability:

1. Mediastinal disease positive on imaging
2. Mediastinal disease negative on imaging with primary tumor characteristics denoting high risk for mediastinal disease
3. Mediastinal disease negative on imaging with primary tumor characteristics denoting low risk for mediastinal disease

The following sections describe the rationale and approach to each of these situations and are summarized in Fig. 6.1.

Mediastinal Disease Positive on Imaging

The goal of pathological assessment of mediastinal lymph nodes is primarily to confirm the diagnosis of N2 or N3 disease beyond doubt so that definitive treatment recommendations may be made. This is particularly true in the case of bulky N2

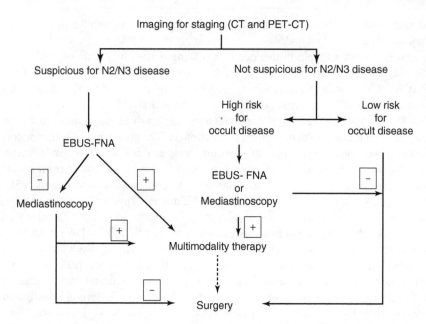

Fig. 6.1 Decision pathway for pathological examination of mediastinum in patients with non-small cell lung cancer. *EBUS-FNA* Endobronchial ultrasound guided fine needle aspiration, *CT* computerized tomography, *PET-CT* positron emission tomography with computerized tomography

lymphadenopathy, multistation N2 lymphadenopathy or N3 lymph node disease, because, in most centers, this warrants non-surgical therapy. Provided all methods of staging with the requisite expertise are available, the current method of choice for obtaining the diagnosis in this setting is EBUS-FNA. Advantages of EBUS-FNA over other modalities include the ability to stage all relevant lymph nodes stations and minimal morbidity. Another distinct advantage of EBUS-FNA in the case of single station N2 disease is the ability to restage the mediastinum after therapy with mediastinoscopy or TEMLA. While small case series demonstrating the safety of redo mediastinoscopy exist, most practitioners avoid this procedure especially if radiation was used. A negative EBUS in this situation should be followed up with mediastinoscopy before initial treatment, as a significant proportion of patients with a mediastinum suspicious on imaging and negative on EBUS will be positive on mediastinoscopy. In case EBUS-FNA is not available in a given center, the procedure of choice is mediastinoscopy.

Mediastinal Disease Negative on Imaging with Primary Tumor Characteristics Denoting High Risk for Mediastinal Disease

High risk criteria are summarized in Table 6.2. In this situation, the mediastinum should be systematically staged in order to identify patients suitable for neo-adjuvant therapy if that is in keeping with the philosophy of the treating

Table 6.2 Criteria for classifying image negative mediastinum as high risk for occult metastases

Criterion	Cut-off
Size	3 cm
Histology	Adenocarcinoma/large cell carcinoma
N1 nodes	Positive on imaging
SUVmax of tumor on PET-CT	High (>5.6)
Location of tumor	Central
Morphology	Cavitation, multicentricity

PET-CT positron emission tomography – computed tomography

multidisciplinary team. EBUS-FNA is the first option in this case, preferably as a separate procedure from the planned resection if the mediastinum is negative. This provides the opportunity for examination of the cell block apart from rapid on site examination. If EBUS is negative, it is reasonable to go ahead with surgical resection. A negative EBUS in this situation does not mandate a mediastinoscopy for confirmation [22]. If EBUS expertise is unavailable, mediastinoscopy can be used in its stead. Mediastinoscopy can be performed at the same time as definitive surgical resection because of the high accuracy of frozen section in this setting [23, 24].

Mediastinal Disease Negative on Imaging with Primary Tumor Characteristics Denoting Low Risk for Mediastinal Disease

In this setting, the pre-test probability of finding occult mediastinal disease is less than 5 %. As such, even if occult N2 disease is found, 5-year survival approaches 27 % with potentially no difference between administration of neoadjuvant vs. adjuvant therapy [25, 26]. Therefore, the surgeon has the option of not performing any pathologic staging of the mediastinum and proceeding directly to resection provided that a systematic lymph node sampling or dissection is performed. If unexpected positive mediastinal nodes are found by VATS lymph node sampling/dissection before resection, some surgeons would delay resection until after induction therapy; however there are insufficient data to determine the appropriateness of this tactic.

Conclusion

Several methods exist for the pathological examination of mediastinal lymph nodes to guide the management of patients with NSCLC. The appropriate use of these techniques depends on the pre-test probability of positivity of mediastinal lymph nodes for cancer as well as the local expertise available. Techniques should be employed in stepwise increasing invasiveness proportionate to the likelihood of finding N2 or N3 disease. The recommendations made in this chapter provide a framework for the rational utilization of available technology for staging the mediastinum.

A Personal View of the Data

Our approach is to use EBUS for patients suspected of having N2 disease and save mediastinoscopy/TEMLA for later to ensure that the mediastinum has responded to induction chemotherapy. I also use mediastinoscopy to exclude occult nodal disease immediately before anatomic resection/lymph node dissection for patients with criteria listed in Table 6.2. If the patient is particularly frail, I use mediastinoscopy more liberally to avoid a futile high-risk resection. Alternatively, for an otherwise healthy patient with a locally aggressive tumor, I use TEMLA to improve superior and contralateral mediastinal nodal recovery thus complementing the transthoracic lymphadenectomy.

Recommendations

- In the presence of mediastinal nodal involvement based on imaging, EBUS-FNA is recommended for initial diagnosis and nodal staging (Evidence quality moderate; weak recommendation).
- A negative EBUS in the presence of nodal involvement based on imaging should be followed up with mediastinoscopy before treatment initiation. (Evidence quality low; weak recommendation).
- Patients who have tumors at high risk for mediastinal nodal involvement in the absence of imaging abnormalities in the mediastinum should have systematic mediastinal staging. (Evidence quality low; weak recommendation)
- In the absence of a high risk tumor or nodal positivity on imaging, pathologic staging of the mediastinum is not required and it is appropriate to proceed directly to resection, provided that a systematic lymph node sampling or dissection is performed intraoperatively. (Evidence quality low; weak recommendation).

References

1. Brozek JL, Akl EA, Alonso-Coello P, Lang D, Jaeschke R, Williams JW, et al. Grading quality of evidence and strength of recommendations in clinical practice guidelines. Part 1 of 3. An overview of the GRADE approach and grading quality of evidence about interventions. Allergy. 2009;64(5):669–77.
2. Lee HS, Lee GK, Kim MS, Lee JM, Kim HY, Nam BH, et al. Real-time endobronchial ultrasound-guided transbronchial needle aspiration in mediastinal staging of non-small cell lung cancer: how many aspirations per target lymph node station? Chest. 2008;134(2):368–74. Epub 2008/02/12.

3. Block MI. Endobronchial ultrasound for lung cancer staging: how many stations should be sampled? Ann Thorac Surg. 2010;89(5):1582–7. Epub 2010/04/27.
4. Yung RC, Otell S, Illei P, Clark DP, Feller-Kopman D, Yarmus L, et al. Improvement of cellularity on cell block preparations using the so-called tissue coagulum clot method during endobronchial ultrasound-guided transbronchial fine-needle aspiration. Cancer Cytopathol. 2012;120(3):185–95. Epub 2011/12/07.
5. Sanz-Santos J, Serra P, Andreo F, Llatjos M, Castella E, Monso E. Contribution of cell blocks obtained through endobronchial ultrasound-guided transbronchial needle aspiration to the diagnosis of lung cancer. BMC Cancer. 2012;12:34. Epub 2012/01/24.
6. Wallace MB, Pascual JM, Raimondo M, Woodward TA, McComb BL, Crook JE, et al. Minimally invasive endoscopic staging of suspected lung cancer. JAMA. 2008;299(5):540–6. Epub 2008/02/07.
7. De Leyn P, Lardinois D, Van Schil PE, Rami-Porta R, Passlick B, Zielinski M, et al. ESTS guidelines for preoperative lymph node staging for non-small cell lung cancer. Eur J Cardiothorac Surg. 2007;32(1):1–8. Epub 2007/04/24.
8. Little AG, Rusch VW, Bonner JA, Gaspar LE, Green MR, Webb WR, et al. Patterns of surgical care of lung cancer patients. Ann Thorac Surg. 2005;80(6):2051–6; discussion 6. Epub 2005/11/25.
9. Cho JH, Kim J, Kim K, Choi YS, Kim HK, Shim YM. A comparative analysis of video-assisted mediastinoscopy and conventional mediastinoscopy. Ann Thorac Surg. 2011;92(3):1007–11. Epub 2011/05/24.
10. De Waele M, Serra-Mitjans M, Hendriks J, Lauwers P, Belda-Sanchis J, Van Schil P, et al. Accuracy and survival of repeat mediastinoscopy after induction therapy for non-small cell lung cancer in a combined series of 104 patients. Eur J Cardiothorac Surg. 2008;33(5):824–8. Epub 2008/03/18.
11. Zielinski M. Video-assisted mediastinoscopic lymphadenectomy and transcervical extended mediastinal lymphadenectomy. Thorac Surg Clin. 2012;22(2):219–25. Epub 2012/04/24.
12. Turna A, Demirkaya A, Ozkul S, Oz B, Gurses A, Kaynak K. Video-assisted mediastinoscopic lymphadenectomy is associated with better survival than mediastinoscopy in patients with resected non-small cell lung cancer. J Thorac Cardiovasc Surg. 2013;146(4):774–80. Epub 2013/06/20.
13. Silvestri GA, Gould MK, Margolis ML, Tanoue LT, McCrory D, Toloza E, et al. Noninvasive staging of non-small cell lung cancer: ACCP evidenced-based clinical practice guidelines (2nd edition). Chest. 2007;132(3 Suppl):178S–201. Epub 2007/10/06.
14. Silvestri GA, Gonzalez AV, Jantz MA, Margolis ML, Gould MK, Tanoue LT, et al. Methods for staging non-small cell lung cancer: diagnosis and management of lung cancer, 3rd ed: American College of Chest Physicians evidence-based clinical practice guidelines. Chest. 2013;143(5 Suppl):e211S–50. Epub 2013/05/10.
15. Li Y, Su M, Li F, Kuang A, Tian R. The value of (1)(8)F-FDG-PET/CT in the differential diagnosis of solitary pulmonary nodules in areas with a high incidence of tuberculosis. Ann Nucl Med. 2011;25(10):804–11. Epub 2011/09/01.
16. Meyers BF, Haddad F, Siegel BA, Zoole JB, Battafarano RJ, Veeramachaneni N, et al. Cost-effectiveness of routine mediastinoscopy in computed tomography- and positron emission tomography-screened patients with stage I lung cancer. J Thorac Cardiovasc Surg. 2006;131(4):822–9; discussion 889. Epub 2006/04/04.
17. Defranchi SA, Cassivi SD, Nichols FC, Allen MS, Shen KR, Deschamps C, et al. N2 disease in T1 non-small cell lung cancer. Ann Thorac Surg. 2009;88(3):924–8. Epub 2009/08/25.
18. Gomez-Caro A, Boada M, Cabanas M, Sanchez M, Arguis P, Lomena F, et al. False-negative rate after positron emission tomography/computer tomography scan for mediastinal staging in cI stage non-small-cell lung cancer. Eur J Cardiothorac Surg. 2012;42(1):93–100; discussion 100. Epub 2012/02/01.
19. Lee PC, Port JL, Korst RJ, Liss Y, Meherally DN, Altorki NK. Risk factors for occult mediastinal metastases in clinical stage I non-small cell lung cancer. Ann Thorac Surg. 2007;84(1):177–81. Epub 2007/06/26.

20. Shafazand S, Gould MK. A clinical prediction rule to estimate the probability of mediastinal metastasis in patients with non-small cell lung cancer. J Thorac Oncol. 2006;1(9):953–9. Epub 2007/04/06.

21. Chen K, Yang F, Jiang G, Li J, Wang J. Development and validation of a clinical prediction model for N2 lymph node metastasis in non-small cell lung cancer. Ann Thorac Surg. 2013;96(5):1761–8. Epub 2013/09/04.

22. Yasufuku K, Pierre A, Darling G, de Perrot M, Waddell T, Johnston M, et al. A prospective controlled trial of endobronchial ultrasound-guided transbronchial needle aspiration compared with mediastinoscopy for mediastinal lymph node staging of lung cancer. J Thorac Cardiovasc Surg. 2011;142(6):1393–400 e1. Epub 2011/10/04.

23. Attaran S, Jakaj G, Acharya M, Anderson JR. Are frozen sections of mediastinoscopy samples as effective as formal paraffin assessment of mediastinoscopy samples for a decision on a combined mediastinoscopy plus lobectomy? Interact Cardiovasc Thorac Surg. 2013;16(6):872–4. Epub 2013/02/22.

24. Sanli M, Isik AF, Tuncozgur B, Akar E, Deniz H, Bakir K, et al. The reliability of mediastinoscopic frozen sections in deciding on oncological surgery in bronchogenic carcinoma. Adv Ther. 2008;25(5):488–95. Epub 2008/06/05.

25. Tsitsias T, Boulemden A, Ang K, Nakas A, Waller DA. The N2 paradox: similar outcomes of pre- and postoperatively identified single-zone N2a positive non-small-cell lung cancer. Eur J Cardiothorac Surg. 2014;45(5):882–7. doi:10.1093/ejcts/ezt478.

26. Darling GE, Allen MS, Decker PA, Ballman K, Malthaner RA, Inculet RI, et al. Randomized trial of mediastinal lymph node sampling versus complete lymphadenectomy during pulmonary resection in the patient with N0 or N1 (less than hilar) non-small cell carcinoma: results of the American College of Surgery Oncology Group Z0030 Trial. J Thorac Cardiovasc Surg. 2011;141(3):662–70. Epub 2011/02/22.

Chapter 7
Preoperative Smoking Cessation for Lung Resection Patients

Alberto de Hoyos and Malcolm DeCamp

Abstract Smoking is the leading cause of preventable death. The prevalence of smoking in the United States remains above 20 % despite intensive cessation programs and awareness of the risks of smoking by the general population. Smoking cessation programs that include counseling and pharmacotherapy have been proven to be effective in achieving long standing abstinence. In lung cancer patients, smoking cessation is associated with significant improvements in quality of life, all cause mortality, life expectancy and postoperative complications. Preoperative smoking cessation prior to a variety of surgical interventions including pulmonary resection reduces the risk of total, respiratory and wound complications. A team approach and adherence to the guidelines for smoking cessation including ongoing assessment, education, pharmacotherapy and referral for additional counseling should become an integrated part of preparing patients for all forms of lung cancer treatment including surgery.

Keywords Nicotine addiction • Nicotine replacement • Behavioral counseling • Smoking • Smoking cessation • Cancer • Lung cancer • Surgery • Pulmonary resection • Thoracic surgery

A. de Hoyos, MD, FACS, FCCP
Division of Thoracic Surgery, Northwestern Memorial Hospital, Northwestern University Feinberg School of Medicine, Chicago, IL USA

M. DeCamp, MD, FACS, FCCP (✉)
Division of Thoracic Surgery, Northwestern Memorial Hospital,
Northwestern University Feinberg School of Medicine,
676 N. St. Clair Street, Suite 650, Chicago, IL 60611, USA
e-mail: mdecamp@nmh.org

M.K. Ferguson (ed.), *Difficult Decisions in Thoracic Surgery*,
Difficult Decisions in Surgery: An Evidence-Based Approach 1,
DOI 10.1007/978-1-4471-6404-3_7, © Springer-Verlag London 2014

Introduction

Tobacco consumption results in more than five million deaths worldwide each year and accounts for nearly 90 % of all lung cancer cases. Smoking is the single greatest cause of disease and premature death in the United States. Despite a decline in tobacco use, nearly one fifth of American adults continue to smoke cigarettes, making it the most important cause of preventable death. Despite the evidence that tobacco is harmful to almost every organ of the body, and the recognition that quitting results in short and long term benefits, there is limited evidence of which smoking cessation techniques and interventions are most effective in patients with lung cancer scheduled to undergo pulmonary resection. In this chapter we review the literature evaluating the effectiveness of smoking cessation strategies among patients with early stage lung cancer, oncology patients and the general population.

Search Strategy

The MEDLINE electronic database and Cochrane CENTRAL were used to identify studies published from January 1, 2000 to September 1, 2013 using the MeSH headings "smoking" or "smoking cessation" and "cancer", "lung cancer" or "surgery", "pulmonary resection" or "thoracic surgery". The study designs included retrospective studies, prospective cohort studies, randomized controlled trials (RCT), systematic reviews and meta-analyses. Search limits were used to exclude non-English language publications.

The Problem: Nicotine Addiction

Nicotine has been recognized as the most highly addictive of all chemical substances commonly abused [1]. A chief impediment for the majority of smokers who try to quit is the neurobiology of tobacco dependence, which is fed by the most efficient delivery device of nicotine that exists – the cigarette. Cigarette smoking delivers high concentrations of nicotine to the central nervous system (CNS) within seconds of each puff. On average a cigarette contains between 13 and 19 mg of nicotine; smoking one cigarette typically delivers 1–2 mg of nicotine. The primary target for nicotine in the CNS, the chemical structure of which resembles that of acetylcholine, is the $cx4\beta2$ nicotinic acetylcholine receptor. When activated by nicotine binding, stimulation results in the release of several neurotransmitters including dopamine, serotonin, noradrenaline, acetylcholine, and beta-endorphins. Release of dopamine in the nucleus accumbens provides the positive reinforcement and feelings of pleasure observed with cigarette smoking. Smoking one cigarette results in a high level of occupancy of the $cx4\beta2$ receptors while consuming three cigarettes completely saturate these receptors for as long as 3 h. Craving results when the receptor occupancy declines over time, and reducing that craving requires achieving virtually complete receptor saturation by smoking the next cigarette, closing the feedback loop.

Smoking Cessation in Cancer Patients

The estimates for the prevalence of smoking at the time of lung cancer diagnosis have ranged from 24 to 60 %, which is up to three times that of the general US adult population. It is estimated that up to 83 % of all active smokers continue to smoke after a diagnosis of lung cancer [2]. Despite encouragement to quit smoking and strong intentions to quit, continued tobacco use after diagnosis of lung cancer remains a problem in this patient population and remains a frustrating circumstance for both patient and physician [3]. Lung cancer diagnosis may be viewed as a "teachable moment" and cessation programs at the time of surgery have been shown to be especially effective [4].

Techniques for assisting smokers to quit include behavioral counseling, cognitive therapy, and referral to quit lines or smoking cessation services and pharmacological interventions [5, 6]. Persistent smoking in the oncology population has a multitude of adverse effects during the treatment of malignancy, increases the risk of recurrence or a second primary tumor and reduces survival. Smoking cessation is a formidable challenge in this complex population as demonstrated by several systematic reviews and meta-analyses [7, 8]. These studies failed to demonstrate a clear benefit of some interventions over usual care. However, interventions in the perioperative period resulted in significantly improved cessation rates.

While the goal of any intervention is permanent tobacco abstinence, this is rarely achieved with a single treatment. Smoking cessation is a dynamic process that involves a sequence of unsuccessful attempts to quit before long term abstinence is achieved. Indeed, relapse is the most likely consequence from any single quit attempt. Health care providers (and patients) need to be aware that most patients will require six or more quit attempts before achieving permanent abstinence and should not view prior attempts as total failures but as practice for the next quit attempt.

Smoking Cessation Before Surgery

Nearly 50 % of patients who smoke at the time of lung cancer surgery continue to smoke afterward [2]. Recent studies from the Society of Thoracic Surgeons General Thoracic Surgery Database have demonstrated that ongoing smoking is associated with increased risk of postoperative complications after lobectomy, pneumonectomy and esophagectomy [9]. The converse, perioperative smoking cessation, has been demonstrated to reduce the risk of total, respiratory and wound complications prior to a variety of surgical interventions. Continued smoking has been associated with an increased risk of all-cause mortality in patients with lung cancer [10].

Several studies and meta-analyses have demonstrated the effectiveness of smoking cessation programs prior to elective surgery [11–14]. Unfortunately, these effects can be short lived and there is a significant risk of relapse during the first 2 months after surgery. Reports from longitudinal studies of patients undergoing surgical treatment for lung cancer, all of whom presumably stopped smoking at least temporarily during hospitalization, suggest that rates of relapse are high in this patient population. Results show that 25–33 % of patients with a smoking history relapse back to smoking by 3 months post-surgery. Nearly 40 % of patients were smoking by 12 months after their potentially curative lung cancer resection [14]. Low household income, exposure to environmental tobacco smoke at home and depression were risk factors associated with returning to smoking. Intensive smoking cessation interventions retained a significant effect on long-term smoking cessation versus brief interventions. Better strategies tailored to the needs of these patients are required to improve long term abstinence in this challenging group of patients

A randomized controlled trail (RCT) in preoperative surgical patients demonstrated a significant improvement in abstinence from smoking (76 %) when the intervention was provided in the pre-operative clinic compared to the control group (56 %) [13]. Among patients with lung cancer undergoing surgery, intensive preoperative cessation pharmacotherapy is recommended as a method of improving abstinence rates [15]. Given the impact of smoking on treatment (surgery, radiation, chemotherapy), a patient's smoking status should be considered part of all treatment decisions. For highly dependent smokers, tailored intensive interventions that combine behavioral interventions with combined pharmacologic cessation aids may be more helpful.

Pharmacotherapy

There is significant evidence that the odds of a smoker quitting are increased by using a multimodality approach that includes counseling and pharmacotherapy [15–18]. All seven first line medications (nicotine replacement therapy (NRT) products: patch, gum, lozenge, nasal spray and inhaler, bupropion slow release (SR) and varenicline), have been shown to reliably increase long-term smoking abstinence rates in the 2008 US Public Health Service (USPHS) clinical practice guideline for treating tobacco use and dependence (Table 7.1) [19–22]. Clinicians should also consider the use of certain combinations of medications identified as effective in the guideline.

Although a broad literature exists guiding behavioral and pharmacological interventions in general surgical populations, there is relative paucity of data guiding medication choices in patients with malignancy [6]. There are only four studies that specifically evaluated the use of pharmacologic therapy among patients with cancer in the perioperative setting and only two were performed in

Table 7.1 Published evidence of a variety of smoking cessation interventions

Intervention	Number of studies	Estimated odds ratio[a] (95 % CI)	Estimated abstinence rate (95 % CI)	Total N
No intervention	–	–	3–5	–
Simple advice vs usual care	17	1.6 (1.4–1.9)	5.2 (3.2–6.5)	15,930
Patient-initiated telephone quit line@vs usual care	9	1.4 (1.2–1.5)	9.0 (8.5–14.1)	18,500
Placebo in medication trials	80	1.0	13.8	14,537
Single agents				
Nicotine gum (6–14 weeks)	13	1.5 (1.2–1.7)	19.0 (16.5–21.9)	662
NRT vs placebo or no treatment	111	1.5 (1.5–1.6)	22.2 (18.7–24.8)	43,000
Nicotine patch (6–14 weeks)	31	1.9 (1.7–2.2)	23.4 (21.3–25.8)	16,625
Nicotine patch (>14 weeks)	6	1.9 (1.7–2.3)	23.7 (21.0–26.6)	5,939
Bupropion SR	45	2.0 (1.8–2.2)	24.2 (22.2–26.4)	13,182
Nicotine inhaler	4	2.1 (1.5–2.9)	24.8 (19.1–31.6)	3,282
Long-term nicotine gum (>14 weeks)	40	2.2 (1.5–3.2)	26.1 (19.7–33.6)	1,500
Nicotine nasal spray	4	2.3 (1.7–3.0)	26.7 (21.5–32.7)	1,126
Varenicline (2 mg/day)	14	3.1 (2.5–3.8)	33.2(28.9–37.8)	5,611
Combination therapy				
Nicotine patch + inhaler	2	2.2 (1.3–3.6)	25.8 (17.4–36.5)	446
Nicotine patch + bupropion SR	6	2.5 (1.9–3.4)	28.9 (23.5–35.1)	1,106
Nicotine patch (>14 weeks) + nicotine@gum or spray	5	3.6 (2.5–5.2)	36.5 (28.6–45.3)	800

Modified from: Fiore et al. [19], Stead et al. [20], Mahvan et al. [21], Stead et al. [22]
Abbreviations: *vs* versus, *SR* sustained release
[a]An odds ratio >1.0 means that patients using the intervention are more likely not to smoke at 6–12 months; larger numbers correlate with greater effectiveness

patients with lung cancer. The other two studies were performed in patients with breast cancer. The study by Park et al. utilized a nonrandomized design to assign 49 smokers with suspected thoracic malignancy to either control group or a 12 week program consisting of varenicline and smoking cessation counseling [23]. Cotinine-confirmed 7 day point prevalence abstinence rates were 28.1 % in the intervention group versus 14.2 % in the control group at 2 weeks, and 34.4 % versus 14.3 % respectively at 12 weeks. Although these differences were not statistically significant in this small pilot study, these data suggest that a successful cessation intervention using varenicline can be delivered around the time of diagnosis and prior to therapy. In another small study of thoracic surgery patients, Kozower et al. described quit rates following a 10 min office-based intervention with a thoracic surgeon. The 40 participants were offered medication and instructed on use of a state-based quit line, used by 50 % and 7.5 % of the participants respectively. Biochemically confirmed abstinence rates at 3-month follow up were 35 %, suggesting that the surgery environment is a powerful place for effecting abstinence [24].

Nicotine Replacement Therapy

Nicotine replacement therapy products contain pure nicotine without other carcinogens and deliver 1/3–2/3 the concentration produced by cigarette smoking. Nicotine replacement therapy is based on the principle that nicotine is the dependence-producing constituent of cigarette smoking and that smoking cessation can be achieved by replacing nicotine without the toxins in cigarette smoke. Although NRT does not completely relieve the withdrawal symptoms, it makes the experience of stopping less unpleasant. All NRTs are nicotinic acetylcholine receptor agonists but compared with smoking a cigarette, the nicotine via NRT products is delivered to the brain much more slowly and at a lower dose. They do not reproduce the rapid and high levels of nicotine achieved through inhalation of cigarette smoke.

A Cochrane review of 132 trials with over 40,000 patients found that all forms of NRTs increase quit rates by one-and-a-half to twofold [25]. The efficacies of the various forms of NRT are generally similar but compliance may be the limiting factor. One study comparing four forms of NRT found comparable 12 week abstinence rates (20–24 %) but compliance varied: 11 % with the inhaler, 15 % with the nasal spray, 38 % with the gum, and 82 % with the patch. In nearly every randomized clinical trial performed to date, the nicotine patch has been shown to be effective compared with placebo, usually with a doubling of the smoking abstinence rate (Table 7.1) [19–22].

It seems possible to improve the efficacy of NRT by combining the transdermal patch (slow release) with an oral formulation (fast release) that permits ad libitum nicotine delivery. NRT is typically started the day of the quit date though pre-cessation treatment is considered safe and may be advantageous for smokers to try NRT prior to the stress of quitting to determine which agent or agents are preferable.

Most patients use NRT for 4–8 weeks but it is safe for longer use if needed to maintain smoking abstinence. The optimal length of treatment has not been determined but longer term treatment (more than 14 weeks) appears to provide benefit over standard lengths of treatment when combining nicotine patches and nicotine gum. Furthermore, long term treatment of up to 6 months with triple combination therapy (nicotine patches, Bupropion, and nicotine vapor inhaler) appears superior to standard dose nicotine patch therapy given over a 10 week period. For the best chance at success with these therapies, they may be used in combination and should be dose-appropriate based on the patient's need.

Non-nicotine Medications

There are two non-nicotine medications which have been proven to be effective as smoking-cessation pharmacotherapy – bupropion and varenicline. Varenicline is considered more effective based on randomized trials. The U.S. Food and Drug Administration (FDA) has issued boxed warnings for both drugs due to reports of increased risks of psychiatric symptoms and suicide. Given the well-established link between smoking and psychiatric disease, there is no easy way to determine whether or not these adverse events are directly related to the medications. Unfortunately these warnings may deter clinicians from discussing or prescribing bupropion and/or varenicline.

Bupropion (Wellbutrin/Zyban)

Bupropion hydrochloride is an atypical slow-acting antidepressant recommended by the FDA as a first-line drug for the treatment of smokers. Bupropion is known to inhibit the reuptake of norepinephrine and dopamine in the nucleus accumbens, a key area for nicotine reinforcement. Additionally, bupropion antagonizes brain nicotine receptors and blocks the reinforcement effects of nicotine. It has been demonstrated to decreases craving and symptoms of withdrawal.

Since it takes up to 2 weeks to take effect, it is advised to establish a definitive quit date 2 weeks after beginning the medication. Bupropion has been shown to double the odds of cessation and appears to have similar effectiveness to NRT. In addition, studies have suggested that a combined approach with bupropion plus a nicotine patch may be even more effective. The dose of bupropion SR is 150 mg tablet per day, preferably upon waking, for 3 days, then increasing to one table twice daily. The doses should be separated by at least 8 h with the second dose as far away from bedtime as possible. The 2008 USPHS guideline recommends the combined use of bupropion SR and nicotine replacement therapy [19]. The length of recommended treatment is at least 3 months. In patients with depressive symptoms attempting to quit, bupropion should be considered in combination with NRT.

Varenicline

Varenicline is a partial nicotinic agonist; it binds to the nicotinic receptors, thereby preventing nicotine binding. This partial agonist activity induces receptor stimulation and reduces withdrawal symptoms during cessation. Varenicline also blocks the dopaminergic stimulation responsible for the reinforcement and reward associated with smoking. This action reduces the craving and the pleasure associated with cigarette smoking.

The effectiveness of varenicline in smoking cessation was demonstrated in six clinical trials. Five of the six studies were RCTs in which varenicline was shown to be superior to placebo in helping people quit smoking. In two of the five placebo controlled studies, varenicline-treated patients were more successful in giving up smoking than patients treated with bupropion [26, 27]. Evidence suggests that using varenicline can increase the chances of successful long-term smoking cessation between two-and threefold compared with pharmacologically unassisted quit attempts. In a 2009 meta-analysis of 101 studies of pharmacotherapy for smoking cessation, varenicline was found to be more effective than bupropion and NRT monotherapy in achieving continuous abstinence rates at 12 and 24 weeks [28]. In a more recent systematic review and multiple treatment meta-analyses, varenicline exhibited the largest and more sustained treatment effects compared to other pharmacotherapies [29]. A recent double-blind, randomized, placebo controlled trial of varenicline, demonstrated its effectiveness in the perioperative setting in patients undergoing a variety of non-thoracic surgical procedure [30]. Varenicline was also found to be slightly more effective than combination NRT and approximately triples the chances of long term abstinence versus placebo.

Varenicline is supplied in a "Starting Month Pack" and a "Continuing Month Pack". Since it takes 1 week to take effect, it is advised to set the quit date 1 week after beginning the medication. The Starting Pack begins with 0.5 mg daily for 3 days, followed by 0.5 mg twice daily for 4 days. The target quit date is day 8 when the maintenance dose of 1 mg twice daily begins. The initial treatment period should be at least 12 weeks (one starting pack plus two continuing packs). The decision to continue past 12 weeks should be individualized, keeping in mind that higher quit rates are seen with longer duration of treatment. From a practical standpoint (as with any cessation medication), longer treatment can be recommended for abstinent smokers who are not secure and are concerned about smoking relapse.

Combination Pharmacotherapy

Data from RCTs suggest that certain combinations of first-line cessation medications are efficacious in promoting long-term abstinence. Improved cessation rates with combination therapy appear to be primarily due to greater craving suppression. As such, the 2008 USPHS clinical practice guideline considers the following regimens to be appropriate first-line therapy in patients attempting to quit smoking [19].

Combination NRT

Combination NRT involves the use of a long-acting formulation (patch) in combination with a short-acting formulation (gum, lozenge, inhaler, or nasal spray). The long-acting formulation, which delivers relatively constant levels of the drug, is used to prevent the onset of severe withdrawal symptoms, and the short-acting formulation, which delivers nicotine at faster rate, is used as needed to control withdrawal symptoms or cravings that may occur during potential relapse situations (for example, after meals, when under stress, or when around other smokers). A recent meta-analysis found that the combination of NRTs was significantly more effective than single agent NRT. The odds of long-term (>6 months) abstinence were 1.4 times better with the combination therapy compared to nicotine monotherapy [19].

NRT and Bupropion

Combination therapy with bupropion SR and NRT has been evaluated in three long-term controlled trials. Patients receiving combination therapy were significantly more likely to quit than were patients randomized to the nicotine patch alone. The odds of long-term (>6 months) abstinence were 1.3 times better with the combination therapy compared to the nicotine patch monotherapy [19].

Although seven first line medications are recommended by the USPHS clinical practice guideline, there is no guidance on how to select a particular form of pharmacotherapy or combination of pharmacotherapy that will be most useful for individual patients or which specific form of pharmacotherapy should be used first. Due to the lack of evidence-based recommendations, clinicians are faced with the problem of selecting pharmacotherapy relying only on patient preference and past experience or familiarity with particular medications. Practitioners can rely on guidance from a panel of experts (Delphi) for making the best use of less than perfect information and utilize their suggested algorithm for tailoring pharmacotherapy to make recommendations [31].

Recommendations and Best Practices for Smoking Cessation

The updated USPHS clinical practice guideline for treating tobacco use and dependence suggests that all clinicians can effectively implement cessation strategies. The guideline endorses a condensed user friendly model for the healthcare provider who does not have the time, inclination or expertise to provide more comprehensive tobacco cessation counseling. The Ask, Advise, and Refer (AAR) approach is an abbreviated format that is easy to use and put into practice by nurses and physicians (Table 7.2) [32]. Cessation interventions as brief as 3 min can significantly increase quit rates. By adopting a simple series of questions taking 1–3 min to complete, heath care professionals can initiate smoking cessation interventions that double or triple the chance of quitting in patients scheduled to undergo a surgical procedure [32]. Integrating these strategies into daily practice provides opportunities to significantly reduce postoperative complications and improve the quality and duration of our patients' lives.

Pharmacotherapy is an essential component of smoking cessation programs and should be offered to all patients attempting to quit. Therapies that have been shown to be effective and are recommended as first-line treatment include the following: NRT products, sustained- release bupropion and varenicline. In addition, NRT combinations or the combination of bupropion and NRT (double therapy) has been demonstrated to be superior to either one alone and can be considered if monotherapy is ineffective. Choosing a combination pharmacotherapy is indicated for patients based on the following factors: failed attempt with monotherapy, patients with breakthrough cravings, level of dependence, multiple failed prior attempts and patients with nicotine withdrawal. When prescribing combinations of pharmacotherapy (double or triple therapy), first select combinations of NRT (nicotine patch plus a nicotine lozenge, inhaler, spray or gum). For more heavily dependent patients, prescribe a combination of NRTs plus bupropion or varenicline. The use of two or more forms of NRT has the strongest evidence base and is the most commonly used form of combination therapy. There is a high level of confidence that this combination can be used safely and effectively. This approach permits optimal titration of

Table 7.2 The "AAR" abbreviated approach to smoking cessation counseling

Tobacco cessation counseling	
1. **Ask**. Ask and document if your patient smokes or uses smokeless tobacco products	Many smokers want to quit and appreciate the encouragement of health professionals
2. **Advise**.	
Give clear advice and emphasize the benefits of quitting:	Personalize the advice
It is the best thing that you can do to improve your health	Link smoking to a current illness (emphysema, lung cancer) and discuss how stopping smoking might help improve health
I understand that stopping smoking can be difficult, but if you want to stop smoking I can help you	The peri-operative examination provides the perfect opportunity to discuss smoking cessation with the patient
Benefits include:	
Decreased risk of a heart attack, stroke, coronary heart disease; lung, oral and pharyngeal cancer	
Decreased risk of postoperative complications	
3. **Refer**	Provide support:
Tell the patient that help is a free phone call away	Healthcare workers able to provide support and medication should do so. Support includes:
	Offering advice
Provide patient with quit line numbers (1-800-QUIT-NOW). Evidence suggests quit line use can more than triple success in quitting	Setting a quit date
	Advising that complete abstinence from smoking is best
Refer to smoking cessation services	Arrange medication to aid the quit attempt
	Nicotine replacement therapy
	Bupropion
	Varenicline
	Combinations

Adapted from Zillich et al. [32]

NRT to meet nicotine needs and can be achieved easily and cheaply [31]. Varenicline is significantly more effective than other pharmacotherapy interventions and should be considered in the development of clinical practice guidelines. A recent systematic review of the effectiveness of relapse prevention intervention found NRT, bupropion and varenicline to be effective in preventing relapse following an initial period of abstinence or an acute treatment episode [33].

The paucity of well design studies in patients with lung cancer, leaves significant gaps in our understanding of the best approaches to treating this particularly vulnerable group.

Conclusion

In the US, about 20 % of adults smoke and tobacco dependence remains the leading avoidable cause of death. Without active treatment only 3–5 % of smokers attempting to quit achieve long-term abstinence. Smoking cessation counseling increases cessation rates over no counseling. Although more intensive interventions yield higher quit rates, even brief advice – as few as 3 min – has been shown to have a critical impact on the likelihood of quitting

The combination of counseling and pharmacotherapy results in improved cessation rates. There are seven FDA-approved first-line medications for smoking cessation: five NRT products as well as bupropion and varenicline. In general, based on meta-analyses, the single agents double the likelihood of abstinence at 6-month follow-up relative to placebo. Varenicline and combination NRT each nearly triple the likelihood of successful cessation. Smoking cessation and counseling should be used together whenever possible since neither by itself is as effective as is combination. Smokers remain at notable risk of relapse for many months after initial abstinence or after lung cancer resection. Ongoing counseling over the course of a year or extending the use of medications (up to 6 months or a year) appear to increase long-term abstinence rates.

The 2008 USPHS clinical practice guideline presents more compelling evidence for the efficacy and cost effectiveness of treatment for tobacco use and dependence. For clinicians, the guideline offers four key conclusions:

- Tobacco dependence is a chronic remitting and relapsing condition. Repeated attempts to quit should be encouraged for all smokers at every opportunity.
- Counseling as brief as 3 min is an effective treatment for tobacco dependence.
- Effective medications and medication combinations are currently available and should be used for all smokers who are motivated to quit.
- Of all the first line medications provided as monotherapy, varenicline appears to have the greatest efficacy after 3–6 months.

Clinicians should take every opportunity to encourage smoking cessation and provide effective treatment. Based on the review of the literature, the ideal smoking cessation intervention should be initiated in the preoperative period prior to surgery and continued in the postoperative period. The ideal cessation strategy should include both nonpharmacologic interventions such as cessation advice (counseling, behavioral support), as well as pharmacological interventions.

Recommendations

Counseling and first line medications (NRTs, bupropion, varenicline) are effective when used by themselves for treating tobacco dependence. However, the combination of counseling and medication is more effective than either alone. Clinicians should encourage all individuals making a quit attempt to use both counseling and medication. The combination of long term patch + ad libitum NRT (gum or spray) is more effective than the nicotine patch alone. Offer telephone counseling as an effective method of stopping smoking. People who smoke can be directed to quit lines (1-800-QUIT-NOW). For lung cancer patients attempting cessation in conjunction with surgical interventions, counseling and pharmacotherapy are recommended at the outset of surgical planning. Reliance on short, low intensity cessation counseling alone does not improve abstinence outcomes. Among lung cancer patients with depressive symptoms, cessation pharmacotherapy with bupropion is recommended as a method to improve abstinence rates, depressive symptoms and quality of life. Among lung cancer patients undergoing surgery, the timing of cessation does not appear to increase the risk of perioperative complications. Cessation interventions should be initiated in the pre-operative period. Delaying surgical procedures in favor of longer abstinence duration is not justified.

A Personal View of the Data

We ask every new and returning patient about their smoking status (active, former, never). For active smokers who need elective surgery, it is important to embrace the "teachable moment" philosophy and mandate a minimum of 3–4 weeks of abstinence coupled with daily aerobic exercise (walking). These are the two things within their control that they can do to get ready for surgery. We encourage them to focus on the short-term goal of decreasing surgical complications, to then celebrate that success and worry about this prior "lifetime" smoking habit thereafter. We offer them counseling with supporting literature of three options; 1-800 Quitline, our institutional cessation counselors who offer group or individual services or an ongoing trial in our cancer center which provides counseling and free varenicline. We discuss pharmacologic aids briefly and typically recommend dual NRT with the patch and gum if they have never tried to quit. If they have previously tried to quit and failed or resumed smoking we recommend and prescribe varenicline with nicotine gum for break through cravings. If they have a prior history of depression, we prescribe bupropion and nicotine gum.

For former smokers who remain abstinent, we acknowledge that accomplishment and congratulate them in recognition of the highly addictive nature of nicotine as a chemical/drug and the social/behavioral addiction to smoking.

For post-op or follow-up patients who have "fallen off the smoking cessation wagon", we point out the reality that the average smoker attempts to quit seven times before he/she is successful. We encourage them to try again and remind them of all the tools we have to help. We remind them that they and their social network need to commit to the cessation goal. If the spouse is a smoker, we encourage them to quit together. If they have a lung cancer diagnosis or significant COPD, we point out to them that their lungs have already been proven to be "fertile soil" for these diseases and that continued smoking is inviting further disease progression and/or recurrence. We then use the similar recommendations detailed above regarding counseling, NRT and/or drugs.

With regard to E&M billing, it is important to add nicotine dependence as a discreet diagnosis in addition to whatever diagnosis code is the primary reason for the encounter (e.g. lung cancer). We have developed some standard language which we incorporate into the office note within the electronic health record to document the time and effort spent on smoking cessation counseling and thereby support the small but real reimbursement codes for this work which in turn get added to the bill for that service.

Recommendations
- Offer counseling, including telephone counseling, as an effective method of stopping smoking. (Evidence quality high; strong recommendation)
- For lung cancer patients attempting cessation in conjunction with surgical interventions, counseling and pharmacotherapy are recommended at the outset of surgical planning. (Evidence quality high; strong recommendation)
- Among lung cancer patients undergoing surgery, the timing of cessation does not appear to increase the risk of perioperative complications. Delaying surgical procedures in favor of longer abstinence duration is not justified. (Evidence quality high; strong recommendation)
- Counseling and first line medications (NRTs, bupropion, varenicline) are effective when used by themselves for treating tobacco dependence. However, the combination of counseling and medication is more effective than either alone. (Evidence quality high; strong recommendation)
- The combination of long term patch + ad libitum NRT (gum or spray) is more effective than the nicotine patch alone. (Evidence quality high; strong recommendation)

References

1. Leone F, Evers-Casey S. Developing a rational approach to tobacco use treatment in pulmonary practice: a review of the biological basis of nicotine addiction. Clin Pulm Med. 2012;19:53–61.
2. Slatore CG, Au DH, Hollingworth W. Cost-effectiveness of a smoking cessation program implemented at the time of surgery for lung cancer. J Thorac Oncol. 2009;4:499–504.
3. Waller LL, Weaver KE, Petty WJ, Miller AA. Effects of continued tobacco use during treatment of lung cancer. Expert Rev Anticancer Ther. 2010;10:1569–75.
4. Shi Y, Warner D. Surgery as a teachable moment for smoking cessation. Anesthesiology. 2010;112:102–7.
5. de Hoyos A, Southard C, DeCamp M. Perioperative smoking cessation. Thorac Surg Clin. 2012;22:1–12.
6. Zaki A, Abrishami A, Wong J, Chung F. Interventions in the preoperative clinic for long term smoking cessation: a quantitative systematic review. Can J Anesth. 2008;55:11–21.
7. Nayan S, Gupta M, Sommer D. Evaluating smoking cessation interventions and cessation rates in cancer patients: a systematic review and meta-analysis. ISRNet Oncol. 2011;2011:ID894023.
8. Nayan S, Gupta M, Strychowsky J, Sommer D. Smoking cessation interventions and cessation rates in the oncology population: an updated systematic review and meta-analysis. Otolaryngol Head Neck Surg. 2013;149:200–11.
9. Mason D, Subramanian S, Nowicki E, Grab J, Murthy S, Rice T, Blackstone E. Impact of smoking cessation before resection of lung cancer: the society of thoracic surgeons general thoracic surgery database study. Ann Thorac Surg. 2009;38:362–71.
10. Parsons A, Daley A, Begh R, Aveyard P. Influence of smoking cessation after diagnosis of early stage lung cancer on prognosis: systematic review of observational studies with meta-analysis. Br Med J. 2010;340:b5569.
11. Cropley M, Theadom A, Pravettoni G, Webb G. The effectiveness of smoking cessation interventions prior to surgery: a systematic review. Nicotine Tob Res. 2008;10:407–12.

12. Villebro T, Moller N. Interventions for preoperative smoking cessation (Review). Cochrane Database Syst Rev. 2010;(7):CD002294.
13. Wolfenden L, Wiggers J, Knight J, Campbell E, Rissel C, Keridge R, Spigelman A, Moore K. A programme for reducing smoking in pre-operative surgical patients: randomized controlled trial. Anesthesia. 2005;60:172–9.
14. Walker M, Vidrine D, Gritz E, Larsen R, Yan Y, Govindan R, Fisher E. Smoking relapse during the first year after treatment for early stage non-small cell lung cancer. Cancer Epidemiol Biomarkers Prev. 2006;15:2370–7.
15. Leone FT, Evers-Casey S, Toll BA, Vachani A. Treatment of tobacco use in lung cancer. Diagnosis and management of lung cancer, 3rd ed: American College of Chest Physicians evidence based clinical practice guideline. Chest. 2013;143 Suppl 5:e61S–77.
16. Reus V, Smith B. Multimodal techniques for smoking cessation: a review of their efficacy and utilization and clinical practice guidelines. Int J Clin Pract. 2008;62:1753–68.
17. Ebbert J, Sood A, Hays T, Dale L, Hurt R. Treating tobacco dependence: review of the best and latest treatment options. J Thorac Oncol. 2007;2:249–56.
18. Chandler M, Rennard S. Smoking cessation. Chest. 2010;137:428–35.
19. Fiore M, Jean C, Baker T, Bailey W, Bemowitz N. Treating tobacco use and dependence update. Rockville: U.S. Dep. Health Human Serv., U.S. Public Health Serv; 2008.
20. Stead L, Perera R, Bullen C, Lancaster D. Nicotine replacement therapy for smoking cessation (Review). Cochrane Database Syst Rev. 2008;CD000146.
21. Mahvan T, Namdar R, Voorhees K, Smith P, Ackerman W. Which smoking cessation interventions work best? J Fam Pract. 2011;60:430–1.
22. Stead L, Perera R, Lancaster T. A systematic review of interventions for smokers who contact quitlines. Tob Control. 2007;16 Suppl 1:i3–8.
23. Park ER, Japuntich S, Temel J, Lanuti M, Pandiscio J, Hilgenberg J, et al. A smoking cessation intervention for thoracic surgery and oncology clinics: a pilot study. J Thorac Oncol. 2011;6:1059–65.
24. Kozower BD, Lau CL, Phillips JV, Burks SG, Jones DR, Stukenborg GJ. A thoracic surgeon-directed tobacco cessation intervention. Ann Thorac Surg. 2010;89:926–30.
25. Stead L, Perera R, Bullen C, Mant D. Lancaster T. Nicotine replacement therapy for smoking cessation. Cochrane Database Syst Rev. 2008;(1):CD000145.
26. Cataldo J, Dubey S, Prochaska J. Smoking cessation: an integral part of lung cancer treatment. Oncology. 2011;78:289–301.
27. Jorenby D, Hays J, Rigotti N, Azoulay S, Watsky E, Williams K, Billing C, Gong J, Reeves K. Efficacy of varenicline, an alpha4beta2 nicotinic acetylcholine receptor partial agonist, vs placebo or sustained release bupropion for smoking cessation. A randomized controlled trial. JAMA. 2006;296:56–63.
28. Mills EJ, Wu P, Spurden D, Ebbert JO, Wilson K. Efficacy of pharmacotherapies for short-term smoking abstinence: a systematic review and meta-analysis. Harm Reduct J. 2009;10:6–25.
29. Mills E, Wu P, Lockhart I, Thorlund K, Puhan M, Ebbert J. Comparisons of high-dose and combination nicotine replacement therapy, varenicline, and bupropion for smoking cessation: a systematic review and multiple treatment meta-analysis. Ann Med. 2012;44:588–97.
30. Wong J, Abrishami A, Yang Y, Zaki A, Friedman Z, Selby P, Chapman K, Chung F. A perioperative smoking cessation intervention with varenicline. A double-blind, randomized, placebo-controlled trial. Anesthesiology. 2012;117:755–64.
31. Bader P, McDonald P, Selby P. An algorithm for tailoring pharmacotherapy for smoking cessation: results from a Delphi panel of international experts. Tob Control. 2009;18:34–42.
32. Zillich AJ, Corelli RL, Hudmon KS. Smoking cessation for the busy clinician. Rx Consult. 2007;16:1–8.
33. Agboola S, McNeil A, Coleman T, Leonardi BJ. A systematic review of the effectiveness of smoking relapse prevention intervention for abstinent smokers. Addiction. 2010;105:1362–80.

Chapter 8
High Tech Exercise Testing in Assessing Candidates for Lung Resection

Alessandro Brunelli and Michele Salati

Abstract We reviewed the most recent evidence regarding high tech exercise test for the physiologic evaluation of candidates to lung resection. The quality of the available evidence ranged from low to moderate. Based on the published information we recommend that cardiopulmonary exercise test be used for preoperative functional evaluation. Patients with VO2max >20 ml/kg/min or 75 % should be regarded low risk for major anatomic lung resection. Patients with VO2max <10 ml/kg/min or 35 % should be regarded high risk for major anatomic lung resection.

Keywords VO2max • Lung resection • Morbidity • Mortality • Cardiopulmonary exercise test

Introduction

During the last 10 years a growing body of evidence proved the effectiveness of high tech cardiopulmonary exercise testing (CPET) in estimating the risk of morbidity and mortality following lung resection. At present, three different published guidelines include CPET in algorithms to stratify the surgical risk of lung resection:

- European Respiratory Society/European Society of Thoracic Surgeons (ERS/ESTS) clinical guidelines on fitness for radical therapy in lung cancer patients (surgery and chemo-radiotherapy)—published in 2009 on behalf of the European Respiratory Society (ERS) and the European Society of Thoracic Surgeons (ESTS) [1]
- Guidelines on the radical management of patients with lung cancer—published in 2010 on behalf of the British Thoracic Society (BTS) and the Society for Cardiothoracic Surgeons of Great Britain and Ireland (SCTS) [2]

A. Brunelli, MD (✉) • M. Salati, MD
Department of Thoracic Surgery, Ospedali Riuniti Ancona,
Via Conca 1, Ancona 60129, Italy
e-mail: brunellialex@gmail.com

M.K. Ferguson (ed.), *Difficult Decisions in Thoracic Surgery*,
Difficult Decisions in Surgery: An Evidence-Based Approach 1,
DOI 10.1007/978-1-4471-6404-3_8, © Springer-Verlag London 2014

- Physiologic evaluation of the patient with lung cancer being considered for resectional surgery—published in 2013 on behalf of the American College of Chest Physicians (ACCP) [3]

As stated in these papers, the use of CPET, following the cardiologic evaluation of the patient and the estimation of the pulmonary function (including measurement of the carbon monoxide lung diffusion capacity), allows definitive assessment of the risk of surgery, particularly in those patients with impaired lung function. In fact, several recent papers have shown that the combination of a poor performance at CPET (usually expressed as a value of maximum oxygen consumption—VO2max <15 ml/kg/min) with low predicted postoperative values of forced expiratory volume in 1 s (ppoFEV1) and carbon monoxide lung diffusion capacity (ppoDLCO) (ppoFEV1 or ppoDLCO <30–40 %) is associated with high morbidity and mortality rates in lung cancer patients considered for anatomic lung resection.

The objective of this chapter is to present a review of the current scientific evidence on the use of high tech exercise testing before lung resection in order to clarify the following points:

- when to perform the CPET evaluation during the preoperative functional assessment
- how to interpret the CPET information for stratifying the risk in case of anatomic lung resection.

Search Strategy

We performed a systematic literature search with the aim of answering the following PICO (Patients, Intervention, Comparator, Outcome) question: "In patients submitted to anatomic lung resection is the VO2max measured during the preoperative cardiopulmonary exercise test predictive of postoperative morbidity and mortality?" The Medical Subject Headings (MeSH) terms used for searching were: "lung resection" AND "cardiopulmonary exercise test" AND ("morbidity" OR "mortality"). The resultant papers were examined by both authors, who selected those to retrieve considering the titles (first exclusion process) and then the abstracts of the remaining studies (second exclusion process). Review papers were also searched for cross-references (Fig. 8.1). We decided to include exclusively those papers written in English language with a date of publication within the last 10 years in order to produce updated recommendations. The search was carried out in August 2013.

Results

The use of CPET in the preoperative evaluation of patients considered for lung resection was proposed more than 30 years ago. Eugene and colleagues highlighted the ability of maximum oxygen consumption (VO2max) (expressed as absolute

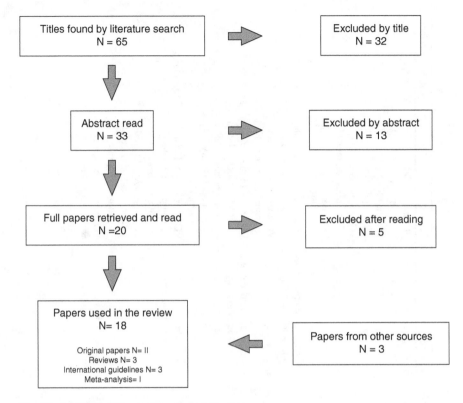

Fig. 8.1 Methods of literature search and selection

value in ml) in predicting the postoperative complications better than the pulmonary function test in a group of 19 patients [4]. Some years later Bolliger and colleagues corroborated these data publishing two different papers in larger cohorts of patients [5, 6]. They emphasized the role of VO2max expressed as percent of predicted value in defining the risk of lung resection. In particular, in a series of 125 surgical candidates for anatomic lung resection submitted to an exhaustive preoperative evaluation including CPET, they found that 90 % of the patients with a VO2max <60 % of predicted values experienced a postoperative complication.

During the last 10 years, many other papers confirmed the role of CPET as the gold standard in the functional preoperative evaluation of lung resection candidates. These papers, as shown in Fig. 8.1 were selected and analyzed for the present review, following the above mentioned criteria. Table 8.1summarizes the original articles studying the association between VO2max measured during CPET and the postoperative risk of morbidity and mortality following lung resection.

In 2005 Win and colleagues [7] published a prospective study on 101 patients evaluated by CPET and then submitted to curative lung surgery. They found that the VO2max expressed as percentage of predicted was the only parameter associated with surgical complications and death and concluded that a VO2max <50 % of predicted should identify a high risk category of patients.

Table 8.1 Original papers on VO2max and postoperative morbidity and mortality

Study	Patients	Evaluation protocol	Outcome	Results	Quality of evidence
Win et al. [7]	101 candidates to anatomic lung resection	Systematic CPET (estimation of VO2max and VO2max%)	Postsurgical complications including mortality	VO2max% >50: complication rate 10 % VO2max% <50: complication rate 67 % VO2max% >60: complication rate 9 % VO2max% <60: complication rate 36 %	Moderate
Bayram et al. [8]	55 candidates to anatomic lung resection	Systematic CPET (estimation of VO2max)	Postsurgical complications including mortality	VO2max >15 ml/kg/min: complication rate 0 VO2max <15 ml/kg/min: complication rate 40 %	Low
Loewen et al. [9]	346 candidates to anatomic lung resection (multiinstitutional)	Systematic CPET (estimation of VO2max and VO2max%)	Postsurgical complications including mortality	VO2max <15 ml/kg/min or <65 % associated with mortality and cardiopulmonary morbidity	Moderate
Brunelli et al. [10]	204 candidates to anatomic lung resection	Systematic CPET (estimation of VO2max and VO2max%)	Cardiopulmonary complications and death	VO2max <12 ml/kg/min: complication rate 33 % and mortality rate 13 %; VO2 max >20 ml/kg/min complication rate: 7 % and mortality rate 0	Moderate
Bobbio et al. [11]	73 candidates to anatomic lung resection	Systematic CPET (estimation of VO2max)	Postsurgical complications including mortality	VO2max not associated with outcome	Low

Study	Population	CPET	Outcome	Findings	Evidence level
Licker et al. [12]	210 candidates to anatomic lung resection (with FEV1 <80 %)	CPET (estimation of VO2max and VO2max%)	Cardiopulmonary complications including mortality	VO2max <10 ml/kg/min: complication rate 65 %; VO2max >10 ml/kg/min: complication rate 17.7 %	Moderate
Kasikcioglu et al. [13]	49 candidates to anatomic lung resection	Systematic CPET (estimation of VO2max and Oxygen uptake kinetics)	Cardiopulmonary complications including mortality	VO2 max and oxygen uptake kinetics associated with poor outcome	Low
Campione et al. [14]	49 candidates to anatomic lung resection (retrospective)	Systematic CPET (estimation of VO2max, HR at peak and Oxygen pulse)	Cardiopulmonary complications including mortality	Only HR at peak and oxygen pulse associated with poor outcome	Low
Torchio et al. [15]	145 selected candidates to anatomic lung resection	CPET (estimation of VO2max, and VE/VCO2 slope)	Cardiopulmonary complications and death	VE/VCO2 slope ≥34: mortality rate 5.5 %; VO2max associated with complications	Moderate
Brunelli et al. [16]	225 candidates to anatomic lung resection	Systematic CPET (estimation of VO2max and VE/VCO2 slope)	Respiratory complications	VE/VCO2 >35: complication rate 22 % and mortality rate 7.2 %	Moderate

CPET Cardiopulmonary exercise test, *HR* heart rate, *VO2max* maximum oxygen consumption, *VE/VCO2* ventilation to carbon dioxide production ratio, *FEV1* forced expiratory volume in 1 s

In 2007, two different studies confirmed the role of VO2max, expressed as ml/kg/min, as a predictor of cardiopulmonary complications including death. Bayram and colleagues [8] in a cohort of 55 patients submitted to major lung resection found a correlation between poor surgical outcome and a VO2max <15 ml/kg/min. They registered no cardiopulmonary morbidity or mortality for patients with a VO2max >15 ml/kg/min. Similarly, Loewen and colleagues reported the data of the Protocol 9,238 of the Cancer and Leukemia Group B investigating the ability of VO2 measurement in predicting the surgical risk in lung resection [9]. Again, they found that the patients with a VO2max <15 ml/kg/min were exposed to a higher risk of postoperative respiratory failure and death.

Brunelli and colleagues in a large mono-institutional series published in 2009 [10] showed that VO2max expressed in ml/kg/min was an independent predictor of complications. They found that a VO2max <12 ml/kg/min was associated with a risk of cardiopulmonary complications and a risk of mortality fivefold and 13-fold higher compared to those with a VO2max >20 ml/kg/min, respectively. A VO2max <12 ml/kg/min was associated with a mortality rate of 13 % whilst no mortality was observed in the group of patients with VO2max >20 ml/kg/min. Notably, only 14 % of the entire population displayed a value of VO2max greater than 20 ml/kg/min reflecting the complex case-mix of patients presenting to a modern thoracic surgical practice.

Unlike previous studies, Bobbio and colleagues [11] failed to demonstrate an association between VO2max and surgical outcome in a cohort of 71 patients submitted to anatomic lung resection (excluding pneumonectomy).

Finally, in 2011, Licker and colleagues [12] published a retrospective analysis on 210 patients submitted to major lung resection with FEV1 <80 % of predicted and evaluated by CPET. They found a fourfold higher risk of cardiopulmonary complications in those patients with a VO2max <10 ml/kg/min, in comparison to the ones with a VO2max >17 ml/kg/min.

Most recently some papers [13–15] suggested other parameters measured during CPET that may be used to refine the preoperative risk assessment. In particular, the oxygen uptake efficiency slope (which represents the rate of increase of VO2 against the minute ventilation volume), the oxygen pulse (which measures the VO2 against the heart rate) and ventilatory inefficiency (which measures the total ventilation against the carbon dioxide production-VE/VCO2 slope) have been demonstrated to be associated with postoperative complications even in those groups of patients in which the VO2max was not a good predictor of morbidity and mortality. In particular, a paper published by Brunelli and colleagues [16] in 2012 in a series of 225 consecutive candidates for anatomic lung resection, demonstrated that the VE/VCO2 slope was the best predictor of respiratory complications and death. A value greater than 35 was proposed as the best threshold discriminating between high and low risk surgical candidates.

During the last 4 years, on the basis of the available evidence mentioned above, additional reviews [17–19] and one meta-analysis [20], three different organizational task forces recommended specific algorithms for the physiologic evaluation of lung resection candidates [1–3]. Taking into account some differences, all these protocols indicated the CPET as the more sophisticated and reliable instrument for defining the risk for pulmonary resection. They consistently recommended a preliminary cardiac evaluation and a subsequent measurement of split lung function and VO2max estimated at CPET to define the risk of surgery. In general, a VO2max >20 ml/kg/min or 75 % indicates a low risk for anatomic lung resection regardless the ppoFEV1 or ppoDLCO values. A VO2max <10 ml/kg/min or 35 % indicates a high risk for anatomic lung resection (i.e. a risk of mortality greater than 10 % and a risk of substantial functional loss or complications after surgery).

Some differences exist among these documents regarding the respective order of the functional tests. The ACCP and the BTS/SCTS recommended performing CPET as a subsequent step after pulmonary function test evaluation and the calculation of the split lung function. The ERS/ESTS protocol proposed a more liberal use of CPET in all patients with either FEV1 or DLCO <80 %. However, logistic and financial issues may limit the applicability of these recommendations in some centers. A recent paper from Novoa and colleagues [21] demonstrated a non-compliancy rate of 26 % in the application of the ERS/ESTS algorithm when it recommends the use of CPET.

Recommendations

Based on the consensus emerged from the recent international guidelines on this topic, the use of the CPET, as a high tech instrument for the physiologic assessment of the patients undergoing to anatomic lung resection, should be considered the gold standard of the functional evaluation (evidence quality moderate).

Based on the available evidence we propose the following recommendations:

- CPET with measurement of VO2max should be used for estimating the risk of candidates to anatomic lung resection, especially in those patients with reduced postoperative respiratory function (ppoFEV1 and or ppoDLCO <30 %).
- Patients with a VO2max >20 ml/kg/min or 75 % of predicted values, regardless their preoperative pulmonary function, should be regarded at low risk for major anatomic lung resection.
- Patients with a VO2max <10 ml/kg/min or 35 % of predicted values should be regarded at high risk for major anatomic lung resection (lobectomy or pneumonectomy). Minor procedures or alternative non-surgical treatments should be recommended in these patients.

A Personal View of the Data

High tech exercise testing is the gold standard for assessing physical fitness before lung resection. It provides a wealth of direct and indirect measurements that can precisely detect a possible deficit in the oxygen transport chain. This may have clinical implications as the defect can be corrected (through medical therapy, coronary revascularization or rehabilitation) and patients brought to surgery in a better physical condition minimizing their surgical risk. However, the widespread use of CPET has been limited in several centers by a lack of culture, logistics and lack of resource utilization.

Moreover, the recent advent of minimally invasive thoracic surgery (i.e. video assisted thoracic surgery lobectomy) may question the traditional operability indicators since this approach has been shown to be particularly effective in reducing morbidity and mortality particularly in high-risk patients. The utility of CPET in this context needs to be carefully evaluated by future investigations as VO2max below critical values may be used to dictate a video assisted thoracic surgery (VATS) approach rather than thoracotomy.

Recommendations

- CPET with measurement of VO2max should be used for estimating the risk of candidates for anatomic lung resection, especially in those patients with reduced postoperative respiratory function (ppoFEV1 and or ppoDLCO <30 %) (evidence quality moderate; strong recommendation).
- Patients with a VO2max >20 ml/kg/min or 75 % of predicted values, regardless their preoperative pulmonary function, should be regarded at low risk for major anatomic lung resection (evidence quality moderate; strong recommendation).
- Patients with a VO2max <10 ml/kg/min or 35 % of predicted values should be regarded at high risk for major anatomic lung resection (lobectomy or pneumonectomy) (evidence quality moderate; strong recommendation). Minor procedures or alternative non-surgical treatments should be recommended in these patients.

References

1. Brunelli A, Charloux A, Bolliger CT, Rocco G, Sculier JP, Varela G, et al. ERS/ESTS clinical guidelines on fitness for radical therapy in lung cancer patients (surgery and chemoradiotherapy). Eur Respir J. 2009;34:17–41.
2. Lim E, Baldwin D, Beckles M, Duffy J, Entwisle J, Faivre-Finn C, et al. Guidelines on the radical management of patients with lung cancer. Thorax. 2010;65:iii1–27.

3. Brunelli A, Kim AW, Berger KI, Addrizzo-Harris DJ. Physiologic evaluation of the patient with lung cancer being considered for resectional surgery. Chest. 2013;143:e166S–90.
4. Eugene J, Brown SE, Light RW, Milne NE, Stemmer EA. Maximum oxygen consumption: a physiological guide to pulmonary resection. Surg Forum. 1982;33:260–2.
5. Bolliger CT, Jordan P, Solèr M, Stulz P, Grädel E, Skarvan K, et al. Exercise capacity as a predictor of postoperative complications in lung resection candidates. Am J Respir Crit Care Med. 1995;151:1472–80.
6. Brutsche MH, Spiliopoulos A, Bolliger CT, Licker M, Frey JG, Tschopp JM. Exercise capacity and extent of resection as predictors of surgical risk in lung cancer. Eur Respir J. 2000;15:828–32.
7. Win T, Jackson A, Sharples L, Groves AM, Wells FC, Ritchie AJ, et al. Cardiopulmonary exercise tests and lung cancer surgical outcome. Chest. 2005;127(4):1159–65.
8. Bayram AS, Candan T, Gebitekin C. Preoperative maximal exercise oxygen consumption test predicts postoperative pulmonary morbidity following major lung resection. Respirology. 2007;12:505–10.
9. Loewen GM, Watson D, Kohman L, Herndon 2nd JE, Shennib H, Kernstine K, et al. Preoperative exercise Vo2 measurement for lung resection candidates: results of Cancer and Leukemia Group B Protocol 9238. J Thorac Oncol. 2007;2:619–25.
10. Brunelli A, Belardinelli R, Refai M, Salati M, Socci L, Pompili C, et al. Peak oxygen consumption during cardiopulmonary exercise test improves risk stratification in candidates to major lung resection. Chest. 2009;135:1260–7.
11. Bobbio A, Chetta A, Internullo E, Ampollini L, Carbognani P, Bettati S, et al. Exercise capacity assessment in patients undergoing lung resection. Eur J Cardiothorac Surg. 2009;35(3): 419–22.
12. Licker M, Schnyder JM, Frey JG, Diaper J, Cartier V, Inan C, et al. Impact of aerobic exercise capacity and procedure-related factors in lung cancer surgery. Eur Respir J. 2011;37: 1189–98.
13. Kasikcioglu E, Toker A, Tanju S, Arzuman P, Kayserilioglu A, Dilege S, et al. Oxygen uptake kinetics during cardiopulmonary exercise testing and postoperative complications in patients with lung cancer. Lung Cancer. 2009;66:85–8.
14. Campione A, Terzi A, Bobbio M, Rosso GL, Scardovi AB, Feola M. Oxygen pulse as a predictor of cardiopulmonary events in lung resection. Asian Cardiovasc Thorac Ann. 2010;18: 147–52.
15. Torchio R, Guglielmo M, Giardino R, Ardissone F, Ciacco C, Gulotta C, et al. Exercise ventilatory inefficiency and mortality in patients with chronic obstructive pulmonary disease undergoing surgery for non-small-cell lung cancer. Eur J Cardiothorac Surg. 2010;38:14–9.
16. Brunelli A, Belardinelli R, Pompili C, Xiumé F, Refai M, Salati M, et al. Minute ventilation-to-carbon dioxide output (VE/VCO2) slope is the strongest predictor of respiratory complications and death after pulmonary resection. Ann Thorac Surg. 2012;93:1802–6.
17. Von Groote-Bidlingmaier F, Koegelemberg VF, Bolliger CT. Functional evaluation before lung resection. Clin Chest Med. 2011;32:773–82.
18. Pichurko BM. Exercising your patients: which test(s) and when? Respir Care. 2012;57: 100–10.
19. Salati M, Brunelli A. Preoperative assessment of patients for lung cancer surgery. Curr Opin Pulm Med. 2012;18:289–94.
20. Benzo R, Kelley GA, Recchi L, Hofman A, Sciurba F. Complication of lung resection and exercise capacity: a meta-analysis. Respir Med. 2007;101:1790–7.
21. Novoa NM, Ramos J, Jiménez MF, González-Ruiz JM, Varela G. The initial phase for validating the European algorithm for functional assessment prior to lung resection: quantifying compliance with the recommendations in actual clinical practice. Arch Bronconeumol. 2012;48(7):229–33.

Chapter 9
Management of Perioperative Anticoagulation in Lung Resection

Jacob R. Moremen and DuyKhanh P. Mimi Ceppa

Abstract The perioperative management of anticoagulation in patients undergoing pulmonary resection encompasses multiple topics, inherent in each being the balance between the risks of surgical bleeding versus the risks of thrombosis. To address this topic, we evaluated the available literature for recommendations regarding (1) the use of anticoagulation for venous thromboembolism (VTE) prophylaxis(2), the management of patients on chronic anticoagulation (history of pulmonary embolism, chronic atrial fibrillation, mechanical heart valve, etc.), and (3) the management of patients on acute or chronic antiplatelet therapy (cardiac stents, peripheral vascular stents, etc.). We summarize the available data and provide recommendations on how to contend with each of these scenarios in patients undergoing pulmonary resection.

Keywords Noncardiac thoracic surgery • Pulmonary resection • Anticoagulation • Deep venous thrombosis prophylaxis • Pulmonary embolism • Atrial fibrillation • Antiplatelet therapy • Cardiac stent • Drug-eluting stent

Introduction

Patients undergoing thoracic surgery, particularly those with cancer, are at least at moderate risk of thromboembolic disease. In addition, many such patients are already taking anticoagulants because of underlying medical conditions. The perioperative management of anticoagulation in patients undergoing pulmonary resection encompasses multiple topics, inherent in each being the balance between the risks of

J.R. Moremen, MD (✉) • D.P. Mimi Ceppa, MD
Division of Cardiothoracic Surgery, Department of Surgery, Indiana University School
of Medicine, 545 Barnhill Drive EH 215, Indianapolis, IN 46220, USA
e-mail: dpceppa@iupui.edu

M.K. Ferguson (ed.), *Difficult Decisions in Thoracic Surgery*,
Difficult Decisions in Surgery: An Evidence-Based Approach 1,
DOI 10.1007/978-1-4471-6404-3_9, © Springer-Verlag London 2014

surgical bleeding versus the risks of thrombosis. We evaluated the available literature for recommendations regarding 1(1) the use of anticoagulation for venous thrombo-embolism (VTE) prophylaxis, 2(2), the management of patients on chronic antico-agulation (history of pulmonary embolism, chronic atrial fibrillation, mechanical heart valve, etc.), and 3(3) the management of patients on acute or chronic antiplate-let therapy (cardiac stents, peripheral vascular stents, etc.). Few large-scale studies have been performed on these topics that are specific to thoracic surgery. Many of the recommendations in the literature have been based on outcomes for other surgical specialties. We summarize the available data and provide recommendations on how to contend with each of these scenarios in patients undergoing pulmonary resection.

Search Strategy

We conducted a focused review of the current guidelines related to medical manage-ment and risks of anticoagulation therapy. We then performed a comprehensive review of the literature related to thoracic surgery and anticoagulation therapy. Literature searches were conducted in the PubMed database using the key words: anticoagulation, deep venous thrombosis, pulmonary embolism, atrial fibrillation, drug-eluting stent, heparin, warfarin, antiplatelet therapy, clopidogrel, pulmonary resection, lobectomy, thoracic surgery, noncardiac thoracic surgery. Searches were limited to the English language, human subjects, and literature published in the last 5 years. Our search returned 400 articles; we critically reviewed 45 articles related to thoracic surgery as well as national guidelines from the American College of Chest Physicians (ACCP) and the American Heart Association (AHA). Emphasis was made on current national guidelines and recommendations.

Prophylaxis for Venous Thromboembolism

Patients undergoing thoracic surgery are considered at least at moderate risk for VTE. In studies of patients undergoing thoracotomy for pulmonary resection, VTE occurred in approximately 1.7 % of patients and pulmonary embolism occurred in 1.2 % of patients despite perioperative prophylaxis [1]. Patients undergoing extended pulmonary resections or pneumonectomy are at even higher VTE risk, with reported rates as high as 7.4 % [2, 3].

Data evaluating the use of VTE prophylaxis in patients undergoing thoracic sur-gery are limited. Two small trials evaluating the use of perioperative VTE prophy-laxis have were published over 20 years ago. The first paper compared the used of differing doses (5,000 units twice daily versus 7,500 units twice daily) of unfrac-tionated heparin (UFH) while the second paper compared the use of UFH with the use of nadroparin [4, 5]. The remaining data on the topic were retrospective reviews, mostly evaluating the use of VTE prophylaxis in patients undergoing extrapleural pneumonectomy, who are considered high risk for VTE (Table 9.1). Mason et al.

Table 9.1 Studies on VTE prophylaxis in patients undergoing thoracic surgery

Study/year	Population	Study type	Number of patients	Prophylaxis	Bleeding complication	Thrombotic complication	Mortality	p	Quality of evidence
Sugarbaker et al. (2004) [3]	Extrapleural pneumonectomy (Mesothelioma)	Retrospective	328	NR	NR	21 (6.4 %) DVT; 5 (1.5 %) PE	6/496 (1.2 %)	N/a	Low
Mason et al. (2006) [2]	Pneumonectomy for malignancy	Retrospective	336	UFH, ICDs	None requiring reoperation	25 (7.4 %) total: 8 (2.3 %) PE	3 (0.8 %)	N/a	Low
Dentali et al. (2008) [6]	Lung malignancy	Retrospective	690	UFH (67 %), LMWH (22 %)	NR	3 (0.4 %) DVT only, 9 DVT/PE (1.3 %)	4 (0.6 %)	NR	Low
Egawa et al. (2009) [7]	Thoracic and cardiovascular surgery	Randomized, consecutive series	A: 1,467; B: 1,389 on protocol	A: NR; B: CS (low risk), CS + chemical proph (high risk)	NR	A: 6 (0.4 %) PE; B: none	None	NR	Low
Girard et al. (2011) [8]	Pulmonary and Thoracic surgery ward	Retrospective	A: 2,989; B: 3,085	A: Enoxaparin; B: Fondaparinux	B > A transfusion 3.1 vs 1.8 %*	A = B	NR	*0.002	Low
Bille et al. (2012) [9]	Extrapleural pneumonectomy (Mesothelioma)	Randomized, consecutive series	A: 10; B: 11	A: LMWH + CS; B: LMWH + CS + warfarin	None	A: 3 PE; 1 fatal; B: none	A: 1 (10 %)	*0.05	Low
Gomez-Hernandez et al. (2013) [10]	Elective thoracic surgery (68 % malignancy)	Retrospective	6,004	LMWH day prior, cont post-op	NR	Total 11 (0.18 %); PE 7 (0.11 %)	3/7 PE (all s/p R pneumonectomy)	N/a	Mod

NR not reported, *DVT* deep vein thrombosis, *VTE* venous thromboembolism, *PE* pulmonary embolism, *UFH* unfractionated heparin, *ICDs* intermittent compression devices, *LMWH* low molecular weight heparin, *CS* compression stockings

reported the results of their review of 336 patients undergoing pneumonectomy for malignancy who were all treated with twice daily dosing of UFH with intermittent compression devices [2]. Five percent of patients were diagnosed with deep venous thrombosis (DVT) while 2.3 % were diagnosed with a pulmonary embolism. Gomez-Hernandez et al. published their retrospective review of over 6,000 patients undergoing elective thoracic surgery [10]. In their study, they followed the ACCP guidelines for VTE risk stratification, prophylaxis, and diagnosis. Patients in whom VTE prophylaxis was recommended received the first dose of low molecular weight heparin (LMWH) prior to surgery with continuation post-operatively without delay. They reported a DVT rate of 0.18 % and pulmonary embolism rate of 0.11 %. Interestingly, three of seven patients who were diagnosed with a pulmonary embolism had a right pneumonectomy. The remaining studies compared LMWH with warfarin, LMWH with fondapurinox, or UFH with LMWH and found no significant differences in treatment [6–9]. The risk of post-operative bleeding was mentioned in only one of these studies and also demonstrated no significant difference in bleeding between treatment groups. Therefore, due to the limited data, VTE prophylaxis guidelines in the setting of thoracic surgery have been inferred from data in patients undergoing general or abdomino-pelvic surgery.

Recommendations

The ACCP 9th edition VTE prophylaxis guidelines recommend the use of UFH, LMWH, or mechanical prophylaxis in patients undergoing thoracic surgery who are at low risk of bleeding [11]. Patients who are undergoing pneumonectomy or extended pulmonary resection UFH or LMWH is recommended once adequate hemostasis has been established. In addition, these patients should have mechanical prophylaxis. Patients who are at high risk of bleeding should undergo mechanical prophylaxis over no prophylaxis.

Management of Patients on Chronic Anticoagulation or Vitamin K Antagonists (VKA)

Patients present to the thoracic surgeon while taking VKAs for several known and frequently unknown indications. It is crucial to ascertain the true indication for treatment with VKAs in order to appropriately manage perioperative anticoagulation. The most common indications for VKA therapy are chronic atrial fibrillation, pulmonary embolism, and presence of a mechanical heart valve. We address each of these clinical scenarios individually. In managing the use of VKAs perioperatively, one must consider each individual patient's risk for thrombosis (particularly in the prothrombotic state induced by surgery) with the patient's risk for bleeding. Most of the data addressing this topic are from studies in patients in a non-operative setting. Therefore, guidelines on the perioperative management of VKAs are inferred from data in non-operative patients and based on risks of thrombus formation.

Atrial Fibrillation

Conditions and comorbidities found to affect VTE risk are congestive heart failure, hypertension, age over 75, diabetes, and prior history of stroke or transient ischemic attack (TIA). As such the risk for VTE in patients with atrial fibrillation is largely based on CHADS$_2$ score (Congestive heart failure, Hypertension, Age >75 years, Diabetes mellitus, prior Stroke or TIA) calculator that assigns risk of VTE according to pre-existing comorbidities [12]. Patients at high risk of VTE include CHADS$_2$ score of 5 or 6, history of stroke or transient ischemic attack within 3 months prior to surgery, or rheumatic valvular heart disease. Patients at a moderate risk patients have a CHADS$_2$ score 3 or 4. Finally, patients at a low risk are defined by CHADS$_2$ score of 0–2 (no prior history of stroke or TIA).

Pulmonary Embolism

Patients with VTE or pulmonary embolism within 3 months of surgery or severe thrombophilia (e.g., protein C, protein S, or antithrombin deficiency; antiphospholipid antibodies) are considered high risk of having a recurrent event. Patients at moderate risk are those who had a VTE or pulmonary embolism 3–12 months prior to surgery, those with mild thrombophilia (e.g., heterozygous factor V Leiden), recurrent VTE, or current malignancy. Finally, patients with a history of VTE or pulmonary embolism more than 1 year ago and no other risk factors are considered to be at low risk of a perioperative thrombotic event.

Mechanical Heart Valve

Patients with any mitral valve prosthesis, any caged-ball or tilting aortic valve prosthesis, or a history of stroke or transient ischemic attack within 6 months prior to surgery are at high risk of a thrombosis. Patients at moderate risk for thrombosis are those with a bileaflet aortic valve prosthesis and one or more of the following risk factors—atrial fibrillation, prior stroke or transient ischemic attack, hypertension, diabetes, congestive heart failure, or age older than 75 years. Low risk patients are those with a bileaflet aortic valve prosthesis without atrial fibrillation and no other stroke risk factors.

Recommendations

The ACCP recommends that in patients who require cessation of VKA on account of risk of bleeding from surgery that warfarin be held 4–5 days prior to operation in patients at low risk for VTE. Patients who are at low risk of thrombosis as delineated above, bridging with either intravenous UFH or LMWH is not recommended. Patients who are at high risk of thrombosis as delineated above should be bridged with either intravenous UFH or subcutaneous LMWH. Patients at moderate risk for thrombosis should be assessed on an individual basis. Finally, patients who require temporary interruption of VKAs should resume VKAs 12–24 h after surgery if there is adequate hemostasis instead of later resumption [13].

Management of Patients on Antiplatelet Therapy for Cardiac Stents

Approximately 600,000 patients undergo coronary artery interventions with either bare metal or drug eluting stents in the United States each year [14]. These patients are maintained on an appropriate antiplatelet regimen, which typically includes aspirin and clopidogrel (Plavix), for a defined period of time. The 2011 American College of Cardiology Foundation (ACCF)/American Heart Association (AHA) guidelines for percutaneous coronary intervention recommend aspirin use indefinitely, and P2Y12 inhibition with clopidogrel, or in certain circumstances, prasugrel or ticagrelor, for a minimum of 1 month. Patients should continue antiplatelet therapy with a P2Y12 inhibitor up to 12 months following implantation of a bare metal stent (BMS). Patients undergoing drug eluting stent (DES) implantation require treatment with an aspirin and P2Y12 inhibition for a minimum of 12 months.

Up to 5 % of patients undergoing percutaneous coronary intervention undergo surgery within the first year after coronary stenting [15]. Moreover, the perioperative morbidity and mortality in patients undergoing surgical procedures following percutaneous coronary intervention (PCI) with stenting are as high as 40 and 20 %, respectively [16, 17]. The risk of early discontinuation of antiplatelet therapy is severe. Discontinuation of clopidogrel therapy within 1 month of DES placement carried a 25 % stent thrombosis rate in one series [18]. In a large observational cohort study of more than 2,000 patients, thrombosis of DES occurred in 29 % of patients in whom antiplatelet therapy was discontinued prematurely (<3 months after sirolimus-eluting stents and <6 months after paclitaxel-eluting stents), with a mortality rate of 45 % [19].

Data on patients with DES <12 months old and BMS <1 month, or high risk patients with either, undergoing thoracic surgery is limited to small case series (Table 9.2). The increased thrombotic risk following surgery is well described. Two small series of 32 and 33 patients demonstrated major adverse cardiac events at rates of 9.3 % and 36 % [20, 21], respectively, when clopidogrel was held 5–7 days

Table 9.2 Studies on dual antiplatelet therapy in thoracic surgery patients

Study/year	Population	Study type	Number of patients	Antiplatelet indication	Management	Bleeding complication	Thrombotic complication	Mortality	Notes	Evidence strength
Brichon et al. (2006) [20]	Major lung resection	Retrospective	32	BMS	Stop clopidogrel 7–10 days prior	Transfusion 3/32 (9.3 %)	Stent thrombosis 3/32 (9.3 %)	1/32 (3 %)		Low
Cerfolio et al. (2010) [21]	Thoracic surgery	Prospective, consecutive series	33	Stent 21 (63 %); Other 11 (33 %)	Continued clopidogrel	2/33 (6 %) return to OR	MI: 0/8 vs control 5/14 (36 %)	No difference	*Lobectomy only p=0.05	Low
Ceppa et al. (2011) [22]	Lung resection	Retrospective	54 (+108 controls)	Stent (74 %), Other cardiac (18.6 %), PVD (5.6 %)	A: bridge w eptifibatide* B: Hold 5 days prior**	Equivalent to controls	Equivalent to controls	3.7 %	*High risk **Low risk	Low
Paul et al. (2013) [23]	Thoracic surgery	Retrospective	165 (64 matched controls)	Varied, most stents	A: Continued B: Held >5d C: ASA bridge	Transfusion*, reoperation** A: 35 %, 5 % B: 3, 1 % C: 11, 4 %	Post-op MI*** A: 0 B: 3 C: 4	1 MI-related death Group B	*A > B, p=0.001 A > C, p=0.004 **NS ***NS	Low
Fernandez et al. (2013) [24]	Major lung resection + stent <1 year	Retrospective (SEER data)	519 (+21,892 controls)	BMS	NR	NR	MACE 9.3 vs. 4.9 % control*	7.7 vs. 4.6 % control**	*p<0.0001 **p<0.0001	Low

BMS bare metal stent, *MI* myocardial infarction, *ASA* aspirin, *PVD* peripheral vascular disease, *NS* non-significant, *MACE* major adverse cardiac event, *SEER* Surveillance, Epidemiology, and End Results

prior to thoracic surgery. A recent review of the SEER (Surveillance Epidemiology and End Results) Medicare data by Fernandez et al. demonstrated a similar rate of 9.3 % major adverse cardiac events versus 4.9 % in controls in over 500 patients who underwent major lung resection within 1 year following the placement of a BMS [24].

When evaluating retrospective series of thoracic patients on clopidogrel we found that management of antiplatelet therapy is varied. However, the most common management is to discontinue antiplatelet therapy preoperatively [20, 22]. Data from the Clopidogrel in Unstable Angina to Prevent Recurrent Events (CURE) trial showed an increased risk for clopidogrel-associated perioperative bleeding in patients with coronary artery disease (CAD) undergoing coronary artery bypass grafting (CABG). This finding was confirmed by Kapetanakis and colleagues [25], showing that patients receiving clopidogrel in the 7 days before off-pump CABG have a fivefold risk of reoperation for bleeding and an increased need for transfusion.

Two recent series provide insight into the bleeding risk of patients taking clopidogrel while undergoing noncardiac thoracic surgery. Cerfolio et al. operated on 32 consecutive patients who presented on clopidogrel for various reasons (63 % recent coronary stent, 33 % CAD or valvular disease) [21]. Antiplatelet therapy was not stopped preoperatively. There were zero thrombotic complications and only two major bleeding events that required return to the operating room. Both of these cases were redo thoracotomies. The breadth of cases in this study included: 11 thoracotomy with lobectomy patients (one robotically assisted lobectomy), six video-assisted wedge resection, four mediastinoscopy, and two Ivor Lewis esophagogastrectomy. A more recent report examined 182 thoracic operations on 165 patients after DES or BMS and measured outcomes based on whether the clopidogrel was held, continued, or bridged with aspirin [23]. There were seven (4.2 %) major adverse cardiac events, with one cardiac-related mortality in the cohort of patients that did not continue clopidogrel perioperatively. In comparing this cohort of patients to case-matched controls, however, the difference in major adverse cardiac events did not reach statistical significance. The authors attributed this finding to the small number of cases included in the retrospective study. They did report a significant difference in the rate of transfusion in the cohort of patients who were continued on clopidogrel perioperatively.

A proposed management strategy is to bridge patients on dual antiplatelet therapy with a shorter-acting antiplatelet inhibitor. Bridging is thought to maintain the protection of the new DES while limiting the irreversible bleeding impact of clopidogrel. The current literature describing perioperative bridging therapy consists of mostly small case series using glycoprotein IIb/IIIa inhibitors tirofiban [25–27] and eptifibatide [22, 28–30] (Table 9.3). Only one of these papers was in the thoracic surgery patient population [22]. Savonitto et al. performed a prospective trial and examined bridging with tirofiban in 30 consecutive patients with DES implantation (<6 months) undergoing urgent cardiac and noncardiac operations [25]. No ischemic events were reported and only two bleeding events among those 30 patients. Rassi et al. found in matched cohorts no significant increase in bleeding events in patients who were bridged with a glycoprotein IIb/IIIa inhibitor [28]. Although there was a trend towards higher returns to the operating room for bleeding, this finding did not reach statistical significance. In the unmatched 100-patient cohort

Table 9.3 Studies on bridging therapy (eptifibatide, tirofiban, cangrelor) while off dual antiplatelet therapy

Study/year	Population	Study type	Duration of stent implant	Number of patients	Bridging medication	Timing of bridge (preop)	Bleeding complication	Thrombotic complication	Mortality	Evidence strength
Broad et al. (2007) [26]	ENT, general surgery	Retrospective	Varied	15	Tirofiban + Heparin	3 days	None	None	None	Low
D'Urbano et al. (2008) [27]	Varied	Case series	<3 month	4	Tirofiban	5 days	None	None	None	Low
Bigalke et al. (2009) [30]	Varied	Case series	<30 days	7	Eptifibatide	72 h	None	None	None	Low
Savonitto et al. (2010) [25]	Major or eye surgery	Prospective	<6 month or <1 year and high risk	30	Tirofiban	5 days	1 TIMI major 1 TIMI minor	None	None	Low
Ceppa et al. (2011) [22]	Major lung resection	Retrospective	<1 year or high risk	7	Eptifibatide	2–3 days	2 transfused	None	None	Low
Morrison et al. (2012) [29]	Noncardiac (NC) Cardiac(Card)	Retrospective	<1 year	6 NC 13 Card	Eptifibatide	4 days	Major: 7 Card, 0 NC Minor: 1 Card, 1 NC	None	None	Low
Angiolillo et al. (2012) [31]	CABG	Randomized, double blind, multicenter,	Variable	210	Cangrelor[a], placebo	2–7 days	Equivalent	Equivalent	NR	Moderate
Rassi, et al. (2012) [28]	Noncardiac (NC) Cardiac(Card)	Retrospective	118 days (median) 100	100	Eptifibatide		34 % 5 or more RBC transfused	MACE: 7 MI: 0	6 %	Low

TIMI thrombolysis in myocardial infarction, *MACE* major adverse cardiac event, *CABG* coronary artery bypass graft

[a]Not commercially available

there were no episodes of stent thrombosis or myocardial infarction. There was, however, a rate of transfusions of five or more units of blood of 34 %. Half of patients requiring post-operative transfusion were redo operations. Additionally, the authors noted that cardiac cases carried a higher transfusion rate than noncardiac cases. Finally, The Bridging Antiplatelet Therapy with Cangrelor in Patients Undergoing Cardiac Surgery (BRIDGE) trial recently examined the use of cangrelor, an intravenous reversible inhibitor of the P2Y12 ADP receptor (not commercially available in the U.S.) [31]. The primary endpoint was a platelet assay (P2Y12 Reaction Units) as a measure of platelet function. In this randomized, double-blinded, multi-institutional trial the authors reported a higher level of platelet inhibition throughout the perioperative period without a significant increase in major bleeding when compared with placebo.

Recommendations

There are no randomized trials comparing various perioperative management strategies of patients with coronary stents on dual antiplatelet therapy. The ACCP recommends the continued perioperative use of aspirin in patients with a moderate to high risk for cardiovascular events requiring noncardiac surgery [13]. Patients who are at low risk of a cardiovascular event may stop aspirin 7–10 days before surgery. Patients who are receiving dual antiplatelet therapy due to a coronary stent should delay surgery at least 6 weeks and 6 months following the placement of a BMS and DES, respectively, when possible. Patients in whom surgery cannot be delayed should continue dual anti-platelet therapy perioperatively in lieu of stopping dual antiplatelet therapy. No formal recommendations regarding the use of bridging patients on dual antiplatelet therapy with UFH, LWMH or glycoprotein IIb/IIIa antagonists (i.e., eptifibatide) were made by the ACCP on account of the scant amount of data available on the topic.

Summary of Recommendations

Prophylaxis for Venous Thromboembolism

The use of UFH, LMWH, or mechanical prophylaxis in patients undergoing thoracic surgery who are at low risk of bleeding is recommended (evidence quality low; weak recommendation). Patients who are undergoing pneumonectomy or extended pulmonary resection UFH or LMWH is recommended once adequate hemostasis has been established (evidence quality low; weak recommendation). In addition, these patients should have mechanical prophylaxis (evidence quality low; weak recommendation). Patients who are at high risk of bleeding should undergo mechanical prophylaxis over no prophylaxis (evidence quality low; weak recommendation).

Management of Patients on Chronic Anticoagulation or VKAs

In patients who require cessation of VKA on account of risk of bleeding from surgery we recommend that warfarin be held 4–5 days prior to operation in patients at low risk for VTE (evidence quality low; weak recommendation). Patients who are at low risk of thrombosis as delineated above, bridging with either intravenous unfractionated heparin (UFH) or subcutaneous low molecular weight heparin (LMWH) is not recommended (evidence quality low; weak recommendation). Patients who are at high risk of thrombosis as delineated above should be bridged with either intravenous UFH or subcutaneous LMWH (evidence quality low; weak recommendation). Patients at moderate risk for thrombosis should be assessed on an individual patient basis. Finally, patients who require temporary interruption of VKAs should resume VKAs 12–24 h after surgery if there is adequate hemostasis (evidence quality low; weak recommendation) instead of later resumption.

Management of Patients on Antiplatelet Therapy for Cardiac Stents

The continued perioperative use of aspirin in patients with a moderate to high risk for cardiovascular events requiring noncardiac surgery is recommended (evidence quality low; weak recommendation). Patients who are at low risk of a cardiovascular event may stop aspirin 7–10 days before surgery (evidence quality low; weak recommendation). Patients who are receiving dual antiplatelet therapy due to a coronary stent should delay surgery at least 6 weeks and 6 months following the placement of a BMS and DES, respectively, when possible (evidence quality low; weak recommendation). Patients in whom surgery cannot be delayed should continue dual anti-platelet therapy perioperatively in lieu of stopping dual antiplatelet therapy (evidence quality low; weak recommendation). Bridging patients on dual antiplatelet therapy with UFH, LWMH or glycoprotein IIb/IIIa antagonists (i.e., eptifibatide) may be considered in patients with extremely high risk of adverse cardiovascular event (evidence quality low; weak recommendation).

Conclusion

We discuss the perioperative management of anticoagulation in the setting of pulmonary resection. While there are few data specific to thoracic surgery, in particular, a significant amount of useful information could be extrapolated from data in the general surgery literature. The recommendations for VTE prophylaxis and perioperative management of VKA are relatively

straightforward. More controversial are the recommendations for the management of patients on dual antiplatelet therapy for recent coronary stents. There
are no high quality data on the topic and the clinical significance of this topic
certainly warrants future randomized trials to further elucidate how to best
manage these patients.

A Personal View of the Data

We routinely use LMWH starting the first post-operative day following a pulmonary
resection. In addition, all patients have mechanical prophylaxis at least until they
are ambulating daily. In patients who are at high risk of bleeding, initiation of VTE
prophylaxis is typically deferred until chest tube output is serosanguinous and
hemoglobin levels are stable. Finally, we treat patients undergoing pneumonectomy
in the same manner as patients undergoing non-pneumonectomy pulmonary
resections.

Pulmonary resections are at high risk of bleeding in the setting of perioperative
antithrombotic drug administration. Therefore, we typically do not bridge patients
with atrial fibrillation who present on VKAs preoperatively, unless the patient is at
high risk of VTE. All patients with a mechanical valve are bridged with LMWH,
unless they are at high risk of thrombosis. Patients with a mechanical valve who are
at high risk of thrombosis are admitted preoperatively for bridging with UFH. We
bridge both moderate- and high-risk patients on VKA for pulmonary embolism with
subcutaneous LMWH with the last dose being administered on the morning of the
day prior to surgery. In patients with acute pulmonary embolism requiring anticoagulation, we prefer to delay surgery for at least 2 weeks prior to pulmonary resection. In the rare event that delay is not possible, we treat patients with intravenous
UFH with cessation of UFH administration 6 h prior to skin incision. Intravenous
UFH is resumed within 6 h of the termination of the surgical procedure provided
there is adequate hemostasis.

At our institution, aspirin is uniformly continued on all patients with coronary
stents regardless of procedure planned. When performing a procedure with a low
risk of bleeding (i.e., pulmonary wedge resection), we continue dual antiplatelet
therapy perioperatively. Patients who are undergoing a moderate to high-risk procedure for bleeding (lobectomy, segmentectomy, pneumonectomy) are continued
on aspirin but clopidogrel is stopped 5–7 days before surgery. Dual anti-platelet
therapy is restarted as soon as possible post-operatively (ideally post-operative
day 1) provided that there is no concern for bleeding. We consider bridging
patients on dual platelet therapy with a glycoprotein IIb/IIIa inhibitor pre-opera-
tively in patients with a high-risk of in-stent thrombosis (high-risk location, bifurcation, long segment stent, <3 months from DES placement). However, this
scenario rarely occurs.

Recommendations for Prophylaxis for Venous Thromboembolism
- The use of UFH or LMWH in patients undergoing thoracic surgery who are at low risk of bleeding is recommended (evidence quality low; weak recommendation).
- Patients who are undergoing pneumonectomy or extended pulmonary resection UFH or LMWH is recommended once adequate hemostasis has been established (evidence quality low; weak recommendation).
- Patients should have mechanical prophylaxis (evidence quality low; weak recommendation).

Recommendations for Management of Patients on Chronic Anticoagulation or VKAs
- In patients who require cessation of VKA on account of risk of bleeding from surgery we recommend that warfarin be held 4–5 days prior to operation in patients at low risk for VTE (evidence quality low; weak recommendation).
- For patients who are at low risk of thrombosis, bridging with either intravenous unfractionated heparin (UFH) or subcutaneous low molecular weight heparin (LMWH) is not recommended (evidence quality low; weak recommendation).
- Patients who are at high risk of thrombosis should be bridged with either intravenous UFH or subcutaneous LMWH (evidence quality low; weak recommendation).
- Patients at moderate risk for thrombosis should be assessed on an individual patient basis.
- Patients who require temporary interruption of VKAs should resume VKAs 12–24 h after surgery if there is adequate hemostasis instead of later resumption (evidence quality low; weak recommendation).

Recommendations for Management of Patients on Antiplatelet Therapy for Cardiac Stents
- The continued perioperative use of aspirin in patients with a moderate to high risk for cardiovascular events requiring noncardiac surgery is recommended (evidence quality low; weak recommendation).
- Patients who are at low risk of a cardiovascular event may stop aspirin 7–10 days before surgery (evidence quality low; weak recommendation).

- Patients who are receiving dual antiplatelet therapy due to a coronary stent should delay surgery at least 6 weeks and 6 months following the placement of a BMS and DES, respectively, when possible (evidence quality low; weak recommendation).
- Patients in whom surgery cannot be delayed should continue dual antiplatelet therapy perioperatively in lieu of stopping dual antiplatelet therapy (evidence quality low; weak recommendation).
- Bridging patients on dual antiplatelet therapy with UFH, LWMH or glycoprotein IIb/IIIa antagonists (i.e., eptifibatide) may be considered in patients with extremely high risk of adverse cardiovascular event (evidence quality low; weak recommendation).

References

1. Kalweit G, Huwer H, Volkmer I, Petzold T, Gams E. Pulmonary embolism: a frequent cause of acute fatality after lung resection. Eur J Cardiothorac Surg. 1996;10(4):242–6. discussion 6–7.
2. Mason DP, Quader MA, Blackstone EH, Rajeswaran J, DeCamp MM, Murthy SC, et al. Thromboembolism after pneumonectomy for malignancy: an independent marker of poor outcome. J Thorac Cardiovasc Surg. 2006;131(3):711–8.
3. Sugarbaker DJ, Jaklitsch MT, Bueno R, Richards W, Lukanich J, Mentzer SJ, et al. Prevention, early detection, and management of complications after 328 consecutive extrapleural pneumonectomies. J Thorac Cardiovasc Surg. 2004;128(1):138–46.
4. Cade JF, Clegg EA, Westlake GW. Prophylaxis of venous thrombosis after major thoracic surgery. Aust N Z J Surg. 1983;53(4):301–4.
5. Azorin JF, Regnard JF, Dahan M, Pansart M. Efficacy and tolerability of fraxiparine in the prevention of thromboembolic complications in oncologic thoracic surgery. Annales de Cardiologie et d'Angeiologie. 1997;46(5–6):341–7.
6. Dentali F, Malato A, Ageno W, Imperatori A, Cajozzo M, Rotolo N, et al. Incidence of venous thromboembolism in patients undergoing thoracotomy for lung cancer. J Thorac Cardiovasc Surg. 2008;135(3):705–6.
7. Egawa N, Hiromatsu S, Shintani Y, Kanaya K, Fukunaga S, Aoyagi S. Prevention of venous thromboembolism in thoracic and cardiovascular surgery. Asian Cardiovasc Thorac Ann. 2009;17(5):505–9.
8. Girard P, Demaria J, Lillo-Le Louet A, Caliandro R, Le Guillou JL, Crespin M, et al. Transfusions, major bleeding, and prevention of venous thromboembolism with enoxaparin or fondaparinux in thoracic surgery. Thromb Haemost. 2011;106(6):1109–16.
9. Bille A, Okiror L, Karenovics W, Pilling J, Lang-Lazdunski L. What is the optimum strategy for thromboembolic prophylaxis following extrapleural pneumonectomy in patients with malignant pleural mesothelioma? Interact Cardiovasc Thorac Surg. 2012;15(2):201–3.
10. Gomez-Hernandez MT, Rodriguez-Perez M, Novoa-Valentin N, Jimenez-Lopez M, Aranda-Alcaide JL, Varela-Simo G. Prevalence of venous thromboembolism in elective thoracic surgery. Arch Bronconeumol. 2013;49(7):297–302.

11. Gould MK, Garcia DA, Wren SM, Karanicolas PJ, Arcelus JI, Heit JA, et al. Prevention of VTE in nonorthopedic surgical patients: antithrombotic therapy and prevention of thrombosis, 9th ed: American College of Chest Physicians evidence-based clinical practice guidelines. Chest. 2012;141(2 Suppl):e227S–77.
12. Gage B, Waterman A, Shannon W. Validation of clinical classification schemes for predicting stroke results from the National Registry of Atrial Fibrillation. JAMA. 2001;285:2864–70.
13. Douketis JD, Spyropoulos AC, Spencer FA, Mayr M, Jaffer AK, Eckman MH, et al. Perioperative management of antithrombotic therapy: antithrombotic therapy and prevention of thrombosis, 9th ed: American College of Chest Physicians evidence-based clinical practice guidelines. Chest. 2012;141(2 Suppl):e326S–50. [Erratum appears in Chest. 2012 ;141(4):1129].
14. Chan PS, Patel MR, Klein LW, Krone RJ, Dehmer GJ, Kennedy K, et al. Appropriateness of percutaneous coronary intervention. JAMA. 2011;306(1):53–61.
15. Vicenzi MN, Meislitzer T, Heitzinger B, Halaj M, Fleisher LA, Metzler H. Coronary artery stenting and non-cardiac surgery–a prospective outcome study. Br J Anaesth. 2006;96(6): 686–93.
16. Kaluza GL, Joseph J, Lee JR, Raizner ME, Raizner AE. Catastrophic outcomes of noncardiac surgery soon after coronary stenting. J Am Coll Cardiol. 2000;35(5):1288–94.
17. Schouten O, van Domburg RT, Bax JJ, de Jaegere PJ, Dunkelgrun M, Feringa HH, et al. Noncardiac surgery after coronary stenting: early surgery and interruption of antiplatelet therapy are associated with an increase in major adverse cardiac events. J Am Coll Cardiol. 2007;49(1):122–4.
18. Jeremias A, Sylvia B, Bridges J, Kirtane AJ, Bigelow B, Pinto DS, et al. Stent thrombosis after successful sirolimus-eluting stent implantation. Circulation. 2004;109(16):1930–2.
19. Iakovou I, Schmidt T, Bonizzoni E, Ge L, Sangiorgi GM, Stankovic G, et al. Incidence, predictors, and outcome of thrombosis after successful implantation of drug-eluting stents. JAMA. 2005;293(17):2126–30.
20. Brichon PY, Boitet P, Dujon A, Mouroux J, Peillon C, Riquet M, et al. Perioperative in-stent thrombosis after lung resection performed within 3 months of coronary stenting. Eur J Cardiothorac Surg. 2006;30(5):793–6.
21. Cerfolio RJ, Minnich DJ, Bryant AS. General thoracic surgery is safe in patients taking clopidogrel (Plavix). J Thorac Cardiovasc Surg. 2010;140(5):970–6.
22. Ceppa DP, Welsby IJ, Wang TY, Onaitis MW, Tong BC, Harpole DH, et al. Perioperative management of patients on clopidogrel (Plavix) undergoing major lung resection. Ann Thorac Surg. 2011;92(6):1971–6.
23. Paul S, Stock C, Chiu YL, Kansler A, Port JL, Lee PC, et al. Management and outcomes of patients on preoperative plavix (clopidogrel) undergoing general thoracic surgery. Thorac Cardiovasc Surg. 2013;61(6):489–95.
24. Fernandez FG, Crabtree TD, Liu J, Meyers BF. Incremental risk of prior coronary arterial stents for pulmonary resection. Ann Thorac Surg. 2013;95(4):1212–8. discussion 9–20.
25. Savonitto S, D'Urbano M, Caracciolo M, Barlocco F, Mariani G, Nichelatti M, et al. Urgent surgery in patients with a recently implanted coronary drug-eluting stent: a phase II study of 'bridging' antiplatelet therapy with tirofiban during temporary withdrawal of clopidogrel. Br J Anaesth. 2010;104(3):285–91.
26. Broad L, Lee T, Conroy M, Bolsin S, Orford N, Black A, et al. Successful management of patients with a drug-eluting coronary stent presenting for elective, non-cardiac surgery. Br J Anaesth. 2007;98(1):19–22.
27. D'Urbano M, Barlocco F, Poli A, Fetiveau R, Vandoni P, Savonitto S, et al. Unplanned surgery after drug eluting stent implantation: a strategy for safe temporary withdrawal of dual oral antiplatelet therapy. J Cardiovasc Med. 2008;9:737–41.

28. Rassi AN, Blackstone E, Militello MA, Theodos G, Cavender MA, Sun Z, et al. Safety of "bridging" with eptifibatide for patients with coronary stents before cardiac and non-cardiac surgery. Am J Cardiol. 2012;110(4):485–90.
29. Ben Morrison T, Horst BM, Brown MJ, Bell MR, Daniels PR. Bridging with glycoprotein IIb/IIIa inhibitors for periprocedural management of antiplatelet therapy in patients with drug eluting stents. Catheter Cardiovasc Interv. 2012;79(4):575–82.
30. Bigalke B, Seizer P, Geisler T, Lindemann S, Gawaz M, May AE. Perioperative antiplatelet therapy in patients at risk for coronary stent thrombosis undergoing noncardiac surgery. Clin Res Cardiol . 2009;98(5):335–9.
31. Angiolillo DJ, Firstenberg MS, Price MJ, Tummala PE, Hutyra M, Welsby IJ, et al. Bridging antiplatelet therapy with cangrelor in patients undergoing cardiac surgery a randomized controlled trial. JAMA . 2012;307(3):265–74.

Chapter 10
Perioperative Arrhythmia Prophylaxis for Major Lung Resection

Arielle Hodari and Zane Hammoud

Abstract Perioperative arrhythmia is one of the most common complications following general thoracic surgery and carries significant morbidity. Although there is no direct cause and effect relationship between development of perioperative supraventricular arrhythmia and other post-operative complications, it has been shown that the development of an arrhythmia is associated with increased length of stay, morbidity, and mortality. The identification of risk factors for perioperative atrial arrhythmias is crucial in order to direct prophylactic measures to the appropriate patients. Amiodarone and diltiazem significantly reduce the rate of postoperative atrial arrhythmias after major lung resection.

Keywords Arrhythmia • Lung resection • Prophylaxis • Morbidity • Thoracic surgery

Introduction

Perioperative arrhythmia is one of the most common complications following general thoracic surgery and carries significant morbidity. The most common types are atrial fibrillation (AF), supraventricular tachycardia, atrial flutter and premature ventricular contractures. The reported incidence of postoperative supraventricular arrhythmias ranges between 4 and 33 %, and onset typically peaks within the first 3 postoperative days [1]. Some consider it a minor, self-limited complication, but perioperative arrhythmia has been shown in multiple studies to be associated with greater numbers of complications, longer hospital stays, and increased overall hospital costs

A. Hodari, MD (✉) • Z. Hammoud, MD, FACS
Department of Thoracic Surgery, Henry Ford Hospital,
K-14, 2799 West Grand Blvd, Detroit, MI 48202, USA
e-mail: ahodari1@hfhs.org

M.K. Ferguson (ed.), *Difficult Decisions in Thoracic Surgery*,
Difficult Decisions in Surgery: An Evidence-Based Approach 1,
DOI 10.1007/978-1-4471-6404-3_10, © Springer-Verlag London 2014

[2–6]. In addition, as arrhythmias persist or recur, the risk of thromboembolic events, including stroke or transient neurological injury increases. In a study of patients undergoing noncardiac thoracic surgery, the incidence of stroke associated with atrial fibrillation was 1.7 % [7]. Several large trials have established that oral antico-agulation with warfarin is associated with a 60–70 % reduction from the 9.2 % over-all risk of ischemic stroke in patients who have persistent or chronic nonvalvular AF not receiving warfarin [8]. However, the need for anticoagulation due to atrial fibril-lation can lead to bleeding complications and increased healthcare expenditures.

Many studies have shown that increased age is strongly associated with increased development of arrhythmias. As the number of elderly patients continues to rise, thoracic surgeons will face the challenge of patient selection and improved perioperative optimi-zation to minimize postoperative complications [4]. As a result, there is growing interest in identifying high-risk patients to implement prophylactic strategies and improve clini-cal outcomes. This chapter addresses the potential benefits for the prevention of periop-erative supraventricular arrhythmias, outlines the known risk factors associated with its development, and reviews the prophylactic regimens available for prevention.

Search Strategy

A literature search of English language publications from 2000 to 2013 was used to identity published data on perioperative arrhythmia prophylaxis after major lung surgery. Databases searched were PubMed, Embase, Science Citation Index/Social sciences Citation Index and Cochrane Evidence Based Medicine. Terms used in the search were "tachycardia, supraventricular/prevention and control," "heart supra-ventricular arrhythmia/prevention/" "atrial fibrillation/prevent and control," "heart atrium fibrillation/prevention," "arrhythmias, cardiac/prevention and control," "heart arrhythmia/prevention," AND ("intraoperative complications" OR "periop-erative complications" OR "postoperative complications"), "thoracic surgical pro-cedures," "thoracic surgery," "lobectomy," and "pneumonectomy." Articles were excluded if they specifically addressed cardiac surgery or treatment of arrhythmias rather than prophylaxis. Four randomized control trials, 11 cohort studies, one guideline, three systematic reviews, and four review articles were included in our analysis. The data was classified using the GRADE system.

Clinical Relevance of Perioperative Supraventricular Arrhythmia

Although there is no direct cause and effect relationship between development of perioperative supraventricular arrhythmia and other post-operative complications, it has been shown that the development of an arrhythmia is associated with increased length of stay, morbidity, and mortality (Table 10.1). Onaitis and colleagues reported

Table 10.1 Incidence of atrial fibrillation and clinical outcome

Author (year)	N	AF					NO AF				Study type (quality of evidence)
		Incidence of AF (%)	Age	LOS	Morbidity (%)	Mortality (%)	Age	LOS	Morbidity (%)	Mortality (%)	
Roselli et al. (2005) [3]	604	19	68	8	30	8	63	5	9	0	Prospective cohort (low)
Passman et al. (2005) [5]	856	17	69	13.5	NR	NR	64	9.2	NR	NR	Prospective cohort (low)
Hollings et al. (2010) [4]	360	18	75	NR	NR	NR	65	NR	NR	NR	Prospective cohort (low)
Vaporciyan et al. (2004) [6]	2,588	12.3	NR	16.6	NR	7.5	NR	8.2	NR	2	Prospective cohort (low)
Amar et al. (2002) [2]	527	15	68	17	22	11	62	10	6	3	Prospective cohort (low)
Wu et al. (2012) [9]	10,563	3.27	60	NR	NR	NR	57	NR	NR	NR	Retrospective cohort (low)
Amar et al. (2005) [10]	131	29	75	9	NR	3	70	7	NR	1	Prospective cohort (low)
Onaitis et al. (2010) [11]	13,906	12.6	NR	8	NR	5.6	NR	5	NR	1.6	Retrospective cohort (low)
Cardinale et al. (2007) [12]	400	18	NR	9	NR	0	NR	6.5	NR	1	Prospective cohort (low)

AF atrial fibrillation, *NR* not reported, *LOS* length of stay

a retrospective review of the STS database and found a 12.6 % incidence of atrial arrhythmia before discharge from the hospital [11]. Patients who had atrial fibrillation had significantly worse hospital outcomes than patients who did not (including higher rates of reintubation, tracheostomy, prolonged ventilation, acute respiratory distress syndrome (ARDS), pneumonia, empyema). Rates of pulmonary, infectious, and cardiovascular complications were significantly higher in the atrial arrhythmia group. Strikingly, patients experiencing atrial fibrillation had a 3.4-fold greater chance of 30-day mortality than did patients remaining in sinus rhythm. In addition, median length of stay was 3 days longer in the atrial arrhythmia group.

Vaporciyan and colleagues in a retrospective review of 2,588 patients undergoing thoracic surgery found an overall incidence of 12.3 % of atrial fibrillation [6]. The development of arrhythmia was associated with a significant increase in hospital stay, mortality, and hospital charges. When patients without any complications were compared with patients with only atrial fibrillation, there was still a significant increase in hospital cost (approximately $6,400 per patient) for the patients who developed an arrhythmia. A propensity score matched study by Roselli and colleagues at the Cleveland Clinic showed similar results [3]. When atrial fibrillation was the only postoperative complication after lung cancer resection, length of stay, in-hospital mortality and hospital costs were significantly higher. All of these studies support the view that arrhythmias are not a complication to be disregarded, and their occurrence has serious consequences.

Risk Factors

The identification of risk factors for perioperative atrial arrhythmias is crucial in order to direct prophylactic measures to the appropriate patients. Several different studies have consistently shown that the single best indicator for the development postoperative atrial fibrillation is advanced age (over 60 in most studies). In other studies major risk factors for postoperative AF include increased age (over 60 years), higher preoperative baseline heart rate, male sex, nonblack race, cancer staging or tumor size, extent of lung resection, history of hypertension, and congestive heart failure [1, 11, 12]. Results from a study by Amar and colleagues demonstrated that in patients receiving major thoracic operations, the incidence of postoperative AF increased with age: 4 % at younger than 50 years; 8 % from 50 to 59 years; 14 % from 60 to 69 years, and 25 % at 70 years or older [13]. In another investigation by Hollings and colleagues, age greater than 50 years was associated with a significant risk in the incidence of postoperative AF [4].

Wu and colleagues reviewed 10, 563 patients and found seven risk factors for developing intraoperative atrial fibrillation: increasing age, male sex, lung cancer, general anesthesia plus paravertebral block, open operation, resection of one or more lobes, and increased operation time [9]. Passman and colleagues sought to derive and validate a clinical prediction rule to risk-stratify patients for postoperative AF [5]. This study had 856 patients with a 17.2 % incidence of atrial fibrillation.

Using logistic regression, they found that male gender, advanced age, and heart rate >72 bpm on preoperative EKG were independent predictors of postoperative atrial fibrillation. A risk score was assigned with male gender and heart rate greater than or equal to 72 beats per minute each receiving 1 point, and age 55–74 and greater than or equal to 75 years receiving 3 and 4 points, respectively. The clinical score developed was predictive of atrial fibrillation risk in both the derivation and validation models. The risk of postoperative AF ranged from 0 % (0 points) to 14 % (4 points), 21 % (5 points), and 32 % (6 points)

There is evidence that the extent of pulmonary resection is a risk factor for arrhythmia. Anatomic pulmonary resections, such as lobectomy, bilobectomy, and pneumonectomy, have been repeatedly associated with increasing relative risk of postoperative arrhythmia compared with non-anatomic and sublobar resections [3, 6, 11, 14]. Vaporciyan et al. found that increasing the volume of lung resected was associated with increased risk of AF [6]. Lobectomy, bilobectomy, and pneumonectomy were associated with progressively increasing relative risk of developing atrial fibrillation (18, 25, 30 % respectively) Using univariate analysis Onaitis found that increasing extent of operation was a predictor of postoperative atrial arrhythmia (pneumonectomy vs. lobectomy, OR 1.71, 95 % CI 1.43–2.04, p = 0.0001 and bilobectomy vs. lobectomy, OR 1.44, 95 % CI 1.16–1.80, p = 0.001) [11]. In multivariate analysis, increasing extent of operation was associated with higher rates of atrial fibrillation (any type pneumonectomy vs lobectomy, OR 1.95 95 % CI 1.52–2.50, p = 0.0001 and bilobectomy versus lobectomy OR 1.69 95 % CI 1.31–2.18 p = 0.0001) Ciriaco and colleagues found an overall rate of atrial fibrillation in patients undergoing lung resection to be 13 % [15]. Patients undergoing pneumonectomy had a rate of 33 %, lobectomy 12 %, and minor resections had a 0 % rate of atrial fibrillation. Seely et al. also found increasing incidence of atrial fibrillation with more volume resected (17.4 % after lobectomy and 22.6 % after pneumonectomy) [16].

As the interest in minimally invasive approaches to anatomic pulmonary resection has increased, some authors have suggested that utilization of video-assisted thoracic surgery (VATS) may reduce the incidence of postoperative supraventricular arrhythmias. This suggestion, however, is controversial. Villamizer et al. reported a significantly lower incidence of atrial fibrillation among 697 patients after a VATS approach compared with 382 patients after thoracotomy (16 % vs 22 %, p = 0.01) [17]. When a propensity score-matched approach was used, the difference persisted among the two groups (13 % vs. 21 %, p = 0.01). By contrast, Park and colleagues found a similar incidence of atrial fibrillation in a group of 122 patients undergoing VATS lobectomy when compared to a group of 122 patients, age and gender matched, undergoing thoracotomy [18]. Atrial fibrillation occurred in 12 % of patients (15/122) undergoing VATS and 16 % (20/122) undergoing thoracotomy (p = 0.36). Whitson and colleagues reported similar results in a systematic review of the existing literature of VATS versus thoracotomy for lobectomy in lung cancer patients [19]. The mean rate of postoperative atrial fibrillation in 1,095 VATS patients was 5.2 % (95 % CI 2.0–8.4) versus 9 % (95 % CI 2.1–15.8) in 294 patients after thoracotomy (p = 0.33). Hollings and colleagues retrospectively reviewed 360 patients who underwent lobectomy and found that AF occurred in 15 of 54 patients (27 %) undergoing VATS versus 39 of 306 patients (16 %) undergoing thoracotomy [4]. This was not statistically significant (P=0.054). Due to discordant data, the type of surgery cannot be used as a predictor for atrial fibrillation until further studies are done.

Prevention Strategies

Table 10.2 shows the results of the studies examining the efficacy of different pharmacologic strategies for the prevention of postoperative atrial fibrillation. Two systematic reviews and one guideline paper have shown that calcium-channel blockers and beta blockers are effective in reducing postoperative supraventricular arrhythmias. Due to their potential adverse effects, their use should be individualized [24–26].

In a randomized, double-blind placebo controlled study of 330 patients prophylactically treated with either diltiazem or placebo after major lung resection, Amar at al demonstrated that diltiazem significantly reduced the overall incidence of postoperative arrhythmias (15 % vs. 25 %, p=0.03) and nearly halved the incidence of clinically significant arrhythmias when compared to placebo (10 % vs. 19 %, p=0.02) [7]. In this report, treatment with diltiazem started immediately after surgery and continued postoperatively for 2 weeks.

A retrospective case-control study by Lanza and colleagues found a significantly reduced risk of AF after orally administered Amiodarone and suggested that a randomized, controlled trial should be performed [22]. A prospective, randomized study evaluating Amiodarone for prevention of atrial fibrillation after pulmonary resection in 130 patients showed a significantly lower incidence of atrial fibrillation in the Amiodarone group than in the controls (13.8 % vs. 32.3 %), with a relative risk reduction of 57 % and a low incidence of adverse events (respiratory complications) [20]. This study was criticized for the lack of a double-blind placebo controlled design that might have led to a bias in the determination as to whether a patient had atrial fibrillation that required treatment.

Riber et al. had similar results with a double blind-randomized placebo controlled study [21]. Their study had 242 patients and the use of Amiodarone had an absolute risk reduction of 23 %. Patients who received Amiodarone had a significantly lower incidence of atrial fibrillation when compared to placebo (9 % vs. 32 %, p=0.001). In this study, treatment began immediately after surgery and continued postoperatively for 5 days. Five patients in each group experienced possible side effects that led to discontinuation of the study medication. There was no difference between the two groups, no side effects could be traced to the active prophylactic regime, and no pulmonary toxicity was found. Khalil and colleagues found a lower incidence of atrial fibrillation in patients receiving Amiodarone or magnesium when compared to a control group (Amiodarone 9.6 %, Magnesium 12.3 %, control 20.1 %, p=0.005) [23]. There was no statistically significant difference between the Amiodarone and magnesium groups.

Table 10.2 Efficacy of prophylaxis for supraventricular arrhythmia

Author (year)	N	Surgery type	Study type (quality of evidence)	Incidence of AF/SVA Treatment (%)	Control (%)	P-value	
Tisdale et al. (2009) [20]	130	Lobectomy/bilobectomy/pneumonectomy	PRCT (moderate)	Amiodarone 13.8	Control 32.3	0.02	RRR 57 %
Riber et al. (2012) [21]	242	Lobectomy/bilobectomy/pneumonectomy	Double-blind, PRCT (high)	Amiodarone 9	Placebo 32	0.001	ARR 23 %
Amar et al. (2000) [7]	330	Lobectomy/pneumonectomy	Double-blind, PRCT (high)	Diltiazem 15	Placebo 25	0.03	RRR 39 %
Lanza et al. (2003) [22]	83	Pulmonary resection	Retrospective cohort study (low)	Amiodarone 9.7	Control 33	0.025	
Khalil et al. (2013) [23]	438	Pulmonary resection	Double-blind, PRCT (moderate)	Amiodarone 9.6 Magnesium 12.3	Control 20.1	0.005	

AF atrial fibrillation, *SVA* supraventricular arrhythmia, *PRCT* prospective randomized controlled trials, *ARR* absolute risk reduction, *RRR* relative risk reduction

Epidural analgesia has been reported as a prophylactic measure for supraventricular arrhythmias after thoracic surgery by creating a partial sympathectomy. The results have varied. Oka and colleagues randomized 50 patients undergoing surgical resection of primary lung cancer to receive either epidural bupivicaine or epidural morphine [27]. Even though postoperative analgesia was not different in the two groups, the incidence of postoperative tachyarrhythmias was significantly less in the bupivicaine group (28 % vs. 4.3 %, p<0.05). The number of patients in this study however was small and the two groups were not well matched for age with the patients in the morphine group being significantly older than those in the bupivicaine cohort (mean age 67 ± 8.6 years vs. 63.6 years ± 7.9 years). Similar results were found in a study by Simeoforidou and colleagues [28]. The study design contained two groups. In group A, postoperative analgesia consisted of thoracic epidural analgesia with levobupivacaine for six postoperative days. In group B, on the third postoperative day this regimen was changed to patient-controlled intravenous morphine. Their results showed that postoperatively decreased cardiac sympathetic outflow continues with epidural analgesia, whereas it is abolished by the change to intravenous patient-controlled morphine. From this point of view, this study showed that the use of local anesthetics with epidural analgesia seems advantageous for decreasing the risk of postoperative AF, and this benefit is lost with their withdrawal. The opposite results were shown in another randomized trial of patient controlled intravenous analgesia with opioids versus patient-controlled epidural analgesia with ropivicaine [29]. In this study, the epidural group had an incidence of postoperative supraventricular tachycardia of 45 % compared to only 14 % in the opioid group (p=0.021).

The level of C-reactive protein (CRP) has been shown to be elevated in patients with atrial fibrillation/flutter (AF) unrelated to surgery, and statins are known to lower the CRP. The use of statins preoperatively has been suggested to have a protective effect against postoperative development of atrial fibrillation. Amar and colleagues found that the use of statins had a threefold reduction in the incidence of atrial fibrillation after major thoracic surgery independent of CRP levels [10]. Larger randomized studies are needed to evaluate the role of inflammation in the development of atrial fibrillation to better target alternative prophylactic measures.

Conclusions and Recommendations

Perioperative supraventricular arrhythmias are associated with higher postoperative morbidity and mortality, prolonged hospital stay, and increased hospital cost. Patients with risk factors including age >60 years, male gender, history of paroxysmal atrial fibrillation, heart rate greater than 72 BPM, major anatomic resections, and intrapericardial procedures are at higher risk of developing atrial fibrillation. There is currently inadequate evidence for routine prophylaxis of atrial fibrillation in all patients undergoing lung surgery. However, for patients at high risk (two or more risk factors) there is evidence for use of prophylactic measures. Amiodarone and diltiazem significantly reduce the rate of postoperative atrial fibrillation after major lung resection with low side effects (evidence quality moderate). Therefore, the use of diltiazem or Amiodarone in high risk patients should be considered. Some small individual studies provide evidence that other prophylactic measures including statins, magnesium, and epidural analgesia may reduce the incidence of postoperative arrhythmia and are safe. We make a weak recommendation for the use of these as prophylaxis against atrial fibrillation.

A Personal View of the Data

Postoperative supraventricular arrhythmia is a frequent complication in patients undergoing thoracic surgery and is associated with increased length of stay, morbidity, mortality, and hospital cost. Identifying patients at highest risk of developing arrhythmias is essential so that appropriate prophylaxis can be administered. While there is ample data regarding the adverse outcomes that result from postoperative atrial arrhythmias, especially atrial fibrillation, to date there have been no studies that evaluate whether prophylactic treatment of perioperative atrial arrhythmias improves clinical outcomes, increases survival, and decreases hospital costs. Nonetheless, given the current evidence, we hypothesize that reducing the incidence of post operative arrhythmias will in turn improve patient outcomes and decrease hospital costs.

Recommendations

- For patients at high risk (two or more risk factors) we recommendations use of prophylactic measures to prevent atrial fibrillation (Evidence quality high; strong recommendations).
- We recommendation the use of diltiazem or Amiodarone in high risk patients (Evidence quality high; strong recommendation).
- Statins, magnesium, and epidural analgesia may be useful as prophylaxis against atrial fibrillation (Evidence quality low; weak recommendation).

References

1. Amar D. Prevention and management of perioperative arrhythmias in the thoracic surgical population. Anesthesiol Clin. 2008;26(2):325–35.
2. Amar D, Zhang H, Roistacher N. The incidence and outcome of ventricular arrhythmias after noncardiac thoracic surgery. Anesth Analg. 2002;95:537–43.
3. Roselli EE, Murthy SC, Rice TW, Houghtaling PL, Pierce CD, Karchmer DP, et al. Atrial fibrillation complicating lung cancer resection. J Thorac Cardiovasc Surg. 2005;130:438–44.
4. Hollings DD, Higgins RS, Faber LP, Warren WH, Liptay MJ, Basu S, et al. Age is a strong risk factor for atrial fibrillation after pulmonary lobectomy. Am J Surg. 2010;199(4):558–61.
5. Passman RS, Gingold DS, Amar D, Lloyd-Jones D, Bennett CL, Zhang H, et al. Prediction rule for atrial fibrillation after major noncardiac thoracic surgery. Ann Thorac Surg. 2005;79(5):1698–703.

6. Vaporciyan AA, Correa AM, Rice DC, Roth JA, Smythe WR, Swisher SG, et al. Risk factors associated with atrial fibrillation after noncardiac thoracic surgery: analysis of 2588 patients. J Thorac Cardiovasc Surg. 2004;127(3):779–86.

7. Amar D, Roistacher N, Rusch VW, Leung DH, Ginsburg I, Shang G, et al. Effects of diltiazem prophylaxis on the incidence and clinical outcome of atrial arrhythmias after thoracic surgery. J Thorac Cardiovasc Surg. 2000;120:790–8.

8. Fuster V, Ryden LE, Cannom DS, Crijns HJ, Curtis AB, Ellenbogen KA, et al. ACC/AHA/ESC 2006 guidelines for the management of patients with atrial fibrillation: executive summary: a report of the American College of Cardiology/American Heart Association Task Force on Practice Guidelines and the European Society of Cardiology Committee for Practice Guidelines and Policy Conferences(Committee to Develop Guidelines for the Management of Patients with Atrial Fibrillation). Circulation. 2006;114:700–52.

9. Wu DH, Xu MY, Mao T, Cao H, Wu DJ, Shen YF. Risk factors for intraoperative atrial fibrillation: a retrospective analysis of 10563 lung operations in a single center. Ann Thorac Surg. 2012;94(1):193–7.

10. Amar D, Zhang H, Heerdt PM, Park B, Fleisher M, Thaler HT. Statin use is associated with reduction in atrial fibrillation after noncardiac thoracic surgery independent t of C-reactive protein. Chest. 2005;128(5):3421–7.

11. Onaitis M, D'Amico T, Zhao Y, O'Brien S, Harpole D. Risk factors for atrial fibrillation after lung cancer surgery: analysis of the Society of Thoracic Surgeons general thoracic surgery database. Ann Thorac Surg. 2010;90(2):368–74.

12. Cardinale D, Colombo A, Sandri MT, Lamantia G, Colombo N, Civelli M, et al. Increase perioperative N-terminal Pro-B-type natriuretic peptide levels predict atrial fibrillation after thoracic surgery for lung cancer. Circulation. 2007;115:1339–44.

13. Amar D, Zhang H, Leung DH, Roistacher N, Kadish AH. Older age is the strongest predictor of postoperative atrial fibrillation. Anesthesiology. 2002;96:352–6.

14. Rena O, Papalia E, Oliaro A, Cascadio C, Ruffini E, Filosso PL, et al. Supraventricular arrhythmias after resection surgery of the lung. Eur J Cardiothorac Surg. 2001;20:688–93.

15. Ciriaco P, Mazzone P, Canneto B, Zannini P. Supraventricular arrhythmia following lung resection for non-small cell lung cancer and its treatment with amiodarone. Eur J Cardiothorac Surg. 2000;18:12–6.

16. Seely AJ, Ivanovic J, Threader J, Al-Hussaini A, Al-Shehab D, Ramsay T, et al. Systematic classification of morbidity and mortality after thoracic surgery. Ann Thorac Surg. 2010;90(3):936–42.

17. Villamizar NR, Darrabie MD, Burfeind WR, Petersen RP, Onaitis MW, Toloza E, et al. Thoracoscopic lobectomy is associated with lower morbidity compared with thoracotomy. J Thorac Cardiovasc Surg. 2009;138:419–25.

18. Park BJ, Zhang H, Rusch VW, Amar D. Video-assisted thoracic surgery does not reduce the incidence of postoperative atrial fibrillation after pulmonary lobectomy. J Thorac Cardiovasc Surg. 2007;133(3):775–9.

19. Whitson BA, Groth SS, Duval SJ, Swanson SJ, Maddaus MA. Surgery for early-stage non-small cell lung cancer: a systematic review of the video assisted thoracoscopic surgery versus thoracotomy approaches to lobectomy. Ann Thorac Surg. 2008;86:2008–18.

20. Tisdale JE, Wroblewski HA, Wall DS, Rieger KM, Hammoud ZT, Young JV, et al. A randomized trial evaluating amiodarone for prevention of atrial fibrillation after pulmonary resection. Ann Thorac Surg. 2009;88(3):886–93.

21. Riber LP, Christensen TD, Jensen HK, Hoejsgaard A, Pilegaard HK. Amiodarone significantly decreases atrial fibrillation in patients undergoing surgery for lung cancer. Ann Thorac Surg. 2012;94(2):339–44.

22. Lanza LA, Visbal AI, DeValeria PA, Zinsmeister AR, Diehl NN, Trastek VF. Low-dose oral amiodarone prophylaxis reduces atrial fibrillation after pulmonary resection. Ann Thorac Surg. 2003;75(1):223–30.

23. Khalil MA, Al-Agaty AE, Ali WG, Abdel Azeem MS. A comparative study between amioda-rone and magnesium sulfate as antiarrhythmic agents for prophylaxis against atrial fibrillation following lobectomy. J Anesth. 2013;27(1):56–61.
24. Sedrakyan A, Treasure T, Browne J, Krumholz H, Sharpin C, van der Meulen J. Pharmacologic prophylaxis for postoperative atrial tachyarrhythmia in general thoracic surgery: evidence from randomized clinical trials. J Thorac Cardiovasc Surg. 2005;129(5):997–1005.
25. Dunning J, Treasure T, Versteegh M, Nashef SA. Guidelines on the prevention and manage-ment of de novo atrial fibrillation after cardiac and thoracic surgery. Eur J Cardiothorac Surg. 2006;30(6):852–72.
26. Shrivastava V, Nyawo B, Dunning J, Morritt G. Is there a role for prophylaxis against atrial fibrillation for patients undergoing lung surgery? Interact Cardiovasc Thorac Surg. 2004;3(4): 656–62.
27. Oka T, Ozawa Y, Ohkubo Y. Thoracic epidural bupivacaine attenuates supraventricular tachyarrhythmias after pulmonary resection. Anesth Analg. 2001;93(2):253–9.
28. Simeoforidou M, Vretzakis G, Bareka M, Chantzi E, Flossos A, Giannoukas A, et al. Thoracic epidural analgesia with levobupivacaine for 6 postoperative days attenuates sympathetic acti-vation after thoracic surgery. J Cardiothorac Vasc Anesth. 2011;25(5):817–23.
29. Jiang Z, Dai JQ, Shi C, Zeng WS, Jiang RC, Tu WF. Influence of patient-controlled i.v. anal-gesia with opioids on supraventricular arrhythmias after pulmonary resection. Br J Anaesth. 2009;103(3):364–8.

Chapter 11
VATS Versus Open Lobectomy for Stage I or II NSCLC

Kezhong Chen, Yun Li, and Jun Wang

Abstract Although there is a lack of randomized controlled trials comparing VATS lobectomy to open techniques, there is growing evidence with consistent data from matched case-control studies, cohort studies, meta-analyses, and outcomes studies demonstrate that VATS is associated with lower operative mortality, fewer complications and better quality of life. These studies also demonstrate at least oncologic equivalence compared with open lobectomy. VATS lobectomy is a safe and effective approach for lobectomy, we make a strong recommendation for VATS lobectomy over open lobectomy for early stage NSCLC.

Keywords Non-small-cell-lung-cancer • Video-assisted thoracoscopic surgery • Lobectomy thoracotomy • Long survival

Introduction

Surgical resection via a standard thoracotomy has been the mainstay of treatment for patients with early-stage non–small-cell lung cancer (NSCLC) for decades. Since the initial clinical reports on video-assisted thoracoscopic surgery (VATS) lobectomy published in the early 1990s, the role of VATS for treatment of NSCLC has been growing. However, VATS lobectomy has suffered from an imprecise definition and unclear safety profile since its inception, making interpretation of the results of some studies difficult. A standardized technique of VATS lobectomy (individual ligation of lobar vessels and bronchus as well as hilar lymph node dissection or sampling using the video screen for guidance, two or three ports, and no

K. Chen, MD • Y. Li, MD • J. Wang, MD (✉)
Department of Thoracic Surgery, Peking University People's Hospital,
Xi Zhi Men South Street No.11, 100044, Beijing, People's Republic of China
e-mail: jwangmd@yahoo.com

M.K. Ferguson (ed.), *Difficult Decisions in Thoracic Surgery*,
Difficult Decisions in Surgery: An Evidence-Based Approach 1,
DOI 10.1007/978-1-4471-6404-3_11, © Springer-Verlag London 2014

retractor use or rib spreading) in the treatment of NSCLC was demonstrated to be feasible and safe for selected patients in the Cancer and Leukemia Group B (CALGB) 39802 trial [1]. Currently, most minimally invasive thoracic surgeons consider VATS lobectomy to adhere to this definition.

Over the last two decades, growing evidence has suggested that VATS lobectomy is an alternative approach for early stage NSCLC patients and demonstrates superior short- and long-term outcomes. However, most of the data come from nonrandomized comparisons; only three early small RCTs have been conducted [2–4], which demonstrated equivalent outcomes but were too small to demonstrate this in a statistically robust manner. In addition, the use of rib-spreading in these studies would exclude them from being 'true' VATS lobectomies according to the currently accepted definition. Attempts at performing well-powered, multi-institutional, randomized clinical trials to compare outcomes after open and VATS lobectomy for early stage NSCLC were impaired by poor accrual rates. Since paucity of robust clinical data in the form of large randomized controlled trials, the safety and long-term oncological outcomes of VATS are still the concern of thoracic surgeons.

A large, prospective, randomized, multi-institutional trial of open versus VATS lobectomy will likely never take place [5], leaving us to rely on the best available current evidence to draw meaningful clinical conclusions. We are dependent on the herein summarized information to draw clinically applicable conclusions. We review the most current available information comparing VATS lobectomy with open lobectomy for early stage NSCLC from perioperative, oncologic and immunologic effects. It's worth noting that most of these studies involved a mixture of stages, but the large majority of patients were stage I or stage I and II, and a few of them specifically addressed stage II NSCLC [6]. It's difficult to separate outcomes for stage I and II NSCLC.

Search Strategy

Electronic searches were performed using the Medline, Embase, and ScienceDirect databases for eligible studies incorporating the index terms ["non small cell lung cancer" or "Lung cancer"] and ["video-assisted thoracic surgery" or "VATS" or "thoracoscopic surgery" or "minimal invasive"] and ["open" or "thoracotomy"] was used to review the literature between January 1, 1992 and September 1, 2013 published in the English language. Related articles on the reference lists of the manuscripts were also searched for further relevant studies. Abstracts, case reports, and conference presentations were excluded.

Available data in the literature included one prospective cooperative group feasibility study (CALGB 39802), three small randomized controlled trials, a number of single institution case-series and cohort studies, two multi-institutional retrospective studies, and several systematic reviews and meta-analyses.

Perioperative Outcomes

Surgery Time

Yan et al. (which included 1,391 VATS patients and 1,250 thoracotomy patients with early stage NSCLC) indicated that the operating room time for VATS lobectomy (median 3.7 h; range 1.3–4.8) and open lobectomy (median 3.6 h; range 1.4–4.9) for early stage NSCLC are similar [7]. A recent meta-analysis by Chen also showed that no statistical difference was found in the operation time between two groups (95 % confidence interval [CI], −4.68 to 34.03, p=0.14) [8]. However, a retrospective multi-institutional database analysis by Swanson et al. indicated that surgery duration was shorter for open procedures at 3.75 versus 4.09 h for VATS (p<0.001). Since the database provided very large numbers of patients, surgeons, and procedures on a nationwide scale, the result may due to the dissemination of the technical skills necessary to perform VATS lobectomy among practicing surgeons, many of whom may not receive sufficient instruction in the VATS approach as part of their fellowship training [9].

Blood Loss

The systematic review by Yan et al. indicated that the estimated blood loss during VATS lobectomy (median 146 mL; range 72–253) was comparable to (or possibly lower than) open lobectomy (median 235 mL; range 82–443) [7]. There were total of 287 patients in the VATS group and 391 in thoracotomy group in Chen's meta-analysis, and the result showed blood loss was less in VATS group than thoracotomy group in the combined analysis of six studies (95 % CI, −79.32 to −45.66, p<0.01) [8].

Conversion Rate

Based on data from large series, the conversion rate from VATS to thoracotomy is low. Rueth et al. reviewed retrospective studies on VATS lobectomy that included 100 patients or more and showed the conversion rate from VATS to thoracotomy was low (0–22.5 %) [5]. Fourteen studies reported VATS to open lobectomy conversion rate in the meta-analysis by Yan et al. which ranged from 0 % to 15.7 % (median, 8.1 %). Sixty-nine (8.0 %) of 858 patients were reported to have been converted to open lobectomy for the following reasons: technical difficulties, extent of tumor, hilar lymph node metastasis, uncontrollable bleeding, completely fussed fissure, others, and did not specify [7]. Thresholds for conversions vary among surgeons, and these factors change over time as the surgeon gains more experience with the procedure.

Operative Mortality

A recent meta-analysis of propensity score-matched patients showed the operative mortality rates after VATS lobectomy (1.4 %) and open lobectomy (2.0 %) are not statistically different (p=0.28) [10]. Similar results were also demonstrated in Yan and Cheng's meta-analyses [7, 11].

Postoperative Morbidity

The CALGB 39802 prospective, multi-institutional study examined the feasibility of standardized VATS lobectomy for early stage NSCLC and demonstrated that this technique was associated with a low complication rate. Four meta-analyses all showed the overall complication rates was lower in the VATS groups than the thoracotomy groups [7, 8, 10, 11]. In Whitson's study, the rates of atrial fibrillation, pneumonia, and persistent air leak were similar after VATS compared with thoracotomy [12]. Yan et al. had a similar result [7]. However, the results of that study may be confounded by covariates that were not assessed.

Cao et al. noted the overall postoperative morbidity was significantly lower in patients who underwent VATS when compared with propensity score-matched patients who underwent open thoracotomy (24.9 vs 20.2 %; RR, 0.67; 95 % CI 0.56–0.82; p < 0.0001). One meta-analysis identified significantly lower incidences of prolonged air leak (8.1vs 10.4 %; RR, 0.78; 95 % CI 0.63–0.96; p=0.02), pneumonia (3.2 vs 5.0 %; RR, 0.65; 95 % CI 0.47–0.89; P=0.008), atrial arrhythmia (7.3 vs 11.7 %; RR, 0.62; 95 % CI 0.51–0.77; p < 0.00001) and renal failure (0.9 vs 3.0 %; RR, 0.32; 95 % CI 0.12–0.88; p=0.03) for patients who underwent VATS when compared with propensity score-matched patients who underwent open thoracotomy. There were no significantly different incidences of pulmonary embolism, myocardial infarction, significant bleeding and empyema/sepsis between the two treatment groups [10].

The meta-analysis by Chen included nine studies with 1,790 patients and no significant statistical heterogeneity was found. The results revealed the incidence of complications in VATS group was lower than thoracotomy group (OR 0.61, 95 % CI, 0.49–0.76, p < 0.01). Individual common complications were also analyzed. There was no statistical difference in the incidence of prolonged air leak, atrial fibrillation, myocardial infarction and chylothorax between the two groups (p > 0.05). However, the pneumonia incidence in VATS group was lower than thoracotomy group (OR 0.43, 95 % CI, 0.20–0.93, p < 0.05) [8]. According to the literature, less postoperative pain, better conservation of pulmonary function and less inflammatory response by minimally invasive approaches may be the reason for reduced postoperative pneumonia.

Chest Tube Duration and Hospital Length of Stay

Several meta-analyses demonstrated that both the drainage time and length of stay (LOS) of VATS group was consistently shorter than thoracotomy group (Table 11.1). Considering that comparison in the meta-analyses may be confounded by differences in patient factors that were not assessed. Cao et al. presented a meta-analysis involving propensity score-matched patients, in which patients were balanced in all observed significant covariates, making the assessment of the intervention more accurate by minimizing the potential bias between the comparative groups. The result showed the duration of hospitalization was also significantly shorter after VATS [10].

Costs

Swanson et al. analyzed a large, nationally representative database including more than 600 hospitals that included a total of 3,961 patients underwent a lobectomy by a thoracic surgeon by an open (n=2,907) or VATS (n=1,054) approach. Hospital costs were higher for open ($21,016) versus VATS ($20,316) (p=0.027). Adjustment for surgeon experience with VATS over the 6 months prior to each operation showed a significant association between surgeon experience and cost. Average costs ranged from $22,050 for low volume surgeons to $18,133 for high volume surgeons. For open lobectomies, cost differences by surgeon experience were not significant and both levels were estimated at $21,000. This indicates that VATS compared with an open technique offers economic advantages, particularly when an experienced surgeon performs the procedure [9].

Casali's single-institution retrospective cost analysis confirmed that only the operating room related cost in VATS lobectomy is more expensive than a conventional thoracotomy, and this cost is counterbalanced by the significantly shorter hospital stay and the reduced length of stay related costs. The total cost of VATS lobectomy is less expensive than conventional lobectomy [13].

Quality of Life

A number of studies have demonstrated that VATS lobectomy, as compared with open lobectomy, is associated with subjective and objective improvements in surgery-related quality-of-life [14]. Improved pain control seems to be the most commonly

Table 11.1 Systematic reviews and meta-analysis of VATS vs Open lobectomy for perioperative outcomes

Author, year	Quality	Surgery time (h)	Blood loss (ml)	Chest tube duration (days)	Length of stay (days)	Perioperative mortality (%)	Overall complication rates (%)	Air leak (%)	Pneumonia (%)	Arrhythmia (%)
Cheng et al. [11] (2007)	Moderate	VATS > Open WMD:16.17 $P=0.02$	VATS < Open WMD: −79.11 $P<0.00001$	VATS < Open WMD: −0.96 $P=0.002$	VATS < Open WMD: −2.60 $P=0.007$	VATS = Open OR: 0.79 $P=0.53$	VATS < Open OR: 0.48 $P=0.0002$	VATS = Open OR: 1.67 $P=0.09$	VATS = Open OR: 0.56 $P=0.14$	VATS= Open OR: 0.82 $P=0.09$
Whiston et al. [12] (2008)	Low	–	–	VATS: 4.2 Open: 5.7 $P=0.025$	VATS: 8.3 Open: 13.3 $P=0.016$	–	VATS: 16.4 % Open: 31.2 %, $P=0.018$	VATS: 5 % Open:8.8 % $P=0.27$	VATS: 2.7 % Open: 6.0 % $p=0.4$	VATS: 5.2 % Open: 9.0 % $P=0.33$
Yan et al. [7] (2009)	Moderate	VATS: 3.7 (1.3~4.8) Open: 3.6 (1.4~4.9)	VATS:146 (72–253) Open: 235 (82–443)	VATS: 4.5 (1.2–8.0) Open: 5.5 (1.5–10)	VATS: 11.6 (4.1–24) Open: 13.4 (5.3–24.9)	VATS = Open RR: 0.49 $P=0.49$	–	VATS= Open $P=0.71$	VATS = Open $P=0.09$	VATS = Open $P=0.86$
Cao et al. [10] (2012)	Moderate	–	–	–	VATS < Open (95 % CI, = −0.51 to −0.22, $P<0.00001$)	VATS: 1.4 % Open: 2.0 % $P=0.28$	VATS: 20.2 % Open: 24.9 % $P<0.0001$	VATS: 8.1 % Open: 10.4 % $P=0.02$	VATS: 3.2 % Open: 5.0 % $P=0.008$	VATS: 7.3 % Open: 11.7 % $P<0.00001$

Chen et al. [8] (2013)	Low	VATS = Open (95 % CI=4.68–34.03, P=0.14)	VATS < Open (95 % CI= −79.32 to −45.66, p<0.01)	VATS < Open (95% CI= −0.69 to −0.09, P=0.01)	VATS < Open (95 % CI= −2.20 to −1.28, P<0.01)	–	VATS < Open (95 % CI= 0.49–0.76, P<0.01)	VATS = Open (95% CI= 0.49–1.08, P=0.11)	VATS < Open (95% CI= 0.20–0.93, P=0.03)	VATS = Open (95% CI= 0.58–1.09, P=0.15)

WMD Weighted mean differences, *VATS* video-assisted thoracoscopic surgery '<' indicates statistically lower rate or duration according to meta-analysis. "=" indicates no statistically difference. '>' indicates statistically higher rate or duration according to meta-analysis

demonstrated benefit. The main cause of postoperative pain is direct injury to the chest wall and intercostal nerves. Rib spreading in a thoracotomy can cause uncontrolled rib fractures and impingement on intercostal nerves. The diminished surgical trauma to the chest wall from VATS lobectomy is reflected in diminished levels of postoperative pain. The shorter duration of chest tube drainage after VATS lobectomy may also contribute to the lower pain levels. More than 80 % of patients still require narcotic analgesics 3 weeks after an open lobectomy compared with fewer than 40 % patients after a VATS lobectomy. Reduced pain levels may contribute to the observed improved quality of life (QOL) after a VATS resection, and this drives secondary enhancements of QOL scores of performance and symptom control [15]. Tajiri et al. demonstrated that, compared with open lobectomy, VATS lobectomy is associated with lower analgesics requirements and less pain at 1 day, 2 weeks, 4 weeks, 6 months, and 1 year postoperatively [16]. A prospective study by Balduyck et al. analyzed 100 patients after lung cancer surgery and showed more favorable physical function for VATS over thoracotomy at 6 months (p < 0.01) [17].

Many studies have shown objective measurements to suggest that QOL is improved for VATS. Some effects are immediate, and others are more prolonged. Most of the literature has documented a substantial reduction in pain control measures and better physical recovery documented by faster return to work or other equivalents of preoperative functioning [15]. A retrospective study of 204 patients by Kaseda indicated that the postoperative to preoperative ratio of pulmonary function tests (vital capacity and forced expiratory volume in 1s(FEV1)) were better in video-assisted thoracic surgery lobectomy than in open thoracotomy(FEV1 0.848 vs 0.712) (p < 0.0001) [18].

Demmy provided a comprehensive review of subjective and objective QOL measures after VATS lobectomy. They reviewed 97 papers and concluded that QOL was improved after VATS compared with open surgery, and this improvement was demonstrated by better scores on standardized QOL instruments, improved physical activity after surgery, and an earlier return to work [15].

A meta-analysis by Cheng et al. indicated pain measured via visual analog scales (10-point VAS) was significantly reduced by <1 point on day 1, by >2 points at 1 week, and by <1 point at weeks 2–4. Similarly, analgesia requirements were significantly reduced in the VATS group. Postoperative vital capacity was significantly improved (weighted mean differences (WMD) 20, 95 % CI 15–25), and percent predicted forced vital capacity at 1 year was significantly greater for VATS versus open surgery (WMD 7, 95 % CI 2–12). The incidence of patients reporting limited activity at 3 months was reduced (OR 0.04, 95 % CI 0.00–0.82), and time to full activity was significantly reduced in the VATS versus open surgery group (WMD 1.5, 95 % CI 2.1–0.9), but was reported in only one trial [11].

Adjuvant Chemotherapy

Some patients with early-stage NSCLC, especially those with stage II disease, may require adjuvant chemotherapy. However, patients receiving lobectomy through conventional thoracotomy sometimes have delayed adjuvant therapy due to slow recovery, and not infrequently, discontinue treatment because of worsening of performance status. Because the advantages of VATS lobectomy include remission of post-operative pain, less releasing of inflammatory factor and less effect on pulmonary functions, fewer complications and rapid recovery, VATS lobectomy may increase compliance with planned adjuvant chemotherapy [19].

Through propensity score matching, Lee et al. indicated a higher percentage of VATS group received four cycles of the planned adjuvant chemotherapy (95.9 % versus 82.4 %, p=0.015). There was a trend toward better compliance in VATS group with four cycles of adjuvant chemotherapy without reduced dose (83.8 % versus 73.0 %, p=0.162), and four cycles of adjuvant chemotherapy without delayed or reduced dose (70.3 % versus 62.2 %, p=0.385). The result showed thoracoscopy was associated with better compliance with adjuvant chemotherapy after pulmonary resection for NSCLC [20]. A possible explanation of this seems to be associated with lower postoperative pain, better performance status, and better preserved hematologic function before adjuvant chemotherapy.

Oncologic Efficacy

Mediastinal Lymph Node Dissection

Complete mediastinal lymph node dissection is an important part of NSCLC surgery. Sagawa and colleagues performed a prospective study in 29 patients with clinical stage I NSCLC and demonstrated that a complete mediastinal lymph node dissection is s technically feasible with by VATS. In their study, VATS lobectomy and complete mediastinal lymph node dissection was the first step. In the same anesthesia setting, a second surgeon then performed a thoracotomy and completion mediastinal lymph node dissection to remove any residual lymph nodes. On the right side, the average numbers of resected lymph nodes by VATS and remnant lymph nodes were 40.3 and 1.2, respectively. On the left side, there were 37.1 and 1.2 lymph nodes dissected. None of the residual lymph node tissue contained metastatic disease [21].

A meta-analysis by Zhang et al. showed the mean difference of total lymph node dissection (LND) or lymph node sampling(LNS) numbers between the two groups was not significant (−0.63; 95 % CI: −0.47 to 0.21; p=0.14). The heterogeneity in related studies was at an acceptable level (p=0.10, I^2=44 %). The difference in mediastinal LND or LNS numbers between the two groups was also negligible (−0.51; 95 % CI: −1.58 to 0.56; p=0.35), with significant heterogeneity across studies (p=0.04, I2=65 %). The results suggested that total and mediastinal lymph node (LN) numbers were comparable between the VATS group and the thoracotomy group [22].

Licht and colleagues performed a national study of nodal upstaging after thoracoscopic versus open lobectomy. Their data also demonstrated that the number of lymph node stations dissected was similar for both surgical approaches. But nodal upstaging occurred in 281patients (18.6 %) and was significantly higher after thoracotomy for N1 upstaging (13.1 % vs 8.1 %; p < 0.001) and N2 upstaging (11.5 % vs 3.8 %; p < 0.001). However, the overall survival was not different, indicating that differences in nodal upstaging result from patient selection [23].

Recurrence Rate

Concerns on the possibility of technique-dependent recurrence rate in VATS lobectomy puzzled many surgeons, who considered factors such as cancer dissemination during manipulation (suture line, pleura, and/or skin incision), insufficient surgical margin or LN dissection affected the recurrence rate. Good surgical technique is imperative to reduce the risk of such recurrences. Meticulous technique and use of a specimen retrieval bag are essential. Yan showed that there was no significant statistical difference with loco-regional recurrence, but a significant difference was found with systemic recurrence in the VATS group [7].

Zhang et al.'s meta-analysis showed that both systemic (RR = 0.61; 95 % CI 0.48–0.78; p < 0.01) and loco-regional (RR = 0.66; 95%CI 0.46 to –0.95; p = 0.03) recurrence rates were significantly lower in the VATS group. These results may eliminate some apprehension about the technique-dependent recurrence rate related to VATS [22].

Survival Rate

Several studies on long term survival in VATS lobectomy have been published recently. Whitson and colleagues provided an analysis of 39 studies comparing VATS with open lobectomy. In this study, patients with VATS lobectomy had similar survival at 1, 2, 3, and 5 years after resection when compared with those who underwent open resection; at 4 years, patients who underwent VATS lobectomy had improved survival versus patients with open lobectomy (88.4 % vs 71 %; p = 0.003); however, this particular finding is of questionable clinical relevance [12]. More recently, Yan and colleagues performed a similar systematic review. The authors reported that 5-year survival was significantly improved for patients who undergo VATS lobectomy for early-stage NSCLC (RR 0.72; p = 0.04), further suggesting that VATS lobectomy is at least oncologically equivalent to open lobectomy [7].

In a resent meta-analysis by Zhang, of the 13 articles included, the survival rate demonstrated by the Forest plot was significantly higher (RR = 1.09; 95 % CI 1.03–15; p < 0.01) in the VATS group. The included studies were heterogeneous (p < 0.01, $I^2 = 63$ %). After exclusion of the four studies where the follow-up period was 3 or 4 years, the heterogeneity disappeared (P = 0.08, $I^2 = 44$ %). There was a slight adjustment in overall effect, but the final results remained the same (RR = 1.10; 95 % CI 1.04–1.17; p < 0.01) [22]. In Chen's meta-analysis, a total of 2013 patients reported outcomes of 5 year overall survival. The pooled-analysis showed the 5 year survival rate was higher in VATS group than thoracotomy group (OR 1.82, 95 % CI 1.43–2.31,p<0.01) [8].

Taioli's long-term survival meta-analysis in video-assisted thoracoscopic lobectomy compared to open lobectomy in lung-cancer patients showed 5-year survival ranged from 62 % to 97 % for VATS and from 58 % to 97 % for thoracotomy. There was an advantage in 5-year mortality for patients who underwent VATS compared to patients who underwent thoracotomy (meta difference in survival: 5 %; 95 % CI 3–6 %) with large heterogeneity among studies (Q=42.6; P-value 0.001; I^2=55.7 %). Data were stratified according to the geographical area where the study was conducted. Average difference in survival between lung-cancer patients who underwent VATS and those who underwent thoracotomy was large in studies conducted in Asia in comparison with studies conducted in the USA/Europe (5.5 vs 0.5 %). However, a large heterogeneity was observed among Asian studies. Three studies conducted in the USA/Europe reported follow-ups between 30 and 40 months. When those studies were excluded, the difference in 5-year mortality between VATS studies and thoracotomy studies conducted in western countries was 3.2 %. No heterogeneity was observed in the US/European studies [24].

Cao and colleagues performed a multi-institutional propensity score analysis. After matching patients according to propensity score, 1,458 patients were assigned to each treatment group. This large dataset showed patients who underwent standardized VATS lobectomy had similar long-term survival outcomes when compared with those who underwent open lobectomy (p=0.07) [25].

Currently, growing evidence for long-term outcomes reveals a 5-year survival advantage with VATS lobectomy in comparison with classic thoracotomy (Table 11.2). It is not completely clear why this would be the case, but it may be related to the reduced number of cytokines released and the resultant reduction in perioperative immunosuppression seen in VATS patients.

Immunologic Effects

The available evidence suggests that compared with open lobectomy, thoracoscopic procedures show reduced acute-phase responses and better preservation of cellular immune mechanisms. Some studies showed that VATS lobectomy leads to a reduced inflammatory response (lower interleukin and C-reactive protein levels) [2, 26], and less postoperative reduction in CD4 and natural killer cells [27]. Whitson indicated thoracoscopic surgery lobectomy for NSCLC is associated with less impairment of peripheral blood mononuclear cell (PBMC) cytotoxicity, and more rapid recovery of immune function as compared with thoracotomy [28] (Table 11.3).

Postoperative stress response and immune suppression follows both conventional and minimally invasive surgery, but the impact on the postoperative systemic immune response is less than that seen with the conventional approach. The clinical relevance of differences in the postoperative inflammatory response and differential impairment

Table 11.2 Studies comparing the oncologic outcomes of video-assisted thoracoscopic lobectomy versus open lobectomy for early stage non-small cell lung cancer

Author, year	Quality	Recurrence	Lymph node dissection	Survival
Cheng et al. [11] (2007)	Low	VATS = Open (OR:0.78, 95%CI: 0.58–1.04)	VATS = Open (WMD: −0.2, 95%CI: −0.8–0.5)	Mortality 1-year: VATS = Open OR: 0.78 3-year: VATS = Open OR: 1.09 5-year: VATS < Open OR: 0.67 Max: VATS < Open OR: 0.71 Stage I: VATS = Open OR: 0.85 Stage II: VATS = Open OR: 3.15 P=0.26 Stage III: VATS = Open OR: 0.96 P=0.96
Whitson et al. [12] (2008)	Low	–	–	Overall survival 1-year: VATS: 98.2 %, Open: 93.2 %, P=0.28 2-year: VATS: 91.6 %, Open: 84.9 %, P=0.12 3-year: VATS: 87.2 %, Open: 81.6 %, P=0.18 4-year: VATS: 88.4 %, Open: 71.4 %, P=0.003 5-year: VATS: 80.1 %, Open: 65.6 %, P=0.064
Yan et al. [7] (2009)	Moderate	Local: VATS = Open RR=0.64, P=0.24 Systemic: VATS < Open RR=0.57, P=0.03	–	5-year survival VATS > Open, RR=0.72, P=0.04
Zhang et al. [22] (2013)	Low	Local: VATS < Open RR=0.66, P=0.03 Systemic: VATS < Open RR=0.61, P<0.01	VATS = Open (WMD: −0.63 95%CI: −0.47–0.21 P=0.14)	Survival rate VATS > Open RR=1.10, P<0.01
Taioli et al. [24] (2013)	Moderate	–	–	5-year: VATS: 62–97 % Open: 58–97 % Meta difference in survival: 5 %
Chen et al. [8] (2013)	Low	–	–	5-year: VATS > Open OR: 1.82, P<0.01

WMD Weighted mean differences, *VATS* video-assisted thoracoscopic surgery, '<' indicates statistically lower rate according to meta-analysis, "=" indicates no statistically difference, '>' indicates statistically higher rate according to meta-analysis

Table 11.3 Immunologic impact of VATS lobectomy versus open lobectomy [5]

Author, year	Study type	Procedure	Number	Biologic marker	Result
Yim et al. [26] (2000)	Prospective nonrandomized	VATS Open	18 18	IL-6, IL-8, IL-10	VATS: fewer acute phase reactants
Craig et al. [2] (2001)	Prospective randomized	VATS Open	22 19	IL-6, CRP, WBC ROS	VATS: lower levels of IL-6,CRP, and WBC ROS
Leaver et al. [27] (2000)	Prospective randomized	VATS Open	22 19	Lymphocytes (CD4), NK cells	VATS: less reduction in CD4 and NK cells
Whitson et al. [28] (2008)	Prospective randomized	VATS Open	6 7	Cellular cytotoxicity	VATS: less impairment of cellular cytotoxicity

CRP C-reactive protein, *IL* interleukin, *NK* natural killer, *WBC ROS* White blood cell reactive oxygen species production

of cellular immunity after open and VATS for NSCLC has yet to be determined, but these findings could partially explain why perioperative outcomes of VATS lobectomy are superior to the perioperative outcomes of open lobectomy. Whether these biologic differences translate into a long-term survival advantage is not known.

Summary

No randomized controlled trials comparing 'true' VATS lobectomy as defined by the CALGB criteria versus the open technique. Due to a lack of clinical equipoise and widely reported benefits of the minimally invasive approach, we may have missed the opportunity to conduct such randomized controlled trials. However, growing evidence with consistent data from matched case-control studies, cohort studies, meta-analyses, and outcomes studies demonstrate VATS is associated with lower operative mortality, complications, and length of stay in hospital. These studies also demonstrate at least oncologic equivalence compared with open lobectomy, though the mechanisms underlying the potential survival advantage of VATS lobectomy have yet to be definitively determined.

Recommendations

VATS lobectomy is a safe and effective approach for lobectomy, associated with fewer postoperative complications, improved quality-of-life, and improved survival (evidence quality low to moderate) as compared with open lobectomy. VATS lobectomy is preferred over thoracotomy for early stage NSCLC.

A Personal View of the Data

Taking the lead in developing minimally invasive thoracic surgery in China, we were the first to begin routine VATS lobectomy in China. In our department, we have accomplished more than 2,000 VATS lobectomies. Through increasing experience, we have overcome many technical difficulties, and optimized the technique of VATS lobectomy. A total of three incisions are used (eighth interspace in the posterior axillary line, seventh or eighth interspace in the subscapular line, and an 4 cm anterior incision is made at the fourth or fifth interspace in the anterior axillary line). The major features of our technique are: (1) a special angled suction and electrocautery hook cooperate are crossed through a single incision concurrently; (2) creation of a perivascular tunnel for interlobar fissure division; (3) dividing the bronchial arteries initially; and (4) freeing vessels in their subadventitial plane. In addition, use of modified instruments and excellent team cooperation also contribute to the success of surgery.

Now more than 90 % of stage I or II NSCLC are performed by VATS lobectomy in our department. In our experience, VATS lobectomy can be performed in the majority of cases without compromising the perioperative outcomes and oncologic efficacy. We believe the minimally invasive approach also benefits cases that are more complicated, such as patients with locally advanced cancer (Non-N2), previous surgery, and neoadjuvant chemoradiotherapy. Further studies need to be performed to validate the potential benefits of VATS for these patients.

Recommendation
- VATS lobectomy is a safe and effective approach for lobectomy, and is recommended over thoracotomy for early stage NSCLC. (Evidence quality moderate; weak recommendation).

References

1. Swanson SJ, Herndon 2nd JE, D'Amico TA, Demmy TL, McKenna Jr RJ, Green MR, et al. Video-assisted thoracic surgery lobectomy: report of CALGB 39802 – a prospective, multi-institution feasibility study. J Clin Oncol. 2007;25(31):4993–7.
2. Craig SR, Leaver HA, Yap PL, Pugh GC, Walker WS. Acute phase responses following minimal access and conventional thoracic surgery. Eur J Cardiothorac Surg. 2001;20(3):455–63.
3. Kirby TJ, Mack MJ, Landreneau RJ, Rice TW. Lobectomy–video-assisted thoracic surgery versus muscle-sparing thoracotomy. A randomized trial. J Thorac Cardiovasc Surg. 1995;109(5):997–1001; discussion 1001–2.
4. Sugi K, Kaneda Y, Esato K. Video-assisted thoracoscopic lobectomy achieves a satisfactory long-term prognosis in patients with clinical stage IA lung cancer. World J Surg. 2000;24(1):27–30; discussion 30–1.

5. Rueth NM, Andrade RS. Is VATS lobectomy better: perioperatively, biologically and onco-logically? Ann Thorac Surg. 2010;89(6):S2107–11.
6. Howington JA, Blum MG, Chang AC, Balekian AA, Murthy SC. Treatment of stage I and II non-small cell lung cancer: diagnosis and management of lung cancer, 3rd ed: American College of Chest Physicians evidence-based clinical practice guidelines. Chest. 2013;143(5 Suppl):e278S–313.
7. Yan TD, Black D, Bannon PG, McCaughan BC. Systematic review and meta-analysis of ran-domized and nonrandomized trials on safety and efficacy of video-assisted thoracic surgery lobectomy for early-stage non-small-cell lung cancer. J Clin Oncol. 2009;27(15):2553–62.
8. Chen FF, Zhang D, Wang YL, Xiong B. Video-assisted thoracoscopic surgery lobectomy ver-sus open lobectomy in patients with clinical stage non-small cell lung cancer: a meta-analysis. Eur J Surg Oncol. 2013;39(9):957–63.
9. Swanson SJ, Meyers BF, Gunnarsson CL, Moore M, Howington JA, Maddaus MA. Video-assisted thoracoscopic lobectomy is less costly and morbid than open lobectomy: a retrospec-tive multiinstitutional database analysis. Ann Thorac Surg. 2012;93(4):1027–32.
10. Cao C, Manganas C, Ang SC, Peeceeyen S, Yan TD. Video-assisted thoracic surgery versus open thoracotomy for non-small cell lung cancer: a meta-analysis of propensity score-matched patients. Interact Cardiovasc Thorac Surg. 2013;16(3):244–9.
11. Cheng D, Downey RJ, Kernstine K, Stanbridge R, Shennib H, Wolf R, et al. Video-assisted thoracic surgery in lung cancer resection: a meta-analysis and systematic review of controlled trials. Innovations (Phila). 2007;2(6):261–92.
12. Whitson BA, Groth SS, Duval SJ, Swanson SJ, Maddaus MA. Surgery for early-stage non-small cell lung cancer: a systematic review of the video-assisted thoracoscopic surgery versus thoracotomy approaches to lobectomy. Ann Thorac Surg. 2008;86(6):2008–16; discus-sion 2016–8.
13. Casali G, Walker WS. Video-assisted thoracic surgery lobectomy: can we afford it? Eur J Cardiothorac Surg. 2009;35(3):423–8.
14. Handy Jr JR, Asaph JW, Douville EC, Ott GY, Grunkemeier GL, Wu Y. Does video-assisted thoracoscopic lobectomy for lung cancer provide improved functional outcomes compared with open lobectomy? Eur J Cardiothorac Surg. 2010;37(2):451–5.
15. Demmy TL, Nwogu C. Is video-assisted thoracic surgery lobectomy better? Quality of life considerations. Ann Thorac Surg. 2008;85(2):S719–28.
16. Tajiri M, Maehara T, Nakayama H, Sakamoto K. Decreased invasiveness via two methods of thoracoscopic lobectomy for lung cancer, compared with open thoracotomy. Respirology. 2007;12(2):207–11.
17. Balduyck B, Hendriks J, Lauwers P, Van Schil P. Quality of life evolution after lung cancer surgery: a prospective study in 100 patients. Lung Cancer. 2007;56(3):423–31.
18. Kaseda S, Aoki T, Hangai N, Shimizu K. Better pulmonary function and prognosis with video-assisted thoracic surgery than with thoracotomy. Ann Thorac Surg. 2000;70(5):1644–6.
19. Nicastri DG, Wisnivesky JP, Litle VR, Yun J, Chin C, Dembitzer FR, et al. Thoracoscopic lobectomy: report on safety, discharge independence, pain, and chemotherapy tolerance. J Thorac Cardiovasc Surg. 2008;135(3):642–7.
20. Lee JG, Cho BC, Bae MK, Lee CY, Park IK, Kim DJ, et al. Thoracoscopic lobectomy is asso-ciated with superior compliance with adjuvant chemotherapy in lung cancer. Ann Thorac Surg. 2011;91(2):344–8.
21. Sagawa M, Sato M, Sakurada A, Matsumura Y, Endo C, Handa M, et al. A prospective trial of systematic nodal dissection for lung cancer by video-assisted thoracic surgery: can it be per-fect? Ann Thorac Surg. 2002;73(3):900–4.
22. Zhang Z, Zhang Y, Feng H, Yao Z, Teng J, Wei D, et al. Is video-assisted thoracic surgery lobectomy better than thoracotomy for early-stage non-small-cell lung cancer? A systematic review and meta-analysis. Eur J Cardiothorac Surg. 2013;44(3):407–14.
23. Licht PB, Jørgensen OD, Ladegaard L, Jakobsen E, et al. A national study of nodal upstaging after thoracoscopic versus open lobectomy for clinical stage I lung cancer. Ann Thorac Surg. 2013;96(3):943–50.

24. Taioli E, Lee DS, Lesser M, Flores R. Long-term survival in video-assisted thoracoscopic lobectomy vs open lobectomy in lung-cancer patients: a meta-analysis. Eur J Cardiothorac Surg. 2013;44(4):591–7.
25. Cao C, Zhu ZH, Yan TD, Wang Q, Jiang G, Liu L, et al. Video-assisted thoracic surgery versus open thoracotomy for non-small-cell lung cancer: a propensity score analysis based on a multi-institutional registry. Eur J Cardiothorac Surg. 2013;44:849–54.
26. Yim AP, Wan S, Lee TW, Arifi AA. VATS lobectomy reduces cytokine responses compared with conventional surgery. Ann Thorac Surg. 2000;70(1):243–7.
27. Leaver HA, Craig SR, Yap PL, Walker WS. Lymphocyte responses following open and minimally invasive thoracic surgery. Eur J Clin Invest. 2000;30(3):230–8.
28. Whitson BA, D'Cunha J, Andrade RS, Kelly RF, Groth SS, Wu B, et al. Thoracoscopic versus thoracotomy approaches to lobectomy: differential impairment of cellular immunity. Ann Thorac Surg. 2008;86(6):1735–44.

Chapter 12
Robotic-Assisted Thoracoscopic Surgery (RATS) Versus Video-Assisted Thoracoscopic Surgery (VATS) Lobectomy for Stage I or II Non-small Cell Lung Cancer

Eric Vallières and Peter Baik

Abstract In contrast to other surgical subspecialties, robotics has very slowly made its way into the world of thoracic surgery. One of the arguments slowing down the widespread use of robotics in our field is a lack of evidence that the robotic platform is better than the more seasoned video-assisted thoracoscopic approach to the diseases we treat. Considering the role of robotic lobectomy in the treatment of early stage non-small cell lung cancer (NSCLC), the current level of evidence supports a conditional recommendation for its safety, its effectiveness and oncologic outcomes. However, at this time, when comparing to video assisted thoracic surgery (VATS) lobectomy, the cost to benefit ratio does not favor robotic lobectomy.

Keywords RATS (Robotic assisted thoracoscopic surgery) • RAL (Robotic assisted lobectomy) • CPRL (Completely portal robotic lobectomy) • RVATS (Robotic video-assisted thoracic surgery) • VATS (Video assisted thoracic surgery) • Lobectomy • Segmentectomy • Lung Resection • Lung Cancer

Introduction

Video assisted thoracic surgery (VATS) lobectomy has slowly become an accepted method to surgically treat early stage non-small cell lung cancer (NSCLC). Multiple reports have shown similar or better safety, oncologic outcomes and cost

E. Vallières, MD, FRCSC (✉)
Lung Cancer Program, Swedish Cancer Institute,
1101 Madison Street, Suite 900, Seattle, WA 98104, USA
e-mail: eric.vallieres@swedish.org

P. Baik, DO
Lung Cancer Program, Swedish Medical Center, First Hill,
1101 Madison Street, Suite 900, Seattle, WA 98104, USA
e-mail: peterubaik@yahoo.com

M.K. Ferguson (ed.), *Difficult Decisions in Thoracic Surgery*,
Difficult Decisions in Surgery: An Evidence-Based Approach 1,
DOI 10.1007/978-1-4471-6404-3_12, © Springer-Verlag London 2014

effectiveness when compared to open lobectomy. The adoption of the VATS lobectomy platform for cancer has been surprisingly slow over the last 20 years and the resistance by many has been about the limitations of the VATS two-dimensional visualization, its limited maneuverability and related difficulties, particularly in achieving adequate mediastinal nodal dissection [1, 2]. An analysis of the Premier Perspective Database (Premier INC, Charlotte, NC) database published in 2010 by Swanson et al. [2] reported that only 20 % of lobectomies logged in from 2002 to 2007, had been performed by VATS.

Robotic surgical systems have evolved to overcome the technical disadvantages of VATS primarily by allowing a 3-D visualization and magnification of structures, as well as improved maneuverability and dexterity. Despite very limited initial studies comparing a robotic approach to more conventional alternatives, the utilization of robots has gained wide acceptance in urologic and gynecologic surgeries. To date, the acceptance of robotic thoracic surgery remains limited but marketing efforts are likely to impact this reality.

There are two major platforms to achieve anatomic robotic lung resection. The first is referred to as robotic-assisted thoracic surgery/lobectomy (RATS/RAL) where a utility incision is created de facto to aid in the dissection. This creates an intrathoracic to ambient environment communication thus negating the use of carbon dioxide insufflation. The specimen is removed through the utility incision. Alternatively, a completely portal robotic lung resection (CPRL) involves performing the entire procedure through the ports, allowing and requiring carbon dioxide insufflation. The specimen is extracted through an enlarged port at the conclusion of the procedure.

Before the thoracic community endorses robotic lobectomy in the treatment of early stage NSCLC based solely on marketing efforts and strategies, we should critically review and compare its safety, effectiveness and oncologic outcomes and compare them to the more mature VATS experience. Assuming equivalence to the latter, one must finally address the difference in the costs of the various platforms.

As stated above, there are different techniques when robotic platform is used.

RATS: Robotic assisted thoracoscopic surgery
RAL: Robotic assisted lobectomy
CPRL: Completely portal robotic lobectomy
RVATS: Robotic video-assisted thoracic surgery

For this review, we will use RATS when robotic platform is used, regardless of different robotic techniques.

Search Strategy

A systematic search within the last 20 years was performed using PubMed and EBSCO databases. Once the articles were reviewed, additional articles were retrieved from the reference lists. The following search terms were used: robotic, thoracic, video-assisted thoracoscopic, VATS, thoracoscopic, completely portal, pulmonary, lung, resection, lobectomy and segmentectomy.

To date, there are no randomized, controlled studies that have compared robotic lobectomy to VATS lobectomy in the treatment of early stage NSCLC. All the case control studies that we reviewed were clinical outcomes studies with observations limited to the perioperative period. None to date have described long-term comparison, including recurrence and survival rates.

Results

Case Control Studies

In 2011, Jang et al. [3] from South Korea first reported a retrospective study comparing RATS to VATS performed by a single surgeon in between early 2006 and late 2009. All of the patients were considered to have early stage NSCLC. The first group of 40 patients underwent VATS lobectomy between January 2006 and February 2007 (Initial VATS group). The second group consisted of 40 patients who underwent RATS between February 2009 and October 2009 (RAL group). The third group consisted of 40 patients who underwent VATS during the same time period as the RAL patients (Recent VATS group). The surgeon reports having performed 203 VATS and RATS during the period but only 120 patients are included in the study. Although mean age difference was statistically significant, sex, type of cancer, tumor location and pathologic stages were similar. Table 12.1 shows the outcome of the study. The authors concluded that their early experience in RATS was similar to VATS and that experienced VATS surgeons should easily and successfully be capable of transitioning to the robotic platform. There are two issues with the report: First, the median lengths of stay in the VATS groups, 9 days for

Table 12.1 Comparison of tumor characteristics and postoperative outcomes in the robot-assisted, Initial VATS and recent VATS lobectomy group

	OR time (mins)	Rate of conversion (%)	EBL (mL)	Complications (%)	Median LOS (days)	# of lymph nodes dissected	Lymph node stations biopsied
Initial VATS (n = 40)	257 ± 57	7.5	374 ± 374	32.5	9 (6–34)	29 (15–56)	8 (5–11)
Recent VATS (n = 40)	161 ± 39	5	245 ± 173	17.5	7 (4–16)	26 (12–46)	7.5 (5–10)
RAL (n = 40)	240 ± 62	0	219 ± 123	10	6 (4–22)	22 (7–45)	7 (2–10)

Modified from Jang et al. [3]
VATS video-assisted thoracic surgery, *RAL* robotic assisted lobectomy, *EBL* estimated blood loss, *LOS* length of stay, *OR* operating room

initial VATS and 6 days for recent VATS, is higher than what has been published in the literature (median 4 days) [4]. Second, the report lacks information about inclusion and exclusion criteria to this analysis.

Cerfolio et al. [5], from Birmingham, Alabama, reported a retrospectively matched result of completely portal lobectomy with four arms against nerve- and rib-sparing thoracotomies in 2011. RATS (106 patients) were performed by a single surgeon between February 2010 and April 2011. The propensity matched thoracotomy patients (318 patients) were from their previously collected data set. The statistically significant findings that favored robotics approach over open thoracotomy were estimated blood loss (EBL), chest tube duration, hospital days, morbidity and verbal pain scores 3-weeks postoperatively (Table 12.2). They concluded that robotic lobectomy is safe, allows achieving R0 resection, obtaining adequate numbers of lymph nodes and sampling adequate lymph node stations.

Louie et al. [6] recently published a case-control analysis of consecutive completely portal anatomic (lobectomy or segmentectomy) (CPR) lung resection and VATS anatomic resections performed between May 2009 and October 2011. They included patients with solitary pulmonary metastasis and benign lung conditions (bronchiectasis, congenital malformations and localized fungal infections) for a total of 46 RATS and 34 VATS patients included in the study. The only statistically significant difference in demographics was the Eastern Cooperative Oncology Group (ECOG) performance status which, for unclear reasons, favored RATS. Key clinical outcomes between the two approaches were similar (Table 12.3). The authors concluded that RATS resulted in similar surgical outcomes as VATS and that the two MIS platforms can be seen as complimentary to each other. However, long-term follow-up or potential cost differences were not addressed.

At the Western Thoracic Surgical Association meeting in 2013, Lee et al. [7] from Ridgewood, NJ compared their experience of 20 RATS versus 32 VATS performed by a single surgeon between 2011 and 2012. Neither group required conversion to thoracotomy. The only statistically significant finding was the median operating time for RATS was 153 min versus 130 min in VATS (p=0.02) (Table 12.4). In conclusion, they supported the utilization of robotics in minimally invasive thoracic surgery as an alternative platform to VATS.

A recent report by Deen et al. [8] performed a retrospective cost analysis comparing open, VATS and RATS lobectomies and segmentectomies in 190 patients (71 open, 59 RATS and 60 VATS) performed during a similar period. The operative time was longest in RATS, 223 min, versus 202 min in VATS (p=0.0.045) and 180 min in open (p=<0.001) but RATS had the shortest inpatient days: RATS 4.62 days versus 4.75 days in VATS (p=0.777) and 5.47 days in open (p=0.054). The overall, total and procedure costs per case with RATS approach were 17,011.02, 15,811.02 and 14,650.02 (in US $) respectively. Statistically significant cost differences were shown for overall and total cost when compared to VATS (overall (in US$) 13,829.09 (p=<0.001), total 13,662.60 (p=0.019)). The statistically significant reasons for the higher costs in RATS were shown to be operating room costs and the cost of supplies. The authors observed that to render the RATS costs equivalent to those of VATS, the

Table 12.2 Key clinical outcomes

	EBL (mL, median and SD)	OR time (h, median and SD)	# of N2 nodes and stations removed (median)	# of N1 nodes and stations removed (median)	Chest tube days (median and range)	Hospital days (median and range)	Morbidity	Operative mortality	Verbal pain score 3 weeks postop
Robotic (n=106)	30±26	2.2±1.0	12, 5	5, 3	1.5 (1–6)	2.0 (1–7)	28 (27 %)	0	2.5 (0–7)
Thoracotomy (n=318)	90±22	1.5±0.8	11, 5	4, 3	3.0(1–67)	4.0(1–67)	120 (38 %)	11 (3 %)	4.4 (0–8)
P value	0.03	<0.001	0.906, >0.999	0.89, >0.999	<0.001	0.01	0.05	0.11	0.04

Modified from Cerfolio et al. [5]

EBL estimated blood loss, *SD* standard deviation, *N2* ipsilateral mediastinal node, *N1* ipsilateral hilar node, *OR* operating room

Table 12.3 Key clinical outcomes

Characteristics	Robotic	VATS	P value
Lesion size in cm, median (range)	2.8 (0.9–7.2)	2.3 (0.9–4.9)	0.07
Mean operative time (mins)	213	207	0.61
Length of stay (days), median (range)	4 (2–21)	4.5 (2–22)	0.63
ICU stay (days)	0.92	0.64	0.43
Estimated blood loss (mL)	153	134	0.36

Modified from Louie et al. [6]

ICU intensive care unit, *VATS* video-assisted thoracic surgery

Table 12.4 Key clinical outcomes

	Robotic (n = 20)	VATS (n = 32)	P value
Median operating time	153	130	0.02
Hospital LOS	3	3	
Number of lymph nodes	17.5	15.5	0.28
Morbidity	10	15.6	0.69
Mortality	0	3	0.99
Cost (in US $)	48,116	48,015	0.84

Modified from Lee et al. [7]

LOS length of stay, *VATS* video-assisted thoracic surgery

RATS operating room times needed to be decreased by 68 min per case or the hospital length of stay decreased by 1.86 days. Their conclusion was that VATS, when compared to open and RATS, was the less expensive approach to lobectomy and/or segmentectomy. Their analysis also suggested that for RATS to be financially viable one needed to either significantly reduce operative times or the costs of RATS supplies.

Case Series

Park et al. [9] in 2012 reviewed the long-term oncologic results of robotic lobectomies performed for early stage lung cancer at three separate institutions. They retrospectively reviewed 325 consecutive patients, 95 % had clinical stage I disease and the median follow-up of 27 months. The overall 5-year survival was reported at 80 % with 86 % of patients being free of disease. By pathological stage, the 5-year survival rates for stages IA, IB, and II were 91, 88 and 49 % respectively. This report was the first to suggest that the long-term outcomes of RATS lobectomy are at least equal to those of VATS lobectomy in the management of early stage NSCLC. By design however, this cannot be considered a definitive finding.

Table 12.5 shows the additional case series reported, highlighting the experiences at other institutions [9-16]. These data shows the feasibility of robotic lobectomy and suggests similar clinical outcomes of utilizing a robotic platform to early stage lung cancer resection comparing to published outcomes of VATS lobectomy.

Table 12.5 Case series

Reference ID	Type of study	# of patients	Median age (years)	Pathologic stage	OR time (mins)	Chest tube days	Length of stay	Minor complication	Major complication	Mortality	Tumor location	Rate of conversion
Park et al. [9]	Multicenter	325 (204 M; 121 F)	66 (30–87)	IA 176 / IB 72 / IIA / IIB 21 / IIIA 21	206 (110–383)	3 (1–23)	5 (2–28)	70 (21.5 %)	12 (3.7 %)	1	RUL 92 / RML 29 / RLL 71 / RUL/ML 1 / LUL 75 / LLL 57	27
Jett [10]	Single center	8	72 (50–81)	IA 1 / IB 2 / IIB 2 / IV 2 / Infectious 1	231.4 (144–337)		3.1 (2–4)	4			RUL 3 / RML 1 / RLL 1 / LUL 1 / LLL 1 / RML and RLL 1	1
Pardolesi et al. [11]	Multi center	17 (7 M; 10 F)	68.2 (32–82)		189 (138–240)		5 (2–14)	3 (17.6 %)	0	0	LL superior 4 / RLL superior 3 / Lingula 3 / LUL triseg 2 / LLL basilar 4 / RUL anterior 1	0
Park et al. [12]	Single center	34 (13 M; 21 F)	69 (12–85)	IA 25 / IB 3 / IIA 3 / IIB 1	218 (155–350)	3 (2–12)	4.5 (2–14)	1	2	0	RUL 14 / RML 1 / RLL 4 / LUL 10 / LLL 5	4

(continued)

Table 12.5 (continued)

Reference ID	Type of study	# of patients	Median age (years)	Pathologic stage	OR time (mins)	Chest tube days	Length of stay	Minor complication	Major complication	Mortality	Tumor location	Rate of conversion
Gharagozloo et al. [13]	Single center	100 (42 M; 58 F)	65±8	I 82 II 18	216±27	4 (3–42)		26	7	3	RUL 29 RML 7 RLL 17 LUL 31 LLL 16	0
Augustin et al. [14]	Single center	26 (14 M; 12 F)	65 (47–82)		228 (162–375)	7 (3–15)	11 (7–53)	3	1	0	RUL 8 RLL 8 LUL 4 LLL 6	5
Veronesi et al. [15]	Single center	54			74–513			3	8	0	RUL 16 RML 4 RLL 11 LUL 14 LLL 9	7
Gharagozloo et al. [16]	Single center	23 (14 M; 8 F)	66 (41–74)	IA 21 IIA 2	3.2±0.6	2±1.4	5±1.3	2	1	1	RUL 1 RML 3 RLL 8 LUL 0 LLL 11	2

RUL right upper lobe, *RML* right middle lobe, *RLL* right lower lobe, *LUL* left upper lobe, *LLL* left lower lobe, *OR* operating room

Summary and Recommendations

The limited available studies, although retrospective in nature, have shown rela-tive safety for robotic lobectomy when compared to VATS. Whether a more broad base utilization of the technology will translate in the same observation is yet to be seen. In high volume robotic thoracic surgical practices, robotic lobec-tomy appears to be just as effective as VATS comparing conversion rates, oper-ating room (OR) time, length of stay (LOS), morbidity and mortality as well as the number of lymph node stations sampled. As with the adaption of any new technology, one may hypothesize and hope that the effectiveness of robotic lobectomy may improve as the experience increases and the technology pro-gresses. Only one retrospective study has evaluated the oncologic outcome of robotic lobectomy and in a very limited number of patients. Robotic lobectomy however allows replication of the established principles of lung cancer surgery and potentially may improve the quality of the nodal work when comparing to VATS. As such, if one robotic surgeon adheres to these principles, the oncologic results should be similar. At this time, the costs of acquiring and maintaining the equipment as well as the costs of replacing the needed disposable parts are higher than the costs of the equipment needed for VATS. Considering the equiv-alences noted above, unless the robotic platform can result in shorter OR times or LOS after lobectomy, we cannot recommend robotic lobectomy until its related costs can be lowered by a combination of lowering equipment and main-tenance costs.

A Personal View of the Data

The available data on the utilization of robotics in the surgical treatment of stages I or II lung cancer remains very limited: single institution series, small numbers, and short follow-ups. Although, in the reported series, the safety and effectiveness of robotic lobectomy appears similar to those of the more mature VATS lobectomy experiences, randomized studies are needed to compare the two platforms and even to compare the two minimally invasive surgical approaches to modern day open lobectomy. As long as the robotic surgeon adheres to the established principles of lung cancer resection, the oncologic outcome should be similar to those of VATS lobectomy. Some have questioned whether robotic lobectomy could allow better nodal work over what has been seen in large multi-institutional VATS data sets [17].

On the other hand, at this point in time, the costs of robotic lobectomy do not compare favorably to those of VATS lobectomy in the management of early stage NSCLC. As we embark in an era of optimizing resource utilization, robotic lobectomy cannot be recommended over VATS lobectomy at this conjecture.

Recommendation
- Robotic lobectomy has similar initial clinical outcomes compared to VATS lobectomy and likely has similar oncologic outcomes. However, its routine use for lobectomy is not recommended based on the increased costs associated with its use (Evidence quality low; weak recommendation).

References

1. Scott WJ, Allen MS, Darling G, Meyers B, Decker PA, Putnam JB, McKenna RW, Landrenau RJ, Jones DR, Inculet RI, Malthaner RA. Video-assisted thoracic surgery versus open lobectomy for lung cancer: a secondary analysis of data from the American College of Surgeons Oncology Group Z0030 randomized clinical trial. J Thorac Cardiovasc Surg. 2010; 139(4):976–83.
2. Swanson SJ, Meyers BF, Gunnarsson CL, Moore M, Howington JA, Maddaus MA, McKenna RJ, Miller DL. Video-assisted thoracoscopic lobectomy is less costly and morbid than open lobectomy: a retrospective multiinstitutional database analysis. Ann Thorac Surg. 2012; 93(4):1027–32.
3. Jang HJ, Lee HS, Park SY, Zo JI. Comparison of the early robot-assisted lobectomy experience to video-assisted thoracic surgery lobectomy for lung cancer. Innovations. 2011;6(5):305–10.
4. Paul S, Altorki NK, Sheng S, Lee PC, Harpole DH, Onaitis MW, Stiles BM, Port JL, D'Amico TA. Thoracoscopic lobectomy is associated with lower morbidity than open lobectomy: a propensity-matched analysis from the STS database. J Thorac Cardiovasc Surg. 2010; 139(2):366–78.
5. Cerfolio RJ, Bryant AS, Minnich DJ. Starting a robotic program in general thoracic surgery: why, how, and lessons learned. Ann Thorac Surg. 2011;91(6):1729–37.
6. Louie B, Farivar A, Aye RW, Vallieres E. Early experience with robotic lung resection results in similar operative outcomes and morbidity when compared with matches video-assisted thoracoscopic surgery cases. Ann Thorac Surg. 2012;93(5):1598–605.
7. Lee B, Kletsman E, Korst RJ. Robotic lobectomy versus VATS lobectomy for NSCLC: better or the same? In: Podium presentation at: the 39th Annual Meeting of the Western Thoracic Surgical Association. Coeur d'Alene, Idaho, 26–29 June 2013.
8. Deen SA, Kramer JL, Wilshire CL, Vallières E, Farivar AS, Aye RW, Ely R, Louie BE. Defining the cost of care for lobectomy and segmentectomy: a comparison of open, video assisted thoracoscopic and robotic approaches. Ann Thorac Surg. 2014;97:1000–7.
9. Park BJ, Melfi F, Mussi A, Maisonneuve P, Spaggiari L, Caetao Da Silva RK, Veronesi G. Robotic lobectomy for non–small cell lung cancer (NSCLC): long-term oncologic results. J Thorac Cardiovasc Surg. 2012;143(2):383–9.
10. Jett GK. Thoracic robotics at the Heart Hospital Baylor Plano: the first 20 cases. Proc (Bayl Univ Med Cent). 2012;25(4):324–6.
11. Pardolesi A, Park B, Petrella F, Borri A, Gasparri R, Veronesi G. Robotic anatomic segmentectomy of the lung: technical aspects and initial results. Ann Thorac Surg. 2012;94(3):929–34.
12. Park BJ, Flores RM, Rusch VW. Robotic assistance for video-assisted thoracic surgical lobectomy: technique and initial results. J Thorac Cardiovasc Surg. 2006;131(1):54–9.
13. Gharagozloo F, Margolis M, Tepesta B, Strother E, Najam F. Robot-assisted lobectomy for early-stage lung cancer: report of 100 consecutive cases. Ann Thorac Surg. 2009;88(2):380–4.
14. Augustin F, Bodner J, Wykypiel H, Schwinghammer C, Schmid T. Initial experience with robotic lung lobectomy: report of two different approaches. Surg Endosc. 2011;25(1):108–13.

15. Veronesi G, Galetta D, Maisonneuve P, Melfi F, Schmid RA, Borri A, et al. Four-arm robotic lobectomy for the treatment of early-stage lung cancer. J Thorac Cardiovasc Surg. 2010;140(1):19–25.
16. Gharagozloo F, Margolis M, Tepesta B. Robot-assisted thoracoscopic lobectomy for early-stage lung cancer. Ann Thorac Surg. 2008;85(6):1880–6.
17. Boffa DJ, Kosinski AS, Paul S, Mitchell JD, Onaitis M. Lymph node evaluation by open or video-assisted approaches in 11500 anatomic lung cancer resections. Ann Thorac Surg. 2012;94(2):347–53.

Chapter 13
Lobectomy After Induction Therapy for NSCLC in the Presence of Persistent N2 Disease

Benedict D.T. Daly

Abstract Patients who undergo induction therapy for N2 NSCLC should have histologically documented N2 disease and should be restaged following induction therapy to determine the post-induction status of the mediastinal lymph nodes. Patients who have demonstrable disease need to be stratified to determine if the nodal disease is single station, non-bulky, and macroscopic versus microscopic to determine their potential for cure. Invasive restaging has limited sensitivity and negative predictive indices. Patients with limited single station disease and patients with negative restaging are likely to benefit from surgery. Patients requiring a pneumonectomy should not be offered resection.

Keywords Stage IIIA NSCLC • N2 NSCLC • Post treatment staging • Induction therapy • Neoadjuvant therapy • Lobectomy • pN2 NSCLC

Introduction

Considerable diversity of opinion regarding the management of Stage IIIA-N2 non-small cell lung cancer (NSCLC) was noted in a recent survey of surgeons on the Cardiothoracic Surgery Network [1]. Only 32 % of surgeons surveyed favored neoadjuvant treatment followed by lobectomy, if feasible and if N2 disease had been downstaged. An additional 30 % would favor pneumonectomy if N2 disease had been downstaged. Only 12 % would favor surgery if N2 disease

B.D.T. Daly, MD
Department of Surgery, Boston Medical Center,
Boston University School of Medicine, B-402, 88 East Newton Street,
Boston, MA 02118, USA
e-mail: benedict.daly@bmc.org

M.K. Ferguson (ed.), *Difficult Decisions in Thoracic Surgery*,
Difficult Decisions in Surgery: An Evidence-Based Approach 1,
DOI 10.1007/978-1-4471-6404-3_13, © Springer-Verlag London 2014

had not been downstaged. This diversity of opinion reflects the lack of a cohesive approach to the management of N2 NSCLC especially when persistent N2 disease is present after induction therapy, the focus of this chapter. This not surprising because few studies are comparable in terms of patient selection. For example, most studies do not indicate their percentages of patients with single versus multi-station disease, bulky versus non-bulky disease, or macroscopic versus microscopic disease. The percentage of patients with preoperative histologic proof versus radiologic proof of N2 disease is often missing. Variations in preoperative chemotherapy and drug schedule; absent, concurrent, or sequential radiotherapy; a variable radiation dose with or without hyper fractionation; and no or additional adjuvant therapy make few studies directly comparable. Most of the studies are retrospective reviews and few prospective studies have a control group or a sufficient number of patients from which to draw definitive conclusions. In addition, few studies indicate the number or percentage of patients with preoperative pN2 status but rather focus on the total number of pN2 patients identified following resection. How many of those had recalcitrant N2 disease unsuspected at or prior to operation is not indicated. In many studies patients with pN2 status at restaging are not offered resection.

Search Strategy

The search period was limited to publications after 1990 and in English. The search was limited to Medline and the terms were non-small cell lung cancer, N2 or stage IIIA, induction therapy or neoadjuvant therapy. We selected those studies in which the induction regimen was platinum based, patient selection and the induction regimen clearly defined, and a reasonable number of patients included with a minimum median follow-up of 24 months. The data from the pN2 subset of patients had to be identifiable. When Stage IIIB patients were included in the study, the N2 group had to be separable since N0 patients have a better prognosis. For the purposes of discussing operative mortality, only those studies where the vast majority of the patients had preoperatively identified N2 disease were reviewed since it is likely and is our experience that disease stage influences operative risk. Studies that excluded patients with persistent N2 disease from resection were only included in an analysis of pN2 subsets of patients.

In order to make a judgment regarding resection of pN2 NSCLC, we need to look at the results of treatment (short term and long term survival), the risks associated with those results (operative mortality and morbidity), and the results of alternative treatment. There are no studies meeting our criteria that directly compare patients with preoperatively identified persistent N2 disease after induction therapy treated with and without resection. Our recommendations will, therefore, be made indirectly on the basis of best available evidence.

Results

Survival of Patients with Resected pN2 NSCLC

The results of resection of over 500 patients with pN2 NSCLC are presented in Table 13.1 [2–13]. Five of the studies were prospective and seven were retrospective. The percentage of patients with pN2 NSCLC after induction chemotherapy or chemo-radiotherapy followed by resection varied from a low of 18–61 % with an average of 44 %. Patient selection at the pretreatment level and again after induction therapy may account for some differences. Differences in the induction regimens as well as intra-operative management may compound these differences. For example, complete mediastinal lymph node dissections versus lymph node sampling might produce a higher number of patients with recalcitrant pN2 disease and, therefore, better results according to stage.

Perhaps the gold standard for comparing each of these studies is the Intergroup 0139 study which has the largest number of patients [13]. They were treated in both the academic and community setting by a large number of oncologists, radiation therapists and surgeons. The control arm was definitive chemo-radiation. The median survival of patients with pN2 disease following resection in that report was 26.4 months. The average median survival in the other studies in Table 13.1 was 21 months with a range of 10–28 months. The predicted 5 year survival in INT0139 was 25 % versus an average of 18 % in the other studies. These numbers give us our best approximation of the overall anticipated benefit of operating on patients with pN2 NSCLC after induction therapy. This does not answer the question of what is the best induction chemotherapy regimen, whether radiation should be included in the regimen, or whether postoperative adjuvant therapy should be given. In INT 0139 patients received two cycles of adjuvant chemotherapy. In seven of the 12 studies the induction therapy included radiation.

Survival Following Resection of pN2 Subsets

While the studies in Table 13.1 can be interpreted as showing limited benefit to some patients with pN2 NSCLC, it is important to look at potential subsets of these patients who might have a better or worse prognosis. Studies that exclude patients with known post induction preoperative pN2 disease and report only the results of patients with recalcitrant pN2 have noted significantly better results. In the prospective phase II trimodality trial RTOG 0229, where the induction regimen included concurrent chemotherapy with full-dose (60 Gy) radiation, six of 56 (11 %) patients with mediastinoscopy or thoracoscopy positive pN2 disease after induction therapy were excluded from surgery [14]. Ten additional patients had recalcitrant

Table 13.1 Survival of patients with resected pN2 NSCLC

Author	Year	# Resected (%)	% Pneum	Ch/Ch-R	# pN2 (%) +	Median f/u ++	Median surv	5 years surv	Quality
Albain et al. [2]	1995	57 (76)	33	Ch-R	28 (50)	29 months	10 months	18 %	High
Mathisen et al. [3]	1996	35 (78)	18	Ch-R	21 (60)	4–83 months	26 months		High
Bueno et al. [4]	2000	103	37	Both	49 (48)	Min 4 years	15.9 months	9 %	Moderate
Betticher et al. [5]	2003	75 (83)	49	Ch	26 (35)	32 months	16.2 months	11 % 3 years	High
Steger et al. [6]	2009	55 (100)	47	Ch-R	20 (36)	30 months	19 months	16 %	Moderate
Decaluwe [7]	2009	85	24	Ch	49 (53)	51 months		27 %	High
Albain et al. [8]	2009	155 (77)	35	Ch-R	85 (55)	69.3 months	26.4 months	25 %	High
Stefani et al. [9]	2010	175	45	Ch	107 (61)	32.5 months	24.9 month	22 %	Moderate
Freidel et al. [10]	2010	62	58	Both	18 (18)	93 months	28 months	33 %	Moderate
Paul et al. [11]	2011	136	23	Ch, 10 % R	65 (48)	42 months		21 % L; 19 % P	Moderate
Meacci et al. [12]	2011	161	15	Ch-R	40 (25)	24 months		19 %	High
Shitani et al. [13]	2012	52	17	Ch-R	23 (44)	58 months		0	Moderate

Abbreviations: *NSCLC* non-small cell lung cancer, *Pneum* pneumonectomy, *Ch* induction chemotherapy, *Ch-R* induction chemo-radiotherapy, *pN2* persistent N2 disease after induction therapy,+ *f/u* follow-up, ++for those alive at final analysis, ^includes patients with N1 and N3 disease, ^^Only R0 patients, includes N3 patients mediastinal nodal disease discovered after resection. They had a median survival of 33 months but only a progression free survival of 9 months. These results, however, included the six patients with pN2 disease not offered resection. In another study of patients with Stage IIIA-N2 NSCLC, 198 patients completed neoadjuvant chemoradiation and presented for restaging [15]. Forty-nine (25 %) patients had persistent N2 disease and were excluded from surgery. Fourteen patients who were found to have recalcitrant N2 disease on pathology had a 42 % 5 year survival. In this study, however, patients with upstaged nodal disease discovered at surgery were also not resected. These studies suggest that patients with persistent microscopic disease do better.

Meacci reported on their 40 patients who had persistent N2 involvement following induction therapy and demonstrated the most significant factor associated with mortality was the relative macroscopic vs. microscopic residual tumor in the lymph nodes [11]. Patients with macroscopic residual N2 disease had 2.8 times the risk of death. Their 5 year survival rate in these patients was 12.6 %. Conversely it was 54.6 % with microscopic involvement defined as 1–10 % viable tumor cells in the lymph node. Patients with single level involvement had a better survival than patients with multilevel involvement (39.5 % vs. 10.6 %; $p=0.10$). No patient with extracapsular spread survived. Decaluwe demonstrated a difference in survival between patients with single versus multilevel involvement [12]. Patients with single level pN2 involvement had a 37 % 5 year survival whereas patients with multilevel pN2 involvement had a 0 % 5 year survival. Similarly, Tokeda observed a 34.8 % 5 year survival in 17 resected patients with single station pN2 disease versus no 5 year survivors in 16 patients with multi-station pN2 disease [16]. These few studies suggest that patients with persistent multi-station or bulky mediastinal lymph node involvement should not be offered resection. On the other hand, patients identified with single station or microscopic disease in the mediastinal lymph nodes will likely benefit from surgery.

Post Induction Patient Evaluation

One of the problems in managing patients with Stage IIIA-N2 NSCLC is determining who had a satisfactory response to induction therapy. A minimum requirement for most surgical series is an absence of disease progression by CT and PET. A more important determinant is whether a patient's tumor has sufficiently responded to induction therapy to permit a lobectomy as opposed to a pneumonectomy, and most importantly what the status of the mediastinal lymph nodes is.

Evaluation of Lobectomy vs. Pneumonectomy

Not surprising, in most series reporting on surgery for patients with involved mediastinal lymph nodes, the requirement for pneumonectomy in order to achieve an R0 resection is high even after induction therapy. Very often these patients have central

Table 13.2 Operative mortality following induction therapy for N2 NSCLC

Author	Year	# Pts	Ch/ ch-R	XRT dose	HF^	#Pneum^^ (%)	Op mort L+	Op mort P++	Quality
Albain et al. [2]	1995	57	Ch-R	45 Gy		21 (37)	3.5 %	15.7	High
Mathiesen et al. [3]	1996	35	Ch-R	40 Gy	Y	8 (23)	7.4 %	0	High
Betticher et al. [5]	2003	75	Ch			37 (49)	3 % all pts		High
Cerfolio et al. [17]	2005	96	Ch-R	45–60 Gy		12 (13)	0	16.7	High
Steger et al. [6]	2009	55	Ch-R	45 Gy	Y	26 (47)	3.6 % all pts		Moderate
Decaluwe et al. [7]	2009	92	Ch			20 (24)	2.3 %	0	High
Albain et al. [8]	2009	155	Ch-R	45 Gy		54 (35)	1.0 %	26	High
Meacci et al. [12]	2011	161	Ch-R	50.4 Gy	Y/n	6 (15)	0	3	High

Abbreviations: *NSCLC* non-small cell lung cancer, *Pts* patients, *Ch* chemotherapy, *Ch-R* chemo-radiotherapy, *XRT* radiotherapy,^ *HF* hyper-fractionation, ^^ *Pneum* pneumonectomy,+ *Op Mort L* operative mortality for lobectomy.++ *Op Mort P* operative mortality for pneumonectomy

tumors or involved mediastinal lymph nodes adherent to central structures. In Table 13.1 the percentage of patients with N2 NSCLC requiring a pneumonectomy varied from a low of 15 % to as high as 58 %, the average 33 % and the weighted average 36 %. It is important to know the mortality in patients with N2 disease as opposed to, for example, patients with T3N0 or T4N0 tumors; disease stage impacts operative mortality apart from the technical issues involved, and this has been our own experience. Series reporting on operative mortality for patients undergoing lobectomy or pneumonectomy, who received induction therapy, and who had histologic proof of N2 disease prior to resection are shown in Table 13.2 [2, 3, 5–8, 12, 17]. In this table the operative mortality for lobectomy averages 2.37 % but is 10.23 % for pneumonectomy, a fivefold difference. For patients undergoing induction therapy that included radiation in the induction regimen, the mortality was slightly higher with a range from 0 to 26 %. The highest mortality was observed in the randomized controlled study reported by Albain (INT0139) [2]. This study, as we have already mentioned, was performed in many academic and community hospitals which has the strength of accumulating results from a more diverse population of patients and medical professionals. At the same time it begs the question, particularly with regards to pneumonectomy, whether experience in this type of surgery affects mortality. In this study, the operative mortality for pneumonectomy was sufficiently high as to make operation no better than non-operative management with definitive chemotherapy and radiotherapy, whereas the converse was true for lobectomy. While it is generally accepted that the addition of radiation to the induction regimen improves tumor response and sterilization of the mediastinal lymph nodes, this has not necessarily meant improved survival, particularly when one incorporates the mortality associated with pneumonectomy. When the radiation dose escalates to 60 Gy, the operative mortality associated with pneumonectomy generally increases. In addition, while most series report on 30 day and in-hospital mortality, it is becoming clear that this is arbitrary and does not truly reflect the operative risk. The 90 day mortality may be a better approximation of risk associated with pneumonectomy, the 90 day mortality being approximately twice the 30 day mortality [18, 19]. Furthermore, one needs to factor in the reduced 5 year survival associated with pneumonectomy patients and NSCLC in general to appreciate the true risk associated with the decision to operate on any patient with pN2 NSCLC. It is, therefore, imperative to determine whether an R0 resection can be performed by lobectomy and it also important to make a preoperative decision on whether to abandon resection if the need for pneumonectomy is only determined at operation.

Post Induction Evaluation of the Mediastinal Lymph Nodes

This chapter is not debating the relative merits of one induction regimen over another one. However, it is apparent that in order to assess the potential benefit of operation against the risks, it is imperative to know the status of the mediastinal lymph nodes after the induction phase of treatment. There is a consensus based on the results of virtually every study evaluating induction therapy on patients with N2 NSCLC that sterilization of the mediastinal lymph nodes is the single most important factor affecting survival. While patients with recalcitrant pN2 disease i.e., those found to have persistent microscopic disease on histological assessment, have a reasonable survival, these patients are not identified prior to resection and do not impact decision making. On the other hand, certain subgroups of patients with residual pN2 disease have a dismal prognosis and it is important to discover these patients prior to resection, as they are generally not candidates for surgery.

Every patient undergoing induction therapy gets restaged prior to resection, most with a CT scan, PET scan, and MRI of the brain to exclude metastases and assess the status of the mediastinal lymph nodes. In 2010 Rebollo-Aguierre and colleagues from Spain performed a systematic review of the literature to evaluate the effectiveness of FDG-PET in assessing the impact of induction therapy on NSCLC [20]. Pooling data on restaging of the mediastinal lymph nodes in patients with N2 lung cancer, the overall sensitivity in detecting pN2 disease was 63 % and the specificity was 85 %, with a wide range in the positive and negative predictive values. They concluded that it was unsatisfactory to rely on a FDG-PET as the only tool in evaluating response to therapy. Both false positives and false negatives can adversely affect a patient's course of treatment. Direct evaluation of the mediastinal lymph nodes requires invasive staging and if one believes the degree of involvement may impact decision making then mediastinoscopy or VATS becomes necessary. In a small study (CALGB 39803) the sensitivity of videothoracoscopy for restaging was 67 % and the negative predictive value was 73 % [21]. Importantly, the procedure was unsuccessful in

21 %. On the other hand, repeat mediastinoscopy is controversial after induction therapy, particularly when radiation is included in the induction regimen. However, Marra reported mediastinoscopy was successful in 98 % of 104 patients restaged after chemo-radiation for Stage IIIA/B disease with a sensitivity of 61 %, a specificity of 100 % and a negative predictive value of 85 % [22]. In 2009, Szlubowski and colleagues reported on the usefulness of endobronchial ultrasound-guided needle aspiration (EBUS) to restage the mediastinal lymph nodes in a consecutive group of 61 patients with pathologically proven N2 disease who had completed a course of induction chemotherapy [23]. The results from EBUS were then compared to the results following transcervical extended mediastinal lymphadenectomy (TEMLA). The sensitivity, positive and negative predictive values for EBUS were 67, 91 and 79 %. However, 30 % of the patients with false negative results had multi-station lymph node involvement. At this juncture that there is no clear standard or ideal procedure that will identify all patients with residual pN2 disease or multi-station pN2 disease, and there is no method of quantifying the degree of micrometastatic metastatic involvement short of resection. In an attempt to identify patients with N2 NSCLC during initial staging, EBUS of the mediastinal lymph nodes may be a better first step so that mediastinoscopy or VATS can be available for restaging if N2 nodes are found initially.

Survival of Patients Denied Resection with Persistent N2 Disease Following Induction Therapy

Few studies report the results of potentially operable patients with pN2 disease following induction therapy but who were excluded from surgery based on positive restaging. Cerfolio reported on 45 patients initially considered potentially operable who completed a course of induction chemo-radiotherapy and who were found to have persistent N2 disease after repeat minimally invasive mediastinal staging and were not resected as a result [15]. Their 5 year survival was 17 %. In INT0139, the median survival time for the patients in the surgical arm who were not resected was 9 months, identical to the survival of the five patients in the RTOG0229 trial who had persistent N2 disease following restaging and were not brought to surgery [13, 14]. In assessing survival following the demonstration of persistent disease after a course of chemotherapy or chemo-radiation, it must be remembered that most of these patients will get additional treatment if not brought to surgery. Most patients will get additional chemotherapy, and unless the patients received definitive radiation as part of their induction regimen, patients will get a course of radiation therapy or a radiation boost. Therefore, it should be anticipated that there will be some 5 year survivors. The results of definitive chemo-radiation trials for patients with N2 disease are not germane to this analysis since the long-term survivors in these studies are more likely to be the responders in surgical trials.

Morbidity of Lobectomy Following Induction Therapy

Perhaps the most difficult part of decision making in this subgroup of patients with pN2 disease is weighing the morbidity associated with surgery. In most series 40–50 % of patients will have some complication, although the risk of a major complication is much less. Such complications include pneumonia, respiratory failure, bronchopleural fistula, and pulmonary embolus. The potential for these complications will affect patient selection and will vary from surgeon to surgeon and institution to institution. This subjective part of decision making will modify any of the proposed recommendations.

Recommendations

The following are suggested guidelines. In some patients the histologic confirmation of persistent N2 disease or its extent will not be possible. Clinical judgment is required to select the best treatment for each individual. Every effort should be made preoperatively to document N2 disease histologically. If possible, this should be first attempted with EBUS/EUS. Following induction therapy, patients should be restaged with repeat EBUS/EUS, mediastinoscopy, VATS or a combination whenever feasible in conjunction with CT and PET-CT. If patients have documented multi-station pN2 disease, surgery should not be attempted since the patients will likely do as well as with non-operative management. Patients with bulky and documented persistent N2 disease should be treated similarly. Patients with persistent limited single station disease may benefit from lobectomy, mediastinal lymph node dissection and additional chemotherapy/radiotherapy. Patients in whom persistent N2 disease is not documented should be offered resection depending on the intraoperative findings. A critical part of the evaluation process requires a determination of whether a lobectomy is feasible. A decision whether to abandon resection if the need to perform a pneumonectomy arises at operation should be made ahead of time.

A Personal View of the Data

My own philosophy with regard to the management of advanced lung cancer has always been to assess risk versus benefit, be as aggressive as possible, and if in doubt, to err on the side of surgery. This philosophy has been predicated on my experience that without surgery the chances of cure for patients with advanced lung cancer is small although not zero. I do operate on patients with residual limited N2 disease in a single station and in our hands we have achieved a 5 year survival of 40 % in this subset of patients. These patients receive adjuvant chemotherapy with a different regimen than the one used in the induction protocol. In the face of experience I would no longer operate on a patients with grossly positive mediastinal nodes after induction therapy. I have always been impressed that the percentage of patients whose mediastinal nodes have been sterilized far exceeds the number of patients whose primary tumor has been sterilized so that the persistence of positive nodes in the mediastinum is indeed a marker of bad disease. Furthermore, since we have increased our radiation dose from 59.4 to 66 Gy in the induction regimen, there is no room for additional adjuvant radiation and it is most unlikely that one would achieve a home run with a different chemotherapy regimen after miserably failing a platinum containing induction regimen. The only time I break the "rules" is in the young patient with limited microscopic disease in more than one station in whom I am confident I can achieve an R0 resection and am certain I can do a lobectomy. I have not had a mortality after concurrent high dose radiation and chemotherapy in any patient undergoing a lobectomy. The risk, therefore, is small and in this select subset there may be some salvage benefit, albeit small, as well.

Recommendations

- Every effort should be made preoperatively to document N2 disease histologically (Evidence quality high; strong recommendation).
- Initial mediastinal staging should be first attempted with EBUS/EUS to enable mediastinoscopy after induction therapy (Evidence quality low; weak recommendation).
- Following induction therapy patients should be restaged (repeat EBUS/EUS, mediastinoscopy, VATS or a combination) whenever feasible in conjunction with CT and PET-CT (Evidence quality high; strong recommendation).
- If patients have documented multi-station pN2 disease after induction therapy, surgery should not be attempted since the patients will likely do as well as with non-operative management. Patients with bulky and documented persistent N2 disease should be treated similarly (Evidence quality high; strong recommendation).
- Patients with persistent limited single station disease may benefit from lobectomy, mediastinal lymph node dissection and additional chemotherapy/radiotherapy (Evidence quality moderate; weak recommendation).
- Patients in whom persistent N2 disease is not documented should be offered resection depending on the intraoperative findings (Evidence quality high; strong recommendation).
- A critical part of the evaluation process requires a determination of whether a lobectomy is feasible. A decision whether to abandon resection if the need to perform a pneumonectomy arises at operation should be made ahead of time (Evidence quality high; strong recommendation).

References

1. Veermachaneni NK, Feins RH, Stephenson BJ, Edwards LJ, Fernandez FG. Management of stage IIIA non-small cell lung cancer by thoracic surgeons in North America. Ann Thorac Surg. 2012;94:922–6.
2. Albain KS, Rusch VW, Crowley JJ, Rice TW, Turrisi AT, Weick JK, et al. Concurrent Cisplatin/Etoposide plus chest radiotherapy followed by surgery for stages IIIA (N2) and IIIB non-small cell lung cancer: mature results of Southwest Oncology Group phase II study 8805. J Clin Oncol. 1995;13:18880–92.
3. Mathisen DJ, Wain JC, Wright C, Choi N, Carey R, Hilgenberg A, et al. Assessment of preoperative accelerated radiotherapy and chemotherapy in stage IIIA (N2) non-small cell lung cancer. J Thorac Cardiovasc Surg. 1996;111:123–31.
4. Bueno R, Richards WG, Swanson SJ, Jaklitsch MT, Mentzer SJ, Sugarbaker DJ. Nodal stage after induction therapy for stage IIIA lung cancer determines patient survival. Ann Thorac Surg. 2000;70:1826–31.
5. Betticher DC, Schmitz SH, Totsch M, Hansen E, Joss C, von Briel C, et al. Mediastinal lymph node clearance after Docetaxel-Cisplatin neoadjuvant chemotherapy is prognostic of survival in patients with stage IIIA pN2 non-small cell lung cancer; a multicenter phase II trial. J Clin Oncol. 2003;21:1752–9.
6. Steger V, Walles T, Kosan B, Walker T, Kyriss T, Veit S, et al. Trimodal therapy for histologically proven N2/3 non-small cell lung cancer: mid-term results and indicators for survival. Ann Thorac Surg. 2009;87:1676–83.
7. Decaluwe H, De Leyn P, Vansteenkiste J, Dooms C, Van Raemdonck D, Nafteux P, et al. Surgical multimodality treatment for baseline resectable stage IIIA-N2 non-small cell lung cancer. Degree of mediastinal node involvement and impact on survival. Eur J Cardiothorac Surg. 2009;36:433–9.
8. Albain KS, Swann RS, Rusch VW, Turrisi AT, Shepherd FA, Smith C, et al. Radiotherapy plus chemotherapy with or without surgical resection for stage III non-small-cell lung cancer: a phase III randomized controlled trial. Lancet. 2009;374:379–86.
9. Stephani A, Alifano M, Bobbio A, Grigoriou M, Jouni R, Magdeleinat P, et al. Which patients should be operated on after induction chemotherapy for N2 non-small cell lung cancer? Analysis of a 7-yer experience in 175 patients. J Thorac Cardiovasc Surg. 2010;140: 356–63.
10. Friedel G, Budach W, Dippon J, Spengler W, Eschmann SM, Phannenberg C, et al. Phase II trial of a trimodality regimen for stage III non-small cell lung cancer using chemotherapy as induction treatment with concurrent hyperfractionated chemoradiation with Carboplatin and Paclitaxel followed by subsequent resection: a single-center study. J Clin Oncol. 2010;28: 942–8.
11. Paul S, Mirza F, Port JL, Lee PC, Stiles BM, Kansler AL, Altorki NK. Survival of patients with stage IIIA non-small cell lung cancer after induction therapy: age, mediastinal downstaging, and extent of pulmonary resection as independent predictors. J Thorac Cardiovasc Surg. 2011; 141:48–55.
12. Meacci E, Cesario A, Cusumano G, Lococo F, D'Angelillo R, Dall'Armi V, et al. Surgery for patients with persistent pathological N2 IIIA stage in non-small cell lung cancer after induction radio-chemotherapy: the microscopic seed of doubt. Eur J Cardiothorac Surg. 2011;40:656–63.
13. Shitani Y, Funakoshi Y, Inoue M, Takeuchi Y, Okumura M, Maeda H, et al. Pathological status of mediastinal lymph nodes after preoperative concurrent chemoradiotherapy determines prognosis in patients with non-small cell lung cancer. Ann Thorac Cardiovasc Surg. 2012;18: 530–5.
14. Suntharalingam M, Paulus R, Edelman MJ, Krasna M, Burrows W, Gore E, et al. Radiation Therapy Oncology Group protocol 0229: a phase II trial of neoadjuvant therapy with concurrent chemotherapy and full-dose radiation therapy followed by surgical resection and consolidative therapy for locally advanced non-small cell carcinoma of the lung. Int J Radiat Oncol Biol Phys. 2012;84:456–63.

15. Cerfolio RJ, Maniscalco L, Bryant AS. The treatment of patients with stage IIIA non-small cell lung cancer from N@ disease: who returns to the surgical arena and who survives. Ann Thorac Surg. 2008;86:912–20.
16. Takeda S, Maeda H, Okada T, Ymaguchi T, Nakagawa M, Yokota S, et al. Results of pulmonary resection following neoadjuvant therapy for locally advanced (IIIA–IIIB) lung cancer. Eur J Cardiothorac Surg. 2006;30:184–9.
17. Cerfolio RJ, Bryanbt AS, Spencer SA, Bartolucci AA. Pulmonary resection after high-dose and low-dose chest irradiation. Ann Thorac Surg. 2006;80:1224–30.
18. Kim AW, Liptay MJ, Bonomi P, Warren WH, Basu S, Farlow EC, et al. Neoadjuvant chemoradiation for clinically advanced non-small cell lung cancer: an analysis of 233 patients. Ann Thorac Surg. 2011;92:233–43.
19. Doddoli C, Barlesi F, Trousse D, Robitail S, Yena S, Astoul P, et al. One hundred consecutive pneumoectomies after induction therapy for non-small cell lung cancer: an uncertain balance between risks and benefits. J Thorac Cardiovasc Surg. 2005;130:416–25.
20. Rebollo-Aguirre A, Ramos-Font C, Portero RV, Cook GJR, Elvira JML, Tabares AR. Is FDG-PET suitable for evaluating neoadjuvant therapy in non-small cell lung cancer? Evidence with systematic review of the literature. J Surg Oncol. 2010;101:486–94.
21. Jaklitch MT, Gu L, Demmy T, Harpole DH, D'Amico TA, McKenna RJ, et al. Prospective phase II trial of preresection thoracoscopic mediastinal restaging after neoadjuvant therapy for IIIA (N2) non-small cell lung cancer: results of CALBG Protocol 39803. J Thorac Cardiovasc Surg. 2013;146:9–16.
22. Marra A, Hillejan L, Fechner S, Stamatis G. Remediastinoscopy in restaging of lung cancer after induction therapy. J Thorac Cardiovasc Surg. 2008;135:843–9.
23. Szlubowski A, Herth FJF, Soja J, Kolodziej M, Figura J, Cmiel A, et al. Endobronchial ultrasound-guided needle aspiration in non-small-cell lung cancer restaging verified by transcervical bilateral extended mediastinal lymphadenectomy – a prospective study. Eur J Cardiothorac Surg. 2010;37:1180–4.

Chapter 14
Pneumonectomy After Induction Therapy for Non-small Cell Lung Cancer

Benjamin E. Haithcock and Richard H. Feins

Abstract The authors review current data on pneumonectomy in patients with non-small cell cancer after induction chemotherapy and radiation therapy and make recommendations for treatment: Evaluation by a multidisciplinary team for all advanced stage non-small cell lung cancer cases; parenchymal-conserving R0 resection for patients undergoing therapy for resectable NSCLC; pneumonectomies after induction therapy, done in experienced centers; right pneumonectomy in an experienced center after neoadjuvant therapy - if not feasible, consider referral or treatment with chemo radiotherapy.

Keywords Cancer • Lung cancer • Non-small cell lung cancer (NSCLC) • Pneumonectomy • Induction chemotherapy • Radiation therapy • Mortality • Morbidity

Introduction

Non-small cell lung cancer (NSCLC) survival in patients with locally advanced lung cancer improves with improved operability and resectability. These are observed to improve after induction protocols using concurrent chemotherapy and radiation therapy. There are concerns related to the utility of performing a pneumonectomy in this group of patients owing to the reported significant morbidity and mortality of the surgery.

B.E. Haithcock, MD (✉)
Division of Cardiothoracic Surgery, University of North Carolina at Chapel Hill,
3040 Burnett-Womack Building, CB #7065, Chapel Hill, NC 27599-7065, USA
e-mail: benjamin_haithcock@med.unc.edu

R.H. Feins, MD
Division of Cardiothoracic Surgery, Department of Surgery, University of North Carolina,
3040 Burnett-Womack Building, CB #7065, Chapel Hill, NC 27599-7065, USA
e-mail: rfeins@med.unc.edu

M.K. Ferguson (ed.), *Difficult Decisions in Thoracic Surgery*,
Difficult Decisions in Surgery: An Evidence-Based Approach 1,
DOI 10.1007/978-1-4471-6404-3_14, © Springer-Verlag London 2014

Several observational case studies have examined the results related to pneumonectomy after induction therapy for non-small cell lung cancer. There have also been single institutional studies that have demonstrated limited to no significant differences in pneumonectomy morbidity and mortality in this patient population. However, a randomized controlled trial has demonstrated a significant difference in morbidity and mortality after pneumonectomy in this patient population and advocates for parenchymal conserving surgery.

The goal of this chapter is to review the current data relevant to pneumonectomy in patients after induction chemotherapy and radiation therapy and formulate a recommendation based upon data and experience.

Search Strategy

PubMed and the Cochrane Library were used to initiate the search of relevant papers. The search was performed in August 2013 and included the years 2000–2013. Search terms included non-small cell lung cancer, induction therapy, neoadjuvant chemotherapy, neoadjuvant radiation therapy, pulmonary resection, morbidity, mortality, and cancer free survival. The papers that were included were those in English in which there was a clear explanation of the procedure performed. Other inclusion criteria of papers were the stage of the cancer treated, perioperative morbidity and mortality and long-term survival. Review papers were also analyzed for appropriate cross-references of other articles.

Description of Published Data and Impact on Decision Making

Several studies have evaluated patients undergoing pneumonectomy after neoadjuvant therapy for non-small cell lung cancer. Key studies will be summarized in this section. Using the Lung Cancer Study Group data, the overall baseline mortality rate for pneumonectomy for lung cancer was identified to be 6.2 % [1].

Daly et al. from the Boston Medical Center evaluated their data from 30 patients who received 5,940 cGy of radiation and two concurrent cycles of etoposide and cisplatin [2]. The authors examined morbidity, mortality and survival in this patient population. Eighteen patients underwent right pneumonectomy and 12 underwent left pneumonectomy. Thirty four percent (10/29) of these patients had a complete pathologic response. Fifty percent (3/6) of the patients with N1 nodal disease were node negative after neoadjuvant therapy, and 5/11 patients with N2 disease were down staged. 13.3 % (4/30) died in the postoperative period. Of these four patients, one had undergone a right pneumonectomy and expired from aspiration, myocardial infarction and heart failure. Three patients died who underwent left pneumonectomy; one from pneumonia, one from bronchopleural fistula, and another from a massive pulmonary embolism. Morbidity included 16.7 % (5/30) (all five from pneumonia, three due to aspiration). Median survival was 22 months and 5-year survival was 38 % [2].

The Radiation Therapy Oncology Group (RTOG) led a phase III multi-centered intergroup trial in patients with N2 non-small cell lung cancer (Int 0139). Patients were randomized to either concurrent platin based chemotherapy plus radiation therapy (45 Gy) followed by surgery or chemotherapy with definitive radiotherapy and no surgery. Patients in both arms were offered two additional cycles of chemotherapy. In this study, 16 of the 54 patients who underwent pneumonectomy died (29.6 %), the vast majority of whom had a right pneumonectomy. In addition, 45 % of the patients who underwent pneumonectomy were found to have T0N0 disease at the time of surgery. While the overall survival for the two study groups was not significantly different, there was a significant difference in survival and time to recurrence favoring the surgery arm in those patients who did not undergo pneumonectomy. The authors hypothesized that trimodality treatment might be beneficial if a complete resection could be accomplished without pneumonectomy, especially on the right side [3].

Martin et al. from Memorial Sloan Kettering performed a retrospective evaluation of patients undergoing pulmonary resection after induction chemotherapy or chemo radiation [4]. Of the 470 patients undergoing pulmonary resection, 97 (20.6 %) underwent pneumonectomy and of these, 55 patients underwent a standard pneumonectomy, 1 an extrapleural resection, 38 an intrapericardial resection, 2 a combined extrapleural and intrapericardial operation, and 1 a completion pneumonectomy. The overall mortality for all patients was 3.8 % (18/470). Within the pneumonectomy group, overall mortality was 11.3 % (11/97). In-hospital and late mortality in this group were 6.2 and 5.1 % and all deaths were in the 46 patients who underwent a right pneumonectomy. The overall morbidity in the pneumonectomy group alone was 46.4 % (58.7 % for right pneumonectomy and 35.3 % for left pneumonectomy). Multivariate analysis found right pneumonectomy, increased blood loss, and low FEV to be significant predictors of higher morbidity [4].

D'Amato et al. reported their data from the University of Pittsburgh and Ottawa Hospital in Canada [5]. In a retrospective fashion, the group compared 247 patients who underwent pneumonectomy alone versus 68 patients who underwent induction chemotherapy followed by pneumonectomy. Of these 68 patients, 33 received neoadjuvant radiation with an average dose of 45.6 Gy. The overall operative mortality was 9.2 % (10.5 % for right and 7.0 % for left). There was no significant difference in the overall incidence of bronchopleural fistula/empyema, respiratory failure, pneumonia, or 30-day mortality with regards to the side of the pneumonectomy. When comparing the groups who underwent neoadjuvant therapy versus surgery alone, there was also no significant difference in the incidence of bronchopleural fistula/empyema, respiratory failure, pneumonia, or arrhythmia. However, 30-day mortality in the neoadjuvant group was 21 % versus 6.1 % in the surgery alone group. The incidence of bronchopleural fistula and empyema was higher in patients undergoing neoadjuvant therapy and right pneumonectomy compared to left pneumonectomy (16.2 % versus 0 %) [5].

Maurizi et al. compared bronchial and/or vascular sleeve resection with patients undergoing pneumonectomy [6]. All patients received three cycles of chemotherapy consisting of cisplatin-gemcitabine, carboplatin-vinorelbine, or cisplatin-paclitaxel. Patients who underwent radiotherapy were excluded from this study. Thirty nine patients underwent sleeve lobectomy and 39 patients underwent pneumonectomy (19 right and 20 left). Final pathologic stage in the sleeve resection group was stage I in 17 (46.3 %), stage II in ten (25.6 %), and stage III in eight (20.5 %) patients. Complete pathological response was observed in four (10.3 %) patients. Final pathologic stage in the pneumonectomy group was stage I in six (15.4 %), stage II in 15 (38.5 %), and stage III in 18 (46.1 %) patients. 79.5 % of the sleeve resection group had down staging and 53.8 % of the pneumonectomy group had down staging. The postoperative complication rate in the pneumonectomy group was 33.3 % (13) and in the sleeve resection group was 28.2 % (11). There was one patient death in the pneumonectomy group immediately postoperatively (2.6 %) and none in the sleeve resection group. There was no difference in recurrence rate. The 3 and 5 year survival were 68.3 ± 8 and 64.8 ± 8 % for the sleeve resection group and 59.5 ± 5 and 34.5 ± 8 % for the pneumonectomy group. This may have reflected a much greater percentage of Stage III tumors in the pneumonectomy group. It is important to note that right-sided pneumonectomy did not confer a significant difference in morbidity or mortality [6].

Weder et al. retrospectively reviewed the perioperative mortality, morbidity, and outcome of 176 pneumonectomies done after induction chemotherapy or chemo radiotherapy in patients with locally advanced NSCLC [11]. Chemotherapy alone was given preoperatively to 20 % of the patients. Complete response was identified in 21 % of the patients. Of the 176 pneumonectomies, 49 % were performed on the right. The majority of the patients (138/176 or 78 %) underwent some form of an extended resection that included resection of pericardium (112), left atrium (28), parietal pleura (24), trachea/carina (9), chest wall (8), superior vena cava (8), pulmonary artery truncus (8), diaphragm (7), aorta (4), or esophageal wall (3). Postoperative 90-day mortality was 3 %. The deaths included pulmonary embolism (3), respiratory failure (2), and cardiac failure (1). Postoperative 90-day complication rate was 13 % and included pneumonia/ARDS (6), bronchial pleural fistula (5), empyema without bronchial pleural fistula (5), pulmonary embolism (3), hemothorax requiring reoperation (2), heart failure (1), and gastric herniation from a technical issue (1). Univariate logistics regression demonstrated with induction chemo radiotherapy there were fewer major postoperative complications than with chemotherapy alone. Univariate regression failed to show an influence on morbidity with the side and type of operation. Bronchial fistula occurred in three covered stumps (two right and one left pneumonectomy) and two uncovered stumps (all right pneumonectomy). Univariate regression did not show any difference with bronchopleural fistula and type of induction treatment or side of pneumonectomy. Median survival was 23 months. Three and five year survival was 43 and 38 % [11].

Stefani et al. retrospectively reviewed 175 patients treated with neoadjuvant chemotherapy for N2 NSCLC followed by surgical resection [7]. All chemotherapy regimens contained platinum. Within this cohort of patients, 79 (45 %) underwent pneumonectomy, eight of these were tracheal sleeve pneumonectomies. Within the postoperative period, eight (4.5 %) deaths occurred among all pulmonary resections. Six of these deaths occurred after pneumonectomy (7.6 % of all pneumonectomies). Four of the deaths occurred after right pneumonectomies. Within the study, responders to neoadjuvant chemotherapy undergoing pneumonectomy showed a 5-year survival of 34 % and a median survival time of 35.2 months versus 6 % and 15.4 months for non-responders. This is compared with the entire group that had a response to therapy with persistent N2 disease of 30 % and 29.8 months, patients with response to therapy with nodal down staging of 53 % and 60.5 months and nonresponders of 12 % and 19 months [7].

Gudbjartsson et al. from Sweden retrospectively compared the morbidity and mortality in 130 patients undergoing pneumonectomy [8]. Thirty-five (27 %) underwent preoperative chemotherapy, of whom 27 also received preoperative radiotherapy. Ninety-five patients were operated on without any induction treatment. Chemotherapy consisted of three cycles of mitomycin, vinblastine, and cisplatin; or carboplatin and paclitaxel. The radiation therapy was given in doses of 2 Gy up to 44 Gy. The bronchial stump was covered in 73 (56 %) patients, 25 (71.4 %) in the neoadjuvant group. The most common coverage was parietal pleura (30 patients), pericardial or mediastinal fat (17 patients) azygous vein (14 patients), muscle flaps (7 patients) and tissue glue (7 patients). Serious major complications occurred in five patients in the neoadjuvant group (14.3 %) and ten in the surgery only group (10.5 %); this was not statistically significantly difficult. These complications included bronchopleural fistula (BPF), major intraoperative bleeding, myocardial infarction, and respiratory insufficiency with ARDS. A BPF developed in seven right pneumonectomy patients and one left pneumonectomy patient (p = 0.001). Three of these fistulas were in the neoadjuvant group; this was not a significant increase over the surgery alone group. In six of these BPF patients, the stump was covered. Two patients in the surgery alone group developed cardiac herniation requiring immediate reoperation. Minor complications arose in 14 (40 %) patients in the neoadjuvant group and 31(32.6 %) patients in the surgery alone group. This was not significantly different. The most common minor complications seen were atrial fibrillation and congestive heart failure. Three patients were identified to have an empyema. This was treated with tube thoracostomy and antibiotics. Only one patient in the surgery alone group died within 30 days of surgery secondary to pneumonia and respiratory failure after aspiration. Logistic regression analysis demonstrated that the duration of symptoms and right-sided pneumonectomy were significantly associated with an increased risk of BPF. Neoadjuvant treatment, postoperative radiotherapy, or coverage of the bronchial stump had no effect on the risk of BPF. Median overall survival for the entire group was 28 months and there was no significant difference in survival of the two groups at 1 and 5 years. One and 5 year survival in the neoadjuvant group was 74 and 46 % and 72 and 34 % in the surgery alone group [8].

Cerfolio et al. described the results in two groups of patients with N2 NSCLC who underwent neoadjuvant radiotherapy [9]. One group received low dose radiation therapy at less than 60 Gy while the other group received high-dose radiation therapy at greater than 60 Gy. All patients received carboplatin-based

chemotherapy. In their analysis, they identified 12 patients that underwent pneumonectomy (7 on the right). Major complications combined were seven (58.3 %) (71 %
for right and 40 % for left pneumonectomy). Combined operative mortality was two
(16.7 %) (14 % for right and 20 % for left pneumonectomy. From the results of their
studies, these authors recommend avoiding neoadjuvant radiotherapy in any patient
that is known to require a pneumonectomy, especially a right-sided procedure [9].

Kappers et al. evaluated their stage IIIA NSCLC patients treated with surgery
following induction chemotherapy [10]. Thirty-nine patients underwent surgery
while one patient did not undergo resection. Of those undergoing resection there
were 19 lobectomies and 19 pneumonectomies (9 right). The perioperative morbidity after resection was seven after pneumonectomy and four after lobectomy, which
was not significantly different. The overall postoperative 30-day mortality was 3 %
and 90 day was 5 %. Median disease free survival for all patients was 24 months. In
the pneumonectomy group, this was 15 months. Recurrent disease occurred in 9
lobectomy patients and 13 pneumonectomy patients. The local control rate at
5 years was 58 % after lobectomy and 55 % after pneumonectomy. The 2 and 5 year
overall survival was 56 and 28 %. Survival after lobectomy was 43 % at 5 years and
16 % for the pneumonectomy group. In the lobectomy group, the first year mortality
and second year mortality rates were 11 and 21 % while in the pneumonectomy
group this was 26 and 58 %. The causes of death did not differ between the two
groups. In both univariate and multivariate analyses, lobectomy was associated with
favorable survival. From this study, the authors recommend avoiding pneumonectomy after induction therapy. Those patients requiring pneumonectomy due to a
central tumor should be evaluated for definitive chemoradiotherapy [10].

Alifano et al. analyzed their experience in 118 patients (54 underwent a right sided
procedure) treated with pneumonectomy after neoadjuvant chemotherapy [12]. The
bronchial suture line was protected in 56 patients with either pleural flap (31 patients)
or muscular flap (25 patients). There were no intraoperative deaths. There were seven
(5.9 %) postoperative deaths, four (7.4 %) after a right-sided procedure and three after
left pneumonectomy (4.6 %). Bronchopleural fistula (one patient), empyema without
fistula (one patient), postoperative pneumonia and acute respiratory distress (two
patients), cardiogenic shock (two patients), and rhabdomyolysis with renal failure
(one patient) accounted for the causes of death. Univariate analysis did not identify
side of operation as associated with postoperative death. Ninety-day mortality was
11 %. Median survival was 22 months. Three- and 5-year overall survival was 37.9
and 23.7 %. The authors concluded that pneumonectomy after chemotherapy is safe
with an acceptable rate of operative morbidity and mortality [12].

Recommendations

Based on the studies presented, we suggest that all advanced stage non-small cell
lung cancer cases should be evaluated in a multidisciplinary approach. Patients
undergoing induction or neoadjuvant therapy for resectable non-small cell lung cancer patients should undergo parenchymal conserving R0 resection when feasible.

Pneumonectomies after induction therapy should be performed in experienced centers; further study is necessary to determine what qualifies as a center of excellence for pneumonectomy. Right pneumonectomy after neoadjuvant therapy can be performed safely in experienced centers. If this is not feasible, then referral or treatment with definitive chemoradiotherapy should be strongly considered.

There is a dearth of randomized controlled trials evaluating this topic and therefore a strong recommendation concerning pneumonectomy in patients with non-small cell lung cancer undergoing neoadjuvant therapy cannot be definitively made.

A Personal View of the Data

All patients with possible N2 disease are evaluated for surgery as part of trimodality therapy. Mediastinal lymph nodes are evaluated by EBUS to allow for mediastinoscopy after induction therapy prior to surgery. Based on the randomized intergroup study results (INT 0139), patients with documented N2 disease who are potentially operable are treated with neoadjuvant cisplatin-based chemotherapy and 45 Gy radiation therapy. Patients who would require a right pneumonectomy are usually not considered for surgery and are treated with definitive combined chemotherapy and radiation therapy to 60–65 Gy. Patients who would require a lesser resection or a left pneumonectomy are evaluated approximately 3 weeks after completing induction therapy for progression of disease and operability with PET/CT and physiological testing. If felt to be operable, an EBUS and if necessary a mediastinoscopy is performed, most often at the time of possible exploration. The presence of persistent N2 metastasis is considered a contraindication to resection, and these patients are referred back to radiation oncology.

During resection, all bronchial stumps are covered with tissue using the omentum for left pneumonectomy and a healthy intercostal pedicle or pericardial fat pad for lobectomy.

Lymph nodes are extensively sampled but a full skeletonizing lymphadenectomy is not done as it is felt this may lead to bronchial stump devascularization and breakdown. Care is taken to limit fluid volume during the procedure and excessive pressure on the lung during re-inflation as these are felt to possibly contribute to post-operative ARDS, the most feared of post-operative complications. Although there is no hard evidence for their efficacy in preventing post-operative ARDS, intraoperative steroids are given especially if a pneumonectomy is done.

Post induction surgical resection remains one of the most technically challenging lung resections that a thoracic surgeon will perform. It should be avoided for the most part if a right pneumonectomy is required or N2 disease persists after induction therapy, and entirely if the patient is not robust enough to tolerate a very major procedure. There is some evidence that surgery can safely be performed if the radiation dose is increased to 60-65 Gy which obviates the problem of stopping radiation early for a patient subsequently found to be inoperable.

Recommendations

- All advanced stage non-small cell lung cancer cases should be evaluated using a multidisciplinary approach (Evidence quality low; weak recommendation).
- Patients undergoing induction or neoadjuvant therapy for resectable non-small cell lung cancer patients should undergo parenchymal conserving R0 resection when feasible (Evidence quality low; weak recommendation).
- Pneumonectomies after induction therapy should be performed in experienced centers. Further study is necessary to determine what qualifies as a center of excellence for pneumonectomy (Evidence quality low; weak recommendation).
- Right pneumonectomy after neoadjuvant therapy can be performed safely in experienced centers. If this is not feasible, then referral or treatment with definitive chemoradiotherapy should be strongly considered (Evidence quality low; weak recommendation).

References

1. Ginsberg RJ, Hill LD, Eagan RT, Thomas P, Mountain CF, Deslauriers J, et al. Modern thirty-day operative mortality for surgical resections in lung cancer. J Thorac Cardiovasc Surg. 1983;86(5):654–8. PubMed PMID: 6632940.
2. Daly BD, Fernando HC, Ketchedjian A, Dipetrillo TA, Kachnic LA, Morelli DM, et al. Pneumonectomy after high-dose radiation and concurrent chemotherapy for nonsmall cell lung cancer. Ann Thorac Surg. 2006;82(1):227–31. PubMed PMID: 16798219.
3. Albain KS, Swann RS, Rusch VW, Turrisi 3rd AT, Shepherd FA, Smith C, et al. Radiotherapy plus chemotherapy with or without surgical resection for stage III non-small-cell lung cancer: a phase III randomised controlled trial. Lancet. 2009;374(9687):379–86. PubMed PMID: 19632716.
4. Martin J, Ginsberg RJ, Abolhoda A, Bains MS, Downey RJ, Korst RJ, et al. Morbidity and mortality after neoadjuvant therapy for lung cancer: the risks of right pneumonectomy. Ann Thorac Surg. 2001;72(4):1149–54. PubMed PMID: 11603428.
5. d'Amato TA, Ashrafi AS, Schuchert MJ, Alshehab DS, Seely AJ, Shamji FM, et al. Risk of pneumonectomy after induction therapy for locally advanced non-small cell lung cancer. Ann Thorac Surg. 2009;88(4):1079–85. PubMed PMID: 19766784.
6. Maurizi G, D'Andrilli A, Anile M, Ciccone AM, Ibrahim M, Venuta F, et al. Sleeve lobectomy compared with pneumonectomy after induction therapy for non-small-cell lung cancer. J Thorac Oncol. 2013;8(5):637–43. PubMed PMID: 23584296.
7. Weder W, Collaud S, Eberhardt WE, Hillinger S, Welter S, Stahel R, et al. Pneumonectomy is a valuable treatment option after neoadjuvant therapy for stage III non-small-cell lung cancer. J Thorac Cardiovasc Surg. 2010;139(6):1424–30. PubMed PMID: 20416887.
8. Stefani A, Alifano M, Bobbio A, Grigoroiu M, Jouni R, Magdeleinat P, et al. Which patients should be operated on after induction chemotherapy for N2 non-small cell lung cancer? Analysis of a 7-year experience in 175 patients. J Thorac Cardiovasc Surg. 2010;140(2):356–63. PubMed PMID: 20381815.
9. Gudbjartsson T, Gyllstedt E, Pikwer A, Jonsson P. Early surgical results after pneumonectomy for non-small cell lung cancer are not affected by preoperative radiotherapy and chemotherapy. Ann Thorac Surg. 2008;86(2):376–82. PubMed PMID: 18640300.

10. Cerfolio RJ, Bryant AS, Spencer SA, Bartolucci AA. Pulmonary resection after high-dose and low-dose chest irradiation. Ann Thorac Surg. 2005;80(4):1224–30. discussion 30. PubMed PMID: 16181844.
11. Kappers I, van Sandick JW, Burgers SA, Belderbos JS, van Zandwijk N, Klomp HM. Surgery after induction chemotherapy in stage IIIA-N2 non-small cell lung cancer: why pneumonectomy should be avoided. Lung Cancer. 2010;68(2):222–7. PubMed PMID: 19664843.
12. Alifano M, Boudaya MS, Salvi M, Collet JY, Dinu C, Camilleri-Broet S, et al. Pneumonectomy after chemotherapy: morbidity, mortality, and long-term outcome. Ann Thorac Surg. 2008;85(6):1866–72. discussion 72–3. PubMed PMID: 18498785.

Chapter 15
Resection Versus SBRT for Stage I Non-small Cell Lung Cancer in Patients with Good Pulmonary Function

Michael Lanuti

Abstract Anatomic pulmonary resection with systematic lymph node sampling remains the accepted standard for patients with clinical stage I NSCLC. The widespread use of diagnostic chest computed tomography particularly for lung cancer screening has identified smaller tumors. Stereotactic body radiation therapy (SBRT) has emerged as an alternative for medically inoperable patients harboring stage I NSCLC. Results from phase II prospective clinical trials have demonstrated that SBRT is highly effective at primary tumor control while avoiding serious toxicity. The efficacy of SBRT in operable patients with stage I NSCLC is under investigation and evidence to compare treatment equivalency to surgical resection is lacking.

Keywords Stereotactic body radiotherapy • Stereotactic ablative radiotherapy • Lung cancer • Wedge • Sublobar resection • Lobectomy • Early stage • Surgery • Radiation therapy

Introduction

The cornerstone of treatment for stage I non small cell lung cancer (NSCLC) in good risk patients with preserved pulmonary function has primarily been surgical resection. Lobectomy has been the accepted standard of care based on an historical randomized data from the Lung Cancer Study Group [1]. The identification of smaller tumors by virtue of more widespread use of chest CT (particularly for lung

M. Lanuti, MD
Division of Thoracic Surgery, Massachusetts General Hospital, Harvard Medical School,
55 Fruit Street, Blake 1570, Boston, MA 02114, USA
e-mail: mlanuti@partners.org

M.K. Ferguson (ed.), *Difficult Decisions in Thoracic Surgery*,
Difficult Decisions in Surgery: An Evidence-Based Approach 1,
DOI 10.1007/978-1-4471-6404-3_15, © Springer-Verlag London 2014

cancer screening) has prompted a recalibration of surgical options (i.e., smaller anatomic resections) and consideration of ablative modalities. Sublobar approaches to stage IA (T1a-bN0) NSCLC have been extensively investigated over the past decade with comparable morbidity, reduced mortality, and equivalent cancer specific survival compared to the standard of lobectomy [2–4]. Non-operative strategies for stage I NSCLC such as stereotactic ablative radiotherapy (SABR), also known as stereotactic body radiation therapy (SBRT), have been prospectively evaluated in mostly medically inoperable patients with local control rates approximating 90 %, minimal serious toxicity, and survival rates that approach some surgical series [5–7]. To date there are no published randomized clinical trials comparing SBRT to surgical resection in medically operable patients diagnosed with clinical stage I NSCLC. There is no high level evidence available to address this topic.

Search Strategy

A targeted English language literature review was performed in Medline inclusive of publications from 1995 to 2013 looking at human research studies with abstracts. Search terms included [lobectomy OR segmentectomy OR wedge OR segmental resection OR sublobar resection OR stereotactic body radiation therapy OR stereotactic ablative radiotherapy OR stereotactic radiation treatment or stereotactic radiosurgery] AND [non small cell lung cancer OR carcinoma, non small cell lung] AND [survival OR toxicity] AND [stage I]. Studies with <50 patients or a median follow up <1 year were excluded. The search returned 462 papers of which 79 were clinical trials. Data were extracted and graded on quality and relevance to the subject. Twenty-six papers provided the best evidence to attempt to answer the question.

Description of Published Data

Surgical Approach to Stage I NSCLC

There is little doubt that anatomic resection (segmentectomy or lobectomy) affords the best curative approach for patients with stage I NSCLC with preserved cardiopulmonary function. The origin of this recommendation is derived from a single published RCT trial that indentified increased local recurrence (2.4-fold) with sublobar resection compared to lobectomy [1]. Wedge resections were associated with the largest (threefold) risk of recurrence. Local recurrence in surgical series has included recurrence within the same lobe away from the primary site and sometimes within an ipsilateral non-primary lobe or ipsilateral hilar lymph nodes. This definition becomes very important when interpreting local recurrence in studies using ablative therapies. Worldwide 5-year survival for surgically treated NSCLC derived from the 7th edition International Association for the Study of Lung Cancer staging project approaches 73 % for stage IA (T1a-bN0) NSCLC and 58 % for stage IB (T2aN0) [8].

The need for lobectomy in smaller tumors has been challenged in many publications [4, 9–11] over the past decade where sublobar resections (mostly segmentectomy) have been found to have equivalent locoregional control and freedom from recurrence (Table 15.1). Two phase III randomized trials have been developed to address the question of extent of resection for small tumors. The National Cancer Institute launched a RCT in 2008 (CALGB 140503) to compare lobectomy versus sublobar resection for small (≤2 cm) peripheral NSCLC. The Japan Clinical Oncology Group launched a RCT in 2009 investigating lobectomy and sublobar resection for small-sized carcinoma (mixed solid and ground glass; solid component ≤2 cm). These data will be very important for practice changes, however neither study has reported on results. In a recent meta-analysis examining 11,360 patients from 24 studies, lobectomy was associated with improved overall and cancer specific survival (HR 1.4; 95 % CI (1.15–1.69); p=0.0006) compared to sublobar resection (inclusive of tumors ≤5 cm) for stage I NSCLC. This same analysis showed no difference in survival in the subgroup of patients with T1a (≤2 cm) tumors. Furthermore, the meta-analysis showed no difference in survival when specifically comparing segmentectomy to lobectomy for stage I tumors.

The potential pitfalls associated with wedge resections have prompted many thoracic surgeons to either limit their use to small tumors (in the range of 1 cm) where an adequate margin of normal tissue is easier to obtain or add brachytherapy with iodine-125 (^{125}I) seeds to the wedge margin, a technique in which reported local recurrence rates are in the single digits (about 3.3 %) [12].

Stereotactic Body Radiation Therapy for Stage I NSCLC

SBRT has emerged as the preferred treatment approach for stage I NSCLC in patients with peripheral tumors who refuse surgery or are deemed medically inoperable. Evidence of efficacy in lung cancer has been accumulating since 1995 and mostly comes from retrospective observational series (single and multi-institution) and some prospective phase I/II clinical trials. Many of the trials are populated with patients who refuse surgery and patients who are deemed too high risk for surgery. One of the largest contributions to the SBRT literature (with >5-year follow-up) comes from Japan where investigators reported on 257 patients from 14 different hospitals and showed the importance of dose response. The local recurrence rate was significantly lower for a BED (biologic effective dose) of ≥100 Gy compared with a BED <100 Gy (8.4 versus 42.9 %, p=0.01). Disease specific 5-year survival was 73.2 % in the total cohort where 99 patients were considered operable. The overall 5-year survival rates of medically operable and inoperable patients were 64.8 and 35.0 %, respectively [5]. The improved survival in operable patients treated

Table 15.1 Pulmonary resection

Study	N	Treatment	Results	Median F/U	Quality of evidence
Ginsberg et al. [1] Randomized controlled trial	Stage I = 247 (tumors ≤3 cm)	Lobectomy = 125 vs Limited resection = 122 Segment = 82 Wedge = 40	LR = 6.5 % lobe LR = 17.5 % sublobar 5-year OS and CSS no difference between lobar vs sublobar	NR	High
Fernando et al. [12] Retrospective multicenter	Stage IA = 291	Lobectomy = 167 Sublobar = 124 (60 + Brachytherapy)	LR Sublobar = 17.2 % LR Sublobar + Brachy = 3.3 %	34.5 months	Low
Okada et al. [4] Prospective multicenter	Stage IA = 567	Lobectomy = 262 vs Sublobar = 305 Segment = 230 Wedge = 30	5-years DFS Lobe 83 % 5-years DFS Sublob 86 % 5-years OS Lobe 89 % 5-years OS Sublob 90 %	>60 months	Moderate
Schuchert et al. [9] Retrospective	Stage IA = 325	Lobectomy = 235 Segmentectomy = 178	LRR Lobe = 5.3 % LRR Segment = 5.2 % RFS Lobe = 79 % RFS Segment = 77 %	31.8 months	Low
Fan et al. [10] Meta analysis 24 studies	Stage I = 11,360	Lobectomy versus Sublobar (wedge or segmentectomy)	All tumors: improved OS/CSS with lobectomy HR 1.4 (p=0.0006) Tumors ≤2 cm OS/CSS no difference Lobe vs segment OS/CSS no difference	NR	Moderate
Tsutani et al. [11] Retrospective	Stage IA = 481	Lobectomy = 383 Segmentectomy = 98	3-years RFS 87 % 3-years RFS 91 % p=0.14	43.2 months	Moderate

NR not reported, *OS* overall survival, *CSS* cancer specific survival, *RFS* recurrence free survival, *LRR* locoregional recurrence

with SBRT has been corroborated in other prospective series [13, 14] and likely speaks to the negative influence of medical comorbidities in high risk patients. Data supporting the use of standardized SBRT dosing in stage I NSCLC in North America was examined in strictly medically inoperable patients in a phase II multi-institution study (RTOG 0236) [7]. Fifty-five patients with T1/T2 NSCLC were treated with 54 Gy (three fractions × 18 Gy) and followed for recurrence and survival over 2 years. Four patients failed at the primary site or within the same lobe rendering a 3-year local control rate = 91 %. Combining local and regional failures, the 3-year local-regional control rate was 87 %. Disease-free survival and overall survival at 3 years were 48.3 and 55.8 %, respectively.

The lack of dose uniformity and optimal fractionation of SBRT for stage I NSCLC can be seen in Table 15.2. Many of these studies are also limited by a median follow up ≤36 months. Results from both retrospective and prospective series (Table 15.2) show 3-year OS and DFS approaching 57 and 81 %, respectively [13, 15–17]. Five year overall and cancer specific survival after SBRT treatment are mostly absent in the literature thus making comparisons to surgical series of stage I NSCLC rather limited. Although some of the series have operable patients that refuse surgery [5, 13, 17, 18], there are few data to render conclusions regarding the role of SBRT in patients with preserved lung function. One of the more compelling retrospective series reported on 87 medically operable patients with stage IA (n = 65) or stage IB (n = 22) NSCLC treated with SBRT where 5-year OS = 72 % for stage IA and 62 % for stage IB [19]. These results are very similar to surgical series for stage I NSCLC and have spawned the development of clinical trials to compare SBRT to surgery.

Most trials report no significant change in measured pulmonary function following SBRT. Treatment-related toxicities include fatigue and injury to skin, chest wall, lung, brachial plexus and central thoracic structures (i.e. segmental bronchi or pulmonary vasculature). Toxicity increases with cumulative dose, although high-grade toxicities are uncommon in peripheral tumors and treatment-related deaths are rare. Symptomatic radiation pneumonitis (grade 2–4) has been observed in up to 9 % of patients and can be recognized within a median time of about 3.5 months [20]. Organ volume, previous thoracic radiation, and radiosensitizing chemotherapy increase the risk of toxicity. Timmerman reported an 11-fold increased risk of severe toxicity in the treatment of central tumors compared to peripheral tumors [21]. Among patients experiencing toxicity, the median time to observation was 10.5 months. In more recent series, other investigators have adopted a tailored approach to central tumors with smaller fractions (3–8) greatly reducing observed toxicity [22].

Clinical trials have been developed to address whether SBRT can replace surgery for certain patients, the optimal dose-fractionation scheme, and how best to treat patients having central tumors near the proximal tracheobronchial tree. The American College of Surgeons Oncology Group (ACOSOG) and the Radiation Therapy and Oncology Group (RTOG) are accruing patients to a phase III randomized study (RTOG 1021/ACOSOG Z4099) comparing stereotactic body radiotherapy and sublobar resection (with or without brachytherapy) for high-risk operable

Table 15.2 Stereotactic body radiation therapy

Study	N	Treatment	Results	Median F/U	Quality of evidence
Timmerman et al. [21]	Stage IA = 35 Stage IB = 35	SBRT	Local failure 4.3 % Distant failure 10 %	17.5 months	Low
Prospective		Total dose 60 – 66 Gy (3 fractions)	2-years OS 54.7 %		
Onishi et al. [5]	Stage IA = 164	SBRT (variable dose and schedule)	Local failure 14 % Regional failure 11 % Distant failure 20 %	38 months	Low
Retrospective multicenter	Stage IB = 93 99 medically operable	Median tumor = 2.8 cm	Local failure 8.4 % when BED > 100 5-years DFS 73.2 % 5-years OS 47.2 %		
Lagerwaard et al. [18]	Stage IA = 129 Stage IB = 90	SBRT	Local failure 3 % Regional failure 4 % Distant failure 15 %	12 months	Low
Retrospective	39 medically operable	Total dose 60 Gy (3–8 fractions)	2-years DFS (T1) 81 % 2-years DFS (T1) 54 % 2-years OS 64 %		
Fakris et al. [15]	Stage IA = 34 Stage IB = 36	SBRT	Local failure 5.7 % Regional failure 8.6 % Distant failure 12.9 %	50.2 months	Moderate
Prospective single center observation		Total dose 60 – 66 Gy (3 fractions)	3-years DFS 81.7 % 3-years OS 42.7 %		
Timmerman et al. [7]	Stage IA = 44 Stage IB = 11	SBRT	Local failure 10 % Regional failure 13 % Distant failure 22 %	34.4 months	Moderate
Prospective multicenter phase II trial		Total dose 54 Gy (3 × 18 Gy) Tumor <5 cm	3-years DFS 48.3 % 3-years OS 55.8 %		

Study	Design	Patients	Treatment (dose)	Outcomes	Follow-up	Quality
Haasbeek et al. [17]	Retrospective	Stage IA = 118, Stage IB = 85; 41 medically operable	SBRT; Total dose 60 Gy (3–8 fractions)	Local failure 11 %, Regional failure 8.4 %, Distant failure 21 %; 3-years DFS 72.6 %, 3-years OS 45.1 %	12.6 months	Low
Ricardi et al. [16]	Prospective single center phase II trial	Stage IA = 43, Stage IB = 19; 6 medically operable	SBRT; Total dose 45 Gy (3×15 Gy)	Local failure 3.2 %, Regional failure 6.4 %, Distant failure 24 %; 3-years DFS 72.5 %, 3-years OS 57.1 %	28 months	Low
Onishi et al. [19]	Retrospective multicenter	Stage IA = 65, Stage IB = 22; All medically operable, refused surgery	SBRT; Total dose 45-72 Gy (3–10 fractions)	5-years Local failure T1 = 92 %, T2 = 73 %; 5-years OS stage IA 72 %, 5-years OS stage IB 62 %	55 months	Low
Haasbeek et al. [22]	Retrospective	Hilar = 37 Bordering mediastinal structures = 26	SBRT; Total dose 60 Gy (8×7.5 Gy)	Local failure 7.3 %; 3-years OS 64.3 %	35 months	Low
Shibamoto et al. [13]	Prospective multicenter phase II trial	Stage IA = 128, Stage IB = 52; 60 medically operable	SBRT; Total dose 44-52 Gy (3 fractions)	Operable 3-years OS = 74 %; Inoperable 3-years OS = 59 % (p=0.08); Local failure 14 % tumors <3 cm; Local failure 27 % tumor >3 cm	36 months	Low
Grillis et al. [14]	Prospective multicenter series	Stage IA = 318, Stage IB = 167; 56 medically operable	SBRT; Total dose 18-64 Gy (1–15 fractions)	2-years RFS 89 %, 2-years OS 60 %; Operable 2-years OS = 78 %; Inoperable 2-years OS = 58 % (p=0.006); Biopsy proven local failure = 10 %	15 months	Low

NR not reported, *OS* overall survival, *DFS* disease free survival, *RFS* recurrence free survival

patients with non-small cell lung cancer. Japanese investigators have completed enrollment on a nationally funded phase II trial (Japanese Clinical Oncology group 0403) of SBRT in operable patients and are obtaining prospective patient outcomes. In North America RTOG 0618 completed accrual to a phase II study of SBRT (20 Gy × 3 fractions) in operable patients with stage I or II NSCLC. Eligible patients included peripheral T1 or T2/3 tumors ≤5 cm who are considered reasonable surgical candidates by virtue of pulmonary function and a qualified thoracic surgeon. The results of this study will be available in 2015. Unfortunately, two phase III randomized trials comparing SBRT with surgery have closed due to poor accrual: a randomized trial of either surgery or SBRT for early stage IA lung cancer (ROSEL) in the Netherlands and the Accuray Corporation sponsored Cyberknife worldwide trial.

Several retrospective case-matched series (Table 15.3) comparing SBRT to surgery have been published [23–25]. Loco-regional recurrence was similar in the matched cohorts except for a series comparing VATS lobectomy to SBRT [26] where reduced local recurrence favored SBRT with median follow up = 16 months. Some postulate that SBRT may stimulate an immune response to tumor. Though overall survival was improved in the surgical cohorts compared to SBRT, there was no significant difference in cause-specific survival between the two groups. In high risk patients with stage I NSCLC, SBRT was found to be less costly compared to surgery, but surgery was more cost-effective by virtue of prolonged overall survival [25].

Summary of Published Data and Influence on Clinical Practice

SBRT has revolutionized how lung cancers can be managed. SBRT is a reasonable option for medically inoperable stage I NSCLC by virtue of prospective clinical trials [29]; however, its curative role in good risk operable patients has not been evaluated in phase III clinical trials. Until results from well executed randomized studies become available, patients must be evaluated by a multidisciplinary team including radiation oncologists, thoracic surgeons, and medical oncologists to tailor therapy to individual patients. Several phase III trials were initiated but struggled to accrue since thoracic surgeons have difficulty with non-operative therapy for early stage lung cancer in otherwise healthy patients. Despite local control rates that approach 90 %, SBRT does not offer tumor tissue for genotyping nor regional/mediastinal lymph nodes to uncover occult metastases [28]. Lobectomy remains the appropriate treatment for stage I NSCLC patients in good risk patients with preserved lung function. Sublobar resection can be safely considered in patients with limited pulmonary function where wedge resection is associated with the highest risk of local recurrence. Optimal management of T1a (≤2 cm) stage I NSCLC includes surgical resection where phase III data will contribute to parenchymal sparing strategies (i.e., wedge or segmentectomy) versus lobectomy. SBRT for early stage NSCLC should only be offered to medically operable patients in the setting of a clinical trial.

Table 15.3 SBRT versus surgery

Study	N	Treatment	Results	Median F/U	Quality of evidence
Crabtree et al. [23]	Stage I = 538	Surgery = 462	Surgery 3-years OS = 68 % 3-years CSS = 82 % Local control 94 %	19 months	Low
Retrospective		SBRT = 76	SBRT 3-years OS = 32 % 3-year CSS = 82 % Local control = 89 %		
Grills et al. [24]	Stage I = 124	SBRT = 58	Local failure: NS SBRT 4 % Wedge 20 %	24 months	Low
Retrospective		Wedge = 69	Regional failure: NS SBRT 4 % Wedge 18 % Distant failure: NS SBRT 21 % Wedge 19 % Wedge OS 87 % * SBRT OS 72 %		
Puri et al. [25]	Stage I = 114	SBRT = 57	SBRT 3-year OS = 46 % (NS) 3-year CSS = 87 % (NS)	NR	Low
Retrospective		Sublobar = 57	Surgery 3-year OS = 60 % 3-year CSS = 77.6 %		
		Propensity matched	Surgery more cost effective		
Verstegen et al. [26]	Stage I = 128	VATS lobectomy = 64 SBRT = 64	Lobectomy 3-year LRF = 17 % 3-year PFS = 79 % 3-year OS = 77 %	16 month	Low
Retrospective		Propensity matched	SBRT 3-years LRF = 6 % (p = .04) 3-years PFS = 63 % (p = .09) OS = 80 % (p = 0.8)		

NS not significant, *OS* overall survival, *CSS* cancer specific survival, *LRF* locoregional failure, *PFS* progression free survival

A Personal View of the Data

In good risk patients diagnosed with clinical stage I NSCLC there are no competing threats to their survival except for cancer recurrence. Therapeutic options must control local disease and reduce the risk of locoregional and systemic recurrence. Since 4–15 % of clinical stage I NSCLC are upstaged at the time of pulmonary resection [26, 27], ablative non-operative therapy can be associated with understaging and inadequate cancer treatment in otherwise low risk patients. This phenomenon will challenge clinical equipoise and make it very difficult for surgeons to randomize their patients to a clinical trial investigating SBRT versus pulmonary resection. Tumor size (<2 cm), radiographic appearance (ground glass versus solid) and histology subtype (adenocarcinoma vs squamous cell carcinoma) may become even more important when constructing parameters to randomize good risk patients. In the absence of randomized data, SBRT should be reserved for patients with stage I NSCLC who refuse surgery or are high risk and deemed medically inoperable by a qualified thoracic surgeon. Appropriate lung cancer staging remains paramount even in high risk patients.

Recommendations

- SBRT is a reasonable option for medically inoperable stage I NSCLC. (Evidence quality low; weak recommendation)
- Lobectomy is the appropriate treatment for stage I NSCLC patients in good risk patients with preserved lung function. (Evidence quality high; strong recommendation)
- Sublobar resection can be considered in patients with limited pulmonary function. (Evidence quality low; weak recommendation)

References

1. Ginsberg RJ, Rubinstein LV. Randomized trial of lobectomy versus limited resection for T1 N0 non-small cell lung cancer. Lung Cancer Study Group. Ann Thorac Surg. 1995;60:615–22.
2. Keenan RJ, Landreneau RJ, Maley Jr RH, et al. Segmental resection spares pulmonary function in patients with stage I lung cancer. Ann Thorac Surg. 2004;78:228–33.
3. El-Sherif A, Gooding WE, Santos R, et al. Outcomes of sublobar resection versus lobectomy for stage I NSCLC. Ann Thorac Surg. 2006;82(2):408–15.
4. Okada M, Koike T, Higashiyama M, Yamato Y, Kodama K, Tsubota N. Radical sublobar resection for small-sized NSCLC: a multicenter study. J Thorac Cardiovasc Surg. 2006;132(4):769–75.
5. Onishi H, Shirato H, Nagata Y, et al. Hypofractionated stereotactic radiotherapy for stage I non-small cell lung cancer: updated results of 257 patients in a Japanese multi-institutional study. J Thorac Oncol. 2007;2:S94–100.

6. Baumann P, Nyman J, Hoyer M, et al. Outcome in a prospective phase II trial of medically inoperable stage I non–small-cell lung cancer patients treated with stereotactic body radiotherapy. J Clin Oncol. 2009;27:3290–6.
7. Timmerman R, Paulus R, Galvin J, et al. Stereotactic body radiation therapy for inoperable early stage lung cancer. J Am Med Assoc. 2010;303:1070–6.
8. Goldstraw P, Crowley J, Chansky K, et al. The IASLC Lung Cancer Staging Project: proposals for the revision of the TNM stage groupings in the forthcoming (seventh) edition of the TNM Classification of malignant tumours. J Thorac Oncol. 2007;2(8):706–14.
9. Schuchert MJ, Abbas G, Awais O. Anatomic segmentectomy for the solitary pulmonary nodule and early-stage lung cancer. Ann Thorac Surg. 2012;93(6):1780–5.
10. Fan J, Wang L, Jiang GN, Gao W. Sublobectomy versus lobectomy for stage I non-small-cell lung cancer, a meta-analysis of published studies. Ann Surg Oncol. 2012;19(2):661–8.
11. Tsutani Y, Miyata Y, Nakayama H, et al. Oncologic outcomes of segmentectomy compared with lobectomy for clinical stage IA lung adenocarcinoma: propensity score–matched analysis in a multicenter study. J Thorac Cardiovasc Surg. 2013;146(2):358–64.
12. Fernando HC, Santos RS, Benfield JR, Grannis FW, Keenan RJ, Luketich JD, et al. Lobar and sublobar resection with and without brachytherapy for small stage IA non-small cell lung cancer. J Thorac Cardiovasc Surg. 2005;129:261–7.
13. Shibamoto Y, Hashizume C, Baba F, et al. Stereotactic body radiotherapy using a radiobiology-based regimen for stage I nonsmall cell lung cancer. Cancer. 2012;118(8):2078–84.
14. Grills IS, Hope AJ, Guckenberger M, et al. A collaborative analysis of stereotactic lung radiotherapy outcomes for early-stage non-small-cell lung cancer using daily online cone-beam computed tomography image-guided radiotherapy. J Thorac Oncol. 2012;7(9):1382–93.
15. Fakiris AJ, McGarry RC, Yiannoutsos CT, et al. Stereotactic body radiation therapy for early-stage non-small-cell lung carcinoma: four-year results of a prospective phase II study. Int J Radiat Oncol Biol Phys. 2009;75:677–82.
16. Ricardi U, Filippi AR, Guarneri A, et al. Stereotactic body radiation therapy for early stage non-small cell lung cancer: results of a prospective trial. Lung Cancer. 2010;68:72–7.
17. Haasbeek CJ, Lagerwaard FJ, Antonisse ME, Slotman BJ, Senan S. Stage I non small cell lung cancer in patients aged > or=75 years: outcomes after stereotactic radiotherapy. Cancer. 2010;116:406–14.
18. Lagerwaard FJ, Haasbeek CJ, Smit EF, Slotman BJ, Senan S. Outcomes of risk-adapted fractionated stereotactic radiotherapy for stage I non-small cell lung cancer. Int J Radiat Oncol Biol Phys. 2008;70:685–92.
19. Onishi H, Shirato H, Nagata Y, et al. Stereotactic body radiotherapy (SBRT) for operable stage I non-small-cell lung cancer: can SBRT be comparable to surgery? Int J Radiat Oncol Biol Phys. 2011;81:1352–8.
20. Barriger RB, Forquer JA, Brabham JG. A dose-volume analysis of radiation pneumonitis in non-small cell lung cancer patients treated with stereotactic body radiation therapy. Int J Radiat Oncol Biol Phys. 2012;82(1):457–62.
21. Timmerman R, McGarry R, Yiannoutsos C, et al. Excessive toxicity when treating central tumors in a phase II study of stereotactic body radiation therapy for medically inoperable early-stage lung cancer. J Clin Oncol. 2006;24:4833–9.
22. Haasbeek CJ, Lagerwaard FJ, Slotman BJ, Senan S. Outcomes of stereotactic ablative radiotherapy for centrally located early-stage lung cancer. J Thorac Oncol. 2011;6:2036–43.
23. Crabtree TD, Denlinger CE, Meyers BF. Stereotactic body radiation therapy versus surgical resection for stage I non-small cell lung cancer. J Thorac Cardiovasc Surg. 2010;140(2):377–86.
24. Grills IS, Mangona VS, Welsh R, et al. Outcomes after stereotactic lung radiotherapy or wedge resection for stage I non-small-cell lung cancer. J Clin Oncol. 2010;28:928–35.
25. Puri V, Crabtree TD, Kymes S, et al. A comparison of surgical intervention and stereotactic body radiation therapy for stage I lung cancer in high-risk patients: a decision analysis. J Thorac Cardiovasc Surg. 2012;143(2):428–36.

26. Verstegen NE, Oosterhuis JW, Palma DA, et al. Stage I–II non-small-cell lung cancer treated using either stereotactic ablative radiotherapy (SABR) or lobectomy by VATS: outcomes of a propensity score-matched analysis. Ann Oncol. 2013;24(6):1543–8.
27. Boffa DJ, Kosinski AS, Paul S, Mitchell JD, Onaitis M. Lymph node evaluation by open or video-assisted approaches in 11,500 anatomic lung cancer resections. Ann Thorac Surg. 2012;94(2):347–53.
28. Darling GE, Allen MS, Decker PA, et al. Randomized trial of mediastinal lymph node sampling versus complete lymphadenectomy during pulmonary resection in the patient with N0 or N1 (less than hilar) non-small cell carcinoma: results of the American College of Surgery Oncology Group Z0030 Trial. J Thorac Cardiovasc Surg. 2011;141(3):662–70.
29. Mahmood S, Bilal H, Faivre-Finn C, Shah R. Is stereotactic ablative radiotherapy equivalent to sublobar resection in high-risk surgical patients with Stage I NSCLC? Interact Cardiovasc Thorac Surg. 2013;17(5):845–53.

Chapter 16
Digital Drainage Systems After Major Lung Resection

Gonzalo Varela

Abstract Prolonged air leak after lung resection is the most prevalent complication and a source of other morbidities and considerable expenses. Digital pleural drainage systems have appeared in the market claiming to be useful tools for improved postoperative patients' care and control. To date, there is strong evidence in the literature demonstrating that the use of these devices helps to standardize postoperative care. Other advantages (such are their effect on decreasing hospital staying and costs per procedure or the usefulness of stored data for better understanding the physiology of the pleura after lung resection) are still waiting to be proved.

Keywords Pulmonary lobectomy • Pleural drainage • Pleural suction • Prolonged air leak • Pleural pressure

Introduction

Although a relatively minor issue in Thoracic Surgery, proper pleural drainage technique after major lung resection has to be regarded as crucial since prolonged air leak (PAL) after lung resection other than pneumonectomy is the most frequent postoperative adverse event and a cause of considerable expenses [1]. Years ago, in a randomized clinical trial the use of simple plastic bags incorporating a one way flutter valve was demonstrated to be as effective as water seal drains in terms of

G. Varela, MD, PhD
Thoracic Surgery Service, Department of Thoracic Surgery, Salamanca University Hospital and Medical School, Paseo de San Vicente 58, 37007 Salamanca, Spain
e-mail: gvs@usal.es

M.K. Ferguson (ed.), *Difficult Decisions in Thoracic Surgery*,
Difficult Decisions in Surgery: An Evidence-Based Approach 1,
DOI 10.1007/978-1-4471-6404-3_16, © Springer-Verlag London 2014

patients' mobility and postoperative complications [2]. These inexpensive systems have not gained popularity among thoracic surgeons and nowadays more objective information leading to quicker and more accurate chest tube management is demanded in clinical settings.

One year after the publication in 2006 regarding the AIRFIX®, the first digital system for the quantification of the air flow through chest tubes after lung resection [3], Dernevik et al. [4] published their experience with the first commercialized digital pleural drainage unit allowing clinicians to measure both air flow and pressures in the tubing system. According to the developers [3], AIRFIX® was helpful for the diagnosis and management of the postoperative air leaks, permitting chest tube removal without tentative clamping. For Dernevik et al. [4], the capacity of the device for saving data on air flow and pressure was a useful tool for future research in the field of lung surgery. Currently, three digital drainage systems are available in the market having the capacity to measure air flow from the pleural space; in addition, all these devices incorporate a battery powered portable suction pump. Depending on the model, air flow trends can be visualized in a small display window and, optionally, stored data can be exported to a computer for further analysis[1]. The manufacturers' claim several advantages of digital devices, which can be summarized as follows:

• Standardized postoperative care
• Facilitation of early ambulation
• Decreased length of hospital stay and costs
• Improved knowledge through the analysis of exported data

Obviously, switching from conventional to digital devices in a busy Thoracic Surgery unit represents at least an initial increase in acquisition costs, and the long term clinical or economic advantages should be based on sound scientific evidence. In this chapter we discuss the literature on the advantages of the use of digital drainages in Thoracic Surgery.

Search Strategy

Our search strategy was to use the terms ((("2000"[Date – Publication]: "2013"[Date – Publication])) AND (("controlled clinical trial"[Publication Type] OR "meta analysis"[Publication Type] OR "randomized controlled trial"[Publication Type]))) AND (pleural drainage OR pleural suction) AND (lobectomy OR lung resection) on PUBMED. Due to the low numbers of high evidence papers, some case series were also included.

---

[1] Specific characteristics of each commercially available system are neither reviewed nor discussed in this text. The reader can find more information visiting the corporate web pages at: http://old. atmosmed.com/html/seiten/produkte;products;kat,17;910,en.html?PHPSESSID = 49ed7e-ba9ac21fdb048b52640bc48c32; http://www.redax.it/index.asp?ind = famiglia_2.asp; and http://www.medela.com/US/en/healthcare/products/thoracic-drainage/thopaz.html [cited 19 Aug 2013].

Results

Standardized Postoperative Care

Unwarranted variations in medical care (those that cannot be explained by type or severity of illness or by patient preferences) have become a major concern for health organizations [5] and a source of unjustified expenses and morbidity. In Thoracic Surgery, standardized clinical care has been demonstrated to reduce hospital costs with no compromise of the quality of care [6]. On the other hand, increased hospital length of stay following pulmonary resection is due primarily to prolonged air leaks [7] and also to surgeons' personal practices [8]. Thus, the hypothesis that an objective assessment of the presence and amount of postoperative air leak could decrease variations and hospital staying seems to be justified.

The first part of the hypothesis was demonstrated in a prospective study in which a series of patients undergoing major thoracic procedures were randomly allocated to receive a standard or a digital system for pleural drainage [9]. At morning rounds, two surgeons with comparable experience and blinded one to the other's advice recorded his recommendation on whether or not to remove the chest tubes. After completing a series of cases, the inter observer agreement was calculated. While in the traditional group the *kappa* coefficient was 0.37, in the digital series of cases it was 0.88, allowing us to conclude that differences in clinical judgment disappeared with the use of a digital pleural system.

Our results were reproduced by Brunelli et al. [10]. In their study, discrepancies between surgeons were minimized and additionally it was shown that both time to chest tubes withdrawn and total hospital days were decreased. The effect of digital drainage on hospitalization has been studied also by others and their results are shown below.

Therefore, the hypothesis that the use of digital drainage increases agreement between surgeons and is an effective way of decreasing variations in clinical practice has been demonstrated at least in two randomized clinical studies and a sound recommendation can be stated on this.

Facilitation of Early Ambulation

The second advantage claimed for the use of digital drainage is that, thanks to mobile suction, early ambulation of the patients is warranted. As a consequence, more comfort and less postoperative morbidity is theorized for patients undergoing lung resection, but this is arguable.

The clinical advantages of active pleural suction after lung resection (excluding, of course pneumonectomy) have been compared to passive suction by gravity in several randomized clinical trials [11–16] and the evidence has been reviewed in at least four meta-analysis or systematic reviews of the literature [17–20]. Clinical trials have been aimed ascertaining whether the use of active suction represents an advantage in terms of: occurrence of prolonged air leak, drainage time, length of hospital stay or postoperative pneumothorax. Regarding prolonged air leak, in only one out of six trials [16] did the authors find that active suction decreases the occurrence of the complication. In the rest of the papers, there is unanimity stating that the risk of air leaks is not modified by the suction modality, either active or passive. Nevertheless, the authors of all systematic reviews and meta-analyses warn the reader about the bias and methodological differences among the studies lowering the strength of the recommendation on the use of postoperative suction or not.

Starting November 2002, all patients undergoing major thoracic procedures in our unit were included in intensive chest physiotherapy program including early mobilization. In a retrospective analysis of matched lobectomy patients we have reported [21] an impressive decrease of the risk of pulmonary complications which is directly related to the physiotherapy program. Thus, significant improvements can be gained in perioperative care after lung resection not related at all to the type of pleural drainages or suction modality.

Therefore, no evidence-based recommendation can be drawn from the literature. Obviously, for those surgeons believing that active suction after lung resection represents an advantage for their patients, portable devices facilitate early ambulation but with the current data, the cost-effectiveness of this practice cannot be demonstrated.

Decreased Length of Hospital Stay and Cost

According to manufacturers and sellers, digital pleural devices help to decrease hospital stay after lung resection and, as a direct consequence, hospital costs per procedure are lower. In three published investigations [10, 22, 23] the authors have found reductions in the time of chest tube drainage and in the length of hospitalization in the cohort of patients in which digital devices were used. Since overall morbidity for both cohorts of patients in these papers was comparable, the reported reductions in hospital stay should be a consequence of more standardized chest tube management.

The clinical relevance of the reduction in length of hospitalization should be discussed. In the cited papers, it was less than 1 day and, from there, a decrease in the cost per process was estimated at around 500 € [10]. Thus, the adoption of a policy of routinely using digital systems after lobectomy or segmentectomy has to be well balanced against the expected advantages. Maybe digital devices could be cost-effective if used only in cases with a high probability of a postoperative air leak, but this statement has yet to be demonstrated.

Improved Knowledge Through the Analysis of Exported Data

Some of the digital devices available on the market incorporate electronic systems for recording and exporting data to a computer (usually though an SD card). The analysis of instantaneous data and trending of pleural pressures and air flow is

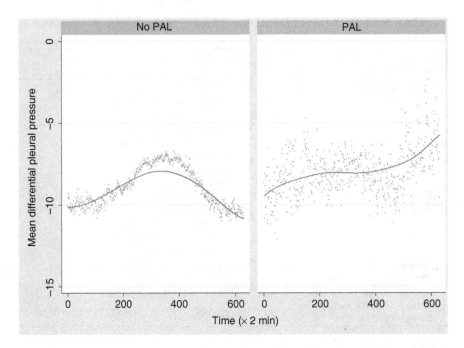

Fig. 16.1 Mean differential pressure trending in the first hours after pulmonary lobectomy. *Left*: patients experiencing prolonged air leak (more than 5 days) through chest tube. *Right*: patients without the complication. Using these data, a mathematical model can be constructed to predict the occurrence of prolonged air leak with the records from the first postoperative hours

proposed as a way for better understanding the pleural mechanics after lung resection for future improvements in postoperative care.

To date, only a few papers analyzing data stored in a digital pleural device have been published. Two papers [24, 25] deal with the analysis of pleural pressure recordings along different segments of the postoperative period and under different situations; these publications have not been followed by clinical applications. The risk of prolonged air leak has been correlated to the pleural pressures in the hours following completion of the surgical procedure. In a series of 136 lobectomy patients [26], we found that the mean expiratory and differential pressures during the second 12 h (between 12 and 24 h) after the operation were consistently associated with PAL (p=0.014) (Fig. 16.1). Thus, measuring the intrapleural pressures with digital devices in the postoperative period could allow us to predict the occurrence of prolonged air leak and implement strategies for early discharge with chest tubes in place for otherwise uncomplicated patients. Similar findings were reported by Brunelli et al. [27]. In their investigation, the level of air leak and pleural pressure through chest tubes at the 6th postoperative hour was associated with the duration of air leak. To my knowledge, these findings have not been applied to early discharge programs after lobectomy.

According to the data in the literature, storing data on the flow of air through chest tubes or on the postoperative pleural pressures still awaits identification of clinical applications and may be interesting only from a theoretical point of view.

Table 16.1 Evidence and recommendations on the use of digital drainage systems after lung resection

Supposed advantage of the use of digital devices	Grade of evidence	Recommendation	Strength of recommendation
Standardized postoperative care facilitated	High	Use digital devices if large variations in clinical practice regarding pleural tubes management are detected	Strong
Early ambulation facilitated	Very low	Not applicable to the general population of thoracic patients. Only in centers routinely using active suction	Weak
Length of hospital stay and costs decreased	Moderate	The effect seems to be a consequence of better standardization. Very small savings (less than 1 day) in hospitalization time	Weak
Improving knowledge on the pleural space after lung resection through the analysis of stored data on pressures and air flow	Very low	Still not applicable to clinical practice. No published benefits for patients	Weak

Conclusions

After the analysis of the related literature, I have found evidence supporting the use of digital systems to facilitate the standardization of postoperative care after lung resection by decreasing variations in clinical practice (Table 16.1). For those surgeons recommending postoperative pleural suction, it is obvious that any smart portable suction device allows early mobilization of the patients, but to date it is not clear if pleural suction is advisable or not as a routine in pulmonary resection.

A Personal View of the Data

In my personal practice, active suction after lobectomy or lesser lung resection is not indicated. All patients undergoing major thoracic procedures are included in an intensive chest physiotherapy program including early mobilization, which is easily achieved because patients are not required to stay on suction. The physiotherapy program is directly related to a substantially reduced risk of pulmonary complications. Thus, significant improvements can be gained in perioperative care after lung resection unrelated to the type of pleural drainage or suction modality.

Recommendations

- Use of digital pleural drainage devices is recommended if large variations in clinical management of pleural tubes are detected, in order to standardize care and reduce costs (Evidence quality high; strong recommendation).
- Use of digital pleural drainage devices is not recommended for the general population of thoracic surgery patients who are managed without active suction (Evidence quality low; weak recommendation).
- Use of digital pleural drainage devices is not recommended as a means to reduce hospital length of stay or costs (Evidence quality low; weak recommendation).

Disclosures The author is an advisor for Atrium Medical (Hudson, NH, USA)

References

1. Varela G, Jiménez M, Novoa N, Aranda JL. Estimating hospital costs attributable to prolonged air leak in pulmonary lobectomy. Eur J Cardiothorac Surg. 2005;27:329–33.
2. Graham AN, Cosgrove AP, Gibbons JR, McGuigan JA. Randomised clinical trial of chest drainage systems. Thorax. 1992;47:461–2.
3. Anegg U, Lidemann J, Matzi V, Mujkic D, Maier A, Fritz L, et al. AIRFIX: the first digital postoperative chest tube airflowmetry: a novel method to quantify air leakage after lung resection. Eur J Cardiothorac Surg. 2006;29:867–72.
4. Dernevik L, Belboul A, Rådberg G. Initial experience with the world's first digital drainage system. The benefits of recording air leaks with graphic representation. Eur J Cardiothorac Surg. 2007;31:209–13.
5. Wennberg JE. Unwarranted variations in healthcare delivery: implications for academic medical centres. BMJ. 2002;325:961–4.
6. Zehr KJ, Dawsin PB, Yang SC, Heitmiller RF. Standardized clinical care pathways for major thoracic cases reduce hospital costs. Ann Thorac Surg. 1998;63:914–9.
7. Bardell T, Petsikas D. What keeps postpulmonary resection patients in hospital? Can Respir J. 2003;10:86–9.
8. Gagarine A, Urschel JD, Miller JC, Bennett WF, Young JEM. Preoperative and intraoperative factors predictive of length of hospital stay after pulmonary lobectomy. Ann Thorac Cardiovasc Surg. 2003;9:222–5.
9. Varela G, Jiménez M, Novoa N, Aranda JL. Postoperative chest tube management: measuring air leak using an electronic device decreases variability in the clinical practice. Eur J Cardiothorac Surg. 2009;35:28–31.
10. Brunelli A, Salati M, Refai M, Di Nunzio L, Xiumé F, Sabbatini A. Evaluation of a new chest tube removal protocol using digital air leak monitoring after lobectomy: a prospective randomised trial. Eur J Cardiothorac Surg. 2010;37:56–60.
11. Prokakis C, Koletsis EN, Apostolakis E, Panagopoulos N, Kouki HS, Sakellaropoulos GC, Filos K, Dougenis DV. Routine suction of intercostal drains is not necessary after lobectomy: a prospective randomized trial. World J Surg. 2008;32:2336–42.
12. Alphonso N, Tan C, Utley M, Cameron R, Dussek J, Lang-Lazdunski L, Treasure T. A prospective randomized controlled trial of suction versus non-suction to the under-water seal drains following lung resection. Eur J Cardiothorac Surg. 2005;27:391–4.

13. Brunelli A, Monteverde M, Borri A, Salati M, Marasco RD, Al Refai M, Fianchini A. Comparison of water seal and suction after pulmonary lobectomy: a prospective, randomized trial. Ann Thorac Surg. 2004;77:1932–7.
14. Cerfolio RJ, Bass C, Katholi CR. Prospective randomized trial compares suction versus water seal for air leaks. Ann Thorac Surg. 2001;71:1613–7.
15. Marshall MB, Deeb ME, Bleier JI, Kucharczuk JC, Friedberg JS, Kaiser LR, Shrager JB. Suction vs water seal after pulmonary resection: a randomized prospective study. Chest. 2002;121:831–5.
16. Leo F, Duranti L, Girelli L, Furia S, Billè A, Garofalo G, Scanagatta P, Giovannetti R, Pastorino U. Does external pleural suction reduce prolonged air leak after lung resection? Results from the AirINTrial after 500 randomized cases. Ann Thorac Surg. 2013;96:1234–9. doi:10.1016/j.athoracsur.2013.04.079.
17. Sanni A, Critchley A, Dunning J. Should chest drains be put on suction or not following pulmonary lobectomy? Interact Cardiovasc Thorac Surg. 2006;5:275–8.
18. Deng B, Tan QY, Zhao YP, Wang RW, Jiang YG. Suction or non-suction to the underwater seal drains following pulmonary operation: meta-analysis of randomised controlled trials. Eur J Cardiothorac Surg. 2010;38:210–5.
19. Coughlin SM, Emmerton-Coughlin HM, Malthaner R. Management of chest tubes after pulmonary resection: a systematic review and meta-analysis. Can J Surg. 2012;55:264–70.
20. Qiu T, Shen Y, Wang MZ, Wang YP, Wang D, Wang ZZ, Jin XF, Wei YC. External suction versus water seal after selective pulmonary resection for lung neoplasm: a systematic review. PLoS One. 2013;8(7):e68087.
21. Novoa NM, Ballesteros E, Jiménez MF, Aranda JL, Varela G. Chest physiotherapy revisited: evaluation of its influence on the overall cardio-respiratory morbidity after pulmonary resection. Eur J Cardiothorac Surg. 2011;40:130–4.
22. Cerfolio RJ, Bryant AS. The benefits of continuous and digital air leak assessment after elective pulmonary resection: a prospective study. Ann Thorac Surg. 2008;86(2):396–401.
23. Filosso PL, Ruffini E, Solidoro P, Molinatti M, Bruna MC, Oliaro A. Digital air leak monitoring after lobectomy for primary lung cancer in patients with moderate COPD: can a fast-tracking algorithm reduce postoperative costs and complications? J Cardiovasc Surg (Torino). 2010;51:429–33.
24. Varela G, Brunelli A, Jiménez MF, Di Nunzio L, Novoa N, Aranda JL, Sabbatini A. Chest drainage suction decreases differential pleural pressure after upper lobectomy and has no effect after lower lobectomy. Eur J Cardiothorac Surg. 2010;37:531–4.
25. Refai M, Brunelli A, Varela G, Novoa N, Pompili C, Jimenez MF, Aranda JL, Sabbatini A. The values of intrapleural pressure before the removal of chest tube in non-complicated pulmonary lobectomy. Eur J Cardiothorac Surg. 2012;41:831–3.
26. Jimenez MF, Varela G, Calvo J, Fuentes MG. Predicting the risk of prolonged air leak after pulmonary lobectomy using intrapleural pressures measured during the first 24 hours. Interact Cardiovasc Thorac Surg. 2012;15 Suppl 1:S55.
27. Brunelli A, Cassivi SD, Salati M, Fibla J, Pompili C, Halgren LA, Wigle DA, Di Nunzio L. Digital measurements of air leak flow and intrapleural pressures in the immediate postoperative period predict risk of prolonged air leak after pulmonary lobectomy. Eur J Cardiothorac Surg. 2011;39:584–8.

Chapter 17
Management of Persistent Post-operative Alveolar Air Leak

Anna L. McGuire and R. Sudhir Sundaresan

Abstract The most common and often frustrating complication for both surgeon and patient following pulmonary resection is persistent alveolar air leak. There are several available management modalities for persistent alveolar air leak. These modalities include: outpatient chest tube drainage, intra-pleural chemical sclerosis, intra-pleural blood patch, topical sealants, pneumoperitoneum, endo-bronchial valves and surgical repair. In this chapter we review the available evidence for use of each of these modalities with the goal of optimal individualized patient care plans for persistent alveolar air leak.

Keywords Persistent alveolar air leak • Intra-pleural chemical sclerosis • Blood patch • Intra-pleural topical sealant • Endo-bronchial valves • Pneumoperitoneum

Introduction

Persistent alveolar air leak following pulmonary resection is the most common complication faced by thoracic surgeons. Despite this, it is one of the most controversial topics with respect to the specific definition of "persistent" and also regarding optimal postoperative management. The definition of post-operative alveolar air leak itself is not controversial: an alveolar-pleural fistula following

A.L. McGuire, MD
Department of Thoracic Surgery, The Ottawa Hospital,
301 Symth Road, Ottawa, ON K4K 1M2, Canada
e-mail: amcguire@toh.on.ca

R.S. Sundaresan, MD (✉)
Department of Surgery, The Ottawa Hospital, University of Ottawa,
501 Smyth Road, Ottawa, ON K1H 8L6, Canada
e-mail: ssundaresan@ottawahospital.on.ca

M.K. Ferguson (ed.), *Difficult Decisions in Thoracic Surgery*,
Difficult Decisions in Surgery: An Evidence-Based Approach 1,
DOI 10.1007/978-1-4471-6404-3_17, © Springer-Verlag London 2014

pulmonary resection. It is distinguished from its more proximal counterpart—the broncho-pleural fistula—by simple anatomy, the latter being a communication between a lobar or segmental pulmonary bronchus and the pleural space. Evidence-based management of post-operative broncho-pleural fistula is beyond the scope of this chapter. "Persistent" or "prolonged" alveolar air leak is variability defined in the literature. The Society of Thoracic Surgeons (STS) database defines an alveolar air leak as persistent if it remains on the 5th postoperative day, as it is unlikely to resolve spontaneously after this time frame. Available reports describe anywhere from postoperative day 2–10 as the benchmark for "persistent". More recently, the "persistent" definition has even been applied to any air leak preventing chest drain removal in a well patient that could otherwise be discharged from hospital.

There is consensus that prevention of alveolar air leak is the best initial management. Prevention includes adherence to meticulous surgical technique, fissureless dissection for lobectomy, use of sealant glue or staple line buttressing material in patients with known risk factors, and minimizing residual pleural space. Surgeon-related technical and patient-related tissue integrity risk factors have been well described in two large retrospective series on prospectively collected data, and include: underlying lung disease (emphysema, pulmonary fibrosis), low predicted forced expiratory volume in 1 s (FEV1), presence of pleural adhesions, corticosteroids and other medications that impair tissue healing, extent and location of resection and resultant size of residual pleural space to fill (upper versus lower, bilobectomy, segmentectomy, wedge resection), expiratory air leak greater than four on postoperative day 1, and immune-compromised state (malnutrition, HIV/AIDS, transplant recipient, recent chemotherapy) [1, 2].

Despite surgeons' best efforts at prevention with risk factor identification and meticulous surgical technique, persistent alveolar air leaks still occur. What then? The objective of this chapter is to review how to manage a persistent alveolar air leak following pulmonary resection, based on the literature available.

Search Strategy

We performed a MEDLINE Ovid literature search for the period 1980–2013. We fused the key terms [air leak] OR [alveolar-pleural fistula] giving an initial 1,472 results. We narrowed the search results by sequentially fusing additional key terms to the initial search in the following manner: AND [pleuodesis] returned 139 articles; AND [endobronchial valve] returned 11 articles; AND [muscle flap] returned 13 articles; AND [postoperative management] returned an additional 6 papers. Titles were read and excluded immediately if not relevant. Abstracts were reviewed to determine further topic relevance. From the above search results, the original reports used to gather the body of evidence-based practice for this chapter appear in Tables 17.1, 17.2, 17.3, 17.4, 17.5 and 17.6.

Table 17.1 Studies reporting efficacy of portable chest drainage systems in outpatient management of persistent air leak

Reference	Study design and period	Population	Definition persistent air leak	Air leak treatment intervention	Duration tube with PAL and intervention	Complications reported	Quality evidence rank
Brunelli et al. [1]	Retrospective review Jan 1995–Jun 2003	n = 558 pulmonary resections n = 32 with persistent air leak discharged on Heimlich valve	>7 days	Heimlich valve	Air leak cessation 13 within 3 weeks 12 within 4 weeks 7 within 2 months	None related to Heimlich	Moderate
Cerfolio et al. [2]	Retrospective review	n = 669 pulmonary resections n = 33 with persistent air leak following lobectomy, segmentectomy, wedge resection	>4 days	Heimlich valve	17 air leak resolved POD#7 and tube removed 9 with airleak at POD#14 admitted for provocative clamping and tube removed POD#15	Prior to discharge 6 pneumothorax and subcutaneous emphysema on Heimlich prior to discharge (all airleaks > 5) After discharge 1 chest tube accidental removal POD#12, remained out	Moderate

(continued)

Table 17.1 (continued)

Reference	Study design and period	Population	Definition persistent air leak	Air leak treatment intervention	Duration tube with PAL and intervention	Complications reported	Quality evidence rank
Cerfolio et al. [3]	Retrospective review Jul 2000–Jul 2007	n = 6,038 pulmonary resections n = 199 with persistent air leak discharged on Heimlich valve	>4 days	Heimlich valve	Follow-up median of 16.5 days from discharge with Heimlich 144 tube removed if no pneumothorax on CXR regardless of air leak 14 with pneumothorax on CXR admitted for provocative clamping regardless of air leak; all tubes removed the next day	None related to Heimlich	Moderate

Study	Design / Dates	Population	Definition	Intervention	Duration	Complications	Level of evidence
Liberman et al. [4]	Retrospective case-control 1997–2006	n=1393 pulmonary resections n=78 with persistent air leak after Lobectomy or bilobectomy by thoracotomy	>5 days	Observation (n=33) Pleurodesis (n=41) Talc (n=30), bleomycin (n=1), doxycycline (n=7), minocycline Heimlich (n=3) Reoperation –muscle flap (n=1)	Mean duration Heimlich not reported Overall mean duration chest tube 11.5 days	1 readmit for pneumothorax 1 empyema with death after talc	Very low (regarding Heimlich) Moderate (regarding chemical pleurodesis)
Rieger et al. [5]	Retrospective review May 2003–Dec 2004	n=457 major thoracic procedures n=36 with persistent air leak after postlobectomy, segmentectomy, wedge resection, pleurodesis, pericardial window, mediastinal dissection or esophagogastrectomy	Not defined	Express mini 500 (Atrium Medical Corp, Hudson, NH)	Mean duration tube 11.2 days	1 readmit for pneumothorax 1 empyema 1 cellulitis 1 underwent talc slurry POD#55 No death No pneumonia	Moderate

(continued)

Table 17.1 (continued)

Reference	Study design and period	Population	Definition persistent air leak	Air leak treatment intervention	Duration tube with PAL and intervention	Complications reported	Quality evidence rank
Tcherveniakov et al. [6]	Retrospective review Nov 2009–Nov 2010	n=74 cases of outpatient tube management; n=43 with persistent air leak following VATS or open lobectomy, wedge, or decortication	Not defined	One-way valve drainage system with soft fluid reservoir	Mean duration tube 19.56 days	6 cellulitis; 4 readmission: 1 tube reinsertion for pneumothorax; 3 Empyema	Moderate
Rahman et al. [7]	Retrospective review	n=98 who underwent bullectomy for recurrent spontaneous pneumothorax; pneumostat applied to all patients regardless of air leak	Not defined	Pneumostat (Atrium Medical Corp, Hudson, NH)	Mean hospital Stay 3.08 days; Mean duration tube 7.5 days	4 cellulitis	Moderate
Lodi and Stefani [8]	Retrospective review Mar 1998–Mar 1999	n=248 pulmonary resections; n=18 with persistent air leak after lobectomy, wedge resection	>6 days	One-way valve drainage system	Mean duration tube 11.5 days	No death; No empyema; No pneumonia; No SC emphysema	Moderate
Ponn et al. [9]	Retrospective review 1990–1997	n=240 cases of outpatient tube management; n=45 outpatient management with persistent air leak after lobectomy, wedge resection	Not defined	Heimlich valve	Mean duration Heimlich 7.5 days	1 admit for suction due to SC emphysema	Moderate
McKenna et al. [10]	Retrospective review Nov 1994–Jul 1995	n=107 LVRS; n=25 with persistent air leak after lung volume reduction surgery	>5 days	Heimlich valve	Mean duration Heimlich 7.7 days	No death; No empyema; No pneumonia	Moderate

POD post-operative day, *CXR* chest x-ray, *VATS* video assisted thoracic surgery, *PAL* persistent alveolar air leak, *LVRS* lung volume reduction surgery

Table 17.2 Studies reporting the efficacy of chemical sclerosis in management of persistent air leak

Reference	Study design and period	Population	Definition persistent air leak	Air leak treatment intervention	Duration tube with PAL and intervention	Complications reported	Quality evidence rank
Liberman et al. [4]	Retrospective case-control 1997–2006	n = 1,393 pulmonary resections	>5 days	Observation (n = 33)	Successful sclerosis in 40 of 41 patients with persistent air leak (97.6 %)	1 readmit for pneumothorax	Moderate
		n = 78 with persistent air leak after Lobectomy or bilobectomy by thoracotomy		Pleurodesis (n = 41)	Mean duration air leak post sclerotherapy was 2.8 days	1 mycocutaneous flap for persistent air leak after talc pleurodesis	
				Talc (n = 30), bleomycin (n = 1), doxycycline (n = 7), minocycline (=1)		1 empyema after talc pleurodesis with death	
				Heimlich (n = 3)	Overall mean duration chest tube 11.5 days		
				Reoperation –muscle flap (n = 1)			

PAL persistent alveolar air leak

Table 17.3 Studies reporting the efficacy of autologous blood patch in management of persistent air leak

Reference	Study design and period	Population	Definition persistent air leak	Air leak treatment intervention	Duration tube with PAL and intervention	Complications reported	Quality evidence rank
Shackcloth et al. [15]	Prospective randomized study over 18 months	n = 319 lobectomy	>5 days	120 mL autologous venous blood pleurodesis	Significant reduction in duration chest tube (6.5 vs 12 days, p<0.001)	1 empyema requiring pleural catheter insertion and antibiotics	Moderate
		n = 20 with persistent air leak after lobectomy			# of pleurodesis sessions to stop air leak 7 required 1 2 required 2 1 required 3 Control group 8 of 10 still had air leak POD#10	No deaths	
Oliveira et al. [16]	Retrospective review	n = 27 with persistent air leak treated with autologous blood	Not defined	Up to 200 ml (depending on pleural cavity size)	23 (85 %) successful pleurodesis	1 empyema (not in patient with history empyema)	Moderate
	Jan 2001–Aug 2008	n = 10 after lobectomy n = 9 after spontaneous pneumothorax n = 4 after bullectomy n = 2 decortication n = 1 after lung biopsy n = 1 empyema		Autologous blood pleurodesis	1 unsuccessful pleurodesis post lobectomy 6 required 2 pleurodesis sessions Mean time to fistula resolution after pleurodesis was 1.5 days	1 fever	

Andreetti et al. [17]	Retrospective case control	n=25 persistent air leak patients after lobectomy	>6 days	Autologous blood pleurodesis	Air leak stopped sooner after pleurodesis than controls; and sooner with 100 ml vs 50 ml (2.3 vs 1.5 days, p=0.005)	No infection	Moderate
		Group A: n=12, 50 ml Group B: n=13, 100 ml Group C: controls, 15 last patients with persistent air leak		n=12, 50 ml n=13, 100 ml	Group C airleak stopped later (12.3 days postop, p=0.0009, and 0.0001)	No deaths No early or late side effects	
Droghetti et al. [18]	Retrospective review Jan 1999–Feb 2006	n=21 persistent air leak after pulmonary surgery	>7 days	50 to 150 ml Autologous Blood pleurodesis	17 (81 %) had air leak resolution rate in the first 24 h of pleurodesis	1 fever (decortication patient)	Moderate
		n=13 lobectomy		N=2, 50 ml N=6, 100 ml	4 required a 2nd pleurodesis 36 h after first	No empyema or other early or late side effects	
		n=1 bilobectomy n=2 decortication for empyema n=5 LRVS		N=13, 150 ml	Chest tubes removed 48 h after air leak cessation		

(continued)

Table 17.3 (continued)

Reference	Study design and period	Population	Definition persistent air leak	Air leak treatment intervention	Duration tube with PAL and intervention	Complications reported	Quality evidence rank
Lang-Lazdunski and Coonar [19]	Retrospective review Jan 2002–Jan 2004	N=196 lung resections N=13 with persistent air leak after lobectomy, bi-lobectomy or wedge	>7 days	N=11 with 50 ml autologous blood pleurodesis N=2 Heimlich valve	All 11 (100 %) air leak cessation -8/11 (72.7 %) within 12 h -3 within 48 h Time to airleak resolution with Heimlich not reported	After pleurodesis Reported no empyema, but 1 pleural fluid culture was *S. aureus* positive 1 pneumonia 2 fever	Moderate
Rivas de Andrés et al. [20]	Retrospective review Jun 1993–Jan 1998	n=6 underwent pleurodesis with autologous blood for persistent air leak after operation	>10 days	50 to 250 ml autologous blood pleurodesis n=2, 50 ml n=1, 250 ml n=3, 100 ml	All 6 (100 %) success 24 h after pleurodesis	No infection No pain No respiratory difficulty No fever No coughing	Low
Dumire et al. [21]	1st 2 cases reported of blood pleurodesis following lobectomy	N=2 cases of autologous blood pleurodesis for persistent air leak following lobectomy	Not defined	50 ml Autologous blood pleurodesis	1st case air leak resolved within 24h of pleurodesis 2nd case air leak decreased in 1st 24h, then resolved	None reported	Very low

PAL persistent alveolar air leak, *LVRS* lung volume reduction surgery

Table 17.4 Studies reporting the efficacy of Thoracoscopy and Fibrin sealants in management of persistent air leak

Reference	Study design and period	Population	Definition persistent air leak	Air leak treatment intervention	Duration tube with PAL and intervention	Complications reported	Quality evidence rank
Suter et al. [22]	Case series	n = 3 with air leak after pulmonary resection (lobectomy, bilobectomy and sleeve lobectomy)	>7 days	Thoracoscopy and fibrin glue	Minimal post-op air leak × 1–2 days Chest tubes removed POD#4 in 2 and POD#3 in 1	None	Very low
Thistlethwaite et al. [23]	Retrospective review	n = 12 with air leak after pulmonary procedure	>10 days	Thoracoscopy and fibrin sealant mixture (20 ml cryoprecipitate and 20 ml 1,000 U/ml thrombin)	Successful air leak sealing in 11 of 12 within 24 h	None	Low
	April 1996–Jan 1997	n = 7 thoracoscopic LVRS, n = 3 lobectomy or bilobectomy, 2 radiologic chest tube insertion for loculated effusion					

PAL persistent alveolar air leak, *LVRS* lung volume reduction surgery

Table 17.5 Studies reporting the efficacy of pneumoperitoneum in management of persistent air leak

Reference	Study design and period	Population	Definition persistent air leak	Air leak treatment intervention	Duration tube with PAL and intervention	Complications reported	Quality evidence rank
Di Giamacomo et al. [24]	Retrospective review Jan 1998–Dec 2000	n=14 with persistent air leak and pleural space problems after pulmonary resection for lung cancer	Not defined	Post-operative pneumoperitoneum mean of 2,100 mL	Obliteration of the pleural space in all after a mean time of 4 days (range, 1–7 days) Air leaks stopped in all after a mean time of 8 days (range, 4–12 days)	None	Low
Cobognani et al. [25]	Retrospective review Jan 1996–Dec 1997	n=12 with persistent air leak and pleural space following lobectomy for cancer	>8 days	Post-operative pneumoperitoneum 1,200–1,300 cm^3	"Immediate reduction in air leaks" Chest drains removed 3–4 days after pneumoperitoneum	None	Low

PAL persistent alveolar air leak

Table 17.6 Studies reporting the efficacy of muscle flaps in management of persistent air leak

Reference	Study design and period	Population	Definition persistent air leak	Air leak treatment intervention	Duration tube with PAL and intervention	Complications reported	Quality evidence rank
Liberman et al. [4]	Retrospective case-control	n = 1,393	>5 days	Observation (n=33)	Successful sclerosis in 40 of 41 patients with persistent air leak (97.6 %)	1 readmit for pneumothorax	Low
	1997–2006	n = 78 with persistent air leak after lobectomy or bilobectomy by thoracotomy		Pleurodesis (n=41)	Mean duration air leak post sclerotherapy was 2.8 days	**1 mycocutaneous flap for persistent air leak after talc pleurodesis**	
				Talc (n=30), bleomycin (n=1), doxycycline (n=7), minocycline (=1)	Overall mean duration chest tube 11.5 days	1 empyema after talc pleurodesis with death	
				Heimlich (n=3)			
				Reoperation – muscle flap (n=1)			
Woo et al. [26]	Retrospective case series	n = 5 with persistent alveolar air leak due to secondary spontaneous pneumothorax	Not defined	Combined latissimus	Chest drains were removed within 5 days post surgery	No complications	Low
	2004–2007			Dorsi-serratus anterior flap		Minor loss of shoulder motion	

(continued)

Table 17.6 (continued)

Reference	Study design and period	Population	Definition persistent air leak	Air leak treatment intervention	Duration tube with PAL and intervention	Complications reported	Quality evidence rank
Backhus et al. [27]	Retrospective review	N = 84 adults received living lobar lung transplant:	Not defined	N = 3 reoperation		1 latissimus dorsi flap necrosed requiring omental transfer	Very low
	Jan 1993—Dec 2003	N = 24 with pleural space problem. N = 9 (38 %) had persistent air leak (3 of these required reoperation)		-2 Latissimus dorsi flaps -Local intercostal muscle pedicle flap N = 6 managed expectantly with chest tubes			

PAL persistent alveolar air leak

Results

We conceptualize management of persistent post-operative alveolar air leak in the following way: outpatient management of the pleural space and the chest drain; and inpatient management with bedside pleurodesis (autologous blood, talc or chemicals) or surgical management, including thoracoscopy with fibrin sealant application, thoracotomy with muscle flap transposition, or pneumoperitoneum. Finally, we conceptualize newer applications of endoscopic management, in particular placement of endobronchial valves.

Outpatient Chest Tube Management with Portable Chest Drainage Devices

The literature search revealed eight retrospective studies reporting experience with outpatient chest tube management, summarized in Table 17.1 [1–10]. Based on the available evidence, outpatient portable chest drainage devices appear efficacious in management of persistent alveolar air leak. This approach facilitates earlier hospital discharge and is safe and acceptable in properly selected patients provided timely access to appropriate medical care and outpatient follow up. Complications are uncommon, the majority of which are infectious in nature. Based on the reports of Cerfolio and colleagues, it is likely most appropriate for patients with expiratory air leaks less than five by the RDJ Cerfolio air leak classification [2, 3]. There is insufficient evidence to recommend one portable chest drainage product over another.

Bedside Pleurodesis

Bedside pleurodesis with intrapleural administration of a sclerosing agent induces a pleural inflammatory response. The goal of this response is to allow pleural space obliteration and air leak cessation. Of the many agents available, the literature for pleurodesis following persistent air leak after lung resection focuses mainly on autologous blood patch. Chemical agents including Talc and doxycyline have been reported for use following pulmonary resection, most notably in the retrospective case-control series by Liberman and colleagues [4]. Other reports focus on the use of these chemicals in the setting of alveolar air leak following primary or secondary spontaneous pneumothorax, and as such may not be generalizable to the lung resection population. Based on the available evidence, bedside pleurodesis does appear to be an efficacious option for management of persistent alveolar air leak with minimal associated complications. From the pleural effusion/pneumothorax literature the known complications of pleurodesis include fever, pain and empyema [11]. Small particle talc has been reported to induce acute respiratory distress syndrome (ARDS) and is no longer used [12, 13]. Talc pleurodesis in the malignant effusion literature is not associated with increased mortality [14]. The results of chemical pleurodesis studies following pulmonary resection are summarized in Table 17.2.

Pleurodesis with autologous blood patch is effective in sealing air leaks after lobectomy and appears to decrease time to chest drain removal and hospital discharge compared to expectant management, as reported in the prospective randomized study by Shackcloth and colleagues [15]. Recommendations cannot be made with respect to what severity of air leak is appropriate for this treatment or comparison of blood with chemical sclerosants. Quantity of autologous blood 100 ml or greater for pleurodesis appears more efficacious then smaller quantities. Similarly, recommendations cannot be made regarding the superiority of one sclerosing agent over another in the setting of postoperative persistent alveolar air leak. Studies on the topic of autologous blood patch pleurodesis are summarized in Table 17.3 [15–21].

Surgical Management of Postoperative Persistent Alveolar Air Leak

Several surgical techniques have been applied for management of persistent alveolar air leak. However, there are no large series addressing surgical management of air leak following pulmonary resection. In general, these authors resorted to surgical management only after the less invasive measures failed to resolve the air leak. There are two small retrospective case series reporting successful management of persistent alveolar air leak following pulmonary resection with thoracoscopic application of fibrin sealant (Table 17.4) [22, 23].

Post-operative pneumoperitoneum involves instillation of air into the peritoneal cavity through a peritoneal dialysis catheter or Veres needle. This approach has also only been reported in small retrospective case series to manage persistent air leak in the setting of a residual pleural space (Table 17.5) [24, 25].

There is slightly more literature available on the use of muscle flaps for concomitant pleural space obliteration and air leak cessation (Table 17.6) [26, 27]. The majority of the data on use of muscle flaps for air leak management is extrapolated from the spontaneous pneumothorax and empyema decortication patient populations. Woo and colleagues suggest consideration for surgical repair of alveolar air leak with myoplasty when the leak is severe (continuous and high volume – requiring suction to maintain equilibrium), there is evidence of pleural dead space, more conservative measures have failed, and finally if the patient has poor reserve secondary to pulmonary disease such as emphysema [26].

Endobronchial Valves

Endobronchial valves were developed as an investigational technique for management of emphysema. We identified three case series reporting use of endobronchial valves in patients with persistent alveolar air leak deemed unsuitable for surgical management. Ideal candidates have a continuous air leak as measured by digital chest drainage device, and identifiable bronchial segmental source of air leak for occlusion. The most recent report by Firlinger and colleagues [28] employed the used of digital chest drainage to accurately quantify volume of air leak pre and post interventions. The limitation of these series is the lack of a control group. As such, it is not conclusive that the air leak improvement is directly related to the valve placement; however the obvious temporal relationship does suggest a therapeutic benefit, with decrease or resolution of the persistent air leaks in the majority of carefully selected patients. The available data are summarized in Table 17.7 [28–30].

Recommendations

The significant majority of the studies cited in this chapter are retrospective reviews [1–3, 5–10, 16, 18–20, 23–25, 27, 29, 30] or retrospective case–control series [4, 17], with very few prospective studies having been completed [15, 28]. We arbitrarily separated the references utilized for this chapter into those published within the past 5 years (ten reports between 2008 – present) and those published prior (23 published before 2008). Interestingly, the ten "recent" reports deal mainly with outpatient chest tube management (four reports) or endobronchial valves (three reports, perhaps reflecting recent enthusiasm in application of this relatively new technology to an old problem); with one report describing chemical and blood pleurodesis each. Consequently the overall quality of the available literature is moderate at best, and it is difficult to cite strong evidence to make definitive statements about optimal management of this problem.

Outpatient management of persistent post-operative air leak appears efficacious in properly selected patients (asymptomatic, adequate lung expansion, airleak severity < 4, minimal pleural fluid drainage, good performance status, social support available, and residence within close proximity to medical care). We make a weak recommendation for use of this treatment modality. Similarly, we make a weak recommendation for the use of chemical sclerosants and blood patch to induce pleural symphysis. The quality of evidence is insufficient to make recommendations for use of pneumoperitoneum, fibrin sealants or endobronchial valves. The available evidence does not allow us to make recommendations with respect to superiority of one treatment modality over another for this clinical problem.

All of these approaches have shown success in management of persistent post-operative air leak, and likely have a role on an individualized case basis. This attitude is reflected in our personal recommendation in the next section.

Table 17.7 Studies reporting the efficacy of endobronchial valve in management of persistent air leak

Reference	Study design and period	Population	Definition persistent air leak	Air leak treatment intervention	Outcomes after intervention	Complications reported	Quality evidence rank
Firlinger et al. [28]	Prospective observational study	N = 19 with persistent air leak monitored with digital chest drainage devices	>7 days	Endobronchial valves used	N = 10 responder (air flow <100 cm³/min)	No adverse events related to the valves were reported	Low
	May 2010–May 2012	N = 13 with identifiable location for continuous leak treated with valve		IBV valve system (Spiration, Inc)	N = 3 no resolution (air flow > 100 cm³/min)		
				Zephyr Endobronchial valve (Pulmonx Co.)	Mean duration tube 7.6 days responders vs 14 non-responders		
Gillespie et al. [29]	Retrospective review	N = 7 with persistent air leak underwent endobronchial valve placement	Not defined	Endobronchial valve	7 (100 %) air leak improvement	None	Low
	Jul 2007–Oct 2008	N = 4 postoperative N = 3 spontaneous pneumothorax		(IBV valve; Spiration, Redmond, WA)	6 resolution 1 reduction Median duration tube 16 days Median duration hospitalization 3 days		

| Travaline et al. [30] | Retrospective review Dec 2002–Jan 2007 | N=40 with persistent air leak N=7 postoperative N=25 spontaneous pneumothorax N=6 iatrogenic N=1 LVRS N=1 trauma | >4 days | Endobronchial valve (Zephyr EBV; Emphasys Medical; Redwood City, CA) | Median duration tube 7.5 days Median duration hospitalization 11 days 19 (47.5 %) resolution 18 (45 %) reduction 2 no change 1 no reported outcome | Adverse events in 6 patients Valve expectoration, malpositioning of the valve requiring redeployment, pneumonia, oxygen desaturation, MRSA colonization | Low |

IBV intra-bronchial valve, *MRSA* methicillin resistant Staphylococcus aureus, *LVRS* lung volume reduction surgery

A Personal View of the Data

There are few more frustrating situations for surgeon and patient alike than the problem of persistent alveolar air leak following a technically sound pulmonary resection. We regard this as an opportunity to rigorously review the technical conduct of the procedure, to identify points for quality improvement in pneumostasis and apply these to future cases, rather than laying blame on patient factors such as poor tissue integrity from emphysema or comorbid conditions affecting tissue healing.

At the Ottawa Hospital our approach to persistent alveolar air leak is as follows. First, we define a persistent leak as one persisting for 5 days after resection. While the management is tailored to individual patient characteristics, there is consensus among the surgeons regarding basic underlying principles.

The first aspect is tube management and suction setting. Patients with air leak are preferentially maintained on a Pleur-evac (Sahara S-1100 Pleur-evac Chest Drainage System; Genzyme Biosurgical, Cambridge, MA) suction-free, so long as the lung remains adequately expanded without signs or symptoms of uncontrolled air leak (dyspnea, dysphonia, important subcutaneous emphysema, pleuritic chest pain). The vast majority of such patients are simply discharged home with their chest drain attached to a portable Pneumostat device (Atrium Medical Corp, Hudson, NH), with weekly follow-up visits in clinic for air leak assessment and chest X-ray. The tube is removed once the air leak has ceased.

Suction is only applied to chest drains at the minimal setting required (range −10 to −40 cm water) to achieve adequate evacuation of air as evidenced by radiographic lung re-expansion and resolution of signs and symptoms. Once the patient is clinically and radiographically stabilized, suction is tapered by −10 cm of water daily until water seal drainage is achieved. In patients who do not tolerate the slow suction wean, suction is maintained for 48 h before a second trial of progressive reduction. If there is significant underlying pulmonary disease (emphysema, pulmonary fibrosis), we continue with weaning suction in addition to adjunctive bedside intrapleural sclerosis with 5 g talc slurry or 500 mg doxycycline. Reoperation is reserved for patients with underlying pulmonary disease *and* a significant residual pleural space. In this fortunately rare situation we involve plastic surgery colleagues for assistance with mobilization of robust pedicled muscle flaps to rotate into the pleural space for obliteration of the residual space and occlusion of the air leak.

We additionally hold the view that digital chest drainage systems have an important role in management of postoperative alveolar air leak (especially for managing "suction-dependent" air leak), and are conducting a prospective randomized trial evaluating its utility. Results of this trial will be forthcoming in 2014.

Recommendations

- Outpatient management of persistent post-operative air leak with indwelling pleural drains appears efficacious in properly selected patients. (Evidence quality moderate; weak recommendation)
- Chemical sclerosants and blood patch are useful to induce pleural symphysis and eliminate air leak. (Evidence quality low; weak recommendation)
- No recommendation can be made for use of pneumoperitoneum, fibrin sealants or endobronchial valves. (Evidence quality very low; no recommendation)
- No recommendation can be made with respect to superiority of one treatment modality over another for persistent postoperative air leak. (Evidence quality low; no recommendation)

References

1. Brunelli A, Monteverde M, Borri A, Salati M, Marasco RD, Fianchini A. Predictors of prolonged air leak after pulmonary lobectomy. Ann Thorac Surg. 2004;77(4):1205–10; discussion 1210.
2. Cerfolio RJ, Bass CS, Pask AH, Katholi CR. Predictors and treatment of persistent air leaks. Ann Thorac Surg. 2002;73(6):1727–30; discussion 1730–1.
3. Cerfolio RJ, Minnich DJ, Bryant AS. The removal of chest tubes despite an air leak or a pneumothorax. Ann Thorac Surg. 2009;87(6):1690–4; discussion 1694–6.
4. Liberman M, Muzikansky A, Wright CD, Wain JC, Donahue DM, Allan JS, et al. Incidence and risk factors of persistent air leak after major pulmonary resection and use of chemical pleurodesis. Ann Thorac Surg. 2010;89(3):891–7; discussion 897–8.
5. Rieger KM, Wroblewski HA, Brooks JA, Hammoud ZT, Kesler KA. Postoperative outpatient chest tube management: initial experience with a new portable system. Ann Thorac Surg. 2007;84(2):630–2.
6. Tcherveniakov P, De Siqueira J, Milton R, Papagiannopoulos K. Ward-based, nurse-led, outpatient chest tube management: analysis of impact, cost-effectiveness and patient safety. Eur J Cardiothorac Surg. 2012;41:1353–6.
7. Rahman M, Ooi Su Min J, Fikri A, Adeeb S, Zamrin D. Pocket-sized Heimlich valve (pneumostat) after bullae resection: a 5-year review. Ann Thorac Surg. 2009;88:979–81.
8. Lodi R, Stefani A. A new portable chest drainage device. Ann Thorac Surg. 2000;69: 998–1001.
9. Ponn RB, Silverman HJ, Federico JA. Outpatient chest tube management. Ann Thorac Surg. 1997;64(5):1437–40.
10. McKenna Jr RJ, Fischel RJ, Brenner M, Gelb AF. Use of the Heimlich valve to shorten hospital stay after lung reduction surgery for emphysema. Ann Thorac Surg. 1996;61(4):1115–7.
11. Brant A, Eaton T. Serious complications with talc slurry pleurodesis. Respirology. 2001;6(3):181–5.
12. Kuzniar TJ, Blum MG, Kasibowska-Kuzniar K, Mutlu GM. Predictors of acute lung injury and severe hypoxemia in patients undergoing operative talc pleurodesis. Ann Thorac Surg. 2006;82(6):1976–81.

13. Baron RD, Milton R, Thorpe JA. Pleurodesis using small talc particles results in an unaccept-ably high rate of acute lung injury and hypoxia. Ann Thorac Surg. 2007;84(6):2136.

14. Shaw P, Agarwal R. Pleurodesis for malignant pleural effusions. Cochrane Database Syst Rev. 2004;(1):CD002916.

15. Shackcloth M, Poullis M, Page R. Autologous blood pleurodesis for treating persistent air leak after lung resection. Ann Thorac Surg. 2001;71(4):1402–3.

16. Oliveira F, Cataneo D, Ruiz R, Cataneo A. Persistent pleuropulmonary air leak treated with autologous blood: results from a University Hospital and Review of Literature. Respiration. 2010;79:302–6.

17. Andreetti C, Venuta F, Anile M, De Giacomo T, Diso D, Di Stasio M, Rendina EA, Coloni GF. Pleurodesis with an autologous blood patch to prevent persistent air leaks after lobectomy. J Thorac Cardiovasc Surg. 2007;133:759–62.

18. Droghetti A, Schiavini A, Muriana P, Comel A, De Donno G, Beccaria M, Canneto B, Sturani C, Muriana G. Autologous blood patch in persistent air leaks after pulmonary resection. J Thorac Cardiovasc Surg. 2006;132:556–9.

19. Lang-Lazdunski L, Coonar AS. A prospective study of autologous 'blood patch' pleurodesis for persistent air leak after pulmonary resection. Eur J Cardiothorac Surg. 2004;26:897–900.

20. de Rivas Andrés JJR, Blanco S, De la Torre M. Postsurgical pleurodesis with autologous blood in patients with persistent air leak. Ann Thorac Surg. 2000;70:270–2.

21. Dumire R, Crobbe MM, Mappin FG, Fontenelle LJ. Autologous 'blood patch' pleurodesis for persistent pulmonary air leak. Chest. 1992;101:64–6.

22. Suter M, Bettschart V, Vandoni RE, Cuttat JF. Thoracoscopic pleurodesis for prolonged (or intractable) air leak after lung resection. Eur J Cardiothorac Surg. 1997;12(1):160–1.

23. Thistlethwaite P, Luketich J, Ferson PF, Keenan RJ, Jamieson SW. Ablation of persistent air leaks after thoracic procedures with fibrin sealant. Ann Thorac Surg. 1999;67:575–7.

24. Di Giamacomo T, Rendina EA, Venuta F, Francioni F, Moretti M, Pugliese F, Coloni GF. Pneumoperitoneum for the management of pleural air apace problems associated with major pulmonary resections. Ann Thorac Surg. 2001;72:1716–9.

25. Carbognani P, Spaggiari L, Solli PG, Tincani G, Bobbio A, Rusca M. Postoperative pneumo-peritoneum for prolonged air leaks and residual spaces after pulmonary resection. J Cardiovasc Surg. 1999;40(6):887–8.

26. Woo E, Tan BK, Lim CH. Treatment of recalcitrant air leaks: the combined latissimus dorsi-serratus anterior flap. Ann Plast Surg. 2009;63(2):188–92.

27. Backhus L, Sievers EM, Schenkel FA, Barr ML, Cohen RG, Smith MA, et al. Pleural space problems after living lobar transplantation. J Heart Lung Transplant. 2005;24(12):2086–90.

28. Firlinger I, Stubenberger E, Muller MR, Burghuber OC, Valipour A. Endoscopic one-way valve implantation in patients with prolonged air leak and the use of digital air leak monitor-ing. Ann Thorac Surg. 2013;95:1243–50.

29. Gillespie CT, Sterman DH, Cerfolio RJ, Nader D, Mulligan MS, Mularski RA, et al. Endobronchial valve treatment for prolonged air leaks of the lung: a case series. Ann Thorac Surg. 2011;91(1):270–3.

30. Travaline JM, McKenna Jr RJ, De Giacomo T, Venuta F, Hazelrigg SR, Boomer M, et al. Treatment of persistent pulmonary air leaks using endobronchial valves. Chest. 2009; 136(2):355–60.

Chapter 18
Surveillance After Resection of Stage I Non Small Cell Lung Cancer

Nathan M. Mollberg

Abstract The results of the National Lung Screening Trial demonstrated a survival benefit for screening high risk patients for the development of lung cancer. However, the yield from surveillance is potentially much higher as patients with a personal history of lung cancer are at highest risk for both recurrence and the development of a metachronous primary lung cancer (MPLC). Surveillance imaging is therefore recommended by many organizations as a means to detect recurrence/MPLC at a time when treatment may lead to long term survival.

Keywords Surveillance • Survival • Stage I non small cell lung cancer

Introduction

Five-year survival in patients with resected stage I non small cell lung cancer (NSCLC) ranges between 55 and 80 %. Tumor recurrence is the most common cause of death, and thus is a major obstacle for long-term survival after resection. While there are a number of reasons to follow patients clinically after curative treatment, the primary goal of surveillance is to detect local recurrence and/or metachronous lung cancers at a time when survival can be prolonged by interventions designed to cure or at least treat the disease more effectively than when discovered later. Currently there is little evidence that early identification of recurrent disease in asymptomatic patients improves long-term survival. However, patients with metachronous tumors detected during follow-up amenable to curative resection

N.M. Mollberg, DO
Department of Cardiothoracic Surgery, University of Washington Medical Center,
1959 NE Pacific Street, Seattle, WA 98195, USA
e-mail: nathan.mollberg@gmail.com

M.K. Ferguson (ed.), *Difficult Decisions in Thoracic Surgery*,   229
Difficult Decisions in Surgery: An Evidence-Based Approach 1,
DOI 10.1007/978-1-4471-6404-3_18, © Springer-Verlag London 2014

have been reported to have favorable long term survival rates. As such, surveillance guidelines and practices vary greatly in imaging interval and modality. However, the existing outcome data on treatment for local recurrence and/or metachronous disease has included patients with higher stage disease in which curative re-resection is less likely to be offered or even possible. Indeed, approximately 80 % of all re-resections reported either for local recurrence or metachronous disease have occurred in patients with initial stage I disease. This chapter will discuss the existing evidence regarding a survival benefit from imaging surveillance for patients who underwent curative resection of stage I NSCLC. This strategy will be discussed in the context of patterns of local recurrence/metachronous tumor development and the ability to undergo a second curative treatment.

Search Strategy

A PubMed search was performed for articles in English 1990–2013 reporting on post-resection outcomes for patients with stage I NSCLC using the mesh search terms "locoregional neoplasm recurrence", "metachronous second primary neoplasms", "prognosis", and "non-small cell lung carcinoma". Articles were selected for review that included information on patients who had undergone resection of pathologic stage I non-small cell lung cancer and that compared surveillance imaging to no surveillance imaging with the outcome of interest being overall survival.

Local Recurrence

Pattern of Local Recurrence for Stage I Patients

Overall crude rates of local/regional recurrence (LRR) for patients with stage I patients vary from 3 to 11 %. This variation is due to a number of factors including the definition of "local recurrence" used, how local followed by distant recurrences are scored, the extent of surgical resection, and the ability to differentiate between a LRR and the development of a second primary lung cancer. Crude rates of local/regional first recurrence of 2.9–6.0 % and estimated 5-year LRR rates of 16–23 % have been reported in studies that define LRR as disease recurrence at the surgical margin, ipsilateral hilum, and/or mediastinum and report on patient cohorts undergoing curative lobar resection or greater without adjuvant therapy [1–4]. Whereas crude rates of 8–11 % and estimated 5-year LRR rates of 10–29 % have been reported using an expanding definition of LRR to include either the supraclavicular or contralateral lymph nodes [2, 5, 6]. Mean disease free intervals of 14.1–19.8 months for local/regional recurrences are similar to those reported for distant metastatic spread [7, 8]. Nearly 80 % of local recurrences occur in the first 2 years [9]. However, two distinct recurrence peaks occur at around 9 and 50 months post-treatment, with a smaller peak occurring around 30 months [10].

Individual Risk Factors for Recurrence in Stage I Patients

The risk of LRR can be influenced by surgical, pathological, and patient factors. The extent of parenchymal resection for early stage lung cancer has an impact on the risk of LRR. The North American Lung Cancer Study Group randomized 276 patients with T1N0 NSCLC to lobar versus adequate sublobar resection (wedge resection or segmentectomy with ≥ 2 cm margins) [3]. Of 247 patients eligible for analysis, 11 % (28/247) of patients were reported to have a LRR. However, patients undergoing sublobar resection had a significantly greater rate of LRR than those undergoing lobar resection (17 % vs. 6 %, p = 0.008). In addition, the effect of sublobar resection on LRR rates applied regardless of the type (wedge or segmentectomy). However, locoregional recurrence rates were higher, possibly as a result of a substantial proportion of large tumors (2–3 cm). Non-randomized trials demonstrate lower locoregional recurrence rates with segmentectomy compared to wedge resection for tumors ≤2 cm. Inadequate nodal assessment (<15 lymph nodes) has been associated with increased local recurrence rates in two prior studies, presumably based on incomplete staging[11, 12]. A third study did not find that the number of resected N1 or N2 nodes was associated with local failure [1]. However, the median number of resected N1 and N2 nodes in their report was two for each station and may have thus confounded their results.

A number of pathologic factors have also been associated with increased risk for LRR. Both increasing size (hazard ratio 2.0) and vascular invasion (HR 2.5) have been reported to be independent predictors of both distant and LRR in stage I patients [1, 7].

Patient factors can also contribute to the risk of LRR. Diabetes (HR 1.8) has been demonstrated to be an independent predictor of LRR in a single report that used an expanded definition of LRR [1]. While a history of smoking in of itself has not been identified as a predictor of LRR, a >20 pack years smoking history has been associated with an increased risk of LRR [12].

Post Recurrence Survival for Stage I Patients

There have been four studies that have reported on postrecurrence survival (PRS) for patients with stage I disease [9, 13–15]. Shimada et al. followed 919 patients to determine factors influencing postrecurrence survival (PRS) and the effect of postrecurrence therapy (PRT) on PRS [13]. Type of recurrence included only local recurrence in 43 patients (25.3 %), distant in 113 (66.5 %), and both in 14 (8.2 %). Of the patients experiencing recurrence, 118 patients (69.4 %) received some form of treatment. However, only 10 % (4/43) with local only recurrence underwent a second intra-thoracic operation. The 1- and 2-year PRS proportions were 73.5 and 51.4 %, respectively. Multivariate analysis demonstrated that receiving any type of PRT was associated with improved PRS; however, being treated with surgery was not. In addition, mode of presentation was not a covariate included in the study multivariate analysis. Nagakawa et al. also evaluated the clinical outcomes of patients with resected lung cancer for postrecurrence prognostic factors [15]. Overall, 22 % (87/397) of patients had a recurrence, of whom 86 % (75/87) had some form of treatment. Reported 1-year and 3-year survival rates were 67.7 and 34.4 %, respectively. There was no significant difference in survival in those patients with local only vs. distant metastases or in those patients that were treated surgically or non-surgically. Once again, receiving some form of treatment was an independent predictor of improved PRS on multivariate analysis. Another study evaluated the prognostic predictors of PRS in patients with local only or local and distant recurrence [9]. Post-recurrence survival in patients with local only recurrence was not significantly different from that in those with both local and distant recurrences. Only treatment for initial recurrence was a significant predictor of post-recurrence survival in multivariate analyses.

In summary, receiving any form of treatment rather than palliation has been identified as a predictor of improved PRS regardless of the pattern of recurrence. However, undergoing surgery has not been demonstrated to improve survival on multivariate analysis, even when comparing surgical vs. non-surgical treatment for LRR. This is likely contributed to by the high re-recurrence rate after local therapies and that LRR may be followed by a distant recurrence in up to 20 % of patients [16]. Therefore receiving systemic rather than local therapy may be of more importance even when considering LRR.

Current Data on Survival Benefit for Post-Resection Surveillance for Local Recurrence

Mode of presentation has been demonstrated in some studies to be a predictor of poor recurrence free survival. This is thought to be as a result of a high association of symptomatic recurrence with distant metastases which would preclude possible curative re-resection. Scheduling frequent follow-up imaging could theoretically identify isolated asymptomatic LRR at a time when curative intent treatment could be provided, however, there is no evidence to support this.

Lamont et al. followed 124 patients using a systematic post-operative surveillance protocol employing CT and CXR. In total 7 % (9/124) developed an isolated local recurrence. Although 89 % (8/9) of isolated local recurrences were asymptomatic at the time of detection, only one of nine was able to be resected [17]. Another study divided patients with resected NSCLC into "intensely" followed versus "non-intensely" followed based on a number of arbitrary criteria [18]. The authors were unable to show any differences between the groups with regard to detection of local recurrences or overall survival. Disease-free and median survival were similar between two groups of curatively resected NSCLC patients followed using a protocol resembling current National Comprehensive Cancer Network (NCCN) guidelines versus follow-up on a symptom oriented basis [19]. Walsh et al. investigated the development of relapse or second primary tumor in patients who experienced recurrence to identify predictors of decreased survival; a disease free interval of ≤12 months was the most significant predictor of decreased survival [20]. Furthermore, when controlling for a disease free interval >12 months, there was no difference in survival for those patients who presented with or without symptoms or based on whether they were treated with palliative or curative intent. This suggests that tumor biology, rather than mode of detection, may be the most important predictor of survival. Westeel et al. prospectively followed patients for the development of recurrence [21]. Compliance was high with scheduled diagnostic procedures/imaging (83–93 %). Univariate analysis demonstrated that disease free interval ≤12 months and symptomatic mode of presentation were associated with decreased survival. However, fiberoptic bronchoscopy accounted for 33 % of asymptomic intra-thoracic recurrences amenable to curative treatment, and about 60 % of their patients underwent pneumonectomy. Resection with pneumonectomy could alter locoregional recurrence rates and exaggerate the importance of bronchoscopy in postresection surveillance. All of the preceding studies, however, have included patient cohorts with both early and late stage disease.

Song et al. examined the clinical outcomes after postoperative recurrence in 475 patients with completely resected stage I NSCLC [14]. Patients were seen in the clinic every 3 months with a CT scan in the first 2 years. Seventy two patients (15 %) experienced recurrence overall, with 50 % of those being distant. Only 18 % of patients had recurrence symptoms. The 1- and 3-year PRS rates were higher than previous reports at 88 and 53 %, respectively. Multivariate analysis revealed that recurrence within 12 months of surgery and a poor response to treatment (based on Response Evaluation Criteria in Solid Tumours guidelines for chemotherapy and a complete resection for surgery) were independent prognostic factors for significantly poor post-recurrence survival, however, the presence of symptoms were not. This suggests that tumor biology, rather than mode of detection, may be the most important predictor of survival.

A beneficial effect of early detection of asymptomatic local recurrence on survival is currently unproven based on the existing literature, as lead and length time bias have been inadequately controlled for. In addition, resection rates for local recurrence are confounded by bias in patient selection and treatment, as well as insufficient reporting of follow-up compliance.

Metachronous Primary Lung Cancer

Incidence and Patterns of Development of Metachronous Tumors

Rice et al. reported the incidence of metachronous primary lung cancer (MPLC) in a large prospective cohort of stage I patients who were followed with chest roentgenogram every 6 months [22]. Overall, 8.6 % (49/569) of patients developed a MPLC, and the overall incidence was two per 100 patient-years. The median interval between surgery for the first primary tumor and the diagnosis of MPLC was 51 months (7.5–108). Another large follow-up study on early stage lung cancer patients (84 % were stage I) reported an increasing hazard rate for second primary cancer over time, with three events per 100 person-years in year 2–6 events per 100 person-years in year 5 [23]. A more recent study demonstrated a smooth increase in metachronous tumor development rate in the first 18–24 months post-treatment, with a constant hazard rate thereafter based on recurrence dynamic modeling [10].

Individual Risk Factors for the Development of Metachronous Primary Lung Cancer

There has been only one study evaluating independent risk factors for the development of MPLCs in stage I patients [22]. Current smokers (HR 1.9) were reported to be at increased risk for the development of a MPLC on multivariate analysis after controlling for age, sex, anatomic versus nonanatomic resection, T stage, tumor location, histology, and smoking status (current vs. former).

Surveillance Imaging for the Development of Metachronous Lung Tumors

Similar to initial primary NSCLC, the stage of the metachronous tumor is the strongest predictor of overall survival [24]. Unlike patients who experience recurrence, post resection survival after resection of MPLC is good with reported 5-year rates as high as 66.0 % [24]. Therefore the ability to discover MPLCs at an early stage may result in the chance for long term survival. A prospective study that followed patients with surveillance chest roentgenogram every 6 months diagnosed only 47 % (23/49) of MPLCs at stage I [22]. This compares poorly to a previous prospective study that followed patients with annual CT scan and diagnosed 84.2 % (16/19) of MPLCs at stage I [17]. These results are similar to other retrospective studies that also employed annual follow-up with CT scan, with 85.0–92.0 % of MPLCs diagnosed at stage I [23, 25].

There has been one formal decision analysis study to predict the cost-effectiveness of annual post-operative surveillance CT scanning of patients with stage IA NSCLC for the development of MPLC [26]. Surveillance with CT scanning was cost-effective in their base case analysis at $47,676 per quality-adjusted life year gained. Assumptions that made surveillance with CT cost-ineffective included a cost of CT >$700 or a false positive rate >14 %, among others. Assumptions on false positive rates were extrapolated from pre-resection screening studies and may not be valid. The only study reporting on the accuracy of CT scan in detecting post-operative recurrence reported a false positive rate of 15 % [27].

Specific Recommendations

Patients with stage I NSCLC should not undergo surveillance imaging in order to detect asymptomatic intra-thoracic recurrences, as a beneficial effect on survival is currently unproven. Patients with stage I NSCLC and enough cardiopulmonary reserve to undergo a second resection should undergo annual surveillance CT to detect early stage metachronous lung cancer.

Summary

The existing data by which to make recommendations regarding post-resection surveillance is comprised of low level observational studies. The data reported suggests that tumor biology is the dominant factor in determining survival after recurrence. Lead time bias confounds studies that demonstrate more frequent surveillance imaging having the effect of discovering more asymptomatic recurrences. Patients with a short disease free interval ($\leq$12 months) will have a poor outcome regardless of treatment. In addition, survival for patients who have local-only intrathoracic recurrences is unlikely to be affected by local treatment alone as a large percentage will go on to have systemic disease and/or fail locally. Patients who have favorable tumor biology that have long disease free intervals are not only more likely to have asymptomatic recurrences detected on annual surveillance imaging, but also are more likely to benefit from treatment as well. The National Lung Screening Trial demonstrated a 20 % relative reduction in lung-cancer specific mortality by screening high-risk individuals with low dose CT (LDCT) scan due in part to stage shift with more early stage cancers being diagnosed. Those patients with a history of lung cancer are at highest risk for developing a MPLC and may also benefit from surveillance with annual LDCT. A number of observational studies have demonstrated that LDCT has the ability to detect a higher percentage of stage I MPLCs which may result in the chance for long term survival with curative intent treatment. However, prospective studies randomizing curatively resected early stage patients to surveillance with annual LDCT vs. standard of care are required before class I recommendations can be made.

A Personal View of the Data

My personal approach to post-resection surveillance includes an annual history and physical exam, along with low dose CT imaging. Patients that develop recurrence within the first year are unlikely to benefit from a survival standpoint by detecting the recurrence at an earlier asymptomatic state. This is thought to be due to aggressive tumor biology as evidenced by a short disease free interval. Tumors with a more favorable biology are not only more likely to have asymptomatic recurrences detected on annual surveillance imaging, but also are more likely to benefit from treatment as well. In addition, annual surveillance imaging can detect second primary lung cancers at an earlier stage and has been demonstrated to be cost-effective in that regard.

Recommendations

- Patients with stage I NSCLC should not undergo surveillance imaging to detect asymptomatic intra-thoracic recurrences, as a beneficial effect on survival is currently unproven. (Evidence quality low; weak recommendation)
- Patients with stage I NSCLC should undergo annual surveillance CT to detect early stage metachronous lung cancer. (Evidence quality low; weak recommendation)

References

1. Varlotto JM, Recht A, Flickinger JC, Medford-Davis LN, Dyer AM, DeCamp MM. Varying recurrence rates and risk factors associated with different definitions of local recurrence in patients with surgically resected, stage I non small cell lung cancer. Cancer. 2010;116(10):2390–400.
2. Martini N, Bains MS, Burt ME. Incidence of local recurrence and second primary tumors in resected stage I lung cancer. J Thorac Cardiovasc Surg. 1995;109:120–9.
3. Ginsberg RJ, Rubinstein LV. Randomized trial of lobectomy versus limited resection for T1 N0 non-small cell lung cancer. Ann Thorac Surg. 1995;60:615–23.
4. Park SY, Lee HS, Jang HJ, Lee GK, Chung KY, Zo JI. Tumor necrosis as a prognostic factor for stage IA non-small cell lung cancer. Ann Thorac Surg. 2011;91(6):1668–73.
5. Saynak M, Veeramachaneni NK, Hubbs JL, Nam J, Qaqish BF, Bailey JE, et al. Local failure after complete resection of N0-1 non-small cell lung cancer. Lung Cancer. 2011;71(2):156–65.
6. Harpole Jr DH, Herndon 2nd JE, Young Jr WG, Wolfe WG, Sabiston Jr DC. Stage I nonsmall cell lung cancer. A multivariate analysis of treatment methods and patterns of recurrence. Cancer. 1995;76(5):787–96.
7. Kelsey CR, Marks LB, Hollis D, Hubbs JL, Ready NE, D'Amico TA, et al. Local recurrence after surgery for early stage lung cancer: an 11-year experience with 975 patients. Cancer. 2009;115(22):5218–27.
8. al-Kattan K, Sepsas E, Fountain SW, Townsend ER. Disease recurrence after resection for stage I lung cancer. Eur J Cardiothorac Surg. 1997;12(3):380–4.
9. Hung JJ, Hsu WH, Hsieh CC, Huang BS, Huang MH, Liu JS, et al. Post-recurrence survival in completely resected stage I non-small cell lung cancer with local recurrence. Thorax. 2009;64(3):192–6.
10. Demicheli R, Fornili M, Ambrogi F, Higgins K, Boyd JA, Biganzoli E, et al. Recurrence dynamics for non-small-cell lung cancer: effect of surgery on the development of metastases. J Thorac Oncol. 2012;7(4):723–30.
11. Sawyer TE, Bonner JA, Gould PM, Deschamps C, Lange CM, Li H. Patients with stage I non-small cell lung carcinoma at postoperative risk for local recurrence, distant metastasis, and death: implications related to the design of clinical trials. Int J Radiat Oncol Biol Phys. 1999;45:315–21.
12. Hung JJ, Jeng WJ, Hsu WH, Chou TY, Huang BS, Wu YC. Predictors of death, local recurrence, and distant metastasis in completely resected pathological stage-I non-small-cell lung cancer. J Thorac Oncol. 2012;7(7):1115–23.

13. Shimada Y, Saji H, Yoshida K, Kakihana M, Honda H, Nomura M, et al. Prognostic factors and the significance of treatment after recurrence in completely resected stage I non-small cell lung cancer. Chest. 2013;143(6):1626–34.
14. Song IH, Yeom SW, Heo S, Choi WS, Yang HC, Jheon S, et al. Prognostic factors for post-recurrence survival in patients with completely resected stage I non-small-cell lung cancer. Eur J Cardiothorac Surg. 2013;45(2):262–7.
15. Nakagawa T, Okumura N, Ohata K, Igai H, Matsuoka T, Kameyama K. Postrecurrence survival in patients with stage I non-small cell lung cancer. Eur J Cardiothorac Surg. 2008;34(3):499–504.
16. Boyd JA, Hubbs JL, Kim DW, Hollis D, Marks LB, Kelsey CR. Timing of local and distant failure in resected lung cancer: implications for reported rates of local failure. J Thorac Oncol. 2010;5(2):211–4.
17. Lamont JP, Kakuda JT, Smith D, Wagman LD, Grannis Jr FW. Systematic postoperative radiologic follow-up in patients with non-small cell lung cancer for detecting second primary lung cancer in stage IA. Arch Surg. 2002;137(8):935–8.
18. Virgo KS, McKirgan LW, Caputo MC, Mahurin DM, Chao LC, Caputo NA, et al. Post-treatment management options for patients with lung cancer. Ann Surg. 1995;222(6):700–10.
19. Younes RN, Gross JL, Deheinzelin D. Follow-up in lung cancer: how often and for what purpose? Chest. 1999;115(6):1494–9.
20. Walsh GL, O'Connor M, Willis KM, Milas M, Wong RS, Nesbitt JC, et al. Is follow-up of lung cancer patients after resection medically indicated and cost-effective? Ann Thorac Surg. 1995;60(6):1563–70; discussion 1570–2.
21. Westeel V, Choma D, Clement F. Relevance of an intensive postoperative follow-up after surgery for non-small lung cancer. Ann Thorac Surg. 2000;70:1185–90.
22. Rice D, Kim HW, Sabichi A, Lippman S, Lee JJ, Williams B, et al. The risk of second primary tumors after resection of stage I non small cell lung cancer. Ann Thorac Surg. 2003;76(4):1001–7.
23. Lou F, Huang J, Sima CS, Dycoco J, Rusch V, Bach PB. Patterns of recurrence and second primary lung cancer in early-stage lung cancer survivors followed with routine computed tomography surveillance. J Thorac Cardiovasc Surg. 2013;145(1):75–81; discussion 81–2.
24. Lee BE, Port JL, Stiles BM, Saunders J, Paul S, Lee PC, et al. TNM stage is the most important determinant of survival in metachronous lung cancer. Ann Thorac Surg. 2009;88(4):1100–5.
25. Haraguchi S, Koizumi K, Hirata T, Hirai K, Mikami I, Kubokura H, et al. Surgical treatment of metachronous nonsmall cell lung cancer. Ann Thorac Cardiovasc Surg. 2010;16(5):319–25.
26. Kent MS, Korn P, Port JL, Lee PC, Altorki NK, Korst RJ. Cost effectiveness of chest computed tomography after lung cancer resection: a decision analysis model. Ann Thorac Surg. 2005;80(4):1215–22.
27. Korst RJ, Kansler AL, Port JL, Lee PC, Altorki NK. Accuracy of surveillance computed tomography in detecting recurrent or new primary lung cancer in patients with completely resected lung cancer. Ann Thorac Surg. 2006;82(3):1009–15.

Chapter 19
Support Therapy for Lung Failure: The Utility of Device Therapy

Christopher Wigfield and Sadeesh Srinathan

Abstract Patients with irreversible lung injury listed for lung transplantation increasingly face the dilemma of requiring a "bridge" to transplantation, which has prompted the development of alternative lung support devices. The utility of extracorporal lung support to improve outcomes for various indications is still in evolution. We review the indications for lung support and the types of extracorporeal support systems and assess the evidence available for device support therapy for respiratory failure. We conclude that device therapy for reversible lung failure should be decided on an individual patient basis. No generic recommendations can currently be made.

Keywords Lung failure • Lung transplantation • Extracorporeal support • Extracorporeal membrane oxygenation

Introduction

Lung failure constitutes the most frequent end organ failure in critical care medicine [1–3]. Mechanical ventilation to augment dysfunctional endogenous gas exchange provided considerable prognostic benefit for over half a century [4–6]. The implementation of protective ventilatory strategies has further reduced the mortality in patients with acute lung injury [7, 8]. Supportive care has been optimized in this patient population, but few patients appear to benefit from pulmonary

C. Wigfield, MD, MD, FRCS (C/TH) (✉)
Department of Surgery, Section of Cardiac and Thoracic Surgery, University of Chicago Medical Center, Chicago, IL, USA
e-mail: cwigfield@surgery.bsd.uchicago.edu

S. Srinathan, MD, MSc, FRCS (C), FRCS (C/TH)
Section of Thoracic Surgery, Winnipeg Health Sciences Centre, Winnipeg, MB, Canada
e-mail: ssrinathan@exchange.hsc.mb.ca

M.K. Ferguson (ed.), *Difficult Decisions in Thoracic Surgery*,
Difficult Decisions in Surgery: An Evidence-Based Approach 1,
DOI 10.1007/978-1-4471-6404-3_19, © Springer-Verlag London 2014

pharmaceutical treatment approaches. More recently, the H1N1 influenza epidemic reemphasized the limitations of mechanical ventilation in severe ARDS [9]. The threat of recurrent epidemics and the incidence of acute respiratory failure second-ary to potentially reversible obstructive, alveolar, vascular or neuromuscular etiolo-gies also underscores the pressure to apply in clinical practice the advances in gas exchange technology to achieve better outcomes [10–12].

In contrast, patients with irreversible lung injury listed for lung transplantation with end-stage respiratory diseases have exceeded the number of suitable donor lungs available for the last decade [13]. Increasingly, these candidates face the dilemma of requiring a "bridge" to transplantation [14]. These factors combined with advances achieved in left ventricular assist devices and perfusion technology prompted the development of alternative lung support devices [15, 16]. While the functionality of some such devices may now be considered superior, the utility of extra-corporal lung support to improve outcomes for various indications is still in evolution.

Our first objective in this review is to provide an overview of the indications for lung support and the types of extracorporeal support systems and discuss the tech-nologies and clinical concepts applied in this setting. Our second objective is to assess the evidence available for device support therapy for respiratory failure on improvement on survival according the indications for the use of these devices.

Clinical Use of Extracorporeal Lung Support

Extracorporeal life support (ECLS), including ventricular assist devices, are fre-quently used to facilitate recovery after major cardiac surgical procedures [17–20]. This technology has since been adapted and evolved for the specific application for respiratory failure and followed several conceptually different approaches (Table 19.1) [21]. Both short term and prolonged ECLS for respiratory failure have now been established in critical care units [22, 23]. Outcomes with the use of these devices appear to have improved over the last decade in these sick patients.

The support system most frequently applied is extracorporeal membrane oxy-genation (ECMO), but technologies developed include several conceptually differ-ent devices. ECMO allows for a "pump system" to pass blood extracorporeally through a membrane gas exchange device and returns it to the patient [24, 25]. The path of the blood flow is determined by the mode of ECMO used, either Veno-Venous (VV) or Veno-Arterial (VA) circulatory support. The designation refers to the site of vascular drainage and perfusion (in and out of the systemic circulation), i.e. the cannulation sites. Both approaches may provide very effective gas exchange support in end-stage respiratory failure, but only VA ECMO provides additional hemodynamic support. VV ECMO predominantly provides oxygenation and CO_2 elimination whereas VA ECMO supports systemic perfusion at the same time. A standard circuit design includes a centrifugal driver or roller pump and a membrane oxygenator with a heparin bonded tubing perfusion system.

Table 19.1 Current methods of support for lung failure

Dysfunction	Clinical example	Devices available	Concept	Benefits	Drawbacks
Respiratory failure	H1N1 infection	vvECMO			
Oxygenation only					
CO_2 only		vv ECMO, NovaLung IVOX	A membrane with inflow from systemic artery (femoral) with return to a systemic vein	No systemic heparinization, allows lung rest as ventilation for CO_2 removal is decreased	Of limited use for oxygenation Requires normal LV function
CO_2 and O_2		vv ECMO va ECMO	Full pulmonary support when sufficient cardiac function to overcome resistance through the membrane (?)	Complete respiratory support, easy (?) to institute, widely available (?)	Requires full anticoagulation….
Combined resp and cardiac failure		v-a ECMO	Full pulmonary and right ventricular support using membrane oxygenator and pump	Full support …	Requires full anticoagulation, limits ability to ambulate and care for patient

There have been significant technological refinements of pump design with centrifugal drive devices being the latest development. An increasingly frequent approach for support for respiratory failure utilizes a dual lumen cannula for institution of VV ECMO via single site percutaneous internal jugular vein insertion. This can greatly facilitate application of ECMO [25, 26].

ECMO systems require a "pump" generating the blood flow to perfuse the oxygenated blood. Alternative designs simplify the approach and have relied on the patient's arterial perfusion pressure to provide extracorporeal gas exchange. The most widely established system in this category is the Novalung® which allows CO_2 elimination via a veno-arterial shunt principle with a polymethylpentene diffusion membrane inter-positioned [14]. In essence this is the same approach as for arterio-venous hemofiltration. In addition to extracorporeal systems, there have been intra-vascular devices for oxygenation such as the diffusion limited oxygenator (IVOX®) [27]. This enables permissive hypercapnia with an indwelling catheter based application.

There are device specific advantages and limitations according to each approach. Few clinical guidelines for application exist and several devices are still in investigational phases and will not be discussed in this chapter. A third category, fully implantable artificial lung devices, are currently experimental in animal models and have not been established in clinical practice outside of such scientific trial protocols. These are not discussed in this review.

Indications for Lung Support Systems

The indications for lung support can be categorized according the reversibility of the lung injury and whether the lung is native or a transplant. The criteria leading to the implementation of lung assist systems may depend on a reversible etiology with a strategy to support to native pulmonary recovery. Non-reversible, i.e. end stage pulmonary disease indications may be present when the patient is considered a candidate for lung transplantation [28]. Essentially three categories exist.

Indications:

A. Reversible injury to the native lungs, i.e. bridge to recovery
B. Reversible injury in a transplanted lung: e.g. acute allograft failure
C. Irreversible injury to native lung, i.e. bridge to transplant

The diagnostic spectrum for lung device support is broad and reflects the specific clinical scenario, few contraindications are generally considered applicable across these scenarios. These include: sepsis and acute sepsis syndromes, irreversible coagulopathy and irreversible injury to damage to other end organ systems without likely chance of recovery. This is particularly pertinent to severe neurological injury from anoxia or stroke.

Respiratory failure encompasses failure in ventilation, oxygenation and CO_2 clearance. This is often combined with a variable degree of cardiac dysfunction, particularly right heart failure. The lung support technologies available address these different components of respiratory failure to a variable extent.

Respiratory Dysfunction (Oxygenation and CO_2 Clearance) and Cardiac Dysfunction

VA ECMO is a modality which removes systemic venous blood and delivers into the central arterial system. It works in parallel to the native pulmonary circulation and is designed to optimize perfusion pressure and oxygen delivery. Driver devices help support mean arterial pressure in addition to improving oxygen saturation. This is measured at the capillary vascular bed with simultaneous monitoring of sufficient preload to maintain left ventricular output. This modality offers near compete cardiopulmonary support.

Respiratory Dysfunction (Oxygen and CO_2) Without Hemodynamic Compromise

VV ECMO is typically used for primary respiratory failure when no significant haemodynamic support is required. Generally, for this approach to be effective, cardiac output is preserved in the patient and specific evaluation shows no likely acute cardiogenic deterioration. Due to the type of VV ECMO support, there are unique considerations for systemic monitoring and daily management when compared with VA ECMO. Blood flow rates for VV ECMO are typically sub-maximal blood flow rates (calculated in L/min for BSA or BMI). This allows for optimized oxygen delivery and CO_2 elimination with reduced peripheral arterial embolic risk as no arterial return cannula is required. In patients with predominant failure of CO_2 clearance but preservation of oxygenation and hemodynamics, the NovaLung® device provides a further alternative.

General Considerations Regarding Indications and Outcomes

Regardless of the primary cause of lung failure, respiratory decompensation is followed by either hypoxia, hypercarbia or both [29, 30]. As described, not all device systems are effective in ameliorating both components of respiratory failure and lung assist technology relies on uncoupling of oxygen delivery versus CO_2 removal primarily to allow for the use of the ventilator with a maximal lung preservation strategy such as minimal lung volumes, ventilation pressures and lower FiO_2 [7]. The ultimate goal with these devices is to allow for resolution of the primary lung injury or to allow time for a transplant (in the case of irreversible lung failure) to occur.

Lung replacement therapy in contrast aims to provide oxygenation and ventilation in a more complete and implantable option. Replacement of other physiological properties of lungs, including metabolic and vascular functions as well as immuno-logic properties do not feature in any of the devices currently available. These two aspects will not be discussed further.

The complexity of the clinical and logistic issues involved imply that ECMO is best provided in dedicated programs. It is reasonable to assume that this is likely associated with optimal outcomes. Resources and manpower requirements ought to be met with adequate protocol provision and procedural guidelines. Interventional lung supplement devices not requiring perfusion services such as the NovaLung® maybe more readily available to critical care units. They nonetheless require spe-cific expertise discerning correct indications and planning destination care with respect to the primary etiology. A detailed evaluation has to rule out all contraindi-cations and other irreversible end-organ failure in particular when patients are selec-tively considered as candidates to bridge to lung transplantation [11, 31].

The second indication in this context is to provide support to recovery after pri-mary graft dysfunction (PGD) in the lung recipient [32, 33]. In this setting lung assist devices may significantly improve outcomes if commenced early after onset of PGD, ideally prior to onset of multi-organ impairment or sepsis [34]. The quality of evidence however is limited by the lack of prospective studies. For lung trans-plant indications, including primary graft dysfunction, it is essential that ECMO support is combined with protective lung ventilation strategies [7, 8]. It is clinically intuitive that the reduction of ventilator induced lung injury (VILI) with low tidal volumes and permissive hypercapnia contribute in these settings. Optimizing sys-temic and respiratory physiotherapy including ambulatory protocols have been introduced with some clinical success, but remain a highly individual indication rather than an evidence based recommendation at present [35].

Results of Use

Determining the quality of evidence supporting the use of lung assist devices is hampered by both the heterogeneous nature of the conditions which constitute the indications as well as the variety of devices available. A further complication is the very rapid development of these technologies which are continually under develop-ment and have not matured sufficiently to undergo trials which produce the high quality evidence which we seek. However, some assessment must still be made to guide clinical care.

Search Strategy

We evaluated the available literature by undertaking a systematic search of the fol-lowing databases: PubMed, EMBASE and the Web of Science. An extensive search strategy was used that yielded 2,012 titles and abstracts. The full text of 157 relevant articles were retrieved and reviewed. To assess the value of these interventions we limited our considerations to mortality as the beneficial outcome and neurological injury as the harm outcome.

We included both observational studies and trials which provided data on mortality and neurological outcome in adult patients were evaluated. We excluded animal studies and studies in children. We considered the evidence according to the clinical indications for use. We have loosely applied the GRADE framework to judge the quality of the evidence supporting the use of these modalities to improve survival [36–38].

Results

Reversible Injury to the Native Lungs—Bridge to Recovery

There were a number of case series but only three clinical trials using ECMO for reversible lung failure. The two older studies published in 1979 (Zapol) and 1994 (Morris) have little applicability to current practice as they used now obsolete ECMO technology and conventional management techniques [21, 39]. The major study informing current practice is the CESAR trial [40]. This trial compared a strategy incorporating ECMO to one without. There were 766 patients screened from 148 centres in the United Kingdom. Of these 180 patients met the inclusion criteria (age 18–65, had Murray score of >3.0 or pH of <7.20 and potentially reversible respiratory failure). Patients were excluded if they had high ventilation pressures or high FiO2 for more than 7 days, intracranial bleeding, contraindication to heparinization or other contraindication for continued active treatment. The patients allocated to the ECMO arm (n=90) were transported to a single ECMO centre, while those allocated to the conventional arm remained in their local hospital or were transferred to a regional centre without ECMO capabilities. Of those who were allocated to the ECMO arm, 68 (75 %) actually received ECMO (venovenous) and in these patients 43 (63 %) survived 6 months without disability. In the 17 patients who did not receive ECMO, 14 survived. The relative risk of death in the overall ECMO arm was 0.69; 95 % CI 0.05–0.97. The overall survival rates in the ECMO arm was 63 % and in the control arm it was 47 %, with an absolute risk reduction of 16 % with number needed to treat 6.25. No neurological injury was noted in either group in this trial. Although this study was a carefully done randomized controlled trial, there are concerns related to the study design such as no limitation on the treatment of the conventional arm and further that randomization necessitated transfer to a centre which not only provided ECMO, but also likely to provide expert non-ECMO ARDS care [41].

A recent systematic review was carried out which combined the results of the CESAR trial with two observational studies with matched patients. The authors concluded that the utility of ECMO is still unclear as their results were very sensitive to reasonable assumptions on the type of analysis and the differences in patient populations where the two recent observational studies were H1N1 patients who were on the whole younger and sicker, but could not be matched and therefore could not be adequately assessed within the study [42, 43].

Although the CESAR RCT could be considered as providing high quality evidence for the use of VV ECMO for reversible lung injury we have reservations about the study design and its applicability our question—does the provision of VV ECMO in itself improve outcome. When considering the inconsistency of results among the two high quality observational studies, we judge that the overall quality of evidence is moderate. Currently, there is an ongoing trial, Extracorporeal Membrane Oxygenation for Severe Acute Respiratory Distress Syndrome (EOLIA) NCT01470703, which may help to clarify this issue further [44].

Review of available Novalung® data revealed a small subset of reports. These studies describe various levels of success with the intervention, but given that they are all observational studies they are considered relatively low quality evidence. Further prospective studies are needed.

Reversible Injury to Transplanted Lung

There are only case series and partial registries which provide information on this cohort of patients as the numbers at any institutions are very small. Fischer et al. were only able to identify 151 patients undergoing ECMO for primary graft dysfunction (PGD) from a multicenter registry [14]. In 93 of the 151 patients support was discontinued due to sufficient lung recovery. Overall 63 patients survived the hospital stay, but a large burden of complications was encountered. The authors conclude from their study, despite its limitations, that ECMO has a clinical role in PGD. Bermudez reported that 39 out of 58 patients were weaned from ECMO support due to lung recovery [26]. Wigfield et al. reported on 22 patients who were placed on ECMO for acute PGD [34]. Successful weaning and survival was associated with early implementation of the support strategy in this cohort. Considering the significant mortality associated with severe (Grade 3) PGD after lung transplantation, this is accepted as a valid indication to improve survival in this setting [45–47].

Irreversible Injury to Native Lung—Bridge to Transplant

Several studies set out to evaluate the impact of ECMO on mortality in patients with acute respiratory failure [41–44]. Mostly uncontrolled or single institution retrospective assessments, the survival rates reported with the institution of ECMO ranged from 50 % to 71 %. These cohorts were compared to historical survival data only. Transfer to an established ECMO center for ventilator or ECMO management was associated with reduced mortality in a study following a cohort with severe H1N1 induced respiratory failure (23.7 v 52.5 % mortality, respectively). Design issues with the study and confounders were acknowledged.

Conclusions

The increasing demand for lung assist devices has resulted in innovative approaches. However, the quality of evidence supporting its use in the clinical setting is limited. This is due in part the wide range of indications for use in disparate populations and the variety of devices available. Overall, we have to judge the quality of evidence supporting the use of these devices as moderate at best for particular indications and low overall. This reflects the nature of the studies available as much as it does the likely effectiveness of the intervention. Considering that lung support is used in gravely ill patients who have no other therapeutic options, it is worth framing this issue in terms of futility. From this perspective we are confident that the quality of evidence suggests that device support in lung failure on the whole is not associated with more harm than the likely alternatives, i.e. continued mechanical ventilatory support. Selected indications and settings may prove to allow for improved outcomes, but conclusive evidence is pending.

Currently, no single approach or system has emerged as "optimal" and given the multifactorial nature of critical care for pulmonary failure this is unlikely to change. The advent of increasingly biocompatible technology as well as tissue engineering and regenerative medicine is likely to yield novel approaches. Further clarification of the indications and contraindications is also likely to improve outcomes. Prospective trials with refined technologies will help us to deliver care for these critically ill patients with more confidence of their utility. Fortunately, there are some studies currently registered which may help to shed light on the appropriate use of these devices.

Recommendations

Device therapy for reversible lung failure should be decided on an individual patient basis. No generic recommendations can currently be made. The best outcomes achieved have been observed in dedicated centers with an experienced service providing this demanding therapeutic option. This is also likely to provide best evidence to support future decision making algorithms and appropriate clinical research regarding this complex topic. It is acknowledged that the pressure to provide a "possible reversibility" often outweighs the probability of full recovery of patients with severe lung failure. In this setting, randomized clinical trials are a formidable task.

A Personal View of the Data

The authors advocate for the decision to support patients with ECMO or similar devices to be made in a multidisciplinary approach. This is particularly true if the goal is recovery from native lung failure where lung transplantation is not a solution. The chance of pulmonary reversibility and systemic recovery ought to be established prior to the institution of ECMO. This may help to avoid unwarranted disrepute of this evolving therapy.

Recommendation

- No generic recommendation for use of extracorporeal support devices in patients with lung failure can be made. (Evidence quality low; no recommendation).

References

1. Mac Sweeney R, McAuley DF, Matthay MA. Acute lung failure. Semin Respir Crit Care Med. 2011;32:607–25.
2. Zilberberg MD, Epstein SK. Acute lung injury in the medical ICU: comorbid conditions, age, etiology, and hospital outcome. Am J Respir Crit Care Med. 1998;157:1159–64.
3. Vincent JL, Akça S, De Mendonça A, Haji-Michael P, Sprung C, Moreno R, Antonelli M, Suter PM, SOFA Working Group Sequential Organ Failure Assessment. The epidemiology of acute respiratory failure in critically ill patients(*). Chest. 2002;121:1602–9.
4. Bernard GR, Artigas A, Brigham KL, Carlet J, Falke K, Hudson L, Lamy M, Legall JR, Morris A, Spragg R, The American-European Consensus Conference on ARDS. Definitions, mechanisms, relevant outcomes, and clinical trial coordination. Am J Respir Crit Care Med. 1994;149:818–24.
5. Sloane PJ, Gee MH, Gottlieb JE, Albertine KH, Peters SP, Burns JR, Machiedo G, Fish JE. A multicenter registry of patients with acute respiratory distress syndrome. Physiology and outcome. Am Rev Respir Dis. 1992;146:419–26.
6. Doyle RL, Szaflarski N, Modin GW, Wiener-Kronish JP, Matthay MA. Identification of patients with acute lung injury. Predictors of mortality. Am J Respir Crit Care Med. 1995;152:1818–24.
7. The Acute Respiratory Distress Syndrome Network. Ventilation with lower tidal volumes as compared with traditional tidal volumes for acute lung injury and the acute respiratory distress syndrome. N Engl J Med. 2000;342:1301–8.
8. Ranieri VM, Suter PM, Tortorella C, De Tullio R, Dayer JM, Brienza A, Bruno F, Slutsky AS. Effect of mechanical ventilation on inflammatory mediators in patients with acute respiratory distress syndrome: a randomized controlled trial. JAMA. 1999;282:54–61.
9. Davies A, Jones D, Bailey M, Beca J, Bellomo R, Blackwell N, Forrest P, Gattas D, Granger E, Herkes R, Jackson A, McGuinness S, Nair P, Pellegrino V, Pettilä V, Plunkett B, Pye R, Torzillo P, Webb S, Wilson M, Ziegenfuss M, Australia and New Zealand Extracorporeal Membrane Oxygenation (ANZ ECMO) Influenza Investigators. Extracorporeal membrane oxygenation for 2009 Influenza A (H1N1) acute respiratory distress syndrome. JAMA. 2009;302:1888–95.
10. Lewandowski K, Rossaint R, Pappert D, Gerlach H, Slama KJ, Weidemann H, Frey DJ, Hoffmann O, Keske U, Falke KJ. High survival rate in 122 ARDS patients managed according to a clinical algorithm including extracorporeal membrane oxygenation. Intensive Care Med. 1997;23:819–35.
11. Hemmila MR, Rowe SA, Boules TN, Miskulin J, McGillicuddy JW, Schuerer DJ, Haft JW, Swaniker F, Arbabi S, Hirschl RB, Bartlett RH. Extracorporeal life support for severe acute respiratory distress syndrome in adults. Ann Surg. 2004;240:595–605; discussion 605–7.
12. Brogan TV, Thiagarajan RR, Rycus PT, Bartlett RH, Bratton SL. Extracorporeal membrane oxygenation in adults with severe respiratory failure: a multi-center database. Intensive Care Med. 2009;35:2105–14.
13. Arcasoy SM, Fisher A, Hachem RR, Scavuzzo M, Ware LB, ISHLT Working Group on Primary Lung Graft Dysfunction. Report of the ISHLT Working Group on Primary Lung Graft Dysfunction part V: predictors and outcomes. J Heart Lung Transplant. 2005;24:1483–8.

14. Fischer S, Hoeper MM, Tomaszek S, Simon A, Gottlieb J, Welte T, Haverich A, Strueber M. Bridge to lung transplantation with the extracorporeal membrane ventilator Novalung in the veno-venous mode: the initial Hannover experience. ASAIO J. 2007;53:168–70.
15. Combes A, Leprince P, Luyt CE, Bonnet N, Trouillet JL, Léger P, Pavie A, Chastre J. Outcomes and long-term quality-of-life of patients supported by extracorporeal membrane oxygenation for refractory cardiogenic shock. Crit Care Med. 2008;36:1404–11.
16. Chen YS, Lin JW, Yu HY, Ko WJ, Jerng JS, Chang WT, Chen WJ, Huang SC, Chi NH, Wang CH, Chen LC, Tsai PR, Wang SS, Hwang JJ, Lin FY. Cardiopulmonary resuscitation with assisted extracorporeal life-support versus conventional cardiopulmonary resuscitation in adults with in-hospital cardiac arrest: an observational study and propensity analysis. Lancet. 2008;372:554–61.
17. Smedira NG, Blackstone EH. Postcardiotomy mechanical support: risk factors and outcomes. Ann Thorac Surg. 2001;71:S60–6; discussion S82–5.
18. Pagani FD, Aaronson KD, Swaniker F, Bartlett RH. The use of extracorporeal life support in adult patients with primary cardiac failure as a bridge to implantable left ventricular assist device. Ann Thorac Surg. 2001;71:S77–81; discussion S82–5.
19. Massetti M, Tasle M, Le Page O, Deredec R, Babatasi G, Buklas D, Thuaudet S, Charbonneau P, Hamon M, Grollier G, Gerard JL, Khayat A. Back from irreversibility: extracorporeal life support for prolonged cardiac arrest. Ann Thorac Surg. 2005;79:178–83; discussion 183–4.
20. Younger JG, Schreiner RJ, Swaniker F, Hirschl RB, Chapman RA, Bartlett RH. Extracorporeal resuscitation of cardiac arrest. Acad Emerg Med. 1999;6:700–7.
21. Zapol WM, Snider MT, Hill JD, Fallat RJ, Bartlett RH, Edmunds LH, Morris AH, Peirce EC, Thomas AN, Proctor HJ, Drinker PA, Pratt PC, Bagniewski A, Miller RG. Extracorporeal membrane oxygenation in severe acute respiratory failure. A randomized prospective study. JAMA. 1979;242:2193–6.
22. Organization, E. E. L. S. ELSO (Extracorporeal Life Support Organization) Guidelines for ECMO Centers. http://www.elso.med.umich.edu/WordForms/ELSO%20Guidelines%20For%20ECMO%20Centers.pdf. Accessed 4 May 2014.
23. Kelly RB, Porter PA, Meier AH, Myers JL, Thomas NJ. Duration of cardiopulmonary resuscitation before extracorporeal rescue: how long is not long enough? ASAIO J. 2005;51:665–7.
24. Peek GJ, Moore HM, Moore N, Sosnowski AW, Firmin RK. Extracorporeal membrane oxygenation for adult respiratory failure. Chest. 1997;112:759–64.
25. Allen S, Holena D, McCunn M, Kohl B, Sarani B. A review of the fundamental principles and evidence base in the use of extracorporeal membrane oxygenation (ECMO) in critically ill adult patients. J Intensive Care Med. 2011;26:13–26.
26. Bermudez CA, Rocha RV, Sappington PL, Toyoda Y, Murray HN, Boujoukos AJ. Initial experience with single cannulation for venovenous extracorporeal oxygenation in adults. Ann Thorac Surg. 2010;90:991–5.
27. Tao W, Zwischenberger JB, Nguyen TT, Tzouanakis AE, Matheis EJ, Traber DL, Bidani A. Performance of an intravenous gas exchanger (IVOX) in a venovenous bypass circuit. Ann Thorac Surg. 1994;57:1484–90; discussion 1490–1.
28. Davis RD, Lin SS. ECMO in lung transplantation. In: Vigneswaran WT, Garrity ER Jr, eds: Lung Transplantation. Informa Healthcare, London, 2010.
29. Rich PB, Awad SS, Kolla S, Annich G, Schreiner RJ, Hirschl RB, Bartlett RH. An approach to the treatment of severe adult respiratory failure. J Crit Care. 1998;13:26–36.
30. Rabin J, Kon Z, Garcia J, Griffith B, Herr D. 1150: successful bridge to transplant after 155 days of VV ECMO. Crit Care Med. 2012;40:1–328.
31. Hämmäinen P, Schersten H, Lemström K, Riise GC, Kukkonen S, Swärd K, Sipponen J, Silverborn M, Dellgren G. Usefulness of extracorporeal membrane oxygenation as a bridge to lung transplantation: a descriptive study. J Heart Lung Transplant. 2011;30:103–7.
32. Shargall Y, Guenther G, Ahya VN, Ardehali A, Singhal A, Keshavjee S, ISHLT Working Group on Primary Lung Graft Dysfunction. Report of the ISHLT Working Group on Primary Lung Graft Dysfunction part VI: treatment. J Heart Lung Transplant. 2005;24:1489–500.
33. Hartwig MG, Davis RD. Surgical considerations in lung transplantation: transplant operation and early postoperative management. Respir Care Clin N Am. 2004;10:473–504.

34. Wigfield CH, Lindsey JD, Steffens TG, Edwards NM, Love RB. Early institution of extracorporeal membrane oxygenation for primary graft dysfunction after lung transplantation improves outcome. J Heart Lung Transplant. 2007;26:331–8.
35. Brain J, Turner D, Rehder K, Smith P, Duane DR, Cheifetz I, et al. 136: Ambulatory ECMO as a bridge to lung transplantation is a more cost effective approach as compared to a non-ambulatory strategy. Crit Care Med. 2012;40:1–328.
36. Group, G. W. Grade Working Group. http://gradeworkinggroup.org/index.htm. Accessed 4 May 2014.
37. McCulloch P. Evidence-based surgery. Surgery (Oxford). 2006;24:272–5.
38. Haynes RB, Devereaux PJ, Guyatt GH. Physicians' and patients' choices in evidence based practice. BMJ. 2002;324:1350.
39. Morris AH, Wallace CJ, Menlove RL, Clemmer TP, Orme JF, Weaver LK, Dean NC, Thomas F, East TD, Pace NL, Suchyta MR, Beck E, Bombino M, Sittig DF, Böhm S, Hoffmann B, Becks H, Butler S, Pearl J, Rasmusson B. Randomized clinical trial of pressure-controlled inverse ratio ventilation and extracorporeal CO_2 removal for adult respiratory distress syndrome. Am J Respir Crit Care Med. 1994;149:295–305.
40. Peek GJ, Mugford M, Tiruvoipati R, Wilson A, Allen E, Thalanany MM, Hibbert CL, Truesdale A, Clemens F, Cooper N, Firmin RK, Elbourne D, CESAR Trial Collaboration. Efficacy and economic assessment of conventional ventilatory support versus extracorporeal membrane oxygenation for severe adult respiratory failure (CESAR): a multicentre randomised controlled trial. Lancet. 2009;374:1351–63.
41. Brindley PG, Cave D, Lequier L. BEST evidence in critical care medicine. Extracorporeal membrane oxygenation (ECMO) in severe adult respiratory distress syndrome. Can J Anaesth. 2010;57:273–5.
42. Noah MA, Peek GJ, Finney SJ, Griffiths MJ, Harrison DA, Grieve R, Sadique MZ, Sekhon JS, McAuley DF, Firmin RK, Harvey C, Cordingley JJ, Price S, Vuylsteke A, Jenkins DP, Noble DW, Bloomfield R, Walsh TS, Perkins GD, Menon D, Taylor BL, Rowan KM. Referral to an extracorporeal membrane oxygenation center and mortality among patients with severe 2009 influenza A(H1N1). JAMA. 2011;306:1659–68.
43. Pham T, Combes A, Rozé H, Chevret S, Mercat A, Roch A, Mourvillier B, Ara-Somohano C, Bastien O, Zogheib E, Clavel M, Constan A, Marie Richard JC, Brun-Buisson C, Brochard L, Network RR. Extracorporeal membrane oxygenation for pandemic influenza A(H1N1)-induced acute respiratory distress syndrome: a cohort study and propensity-matched analysis. Am J Respir Crit Care Med. 2013;187:276–85.
44. Combes A. Clinical trial NCT01470703: extracorporeal membrane oxygenation for severe acute respiratory distress syndrome (EOLIA), 2013. http://clinicaltrials.gov/ct2/show/NCT01470703. Accessed 4 May 2014.
45. Christie JD, Van Raemdonck D, de Perrot M, Barr M, Keshavjee S, Arcasoy S, Orens J, ISHLT Working Group on Primary Lung Graft Dysfunction. Report of the ISHLT Working Group on Primary Lung Graft Dysfunction part I: introduction and methods. J Heart Lung Transplant. 2005;24:1451–3.
46. Christie JD, Carby M, Bag R, Corris P, Hertz M, Weill D, ISHLT Working Group on Primary Lung Graft Dysfunction. Report of the ISHLT Working Group on Primary Lung Graft Dysfunction part II: definition. A consensus statement of the International Society for Heart and Lung Transplantation. J Heart Lung Transplant. 2005;24:1454–9.
47. Barr ML, Kawut SM, Whelan TP, Girgis R, Böttcher H, Sonett J, Vigneswaran W, Follette DM, Corris PA, ISHLT Working Group on Primary Lung Graft Dysfunction. Report of the ISHLT Working Group on Primary Lung Graft Dysfunction part IV: recipient-related risk factors and markers. J Heart Lung Transplant. 2005;24:1468–82.

Chapter 20
Extracorporeal Support for Lung Grafts Prior to Transplantation

Axel Haverich and Christian Kuehn

Abstract Because of the limitations of cold preservation, only optimal donor organs are selected for transplantation; not all potential donor lungs are accepted as suitable for transplantation. Ex-vivo lung perfusion techniques are seeing increased use in lung transplant surgery, the major point of interest being the possibility to recondition marginal donor organs. In addition, a portable organ care system has been developed to completely avoid the use of cold ischemia with its resulting negative consequences. The question of whether this approach will result in a potential benefit to normal lung transplant surgery has yet to be answered.

Keywords Extracorporporeal circulation • Lung transplantation • Ex vivo lung perfusion • Lung preservation

Introduction

Despite a steady improvement in organ donor management and the establishment of standardized methods for preserving donor organs, not all potential donor lungs are accepted as suitable for transplantation. Flushing or rinsing with cold perfusion solution has, for many years, been regarded as the current Gold Standard for preserving lung grafts, as for other solid organs. Despite the fact that there are a number of solutions available for lung transplantation, with the choice of method depending very

A. Haverich, MD (✉) • C. Kuehn, MD
Department of Thoracic, Transplant and Cardiovascular Surgery,
Hannover Medical School, Carl-Neuberg-Str.1, Hannover, 30625, Germany
e-mail: haverich.axel@mh-hannover.de

M.K. Ferguson (ed.), *Difficult Decisions in Thoracic Surgery*,
Difficult Decisions in Surgery: An Evidence-Based Approach 1,
DOI 10.1007/978-1-4471-6404-3_20, © Springer-Verlag London 2014

much on the specific preferences of individual clinics, these solutions do not differ greatly with regard to the post-cold flush perfusion ischemia times achieved. For lungs preserved in this manner, an ischemic limit of 10 h is currently indicated. Harvesting and implantation with subsequent reperfusion should then take place directly, as a more protracted ischemia may lead to a higher risk of primary graft failure and, consequently, a marked decline in the survival rate. Owing to this narrow time frame and the resulting limitations of cold preservation, only optimal donor organs are selected for transplantation. This relatively high rejection rate of potential donor lungs is due to the fear of a less-than-optimal donor organ being additionally damaged by cold preservation, adversely affecting the outcome of transplantation.

Over the last few years, intensive research has been conducted on the development of normothermic perfusion systems for donor lungs. With Ex-vivo Lung Perfusion (EVLP), developed in Sweden in 2007, the donor lung is connected to a system of tubes, similar to a heart-lung machine, and a respirator. With a normothermic system, it is possible to evaluate marginal donor organs and assess organ function using parameters such as oxygen intake, lung elasticity and perfusion and ventilation pressure, to determine their suitability for the transplantation process. Moreover, the cold ischemic time can be reduced through the use of this type of normothermic organ perfusion, thus preventing any potential harm to the donor organ from a lack of oxygen and nutrients.

Search Strategy

We used Medline and PubMed as a database with the search terms "extracorpororeal circulation", "lung transplantation", "ex vivo lung perfusion" and "lung preservation" for relevant literature published until July 1, 2013.

Results

Ex-vivo Reconditioning of Marginal Donor Lungs Using EVLP

Some working groups, particularly those in Lund (Sweden), Toronto (Canada) and Vienna (Austria), already avail of clinical experience in evaluating and improving donor lungs through the use of EVLP and subsequent transplantation [1–4]. In these initial clinical operations, marginal donor lungs which originally appeared to be unsuitable for transplantation were assessed more accurately using normothermic EVLP and successfully transplanted, achieving comparable results to transplants conducted after cold preservation.

The potential to perfuse donor organs with poor oxygenation performance and oedema has also been demonstrated, where the use of a hyperosmolar solution led to significant oedema reduction and a subsequent improvement in oxygenation performance [5]. Normothermic EVLP was thus used not only in the further appraisal of marginal donor lungs but also in the therapeutic application of hyperosmolar solution in the treatment of edematous tissue.

Further thoughts along these lines open up the possibility of reconditioning marginal donor lungs using EVLP in the ex-vivo treatment of a pulmonary oedema and a pulmonary embolism using fibrinolytic agents to apply a surfactant to the airways and administer a high dose of antibiotic therapy for pneumonia, culminating in feasible immunomodulatory therapies [6]. The practical application of this pioneering technology initially requires the conventional removal of the donor lungs after an antegrade perfusion with a quality suitable solution for cold preservation. This preservation can, if necessary, be combined with subsequent retrograde flushing through the pulmonary veins to remove smaller pulmonary emboli. Typically, the standard method of preservation and packing is then to use ice with normothermic EVLP technology, when moving the donor organ to the transplant clinic after transport. The donor organ is surgically prepared for this purpose, using an aseptic technique.

The trachea of the donor and the main stem of the pulmonary artery are then usually connected using a single connector. In some systems, a further connector will be used on the dorsal side of the left atrium to create a closed perfusion circuit. In other cases, the perfusate is drained openly from the pulmonary veins into a reservoir. Additionally, components such as oxygenators, blood pumps, heat exchangers, filters and tubing in the perfusion system are used, similar to what one might expect to find in extracorporeal support. A ventilator is also integrated into the system.

The donor organ is subsequently perfused, via the relevant connection, with a hyperosmolar solution, and this solution can optionally be added to red blood cells, thus facilitating the removal of water from the donor organ. At the same time, the lungs are ventilated using the ventilator, thus oxygenating the perfusate and removing CO_2. To avoid a cumulative effect the powered-up oxygenator drives a gaseous mixture containing low-O_2 and high-CO_2 content around the circuit. Through regular analysis of the blood gas, any improvement or deterioration in the gas exchange capacity of the donor lung can be detected. Once the decision is made to perform transplant surgery after the successful reconditioning of the donor graft, the recipient can be prepared accordingly. The donor lung is then rinsed once again with cold organ-preserving solution and removed from the EVLP system so that no additional warm ischemia is generated during the subsequent transplant operation.

The Role of the Organ Care System (OCS) in Lung Transplantation

The further development of the EVLP can be seen in the standardisation of integrated components in a portable casing. It is precisely for this purpose that Transmedics has developed an integrated unit for transporting donor lungs, containing a blood pump, an oxygenator, an organ chamber, a system of tubing, a heater, a ventilator, a gas tank and a control unit, to be transported by the collection team to the donor hospital, thus eliminating the cold ischaemic time required to transport the donor lung from the donor clinic to the transplant clinic using EVLP.

In other respects, the OCS is applied in a rather similar manner to the stationary EVLP. The lung is removed from the dispenser after an initial flush perfusion and the trachea and pulmonary artery are connected up to the OCS. The OCS has been pre-primed with approx. 1.5 l hyperosmolar perfusion solution, and two red-blood cell concentrates added. The lung is then slowly warmed up and the oxygenation performance of the lung determined in evaluation mode by analysing the blood gas. Transmission times of >8 h running on battery power have been recorded during subsequent transport. During this time, the operating mode, the flow rate of the perfusate and the ventilation parameter can all be checked and adjusted, where necessary, with a mobile monitor. Normothermic perfusion and ventilation of the donor lung can be continued in the transplant clinic until the first lung lobe has been removed from the organ recipient. This is then followed by a cold perfusion of the donor lung to protect it from warm ischemia. Once the two pulmonary lobes have been separated, the transplantation of the first lung lobe can be carried out while the donor organ for the second lung lobe is kept cool.

Clinical Application of EVLP and the OCS

To date, only one randomized, controlled trial has been conducted in which EVLP in the donor lungs and their subsequent transplantation are compared to standard transplantation using extended donor criteria. Cypel and Keshavjee's work, which appeared in the New England Journal of Medicine, describes the application of EVLP in the lung transplantation programme in Toronto, in which a total of 136 lung transplants were performed in the space of little more than a year [6]. These lungs prospectively included an extended donor criteria oxygenation index of <300 mmHg or the presence of an oedema in the EVLP arm (n=23). The ensuing EVLP was conducted in a stationary position for four hours under standard conditions. Only those donor lungs whose initially reduced oxygenation performance improved using EVLP were subsequently transplanted (n=20).

The lung transplants performed over the same period without EVLP were defined as the control group, and the two groups were compared with respect to the primary graft dysfunction (PGD) score after 72 h. The results of this study showed that in the 20 lungs transplanted after EVLP, the oxygenation index rose from 335 mmHg in the donor to 443 mmHg after four hours of EVLP. In addition, there was an incidence of a PGD of two or three in this EVLP group, indicating clinically significant ischemia reperfusion damage of 15 % at 72 h after transplantation, compared to 30 % in the control group which did not have EVLP. In addition to this single randomized trial, there have been just three additional clinical reports with case series of six [5], nine [4] and another six [7] transplants successfully performed after reconditioning marginal donor organs using EVLP. These reports also showed good results after transplantation and after EVLP under static conditions.

To date, the use of the portable OCS system has only been described in an initial pilot trial conducted by our Hannover group in cooperation with colleagues from Madrid [8]. This system was used on 12 patients where the donor organs, following initial cold perfusion as described in the previous section, were connected up to the OCS and transported with warm perfusion and ventilation to the transplant clinic. The donor organs were left in the system for an average of 303 min. No donor organ transplantation was ruled out, and the oxygenation index prior to extraction was 463 mmHg, as compared to 471 mmHg after the OCS was used.

The results of this study have shown that EVLP can also be carried out in a portable system, and that not just marginal donor organs, but also regular donor organs, have been successfully transplanted with a significant reduction in cold ischemia time. Based on these encouraging results with the OCS, an international, multi-centred prospectively-randomized trial involving 200 patients is currently underway to assess whether an improvement in the preservation of donor lungs can be achieved using the OCS, as compared to standard cold ischemia. Transplant surgery is to be performed on one group of patients where donor lungs are to be preserved using conventional flush perfusion and cold ischemia, and in a second group of patients (half) with one lung preserved using the OCS.

Conclusions

Modern EVLP techniques are seeing increased use in lung transplant surgery, the major point of interest being the possibility to recondition marginal donor organs. A randomized clinical trial has been performed with good results, with three additional clinical reports recommending the use of EVLP. Currently, there is an initial prospective randomized clinical trial ongoing in which the portable OCS is employed to avoid the use of cold ischemia with its resulting negative consequences, the results of which are still pending. Despite these recent developments, the question of whether this approach will result in a potential benefit to normal lung transplant surgery has yet to be answered.

A Personal View of the Data

Our personal view of the data and specific recommendations for the current use of extracorporeal support of lung grafts are: in absolute critical donor lung quality, the OCS should be used uniformly. Our personal and institutional experience would also indicate the use of ex vivo lung perfusion in cases with recipient factors, potentially resulting in significantly increased intervals between organ retrieval and transplantation.

Recommendations
- Extracorporeal lung perfusion may be useful in specialized transplant centers to evaluate and possibly recondition marginal donor lungs (Evidence quality moderate; weak recommendation).

References

1. Steen S, Ingemansson R, Eriksson L, Pierre L, Algotsson L, Wierup P, Liao Q, Eyjolfsson A, Gustafsson R, Sjöberg T. First human transplantation of a nonacceptable donor lung after reconditioning ex vivo. Ann Thorac Surg. 2007;83(6):2191–4.
2. Lindstedt S, Hlebowicz J, Koul B, Wierup P, Sjögren J, Gustafsson R, Steen S, Ingemansson R. Comparative outcome of double lung transplantation using conventional donor lungs and non-acceptable donor lungs reconditioned ex vivo. Interact Cardiovasc Thorac Surg. 2011;12(2):162–5.
3. Cypel M, Rubacha M, Yeung J, Hirayama S, Torbicki K, Madonik M, Fischer S, Hwang D, Pierre A, Waddell TK, de Perrot M, Liu M, Keshavjee S. Normothermic ex vivo perfusion prevents lung injury compared to extended cold preservation for transplantation. Am J Transplant. 2009;9(10):2262–9.
4. Aigner C, Slama A, Hötzenecker K, Scheed A, Urbanek B, Schmid W, Nierscher FJ, Lang G, Klepetko W. Clinical ex vivo lung perfusion – pushing the limits. Am J Transplant. 2012;12(7):1839–47.
5. Ingemansson R, Eyjolfsson A, Mared L, Pierre L, Algotsson L, Ekmehag B, Gustafsson R, Johnsson P, Koul B, Lindstedt S, Lührs C, Sjöberg T, Steen S. Clinical transplantation of initially rejected donor lungs after reconditioning ex vivo. Ann Thorac Surg. 2009;87(1):255–60.
6. Cypel M, Yeung JC, Liu M, Anraku M, Chen F, Karolak W, Sato M, Laratta J, Azad S, Madonik M, Chow CW, Chaparro C, Hutcheon M, Singer LG, Slutsky AS, Yasufuku K, de Perrot M, Pierre AF, Waddell TK, Keshavjee S. Normothermic ex vivo lung perfusion in clinical lung transplantation. N Engl J Med. 2011;364(15):1431–40.
7. Zych B, Popov AF, Stavri G, Bashford A, Bahrami T, Amrani M, De Robertis F, Carby M, Marczin N, Simon AR, Redmond KC. Early outcomes of bilateral sequential single lung transplantation after ex-vivo lung evaluation and reconditioning. J Heart Lung Transplant. 2012;31(3):274–81.
8. Warnecke G, Moradiellos J, Tudorache I, Kühn C, Avsar M, Wiegmann B, Sommer W, Ius F, Kunze C, Gottlieb J, Varela A, Haverich A. Normothermic perfusion of donor lungs for preservation and assessment with the organ care system lung before bilateral transplantation: a pilot study of 12 patients. Lancet. 2012;380(9856):1851–8.

Chapter 21
Pulmonary Metastasectomy

Trevor Williams

Abstract Resecting pulmonary metastases is a common thoracic procedure but is poorly studied. Five-year survival rates range from 20 to 50 % after complete resection for various tumor cell types with colorectal carcinoma being at the higher end and melanoma at the lower end. Incomplete resection uniformly portends a poor survival, as does thoracic lymph node involvement. Many studies also identify shorter disease free interval and increasing numbers of metastases as poor prognostic factors but no convincing cutoffs exist to deter resection. Manual palpation detects more malignant nodules than imaging but their resection does not improve survival. Thoracoscopic resection is recommended for limited disease and some subsets of tumors may benefit from resection of two or three nodules.

Keywords Pulmonary metastases • Colorectal cancer • Breast cancer • Sarcoma • Melanoma • Survival • Thoracic lymph nodes

Introduction

Some 50 years ago resection of pulmonary metastases gained popularity in the face of uniformly fatal metastatic osteosarcoma. Repeated resection of pulmonary metastases allowed for some long-term survivors [1, 2]. The indications for surgery were at first strict: control of primary tumor, no extrapulmonary involvement, a disease free interval of at least 12 months and a tumor doubling time of at least 20 days. As chemotherapy improved however, thoracic surgeons became more

T. Williams, MD, MPH
Department of Surgery, Section of Cardiac and Thoracic Surgery, University of Chicago,
5841 South Maryland Ave. Rm E-500, MC5040, Chicago, IL 60637, USA
e-mail: trevor.williams@uchospitals.org

M.K. Ferguson (ed.), *Difficult Decisions in Thoracic Surgery*,
Difficult Decisions in Surgery: An Evidence-Based Approach 1,
DOI 10.1007/978-1-4471-6404-3_21, © Springer-Verlag London 2014

aggressive and the criteria decreased in number, making pulmonary metastasectomy one of the thoracic surgeons primary operations [2, 3].

The literature is replete with studies of patients with pulmonary metastases who have surgery but are not compared to similar non-operated patients; there is no control group. Prognostic factors are derived from surgical groups only; the actual benefit of surgery itself is never shown by direct comparison. If a control group is used, selection bias is uniformly present as the studies are retrospective evaluations of patients selected or not for surgery, which is related to their chance of a better outcome. As we await the results of the first randomized trial on the subject we are limited to making suboptimal comparisons to determine the benefit of this very common therapy [4].

Given the assumption that surgery provides survival benefit, how aggressive should resection be? What survival benefit can be expected? How should the thoracic lymph nodes be managed? What approach is most appropriate? How much parenchyma should be removed to treat the disease?

Search Strategy

A pubmed search with the keyword terms "lung" and "metastasectomy" was performed, limited to the English language. Given the large volume of literature, article citations were systematically reviewed from January 2010 to June 2013. Among these titles, 140 abstracts were reviewed, adding apparently important/relevant papers from reference lists of selected papers. Systematic reviews and larger studies were preferentially included. No randomized data is available and there is mostly no comparison group. Only the more common and studied tumors were included in the selection of papers.

Description of Published Data

Overall Survival (Table 21.1)

No discussion of pulmonary metastasis would be complete without discussing Pastorino's study from the International Registry of Lung Metastases. Between 1991 and 1995, 5,290 patients were enrolled from 18 centers in nine counties across Europe and America, dating back to 1945, with Memorial Sloan Kettering providing the largest series, 1,075 patients. Forty-three percent of metastases were from an epithelial tumor and 42 % from sarcoma. This study demonstrated an actuarial 5-year survival of 36 % across all tumor types, after complete resection. Five-year survival after incomplete resections was only 13 %. Multivariate analysis identified germ cell histology, disease-free interval of 36 months or more and a single metastasis as favorable prognostic factors (Table 21.2). Metastases to hilar/mediastinal lymph nodes was not routinely or systematically performed and therefore, fell out of analysis (<9 % of patients) [5, 6].

Table 21.1 Survival data from reviews

Author (year)	Study date range	# studies/ # patients	Histology	5-year survival	Prognostic factors
Gonzales (2013) [11]	2000–2011	25/2,925	Colorectal carcinoma	R0 27–68 %	Disease free interval, number of pulmonary mets, thoracic lymph node involvement and elevated CEA
Salah (2012) [12]	2000–2012	8/927	Colorectal carcinoma	54.3 %	Disease free interval >36 months, number of pulmonary metastasis 1 vs. >1 and CEA >5 ng/ml
Fiorentino (2010) [9]	1971–2007	51/3,504	Colorectal carcinoma	50 % ± 5 %	n/a
Treasure (2012) [15]	1991–2010	18/1,357	Sarcoma	Bone 34 % Soft tissue 25 %	n/a
Ruiterkamp (2011) [16]	2002–2010	9/?	Breast cancer	31–54 %	Disease free interval >36 months, positive hormone receptor status, stage one cancer initially, small size and <4 mets
Caudle (2011) [18]	1992–2007	6/?	Melanoma	20–33 %	Complete resection, disease free interval >36 months, <3 nodules, no history of extra-thoracic disease, prior response to chemo/ immunotherapy and no nodal disease

Table 21.2 Registry prognostic factors [5]

Disease-free interval	5-year survival (%)
0–11 months	33
12–35 months	31
>36 months	45
Number of metastases	
1	43
2–3	34
>3	27
>10	26

Fifty-three percent of patients had a recurrence, with a median time to recurrence of 10 months (8 months for sarcoma and 12 months for epithelial tumors). Intra-thoracic recurrence was common in sarcoma (66 %) whereas extra-thoracic recurrence was common in melanoma (73 %). A longer 5-year survival of 44 % occurred after a second metastasectomy. Germ cell tumors were outliers. These tumors had multiple metastases in 57 % of patients and a 5-year survival of 68 %, much higher than the 30 % seen with other tumors. They only accounted for seven percent of tumors in the registry, however.

As part of the European Society of Thoracic Surgery Workgroup on pulmonary metastasis, Pfannschmidt reviewed studies concerning non-seminomatous germ cell tumors. They reported an overall survival between 73 and 94 %. First line therapy for this malignancy is chemotherapy, which is highly effective. Surgery has a role in diagnosis of residual nodules, salvage therapy for those that become unresponsive and resecting benign enlarging teratomatous elements. Often residual nodules are only necrosis and the decision to resect may not always be clear. Salvage surgery still has a relatively good 42 % 5-year survival [7].

Colorectal cancer is the most common of the tumors that metastasize to the lungs, though very few patients come to resection. Wade evaluated outcomes of metastatic colorectal cancer in the Veterans Administration hospital system and found that 12 % (2,659/22,715) of patients undergoing colectomy develop pulmonary metastases and of these, only 2.9 % (76/2,659) had pulmonary resection [8]. Fiorentino, as part of a group planning for a clinical trial, analyzed 51 papers of colorectal pulmonary metastases with series having mid-point dates from 1965 to 2000, 3,504 patients. Twenty-five papers gave 5-year survival data after a single pulmonary metastasectomy allowing these authors to estimate a 50 % ± 5 % 5-year survival. They found that elevated CEA correlated with shorter survival and that increasing numbers of patients over the 35 years were undergoing metastasectomy who had bilateral disease or previous pulmonary and hepatic metastasectomy. They concluded that, without a control group, no judgment can be made as to whether surgery actually prolongs survival and performing further small, uncontrolled studies is without merit [9]. This resonates with an earlier systematic review performed by Pfannschmidt wherein predictors of survival were not pooled as disease-free interval and number of pulmonary metastases were significant on multivariate analysis in only two and five of nineteen studies, respectively [10].

Gonzalez and Salah performed more recent analyses. Gonzalez performed a meta-analysis of all studies from 2000 to 2011, with more than 40 patients each; 25 studies were included, totaling 2,925 patients. Seventy-five percent of patients had a solitary pulmonary metastasis; 5-year survival for an R0 resection varied widely from 27 to 68 %. Hazard ratios (HR) were calculated for significant prognostic factors that came from a variable number of studies included: higher number of metastases—HR 2.04 (95 % CI 1.74–2.4); elevated CEA—HR 1.91 (95 % CI 1.57–2.32); positive mediastinal/hilar lymph nodes—HR 1.65 (95 % CI 1.38–2.02), disease free interval—HR 1.59 (95 % CI 1.27–1.98). Previous liver metastases resection did not portend a poor survival [11].

Salah collected data from eight studies (the number they were able to collect data from) published 2000 to 2012 with more than 20 patients/study, R0 resections and isolated lung metastases, totaling 927 patients. Calculated 5-year survival was 54.3 %. Multivariate analysis revealed similar independent prognostic factors: two or more metastases—HR 2.05 (95 % CI 1.58–2.65), pre-thoracotomy CEA >5 ng/ ml— HR 1.84 (95 % CI 1.43–2.38); disease-free interval <36 months—1.39 (95 % CI 1.03–1.86). The authors divided patients into low, intermediate and high risk groups based on the presence of 0–1, 2 or three risk factors, giving 5-year survivals of 68.2, 46.4 and 26.1 % respectively [12]. More complex nomograms for survival after resection of colorectal cancer pulmonary metastasis using these variables exist with external validation [13].

Fiorentino presented a provoking math "thought experiment" demonstrating the possibility of elevated survival data being due to selection bias. Given a 5 % 5-year survival in stage IV disease, 50 patients out of 1,000 patients would be alive at 5 years. If we exclude half of patients over three separate rounds of selection for surgery based on favorable prognostic factors and are able to retain the 50 long-term survivors in the surgery group, we get 50/500, 50/250, 50/125 with 10, 20 and 40 % 5-year survivorship [14].

Treasure's group systematically reviewed all English language articles published 1990 and 2011 evaluating outcomes of pulmonary resection for bone and soft tissue sarcoma metastases with over 20 patients/study. A total of 115 studies were found but only 18 studies qualified for analysis, totaling 1,357 patients. The proportion of sarcoma patients who develop pulmonary metastasis varied from 18 to 50 %, while the proportion of patients with pulmonary metastasis who had metastasectomy ranged from 5 to 88 %. The population base from which patients derived varied considerably between studies. Five-year survival for bone sarcoma was calculated as 34 % (range 23–38 %) and for soft tissue sarcoma 25 % (range 18–44 %). Though not directly compared, cancer registry 5-year survival data for all stage four patients is given for perspective: bone 25 %, soft tissue sarcoma 15 %. Prognostic factors were not addressed and much of the paper discusses the issue of survivor bias and inappropriate interpretation of data [15].

Ruiterkamp's recent extensive review of stage IV breast cancer included a review of seven studies regarding metastasectomy for breast cancer lung metastasis covering patients treated 1960–2007. Five-year survival rates ranged 31–54 % with recurrence rates of 60 % (13–28 % intra-thoracic). Prognostic factors for survival were disease-free interval >36 months, < four metastases, hormone receptor positive tumor, stage I cancer and small size of metastasis. One of the included studies compared surgical to non-operated patients with less than four metastases. Non-operated patients were either not offered or refused surgery. Follow-up was 50 months. Four-year survival was 82.1 % in the surgery group and 31.6 % in chemotherapy/hormonal therapy only group. Though all patients had limited metastatic disease, 73 % of the surgery group and only 33 % of the medical group has solitary pulmonary nodules [16]. Diaz-Canton studied the MD Anderson experience of patients with metastatic breast cancer isolated to lung and treated only with chemotherapy (88 patients). Disease burden was quantified as minimal, moderate or extensive with long-term survivors in each category. Thirty-seven percent of patients had a complete response. While 5- and 10-year survivals were 15 % and 9 %, respectively, four of ten patients with minimal disease were alive at 10 years [17].

Resection of pulmonary metastasis from melanoma has a lower survival. Caudle reviewed six studies reporting 5-year survivals between 20 % and 33 %. Incomplete resection has a similar survival to those not undergoing resection, 0–4 % 5- year survival. Prognostic factors included: complete resection, disease free interval >36 months, two or fewer nodules, prior response to chemo/immunotherapy and no nodal disease [18].

Thoracic Lymph Node Involvement

There is uncertainty about the origin and significance of metastases to thoracic lymph nodes. Either they represent systemic disease that is already extensive portending a worse prognosis or they are a result of lymphatic spread of previously established pulmonary metastases thus making it more important to try and eradicate all pulmonary nodules early and prevent their subsequent spread.

Garcia-Yuste, as part of the European Workgroup analyzed six studies, finding a prevalence ranging from 14 to 32 %, giving a weighted average of 22 %. Tumors were of varied types but colorectal carcinoma was most represented. Five studies gave survival data. Node negative patients achieved 5-year survivals of 36–49 %. Node positive disease had 10–19 % 5-year survival, though two studies did not give 5-year survival data and stated survival was 6 months. A paper by Pfannschmidt reported a median survival of 63.9 months with hilar nodes vs. 32.7 months with mediastinal nodes. Welter, found intra-pulmonary nodes to be more favorable than hilar or mediastinal nodes [6].

A French group recently reviewed seven studies evaluating mediastinal lymphadenectomy in renal cell carcinoma. Prevalence of involved nodes ranged from 10 to 38 % (averaging 30 %), with approximately half of these being mediastinal. Increasing number of involved lymph nodes correlated with progressively reduced survival as did N2 vs. N1 disease. Five-year survival was approximately 50 % in lymph node negative disease. Lymph node positive disease had no 5-year survivors in two studies [19].

The Mayo clinic recently examined their experience over 24 years with colorectal cancer metastasis. Three hundred ten of 518 patients received lymph node dissections, 40 of these had positive nodes (40/310=13 %). Five-year survival for negative lymph nodes was 48.3 %, it was 20.7 % for lymph node positive disease and interestingly 49.3 % in patients without lymph node dissection. A selection bias is certainly present and likely a small proportion of patients in the non-dissected group had positive lymph nodes. Of note, three long-term survivors had a positive N2 node, hinting at a possible therapeutic role of lymph node dissection [20].

There is a consistent and strong association with positive lymph nodes and death. The link seems causal given the plausibility, magnitude of effect and biologic gradient. It seems logical, though unproven, that thoracic lymph nodes represent metastases from pulmonary metastases given the same survival patterns with N1 vs. N2 disease as seen with lung cancer.

Surgical Approach

The issues of imaging, surgical approach and extent of resection were recently addressed by the European workgroup [21–23]. Their conclusions were that helical CT scanning should be performed with 3–5 mm slice thickness, a repeat scan should be obtained 4–6 weeks post-metastasectomy as a baseline, then at intervals depending on doubling time; thoracoscopy (VATS) was not preferred due to the need for palpation to assess for additional metastases; complete resection of all disease should be performed though pneumonectomy was not advised due to the controversial risk- benefit ratio.

Debate in the surgical literature exists over whether pulmonary metastases should be removed by a thoracoscopic approach or thoracotomy due to the high rate of non-imaged metastases. Cerfolio found 34 % of 152 patients had non-imaged pulmonary nodules detected by palpation, almost half of these nodules were malignant. Surprisingly, they report a median resected nodule size of 0.7–0.9 cm in nodules that were not imaged using a 64 slice helical CT scanner with 5-mm cuts [24]. Eckardt prospectively evaluated 37 patients who underwent VATS, followed by thoracotomy, wherein an additional 29 of total 84 nodules were resected (35 % non-imaged nodules). Of non-imaged resected nodules, 28 % were malignant [25].

The argument for palpation is strong if we assume that pulmonary metastases can metastasize, given their high prevalence (20–30 % involvement of thoracic lymph nodes) and the reduced survival seen with incomplete resections. Evidence for a survival benefit is absent however. Molnar reviewed seven studies providing outcome data comparing VATS to thoracotomy with no survival difference between groups in six studies, one found higher recurrence free survival in the VATS group [22]. These authors admitted to disagreement within the working group but still concluded lung palpation was necessary.

In a prospective study of 27 patients undergoing 1 mm cut 16-channel multi-detector row CT and lung resection by thoracotomy after palpation, 198 nodules were resected of a total 117 detected. The average number of nodules resected was 5.8 (range 1–22). Osteosarcoma had a poor sensitivity of 34 %, possibly due to the high number and small size (average 3.7 mm) of nodules but in the 24 non-osteosarcoma patients, sensitivity was 97 % (specificity 54 %). Two nodules were missed in one patient (renal cell carcinoma) with multiple nodules. Different computer programs are now available to increase the radiologist's nodule detection rate and this technology is likely to improve [26].

Han retrospectively studied a population of patients with solitary pulmonary metastases on imaging, and then confirmed pathologically to be solitary, who had undergone resection by a combination of VATS (62 patients) and thoracotomy (43 patients). Both groups had a 25 % intra-thoracic recurrence, repeat surgery was performed and overall survival did not differ [27]. There certainly can be no assured "complete resection" as tumors exist that are small enough to neither feel nor image.

Extent of Resection

Migliore's review found seven reports addressing pneumonectomy for metastatic disease, five of which reported completion pneumonectomy. Operative mortality rates ranged 0–11 % (19 % in one study with R1 resections) and 5-year survival ranged 10–41 %. Seven studies reviewed the issue of repeat metastasectomy with 5-year survivals ranging from 19 to 53.8 %. Thirty percent to 40 % 5-years survivals are reported after a third or fourth thoracotomy. Resectability was an independent prognostic factor for survival after each subsequent thoracotomy but the chance of being resectable decreases after each thoracotomy as does the chance for permanent control. After patients are determined to be unresectable, median survival was 8 months (19 % 2-year survival) [23].

Recommendations

Surgical resection of pulmonary metastasis can improve survival in well-selected patients. Resecting a single pulmonary metastasis is recommended, but higher numbers of metastases with short disease free intervals, especially in patients with melanoma, is not advised.

Thoracic lymph node involvement portends a decreased survival. There is no evidence to support resecting thoracic lymph nodes for survival benefit, but lymph nodes are involved 20–30 % of the time and give prognostic information. Mediastinal lymph node sampling is recommended when it may change treatment. The question of therapeutic benefit form thoracic lymph node dissection remains unanswered.

Manual palpation detects non-imaged nodules, some malignant, but recurrence rates are high regardless of operative approach and survival is unaffected by operative approach. Thoracoscopic surgery is an acceptable approach and follow-up imaging is required regardless of operative approach, given the high recurrence rates.

Complete resection gives a survival advantage over incomplete resection. Incomplete resection does not confer benefit. Pneumonectomy may have a role in highly selected patients with very limited disease.

A Personal View of the Data

It is frustrating to know that surgical intervention can have a beneficial impact on oligo-metastatic disease but not know which patients will benefit. We cannot operate on everyone and say we provide benefit without knowing how the un-operated patient fairs. Thomas Treasure is admirable in pursuit of evidence, where there is none, and hopefully his trial will help delineate a population in whom surgery is clearly recommended or not.

We believe we benefit the patient but is it reasonable to perform thoracotomies and resect all abnormal tissue when the recurrence rates are so high? Is risking more chronic pain and sacrificing more benign parenchyma warranted? The CT scanner and the surgeon's fingers both miss hundreds of cells between 50 and 1,000 μm. The risk of metastases metastasizing is real but how much of that is the uncontrollable biology of the tumor regardless of our intervention and over what time course must we intervene? Repeat thoracoscopic surgery with interval imaging based on doubling time, if possible, is more palatable for patient and surgeon and likely to provide equivalent, if not improved, outcomes with less morbidity.

My personal approach is to perform an R0 resection on any patient with a solitary pulmonary metastasis provided no obvious thoracic lymph nodes are involved; resection in oligometastatic disease may offer a chance for long-term survival. Resecting two to three metastases is indicated for colorectal and breast cancer given improved survival and effective chemotherapy but is less fruitful for melanoma or sarcoma and this is therefore not recommended. Thoracic lymph nodes should be sampled as they are commonly involved and offer significant prognostic information. Thoracoscopic resection is preferred with interval imaging and possible repeat resection.

Recommendations
- Resecting a single pulmonary metastasis is recommended. (Evidence quality low; weak recommendation)
- Mediastinal lymph node sampling is recommended when it may change treatment plans. (Evidence quality low; weak recommendation)
- Thoracoscopic resection of isolated metastases is an acceptable approach. (Evidence quality low; weak recommendation)
- Incomplete resection does not confer a survival benefit and is not recommended. (Evidence quality low; weak recommendation)

References

1. Martini N, Huvos AG, Miké V, Marcove RC, Beattie Jr EJ. Multiple pulmonary resections in the treatment of osteogenic sarcoma. Ann Thorac Surg. 1971;12(3):271–80.
2. Pastorino U, Treasure T. A historical note on pulmonary metastasectomy. J Thorac Oncol. 2010;5(6 Suppl 2):S132–3.
3. Skinner KA, Eilber FR, Holmes EC, Eckardt J, Rosen G. Surgical treatment and chemotherapy for pulmonary metastases from osteosarcoma. Arch Surg (Chic III 1960). 1992;127(9):1065–70; discussion 1070–1.
4. Treasure T, Fallowfield L, Lees B, Farewell V. Pulmonary metastasectomy in colorectal cancer: the PulMiCC trial. Thorax. 2012;67(2):185–7.
5. Pastorino U, Buyse M, Friedel G, Ginsberg RJ, Girard P. Long-term results of lung metastasectomy: prognostic analyses based on 5206 cases. The International Registry of Lung Metastases. J Thorac Cardiovasc Surg. 1997;113(1):37–49.
6. García-Yuste M, Cassivi S, Paleru C. Thoracic lymphatic involvement in patients having pulmonary metastasectomy: incidence and the effect on prognosis. J Thorac Oncol. 2010;5 (6 Suppl 2):S166–9.
7. Pfannschmidt J, Hoffmann H, Dienemann H. Thoracic metastasectomy for nonseminomatous germ cell tumors. J Thorac Oncol. 2010;5(6 Suppl 2):S182–6.
8. Wade TP, Virgo KS, Li MJ, Callander PW, Longo WE, Johnson FE. Outcomes after detection of metastatic carcinoma of the colon and rectum in a national hospital system. J Am Coll Surg. 1996;182(4):353–61.
9. Fiorentino F, Hunt I, Teoh K, Treasure T, Utley M. Pulmonary metastasectomy in colorectal cancer: a systematic review and quantitative synthesis. J R Soc Med. 2010;103(2):60–6.
10. Pfannschmidt J, Dienemann H, Hoffmann H. Surgical resection of pulmonary metastases from colorectal cancer: a systematic review of published series. Ann Thorac Surg. 2007;84(1): 324–38.
11. Gonzalez M, Poncet A, Combescure C, Robert J, Ris HB, Gervaz P. Risk factors for survival after lung metastasectomy in colorectal cancer patients: a systematic review and meta-analysis. Ann Surg Oncol. 2013;20(2):572–9.
12. Salah S, Watanabe K, Welter S, Park JS, Park JW, Zabaleta J, et al. Colorectal cancer pulmonary oligometastases: pooled analysis and construction of a clinical lung metastasectomy prognostic model. Ann Oncol. 2012;23(10):2649–55.
13. Kanemitsu Y, Kato T, Komori K, Fukui T, Mitsudomi T. Validation of a nomogram for predicting overall survival after resection of pulmonary metastases from colorectal cancer at a single center. World J Surg. 2010;34(12):2973–8.
14. Primrose J, Treasure T, Fiorentino F. Lung metastasectomy in colorectal cancer: is this surgery effective in prolonging life? Respirology. 2010;15(5):742–6.
15. Treasure T, Fiorentino F, Scarci M, Møller H, Utley M. Pulmonary metastasectomy for sarcoma: a systematic review of reported outcomes in the context of Thames Cancer Registry data. BMJ Open. 2012;2(5).
16. Ruiterkamp J, Ernst MF. The role of surgery in metastatic breast cancer. Eur J Cancer. 2011;47 Suppl 3:S6–22. Oxf Engl 1990.
17. Diaz-Canton EA, Valero V, Rahman Z, Rodriguez-Monge E, Frye D, Smith T, et al. Clinical course of breast cancer patients with metastases confined to the lungs treated with chemotherapy. The University of Texas M.D. Anderson Cancer Center experience and review of the literature. Ann Oncol. 1998;9(4):413–8.
18. Caudle AS, Ross MI. Metastasectomy for stage IV melanoma: for whom and how much? Surg Oncol Clin N Am. 2011;20(1):133–44.
19. Renaud S, Falcoz P-E, Olland A, Massard G. Should mediastinal lymphadenectomy be performed during lung metastasectomy of renal cell carcinoma? Interact Cardiovasc Thorac Surg. 2013;16(4):525–8.

20. Hamaji M, Cassivi SD, Shen KR, Allen MS, Nichols FC, Deschamps C, et al. Is lymph node dissection required in pulmonary metastasectomy for colorectal adenocarcinoma? Ann Thorac Surg. 2012;94(6):1796–800.
21. Detterbeck FC, Grodzki T, Gleeson F, Robert JH. Imaging requirements in the practice of pulmonary metastasectomy. J Thorac Oncol. 2010;5(6 Suppl 2):S134–9.
22. Molnar TF, Gebitekin C, Turna A. What are the considerations in the surgical approach in pulmonary metastasectomy? J Thorac Oncol. 2010;5(6 Suppl 2):S140–4.
23. Migliore M, Jakovic R, Hensens A, Klepetko W. Extending surgery for pulmonary metastasectomy: what are the limits? J Thorac Oncol. 2010;5(6 Suppl 2):S155–60.
24. Cerfolio RJ, Bryant AS, McCarty TP, Minnich DJ. A prospective study to determine the incidence of non-imaged malignant pulmonary nodules in patients who undergo metastasectomy by thoracotomy with lung palpation. Ann Thorac Surg. 2011;91(6):1696–700; discussion 1700–1.
25. Eckardt J, Licht PB. Thoracoscopic versus open pulmonary metastasectomy: a prospective, sequentially controlled study. Chest. 2012;142(6):1598–602.
26. Kang MC, Kang CH, Lee HJ, Goo JM, Kim YT, Kim JH. Accuracy of 16-channel multidetector row chest computed tomography with thin sections in the detection of metastatic pulmonary nodules. Eur J Cardiothorac Surg. 2008;33(3):473–9.
27. Han KN, Kang CH, Park IK, Kim YT. Thoracoscopic resection of solitary lung metastases evaluated by using thin-section chest computed tomography: is thoracoscopic surgery still a valid option? Gen Thorac Cardiovasc Surg. 2013;61(10):565–70.

Part III
Esophagus

Chapter 22
Optimal Therapy for Barrett High Grade Dysplasia

Gabriel D. Lang and Vani J.A. Konda

Abstract The management of Barrett's esophagus with high-grade dysplasia has undergone an evolution from prophylactic esophagectomy to an organ sparing approach based on endoscopic therapies that have emerged over the recent years. Esophagectomy is now reserved only for selected cases of patients with high-grade dysplasia and intramucosal carcinoma in Barrett's esophagus. This chapter outlines terminology, the appropriate assessment, the management strategy, and the options of therapy for patients with Barrett's esophagus with high-grade dysplasia.

Keywords Barrett's esophagus • High grade dysplasia • Esophagectomy • Endoscopic mucosal resection • Ablation

Abbreviation

BE	Barrett's esophagus
CT	Computed tomography
EUS	Endoscopic ultrasound
GI	Gastrointestinal
HGD	High-grade dysplasia
IMC	Intramucosal carcinoma
LNM	Lymph node metastasis

G.D. Lang, MD
Department of Gastroenterology, Hepatology, and Nutrition, University of Chicago,
5841 S. Maryland Avenue, MC 4076, Chicago, IL 60637, USA

V.J.A. Konda, MD (✉)
Section of Gastroenterology, Department of Medicine, University of Chicago Medical Center,
5841 S. Maryland Avenue, MC #4076, Chicago, IL 60637-1463, USA
e-mail: vkonda@medicine.bsd.uchicago.edu

M.K. Ferguson (ed.), *Difficult Decisions in Thoracic Surgery*,
Difficult Decisions in Surgery: An Evidence-Based Approach 1,
DOI 10.1007/978-1-4471-6404-3_22, © Springer-Verlag London 2014

Introduction

Esophageal adenocarcinoma (EAC) is an increasingly prevalent cancer and caries a dismal prognosis when diagnosed at advanced stages, on the order of 20 % 5-year survival [1, 2]. Barrett's esophagus (BE) is a risk factor for EAC, and is rapidly increasing in incidence throughout the United States [3]. BE occurs when the normal squamous lining of the esophagus undergoes conversion to specialized intestinal, columnar epithelium. Given the 30-fold increase in risk over the general population [4], patients with BE have been targeted for surveillance programs. The detection of high-grade dysplasia (HGD) in patients with BE offers the best marker to identify who is at risk for EAC and represents a point of intervention to cure or prevent EAC. The standard of care has shifted from managing these patients with prophylactic esophagectomy to esophageal sparing approaches that have incorporated emerging endoscopic therapies. This chapter will outline relevant classification terminology, appropriate assessment, management strategies, and options for therapy for patients with BE with HGD.

Search Strategy

This chapter is based on a search of the literature with Medline, PubMed, and selected references using key words Barrett's esophagus, high-grade dysplasia, endoscopic mucosal resection, esophagectomy, and ablation from the years 1988 to 2013. The patient population is focused on patients with Barrett's esophagus with HGD. There is also attention given to patients with intramucosal carcinoma (IMC) as some studies have incorporated both patient populations and HGD and IMC have some similarities in management. Interventions investigated include esophagectomy, endoscopic mucosal resection, radiofrequency ablation, photodynamic therapy, and cryotherapy. Outcomes were based on survival and remission of neoplasia.

Background

Classification

BE is an endoscopic and pathologic diagnosis. Endoscopically, the squamo-columnar junction is detected proximal to the top of the gastric folds with the observation of salmon colored mucosa seen in the tubular esophagus. In the United States BE is defined any length of columnar lined esophagus with intestinal metaplasia, yet there is lack of universal agreement on whether intestinal metaplasia (defined by the presence of goblet cells) is necessary for a diagnosis of BE. In Britain and Japan, the presence of goblet cells is not necessary for a diagnosis of BE. Furthermore a small percentage of adult patients with columnar metaplasia do not contain goblet cells, the chances of detecting goblet cells is proportional to the length of columnar mucosa sampled, sampling error exists, and the presence of goblet cells can wax and wane over the course of BE [5].

The histopathologic diagnosis of BE may be classified into three categories: BE without dysplasia, BE with low-grade dysplasia (LGD), and BE with HGD. Dysplasia is defined as neoplastic cytological and architectural atypia without evidence of invasion past the basement membrane. Carcinoma in situ and HGD are equivalent, and for the purposes of this discussion, the term HGD will be used. Unfortunately, interobserver agreement between expert pathologists is suboptimal due to small biopsy size, lack of consensus on boundaries demarcating degrees of dysplasia, and difficulty discerning dysplasia from inflammation [6].

IMC is defined as neoplasia that extends beyond the basement membrane and into the lamina propria. IMC carries a minimal nodal metastasis risk of less than 5 % [7–9]. The risk of lymph node metastasis relates to differentiation, depth of tumor, lymphatic, vascular, or neural involvement. Submucosal carcinoma invades the submucosa, but not the muscularis propria, and carries a >20 % lymph node metastasis risk [8]. A peculiarity to Barrett's esophagus is the presence of duplicated muscularis mucosa. If not recognized or accounted for, this may lead to overstaging of tumor that may involve the superficial bundle of muscularis mucosa but not the deeper bundle as submucosal carcinoma when it may only be IMC [10, 11]. The identification of BE in the stages of intestinal metaplasia, LGD, HGD, IMC and submucosal carcinoma has profound treatment implications based on their dramatically different prognostic profiles [12].

Appropriate Assessment of Patients with Barrett's Associated Neoplasia

It is critical to confirm all dysplasia with an expert gastrointestinal pathologist as considerable disagreement in the diagnosis of dysplastic BE exists, and this diagnosis has profound treatment and outcome implications. Curvers et al. found that 85 % of patients diagnosed with LGD in six non-university hospitals between 2000 and 2006 were down-staged to non-dysplastic BE or indefinite for dysplasia after histology review by two expert pathologists. After a mean follow up of 51 months, the patients with confirmed LGD in this study had a cumulative risk of progressing to HGD or EAC of 85 % at 109.1 months compared to 4.6 % in 107.4 months for patients down-staged to non-dysplastic BE [13].

A careful endoscopic examination of the Barrett's segment is paramount to detect dysplasia. Visible lesions in the setting of HGD are at high risk of harboring cancer. Visible lesions may be obvious in the cases of protruding lesions or ulcers, but may also be subtler in nature with slight elevations, depressions, or flat appearing mucosa. The traditional surveillance strategy for BE is the Seattle protocol, with targeted biopsies of all visible lesions followed by four quadrant random biopsies every 1–2 cm of the Barrett's segment [14, 15]. However, dysplastic lesions can still be missed on biopsy given the patchy and focal nature of dysplasia, sampling error, and poor adherence to the Seattle protocol, which increases sampling error and risk of missed dysplasia [16]. A detailed exam utilizing high definition white light endoscopy (WLE) is essential in the recognition of lesions. Additional imaging modalities which may improve the detection of neoplasia include magnification endoscopy [17], chromoendoscopy [18], narrow band imaging [19] and confocal laser endomicroscopy [20].

Any mucosal irregularity warrants an endoscopic mucosal resection (EMR), since endoscopically visible lesions in the setting of HGD are associated with a high risk of occult cancer. Mucosal resection of visible lesions provides accurate depth staging and visualization of lateral margins. Chennat et al. found that 14 % of cases were upstaged and 31 % down-staged after endoscopic mucosal resection compared to pre-treatment biopsies [21]. Endoscopically resected specimens allow for greater interobserver agreement between pathologists than standard biopsy specimens [22].

Endoscopic ultrasound and CT help determine tumor depth and regional lymph node metastasis. EUS has improved accuracy for tumor depths at more advanced stages, but has difficulty distinguishing between IMC and submucosal cancer [23]. Therefore, for superficial Barrett's associated neoplasia, EMR is used for depth staging and the role of EUS with fine needle aspiration focuses on detection of nodal metastasis [24].

Rationale for Intervention

The incidence of EAC in patients with non-dysplastic BE was previously thought to be 0.5 % per person per year, but now appears closer to 0.3 % per person per year [25]. HGD is the best marker to identify which patients with BE are at risk of progressing to EAC. It is estimated that 6–20 % of patients with HGD develop EAC within 17–35 months of follow up based on a prospective study [26]. Rastogi et al. found that patients with HGD developed EAC with an average incidence of 6 of every 100 patients per year during the first 1.5–7 years of endoscopic surveillance [27].

There has been an evolution in management strategy for patients with Barrett's associated neoplasia. Traditionally, patients without dysplasia or LGD underwent surveillance. Patients with cancer underwent esophagectomy and/or systemic therapy, and patients with HGD had two radically different options, surveillance or esophagectomy. The surgical literature reported rates of prevalent occult cancer among patients who underwent a prophylactic esophagectomy for the management of HGD ranging from 0 to 73 % [28–30], with an assumed risk of patients with HGD harboring occult invasive EAC estimated to be 40 % [31]. This high risk of prevalent occult cancer supported the rationale for prophylactic esophagectomy in patients with HGD.

A systematic review analyzed the risk of EAC in 441 patients with HGD who underwent esophagectomy and found that, while the pooled average rate of occult adenocarcinoma was 39.9 %, the rate of proven invasive cancer (defined by submucosal invasion or beyond) was only 12.7 % [9]. Most patients in this study were found to have IMC, which carries a 3 % risk of nodal metastasis and is amenable to endoscopic therapy [8, 9, 32]. It is estimated that 80–100 % of patients with HGD can be successfully treated with endoscopic eradication therapy [33] and complete removal of BE with intestinal metaplasia occurs in >75 % of cases [34]. Given that the risk of mortality after esophagectomy is 3–4 % [35], the pursuit of endoscopic therapy may offer an appropriate balance of risks and benefits.

Endoscopic Treatment Approaches

Endoscopic treatment of BE begins with endoscopic resection of visible lesions in the setting of neoplasia, followed by treatment of the remainder of the Barrett's epithelium. These treatment modalities are divided into tissue acquiring and non-tissue acquiring modalities. Tissue acquiring methods include focal EMR, circumferential EMR, and endoscopic submucosal dissection (ESD). Non-tissue acquiring modalities include photodynamic therapy, radiofrequency ablation, and cryotherapy. Visible lesions in patients with BE should be treated with a tissue acquiring modality so that lesions can be appropriately staged and resected. After all areas of localized neoplasia are removed, the remainder of the Barrett's epithelium can be eradicated by non-tissue acquiring modalities in order to treat metachronous or synchronous lesions.

Tissue-Acquiring Ablative Therapies

Endoscopic Resection

EMR removes affected mucosa through the deeper part of the submucosa in a piece-meal or en bloc fashion. It can be performed via band ligation, free hand, lift-and-cut, or cap technique. The primary functions of EMR are to obtain a specimen that allows for accurate histopathologic staging/grading as well as endoscopic treatment. EMR can be performed focally or for the entirety of Barrett's epithelium. Focal EMR is an acceptable technique for patients with low-risk and early lesions with complete remission rates of 97–100 % [36]. Unfortunately, focal EMR, when used a sole modality, has high recurrence rates (14–47 %) [37]. Circumferential EMR, on the other hand, eradicates the entire length of Barrett's epithelium and has complete response rates of 76–100 % [21, 38]. Complications of EMR include bleeding, perforation, and stricture formation.

ESD is a technique in which dissection along the submucosal layer is performed with an endoscopic knife, allowing for resections of larger lesions (over 1.5 cm) and more accurate histopathological assessments. En bloc resection rates associated with ESD are greater than 90 %, and local recurrence rates after ESD are low (0–3.1 %) [39]. This compares favorably with the local recurrence rates of EMR which are approximately 20 %, likely secondary to piecemeal resections [40]. ESD remains a technically challenging procedure requiring specialized training that is not yet performed with great frequency outside of east Asian nations.

Non-tissue Acquiring Modalities

Radiofrequency Ablation

RFA applies direct thermal energy to the mucosal lining circumferentially with a balloon catheter or in a focal fashion. During the procedure, areas of mucosa are directly applied with thermal energy via electrodes embedded on the balloon or focal device. In a randomized trial performed by Shaheen et al. patients with HGD treated with RFA had an 81 % complete eradication rate compared to 19 % of controls that received a sham procedure. 77.4 % of patients in the ablation group had complete eradication of intestinal metaplasia, compared with 2.3 % in controls. The RFA group had lower rates of progression (3.6 % vs. 16.3 %) and fewer cancers (1.2 vs. 9.3 %). Complete remission of intestinal metaplasia was persistent in 92 % of patients at 5 years [41]. Complications include non-cardiac chest pain, lacerations, and stenosis. RFA has decreased complication rates of bleeding and stenosis compared to EMR. Expert opinion suggests that RFA is the best available ablation technique for the treatment of flat HGD and for eradication of residual BE after focal EMR [34].

Cryotherapy

Cryotherapy uses a low-pressure spray catheter to deliver liquid nitrogen to a targeted area in order to freeze the epithelium to a depth of 2 mm. The freezing and subsequent thawing causes ischemic necrosis. Sessions can be repeated every 4–6 weeks and requires a decompression tube in the esophagus to prevent over-inflation and perforation. Recent studies showed initial success with regression of HGD in 94–97 % [42, 43]. Cryotherapy was also studied in 30 patients with HGD and IMC who were not surgical candidates, resulting in a 90 % rate of histologic down staging and 30–40 % of patients experiencing complete resolution of dysplasia. At 1-year, elimination of cancer or down staging was achieved in 68 % of HGD and 80 % of IMC patients [44].

Photodynamic Therapy

In photodynamic therapy (PDT) an intravenous photo sensitizer binds to dysplastic tissue and 2–3 days later an endoscopic delivery of laser light occurs, which produces oxygen radicals and triggers cell death [45]. A retrospective analysis of patients with HGD who received PDT or esophagectomy revealed no significant differences in mortality or long-term survival based, yet found that management of IMC with PDT is less efficacious than other treatment modalities [35]. Complications of PDT include decreased efficacy compared to newer therapies due to the presence of buried glands containing foci of BE after therapy, cutaneous photo-toxicity, and stricture formation. These drawbacks have limited the use of PDT in the current era.

Hybrid Therapy

Hybrid therapy of EMR and RFA, with resection of visible mucosal irregularities via EMR followed by ablation of all intestinal metaplasia with RFA, may be the endoscopic modality of choice. A study performed by Kim et al. including 169 patients with BE and advanced neoplasia, found that EMR followed by RFA achieved complete eradication of dysplasia and complete eradication of intestinal metaplasia in 94 and 88 % of patients respectively, compared with 82.7 and 77.6 % of patients in the RFA only group. The complication rates between both groups were also similar [46].

Follow up

While complete eradication of BE possible, life-long surveillance with biopsies throughout the entire eradicated area is required to monitor for buried glands and the recurrence of neoplasia. Surveillance occurs with targeted biopsies of every suspicious lesion followed by 4-quadrant biopsies every 1–2 cm [34]. The cumulative incidence of recurrent intestinal metaplasia is nearly 32 % following complete eradication of Barrett's epithelium by RFA [47–49]. While median disease free survival for endoscopic therapy and esophagectomy appear equal, higher rates of metachronous and synchronous lesions are found following endoscopic therapy, again highlighting the importance of frequent endoscopic surveillance [50].

Biopsy intervals are typically based on the highest degree of dysplasia prior to ablation. Risk factors for recurrence include long segment BE, piecemeal resection by EMR, and multifocal disease [51]. All endoscopic therapy of BE is accompanied by concomitant lifelong PPI therapy.

Esophagectomy

Until the past decade, esophagectomy was the standard of care for BE with HGD or IMC, but now is reserved for select individuals with submucosal invasion, which carries an approximate 20 % risk of nodal metastasis [52], evidence of lymph node metastasis, or unsuccessful endoscopic therapy. Selected patients with HGD or IMC with high-risk features may also benefit from surgery [53]. High-risk features may include gross characteristics including ulcerated/polypoid lesions, long segment BE, and lesions larger than 2 cm or histological characteristics including poor tumor differentiation, vascular, neural, lymphatic invasion, or multifocal HGD [53, 54].

The most important rationale for esophagectomy is its ability to completely resect the affected area, remove all associated lymph nodes, and afford a potential curative measure. Surgery allows for the most accurate staging and assessment of adequacy by looking for negative margins and lymph nodes. Complete resection minimizes the risk of metachronous lesions, which develop in residual Barrett's. With surgical resection, patients with HGD experience 5 year survival rates of over 90 % [55, 56].

The mortality rate associated with esophagectomy ranges between 1.5 and 15 %, while morbidity is as high as 50 % [57–60] When outcomes were controlled by hospital volume, institutions performing more than ten procedures per year had a significant difference in both post-operative mortality and post-operative complications. High volume centers with greater surgical expertise have decreased mortality rates of approximately 2–3 %, yet morbidity remains high [61, 62].

The complications experienced by 30–50 % of patients undergoing esophagectomy include dumping, anastomotic structuring, hemorrhage, anastomotic leak, infection, nerve palsy, pulmonary complications, regurgitation, diarrhea, and reflux [63, 64]. Both transhiatal and transthoracic esophagectomy techniques are performed in the United States. Transhiatal resections without thoracotomy can prevent respiratory compromise [65]. Transthoracic approaches may provide improved lymph node retrieval [66].

Minimally invasive, vagal sparing esophagectomy carries decreased perioperative morbidity, lower incidence of pulmonary complications, faster postoperative recovery, and shorter hospital stay when compared to transhiatal or en bloc esophagectomy. Unfortunately, the lymph node retrieval is inferior for this procedure. Peyre et al. demonstrated lower infectious, respiratory, and anastomotic complications in patients with HGD or IMC undergoing this procedure compared with transhiatal esophagectomy. The reduced post-vagotomy dumping and diarrhea, as well as shorter hospital stay appear to translate to improved quality of life [67].

It must also be noted that most studies describe outcomes after surgery for cancer and not HGD. Patients with cancer tend to be more debilitated preoperatively, and comorbid diseases are less frequent in patients with HGD alone [68]. Esophagectomy performed specifically for HGD has a pooled mortality of 1 % [68], making it a significantly lower risk procedure than when performed for EAC.

Endoscopic therapy for patients with HGD/IMC has a long-term survival similar to esophagectomy [35]. A retrospective study performed by Zehetner et al. compared 40 patients with HGD/IMC and 61 esophagectomy patents, and found that endoscopic therapy was associated with lower morbidity and similar 3-year survival rates, although multiple endoscopic procedures were necessary [69]. A retrospective study investigating 132 endoscopically treated patients and 46 surgically treated patients at the Mayo Clinic revealed similar mortality rates (17 and 20 % respectively), as well as overall survival. There was an increased rate of recurrent carcinoma in the endoscopically treated cohort, yet all of these patients were successfully re-treated without impact on overall survival [70]. Additional long-term data and comparative data for minimally invasive surgical approaches and endoscopic approaches are needed for the indication of HGD/IMC to better determine what role esophagectomy should play for these patients.

Recommendations

The presence of dysplasia should be confirmed by a gastrointestinal pathologist. Endoscopic resection of mucosal irregularities in the setting of dysplasia in Barrett's esophagus should be performed for accurate T staging of neoplasia. Patients with Barrett's esophagus with high-grade dysplasia should be managed with endoscopic eradication therapy rather than surveillance. Esophagectomy should be reserved for patients with Barrett's associated neoplasia with submucosal invasion, lymph node metastasis, or failure of endoscopic therapy. Esophagectomy should be performed at high volume centers.

Conclusions

Barrett's associated neoplasia has undergone a paradigm shift in recent years. Figure 22.1 demonstrates the current standard approach that applies to most patients with Barrett's associated neoplasia. It is critical to confirm dysplasia with an expert GI pathologist and accurately stage superficial lesions with endoscopic resection. Most experts agree that HGD poses a sufficient risk for malignancy that intervention is warranted [33]. Given these intermediate term results and the minimal lymph node metastasis risk, endoscopic treatment is now standardly offered to patients with HGD and IMC. Currently, the American Gastroenterological Association and American Society for Gastrointestinal Endoscopy both recommend that endoscopic eradication therapy is preferred over surveillance for patients with confirmed HGD and IMC [34]. Given the mortality and morbidity of esophagectomy, surgical resection should be reserved for submucosal invasion, lymph node metastasis, and failure of endoscopic therapy. There may also be selected individuals with high-risk features of Barrett's associated neoplasia that may benefit from esophagectomy over endoscopic therapy; however future studies, longer-term data, and development of risk stratification approaches are required to further define that subset. Patients with Barrett's associated neoplasia should be counseled on all available options, and some may benefit from counseling by both a surgeon and an endoscopist. Ultimately, patients with HGD and IMC in Barrett's esophagus benefit from a multidisciplinary team approach where surgeons, endoscopist and pathologists are working in concert to leverage diagnostic accuracy, treatment efficacy, mitigation of risks and quality of life for patients with Barrett's associated neoplasia.

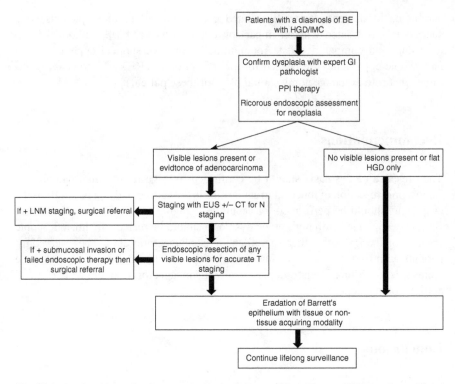

Fig. 22.1 An algorithm reflecting current standard approach for patients with Barrett's associated neoplasia

A Personal View of the Data

My approach systematically begins with counseling patients on all options of therapy and confirming the diagnosis of dysplasia with our gastrointestinal pathologists. I treat patients with high dose proton pump inhibitors twice daily. I standardly begin with a thorough endoscopic evaluation followed by endoscopic therapy. I utilize advanced imaging modalities that include narrow band imaging and/or confocal laser endomicroscopy to enhance my endoscopic examination to improve my diagnostic yield for biopsies and resections. Treatment for patients with high-grade dysplasia first begins with focal endoscopic mucosal resection of any visible lesions. Then, I treat the remainder of Barrett's mucosa radiofrequency ablation. Long segments are first treated with circumferential RFA with the balloon device. I treat shorter segments and residual areas with focal RFA. After treatment is completed, I perform surveillance endoscopies with biopsies yearly. I prepare patients with the knowledge that endoscopic treatment may require multiple modalities, multiple sessions, and indefinite surveillance.

Recommendations

- The presence of dysplasia should be confirmed by a gastrointestinal pathologist. (Evidence quality moderate; weak recommendation)
- Endoscopic resection of mucosal irregularities in the setting of dysplasia in Barrett's esophagus should be performed for accurate T staging of neoplasia. (Evidence quality low; weak recommendation)
- Patients with Barrett's esophagus with high-grade dysplasia should be managed with endoscopic eradication therapy rather than surveillance. (Evidence quality moderate; weak recommendation)
- Esophagectomy should be reserved for patients with Barrett's associated neoplasia with submucosal invasion, lymph node metastasis, or failure of endoscopic therapy (Evidence quality high; strong recommendation)
- Esophagectomy should be performed at high volume centers. (Evidence quality moderate; weak recommendation)

References

1. Gillison EW, Powell J, McConkey CC, Spychal RT. Surgical workload and outcome after resection for carcinoma of the oesophagus and cardia. Br J Surg. 2002;89(3):344–8. PubMed PMID: 11872061.
2. Liu JF, Wang QZ, Hou J. Surgical treatment for cancer of the oesophagus and gastric cardia in Hebei, China. Br J Surg. 2004;91(1):90–8. PubMed PMID: 14716801.
3. Modiano N, Gerson LB. Barrett's esophagus: incidence, etiology, pathophysiology, prevention and treatment. Ther Clin Risk Manag. 2007;3(6):1035–145. PubMed PMID: 18516262, Pubmed Central PMCID: 2387291.
4. Fitzgerald RC, Lascar R, Triadafilopoulos G. Review article: Barrett's oesophagus, dysplasia and pharmacologic acid suppression. Aliment Pharmacol Ther. 2001;15(3):269–76. PubMed PMID: 11207503.
5. Riddell RH, Odze RD. Definition of Barrett's esophagus: time for a rethink–is intestinal metaplasia dead? Am J Gastroenterol. 2009;104(10):2588–94. PubMed PMID: 19623166.
6. Tan A, Macrae F. Management of cancer risk in Barrett's esophagus. J Gastroenterol Hepatol. 2011;26(10):1485–92. PubMed PMID: 21592226.
7. Spechler SJ. Barrett's esophagus: the American perspective. Dig Dis. 2013;31(1):10–6. PubMed PMID: 23797117.
8. Paraf F, Flejou JF, Pignon JP, Fekete F, Potet F. Surgical pathology of adenocarcinoma arising in Barrett's esophagus. Analysis of 67 cases. Am J Surg Pathol. 1995;19(2):183–91. PubMed PMID: 7832278.
9. Konda VJ, Ross AS, Ferguson MK, Hart JA, Lin S, Naylor K, et al. Is the risk of concomitant invasive esophageal cancer in high-grade dysplasia in Barrett's esophagus overestimated? Clin Gastroenterol Hepatol. 2008;6(2):159–64. PubMed PMID: 18096439.
10. Abraham SC, Krasinskas AM, Correa AM, Hofstetter WL, Ajani JA, Swisher SG, et al. Duplication of the muscularis mucosae in Barrett esophagus: an underrecognized feature and its implication for staging of adenocarcinoma. Am J Surg Pathol. 2007;31(11):1719–25. PubMed PMID: 18059229.
11. Lewis JT, Wang KK, Abraham SC. Muscularis mucosae duplication and the musculo-fibrous anomaly in endoscopic mucosal resections for Barrett esophagus: implications for staging of adenocarcinoma. Am J Surg Pathol. 2008;32(4):566–71. PubMed PMID: 18300796.

12. Chennat J, Konda VJ, Waxman I. Endotherapy for Barrett's esophagus: which, how, when, and who? Gastrointest Endosc Clin N Am. 2011;21(1):119–33. PubMed PMID: 21112502.
13. Curvers WL, ten Kate FJ, Krishnadath KK, Visser M, Elzer B, Baak LC, et al. Low-grade dysplasia in Barrett's esophagus: overdiagnosed and underestimated. Am J Gastroenterol. 2010;105(7):1523–30. PubMed PMID: 20461069.
14. Levine DS, Blount PL, Rudolph RE, Reid BJ. Safety of a systematic endoscopic biopsy protocol in patients with Barrett's esophagus. Am J Gastroenterol. 2000;95(5):1152–7. PubMed PMID: 10811320.
15. Reid BJ, Blount PL, Feng Z, Levine DS. Optimizing endoscopic biopsy detection of early cancers in Barrett's high-grade dysplasia. Am J Gastroenterol. 2000;95(11):3089–96. PubMed PMID: 11095322.
16. Peters FP, Curvers WL, Rosmolen WD, de Vries CE, Ten Kate FJ, Krishnadath KK, et al. Surveillance history of endoscopically treated patients with early Barrett's neoplasia: nonadherence to the Seattle biopsy protocol leads to sampling error. Dis Esophagus. 2008;21(6):475–9. PubMed PMID: 18430186, Off J Int Soc Dis Esophagus.
17. Singh R, Anagnostopoulos GK, Yao K, Karageorgiou H, Fortun PJ, Shonde A, et al. Narrow-band imaging with magnification in Barrett's esophagus: validation of a simplified grading system of mucosal morphology patterns against histology. Endoscopy. 2008;40(6):457–63. PubMed PMID: 18459090.
18. Kara MA, Peters FP, Rosmolen WD, Krishnadath KK, ten Kate FJ, Fockens P, et al. High-resolution endoscopy plus chromoendoscopy or narrow-band imaging in Barrett's esophagus: a prospective randomized crossover study. Endoscopy. 2005;37(10):929–36. PubMed PMID: 16189764.
19. Mannath J, Subramanian V, Hawkey CJ, Ragunath K. Narrow band imaging for characterization of high grade dysplasia and specialized intestinal metaplasia in Barrett's esophagus: a meta-analysis. Endoscopy. 2010;42(5):351–9. PubMed PMID: 20200809.
20. Sharma P, Meining AR, Coron E, Lightdale CJ, Wolfsen HC, Bansal A, et al. Real-time increased detection of neoplastic tissue in Barrett's esophagus with probe-based confocal laser endomicroscopy: final results of an international multicenter, prospective, randomized, controlled trial. Gastrointest Endosc. 2011;74(3):465–72. PubMed PMID: 21741642, Pubmed Central PMCID: 3629729.
21. Chennat J, Konda VJ, Ross AS, de Tejada AH, Noffsinger A, Hart J, et al. Complete Barrett's eradication endoscopic mucosal resection: an effective treatment modality for high-grade dysplasia and intramucosal carcinoma–an American single-center experience. Am J Gastroenterol. 2009;104(11):2684–92. PubMed PMID: 19690526.
22. Wani S, Mathur SC, Curvers WL, Singh V, Herrero LA, Hall SB, et al. Greater interobserver agreement by endoscopic mucosal resection than biopsy samples in Barrett's dysplasia. Clin Gastroenterol Hepatol. 2010;8(9):783–8. PubMed PMID: 20472096, Off Clin Pract J Am Gastroenterol Assoc.
23. Yoshinaga S, Oda I, Nonaka S, Kushima R, Saito Y. Endoscopic ultrasound using ultrasound probes for the diagnosis of early esophageal and gastric cancers. World J Gastrointest Endosc. 2012;4(6):218–26. PubMed PMID: 22720122, Pubmed Central PMCID: 3377863.
24. Fernandez-Sordo JO, Konda VJ, Chennat J, Madrigal-Hoyos E, Posner MC, Ferguson MK, et al. Is Endoscopic Ultrasound (EUS) necessary in the pre-therapeutic assessment of Barrett's esophagus with early neoplasia? J Gastrointest Oncol. 2012;3(4):314–21. PubMed PMID: 23205307, Pubmed Central PMCID: 3492480.
25. Wani S, Falk G, Hall M, Gaddam S, Wang A, Gupta N, et al. Patients with nondysplastic Barrett's esophagus have low risks for developing dysplasia or esophageal adenocarcinoma. Clin Gastroenterol Hepatol. 2011;9(3):220–7; quiz e226. PubMed PMID: 21115133.
26. Weston AP, Sharma P, Topalovski M, Richards R, Cherian R, Dixon A. Long-term follow-up of Barrett's high-grade dysplasia. Am J Gastroenterol. 2000;95(8):1888–93. PubMed PMID: 10950031.
27. Rastogi A, Puli S, El-Serag HB, Bansal A, Wani S, Sharma P. Incidence of esophageal adenocarcinoma in patients with Barrett's esophagus and high-grade dysplasia: a meta-analysis. Gastrointest Endosc. 2008;67(3):394–8. PubMed PMID: 18045592.

28. Rice TW, Falk GW, Achkar E, Petras RE. Surgical management of high-grade dysplasia in Barrett's esophagus. Am J Gastroenterol. 1993;88(11):1832–6. PubMed PMID: 8237928.
29. Reid BJ, Weinstein WM, Lewin KJ, Haggitt RC, VanDeventer G, DenBesten L, et al. Endoscopic biopsy can detect high-grade dysplasia or early adenocarcinoma in Barrett's esophagus without grossly recognizable neoplastic lesions. Gastroenterology. 1988;94(1):81–90. PubMed PMID: 3335302.
30. Levine DS, Haggitt RC, Blount PL, Rabinovitch PS, Rusch VW, Reid BJ. An endoscopic biopsy protocol can differentiate high-grade dysplasia from early adenocarcinoma in Barrett's esophagus. Gastroenterology. 1993;105(1):40–50. PubMed PMID: 8514061.
31. Ferguson MK, Naunheim KS. Resection for Barrett's mucosa with high-grade dysplasia: implications for prophylactic photodynamic therapy. J Thorac Cardiovasc Surg. 1997;114(5):824–9. PubMed PMID: 9375613.
32. Konda VJ, Dalal K. Optimal management of Barrett's esophagus: pharmacologic, endoscopic, and surgical interventions. Ther Clin Risk Manag. 2011;7:447–58. PubMed PMID: 22162921, Pubmed Central PMCID: 3233528.
33. Spechler SJ, Sharma P, Souza RF, Inadomi JM, Shaheen NJ, American Gastroenterological A. American Gastroenterological Association technical review on the management of Barrett's esophagus. Gastroenterology. 2011;140(3):e18–52; quiz e13. PubMed PMID: 21376939. Pubmed Central PMCID: 3258495.
34. Bennett C, Vakil N, Bergman J, Harrison R, Odze R, Vieth M, et al. Consensus statements for management of Barrett's dysplasia and early-stage esophageal adenocarcinoma, based on a Delphi process. Gastroenterology. 2012;143(2):336–46. PubMed PMID: 22537613.
35. Prasad GA, Wang KK, Buttar NS, Wongkeesong LM, Krishnadath KK, Nichols 3rd FC, et al. Long-term survival following endoscopic and surgical treatment of high-grade dysplasia in Barrett's esophagus. Gastroenterology. 2007;132(4):1226–33. PubMed PMID: 17408660, Pubmed Central PMCID: 2646409, Epub 2007/04/06. eng.
36. Ell C, May A, Pech O, Gossner L, Guenter E, Behrens A, et al. Curative endoscopic resection of early esophageal adenocarcinomas (Barrett's cancer). Gastrointest Endosc. 2007;65(1):3–10. PubMed PMID: 17185072.
37. Konda VJ, Waxman I. Endotherapy for Barrett's esophagus. Am J Gastroenterol. 2012;107(6):827–33. PubMed PMID: 22488078.
38. Lopes CV, Hela M, Pesenti C, Bories E, Caillol F, Monges G, et al. Circumferential endoscopic resection of Barrett's esophagus with high-grade dysplasia or early adenocarcinoma. Surg Endosc. 2007;21(5):820–4. PubMed PMID: 17294308.
39. Honda K, Akiho H. Endoscopic submucosal dissection for superficial esophageal squamous cell neoplasms. World J Gastrointest Pathophysiol. 2012;3(2):44–50. PubMed PMID: 22532931, Pubmed Central PMCID: 3334390.
40. Katada C, Muto M, Manabe T, Ohtsu A, Yoshida S. Local recurrence of squamous-cell carcinoma of the esophagus after EMR. Gastrointest Endosc. 2005;61(2):219–25. PubMed PMID: 15729229.
41. Shaheen NJ, Overholt BF, Sampliner RE, Wolfsen HC, Wang KK, Fleischer DE, et al. Durability of radiofrequency ablation in Barrett's esophagus with dysplasia. Gastroenterology. 2011;141(2):460–8. PubMed PMID: 21679712, Pubmed Central PMCID: 3152658.
42. Shaheen NJ, Greenwald BD, Peery AF, Dumot JA, Nishioka NS, Wolfsen HC, et al. Safety and efficacy of endoscopic spray cryotherapy for Barrett's esophagus with high-grade dysplasia. Gastrointest Endosc. 2010;71(4):680–5. PubMed PMID: 20363409, Pubmed Central PMCID: 3094022.
43. Greenwald BD, Dumot JA, Horwhat JD, Lightdale CJ, Abrams JA. Safety, tolerability, and efficacy of endoscopic low-pressure liquid nitrogen spray cryotherapy in the esophagus. Dis Esophagus. 2010;23(1):13–9. PubMed PMID: 19515183, Pubmed Central PMCID: 3144029.
44. Dumot JA, Vargo 2nd JJ, Falk GW, Frey L, Lopez R, Rice TW. An open-label, prospective trial of cryospray ablation for Barrett's esophagus high-grade dysplasia and early esophageal cancer in high-risk patients. Gastrointest Endosc. 2009;70(4):635–44. PubMed PMID: 19559428.

45. Petersen BT, Chuttani R, Croffie J, DiSario J, Liu J, Mishkin D, et al. Photodynamic therapy for gastrointestinal disease. Gastrointest Endosc. 2006;63(7):927–32. PubMed PMID: 16733105.
46. Kim HP, Bulsiewicz WJ, Cotton CC, Dellon ES, Spacek MB, Chen X, et al. Focal endoscopic mucosal resection before radiofrequency ablation is equally effective and safe compared with radiofrequency ablation alone for the eradication of Barrett's esophagus with advanced neoplasia. Gastrointest Endosc. 2012;76(4):733–9. PubMed PMID: 22732872.
47. Vaccaro BJ, Gonzalez S, Poneros JM, Stevens PD, Capiak KM, Lightdale CJ, et al. Detection of intestinal metaplasia after successful eradication of Barrett's esophagus with radiofrequency ablation. Dig Dis Sci. 2011;56(7):1996–2000. PubMed PMID: 21468652, Pubmed Central PMCID: 3144139.
48. Orman ES, Li N, Shaheen NJ. Efficacy and durability of radiofrequency ablation for Barrett's esophagus: systematic review and meta-analysis. Clin Gastroenterol Hepatol. 2013;11(10):1245–55. PubMed PMID: 23644385.
49. Orman ES, Kim HP, Bulsiewicz WJ, Cotton CC, Dellon ES, Spacek MB, et al. Intestinal metaplasia recurs infrequently in patients successfully treated for Barrett's esophagus with radiofrequency ablation. Am J Gastroenterol. 2013;108(2):187–95; quiz 196, PubMed PMID: 23247578.
50. Das A, Singh V, Fleischer DE, Sharma VK. A comparison of endoscopic treatment and surgery in early esophageal cancer: an analysis of surveillance epidemiology and end results data. Am J Gastroenterol. 2008;103(6):1340–5. PubMed PMID: 18510606.
51. Esaki M, Matsumoto T, Hirakawa K, Nakamura S, Umeno J, Koga H, et al. Risk factors for local recurrence of superficial esophageal cancer after treatment by endoscopic mucosal resection. Endoscopy. 2007;39(1):41–5. PubMed PMID: 17252459.
52. Leers JM, DeMeester SR, Oezcelik A, Klipfel N, Ayazi S, Abate E, et al. The prevalence of lymph node metastases in patients with T1 esophageal adenocarcinoma a retrospective review of esophagectomy specimens. Ann Surg. 2011;253(2):271–8. PubMed PMID: 21119508.
53. Konda VJ, Ferguson MK. Esophageal resection for high-grade dysplasia and intramucosal carcinoma: when and how? World J Gastroenterol. 2010;16(30):3786–92. PubMed PMID: 20698041, Pubmed Central PMCID: 2921090.
54. Luna RA, Gilbert E, Hunter JG. High-grade dysplasia and intramucosal adenocarcinoma in Barrett's esophagus: the role of esophagectomy in the era of endoscopic eradication therapy. Curr Opin Gastroenterol. 2012;28(4):362–9. PubMed PMID: 22517568.
55. Tseng EE, Wu TT, Yeo CJ, Heitmiller RF. Barrett's esophagus with high grade dysplasia: surgical results and long-term outcome–an update. J Gastrointest Surg. 2003;7(2):164–70; discussion 170–1, PubMed PMID: 12600440.
56. Headrick JR, Nichols 3rd FC, Miller DL, Allen MS, Trastek VF, Deschamps C, et al. High-grade esophageal dysplasia: long-term survival and quality of life after esophagectomy. Ann Thorac Surg. 2002;73(6):1697–702; discussion 702–3, PubMed PMID: 12078755.
57. Swisher SG, Deford L, Merriman KW, Walsh GL, Smythe R, Vaporicyan A, et al. Effect of operative volume on morbidity, mortality, and hospital use after esophagectomy for cancer. J Thorac Cardiovasc Surg. 2000;119(6):1126–32. PubMed PMID: 10838528.
58. van Lanschot JJ, Hulscher JB, Buskens CJ, Tilanus HW, ten Kate FJ, Obertop H. Hospital volume and hospital mortality for esophagectomy. Cancer. 2001;91(8):1574–8. PubMed PMID: 11301408.
59. Bailey SH, Bull DA, Harpole DH, Rentz JJ, Neumayer LA, Pappas TN, et al. Outcomes after esophagectomy: a ten-year prospective cohort. Ann Thorac Surg. 2003;75(1):217–22; discussion 222, PubMed PMID: 12537219.
60. Connors RC, Reuben BC, Neumayer LA, Bull DA. Comparing outcomes after transthoracic and transhiatal esophagectomy: a 5-year prospective cohort of 17,395 patients. J Am Coll Surg. 2007;205(6):735–40. PubMed PMID: 18035255.

61. Birkmeyer JD, Stukel TA, Siewers AE, Goodney PP, Wennberg DE, Lucas FL. Surgeon volume and operative mortality in the United States. N Engl J Med. 2003;349(22):2117–27. PubMed PMID: 14645640.
62. Law S. Esophagectomy without mortality: what can surgeons do? J Gastrointest Surg. 2010;14 Suppl 1:S101–7. PubMed PMID: 19774427.
63. Pohl H, Sonnenberg A, Strobel S, Eckardt A, Rosch T. Endoscopic versus surgical therapy for early cancer in Barrett's esophagus: a decision analysis. Gastrointest Endosc. 2009;70(4):623–31. PubMed PMID: 19394011.
64. Ng T, Vezeridis MP. Advances in the surgical treatment of esophageal cancer. J Surg Oncol. 2010;101(8):725–9. PubMed PMID: 20512949.
65. Hulscher JB, van Sandick JW, de Boer AG, Wijnhoven BP, Tijssen JG, Fockens P, et al. Extended transthoracic resection compared with limited transhiatal resection for adenocarcinoma of the esophagus. N Engl J Med. 2002;347(21):1662–9. PubMed PMID: 12444180.
66. Wolff CS, Castillo SF, Larson DR, O'Byrne MM, Fredericksen M, Deschamps C, et al. Ivor Lewis approach is superior to transhiatal approach in retrieval of lymph nodes at esophagectomy. Dis Esophagus. 2008;21(4):328–33. PubMed PMID: 18477255.
67. Peyre CG, DeMeester SR, Rizzetto C, Bansal N, Tang AL, Ayazi S, et al. Vagal-sparing esophagectomy: the ideal operation for intramucosal adenocarcinoma and Barrett with high-grade dysplasia. Ann Surg. 2007;246(4):665–71; discussion 671–4, PubMed PMID: 17893503.
68. Fernando HC, Murthy SC, Hofstetter W, Shrager JB, Bridges C, Mitchell JD, et al. The Society of Thoracic Surgeons practice guideline series: guidelines for the management of Barrett's esophagus with high-grade dysplasia. Ann Thorac Surg. 2009;87(6):1993–2002. PubMed PMID: 19463651.
69. Zehetner J, DeMeester SR, Hagen JA, Ayazi S, Augustin F, Lipham JC, et al. Endoscopic resection and ablation versus esophagectomy for high-grade dysplasia and intramucosal adenocarcinoma. J Thorac Cardiovasc Surg. 2011;141(1):39–47. PubMed PMID: 21055772.
70. Prasad GA, Wu TT, Wigle DA, Buttar NS, Wongkeesong LM, Dunagan KT, et al. Endoscopic and surgical treatment of mucosal (T1a) esophageal adenocarcinoma in Barrett's esophagus. Gastroenterology. 2009;137(3):815–23. PubMed PMID: 19524578.

Chapter 23
Preoperative Chemo Versus Chemoradiotherapy for Regionally Advanced Esophageal Adenocarcinoma

Basil S. Nasir and Moishe Liberman

Abstract The role of neoadjuvant therapy in patients with resectable locally advanced esophageal cancer has been the focus of multiple trials in the past two decades. This is due to the poor results of surgery alone in this patient population, as well as the disappointing results of trials addressing postoperative adjuvant therapy. The optimal regime, be it preoperative chemotherapy or chemoradiation, has been the subject of debate amongst physicians involved in the care of patients with esophageal cancer. The published data concerning options for neoadjuvant therapy is discussed in detail.

Keywords Esophageal neoplasm • Gastroesophageal junction neoplasm • Preoperative therapy • Neoadjuvant therapy • Chemotherapy • Chemoradiation • Combined modality therapy

Introduction

The treatment of esophageal cancer includes surgery, radiotherapy and chemotherapy, or some combination of these modalities. The treatment for early stage esophageal cancer limited to the mucosa (T1) or the submucosa (T2) has been resection. Once the tumor invades through the muscularis propria (T3), the incidence of lymphatic and distant metastases rises dramatically. In the absence of distant metastatic disease, this stage of tumor progression is commonly referred to

B.S. Nasir, MBBCh • M. Liberman, MD, PhD (✉)
Division of Thoracic Surgery, CHUM Endoscopic Tracheobronchial and Oesophageal Center
(C.E.T.O.C.), University of Montreal, 1560 Sherbrooke Street East, 8e CD – Pavillon
Lachapelle, D-8051, Montreal, QC H2L 4 M1, Canada
e-mail: basilsnasir@gmail.com; moishe.liberman@umontreal.ca

M.K. Ferguson (ed.), *Difficult Decisions in Thoracic Surgery*,
Difficult Decisions in Surgery: An Evidence-Based Approach 1,
DOI 10.1007/978-1-4471-6404-3_23, © Springer-Verlag London 2014

as locally- or regionally-advanced esophageal cancer. Surgical resection has been the mainstay of therapy for patients with adequate reserve to tolerate such a formidable operation; however, unsatisfactory oncologic results have led to investigations of the efficacy of combined modality therapy in this patient population. The most recent National Comprehensive Cancer Network (NCCN) guidelines show that in medically fit patients with non-cervical esophageal cancer, regardless of histology, a combined modality strategy of neoadjuvant chemotherapy or chemoradiation followed by esophagectomy is the best approach [1]. There exists some controversy about the best option for neoadjuvant therapy, be it preoperative chemotherapy alone or chemoradiation. In this chapter, we will examine the evidence for both approaches. We will exclude cervical esophageal cancer and limit the discussion to cancer of the mid and distal esophagus, including tumors of the gastroesophageal junction (GEJ).

Search Strategy

We performed a Medline search for studies published since January, 1993. We used the following search terms: "esophageal neoplasms", "esophageal cancer", "gastroesophageal junction neoplasms", "gastro-esophageal junction cancer", "antineoplastic agents", "chemotherapy", "radiotherapy", "surgery", "neoadjuvant" and "esophagectomy". The computer search was supplemented with manual searches of reference lists for all available review articles, primary studies, and bibliographies of books. Searches were restricted to databases citing articles in English. We limited the data set to randomized controlled trials.

Summary of the Literature

Historically, surgical resection was considered the mainstay of therapy for patients with early and locally-advanced esophageal cancer. However, even after an 'R0 resection' at the initial operation, patients with stage I-III esophageal cancer have progression of disease and 5-year survival rarely exceeds 30 %. Multiple trials evaluating the role of adjuvant postoperative chemotherapy and radiation have showed no major benefit. This is, in part, because of the difficulties of administering additional therapy soon after undergoing a morbid surgical intervention with a significant postoperative morbidity. Therefore, focus has turned to neoadjuvant treatment.

The concept of neoadjuvant chemotherapy is attractive for several reasons. First, patients who respond to preoperative therapy may theoretically have reduced tumor burden and higher likelihood of attaining a complete resection. Second, distant failure is attributed to areas of micrometastases that were missed by the preoperative evaluation, and eradication of these areas with systemic therapy is thought to be more efficacious due to the small size of these deposits. Also, restaging of patients following neoadjuvant therapy may identify patients with biologically unfavorable tumors that progress rapidly and would have done poorly with surgery. Third, the delivery rate of adjuvant therapy may be higher in the preoperative state, before a major intervention such as esophagectomy.

Neoadjuvant Chemotherapy

Multiple studies, including randomized trials, have been performed to assess the role of neoadjuvant chemotherapy plus surgery versus surgery alone. Table 23.1 includes a summary of the most quoted randomized trials that compared a group of patients undergoing neoadjuvant chemotherapy plus surgery versus surgery alone over the last 15 years [2–7]. In addition to these trials, there have been several meta-analyses published with various results, which are also included in Table 23.2 [8–10].

The United Kingdom Medical Research Council (MRC) OEO2 trial was published in 2002 and subsequently was updated in 2009. This trial is the largest single trial addressing neoadjuvant chemotherapy published (802 patients) to date [3]. Patients with esophageal tumors of the upper, middle or lower third of the esophagus, including tumors of the cardia, were enrolled. Almost two thirds of the patients had adenocarcinoma, whereas 31 % has squamous cell carcinoma (SCC) and 3 % had undifferentiated histology. The study group included patients that received two cycles of preoperative cisplatin (CDDP) and 5-fluorouracil (5FU) followed by surgery versus the control group that underwent surgery only. There were 434 patients in the study group versus 437 patients in the control group. Two-year survival was significantly better in the chemotherapy arm at 43 % versus 34 % in the surgery only group. In a later update, this advantage extended to 5- years, with an overall survival rate of 23 % in the chemotherapy group versus 17 % in the surgery group. Progression-free survival was also improved in the chemotherapy arm. One major peculiarity about this trial is the exclusion of 69 patients from one site due to unclear reasons.

The second largest trial by Kelsen et al., known as the Intergroup Trial 113, was published in 1998, 4 years prior to the MRC OEO2 trial [2]. The patient population was similar, including both adenocarcinoma and SCC of the mid and distal esophagus, but excluding tumors of the cardia and tumors proximal to 18 cm from the incisors on endoscopy. The chemotherapy group included 213 patients, and in this group the treatment included 3 cycles of CDDP and 5-FU followed by surgery. Patients who responded were eligible to receive an additional 2 cycles of postoperative chemotherapy. The control group received surgery only and included 227 patients. This trial did not demonstrate the same benefit seen in the MRC OEO2 trial with an overall survival of 23 % at 3 years in the study group versus 26 % in the surgery only group. One of the main criticisms received by this trial is that only 71 % of patients were able to complete the recommended dose of chemotherapy compared with a greater than 90 % completion rate in other trials. This is may be an important confounding variable that may have masked a small, but important advantage in favor of neoadjuvant chemotherapy.

Table 23.1 Selected studies of surgery with or without neoadjuvant chemotherapy

Study	Histology	Treatment	No. of patients	% pCR	Treatment related mortality (%)	Survival	Quality of evidence
Kelsen et al. [2]	SCC 59.7 %	CDDP+5FU + S	213	2.5	6.4	23 % at 3 years	Moderate
		S	227		4	26 % at 3 years	
MRC OEO2 [3]	*SCC 31%*	*CDDP+5FU + S*	*434*	*4*	*N/A*	*23% at 5 years*	*Moderate*
		S	*437*		*N/A*	*17% at 5 years*	
Cunningham et al. (MAGIC) [4]	*ACA 100%*	*Perioperative ECF + S*	*250*			*36.3% at 5 years*	*Low*
		S	*253*			*23% at 5 years*	
Ychou et al. [5]	*ACA 100%*	*Perioperative CDDP+5FU + S*	*113*		*4.6*	*38% at 5 years*	*Moderate*
		S	*111*		*4.5*	*24% at 5 years*	
Ancona et al. [6]	SCC 100 %	CDDP+5FU + S	48	12.8	4.2	22 % at 5 years	Moderate
		S	48		4.2	34 % at 5 years	
Boonstra et al. [7]	*SCC 100%*	*CDDP + etoposide + S*	*85*	*7*	*5*	*26% at 5 years*	*Moderate*
		S	*84*		*4*	*17% at 5 years*	

Rows in italics indicate a statistically significant difference in outcomes

Abbreviations: *ACA* adenocarcinoma, *CDDP* cisplatin, *ECF* epirubicin, cisplatin, 5-fluorouracil, *MRC OE2* Medical Research Council Oesophageal Cancer working party, *pCR* complete pathologic response, *S* surgery, *SCC* squamous cell carcinoma, *5-FU* 5-fluorouracil

Table 23.2 Selected meta-analysis of surgery with or without neoadjuvant therapy

Study	Treatment	No. of patients	Treatment related mortality (95%CI)[a]	Overall survival (95%CI)[a]
Neoadjuvant chemotherapy and surgery versus surgery only				
Urschel et al. [8]	CS	NS	0.94 (0.66–1.35, p=0.76)	1 year: 1.00 (0.76–1.3; p=0.98) 2 year: 0.88 (0.62–1.24; p=0.45) 3 year: 0.77 (0.37–1.59; p=0.48)
	S	NS		
Kaklamanos et al. [9]	CS	845	Difference in mortality 1.7 % (−0.9 to 4.3, p=0.38)[b]	ARR for mortality at 2 years by 4.4 % (0.3–8.5; p=0.07)[b]
	S	838		
Neoadjuvant chemoradiation and surgery versus surgery only				
Sjouquist et al. [10]	*CS*	*1,046*	*Not stated*	*0.87 (0.79–0.96; p=0.005)*
	S	*1,016*		
Urschel et al. [19]	CRS	NS	1.72 (0.96–3.07; p=0.07)	1 year: 0.79 (0.59–1.06; p=0.12) 2 year: 0.77 (0.56–1.05; p=0.1) 3 year: 0.66 (0.47–0.92 p=0.016)
	S	NS		
Kaklamanos et al. [9]	CRS	289	Difference in mortality 3.4 % (95%CI −0.1 to 7.3; p=0.2)[b]	ARR for mortality at 2 years by 6.4 % (95%CI 1.2–14.0; p=0.86)[b]
	S	280		
Fiorica et al. [20]	*CRS*	*385*	*2.10 (1.18–3.73; p=0.01)*	*0.53 (0.32–0.89; p=0.02)*
	S	*379*		
Jin et al. [21]	*CRS*	*659*	*1.68 (1.03–2.73, p=0.04)*	*1 year 1.28 (1.01–1.64, p=.05) 3 year 1.78 (1.2–2.66 p=0.02) 5 year 1.46 (1.07–1.99, p=0.02)*
	S	*649*		
Sjouquist et al. [10]	*CS*	*980*	*Not stated*	*0.78 (0.70–0.88; p<0.0001).*
	S	*952*		

Rows in italics indicate a statistically significant difference in outcomes

Abbreviations: *ARR* absolute risk reduction, *CRS* neoadjuvant chemoradiation and surgery, *CS* neoadjuvant chemotherapy and surgery, *HR* hazard ratio, *NS* not stated, *S* surgery, *95%CI* 95 % confidence interval

[a]Hazard ratio (95 % confidence interval [95%CI]; P value), expressed as chemotherapy and surgery versus surgery alone (treatment versus control; values <1 favor neoadjuvant therapy-surgery arm)

[b]Results from the meta-analysis by Kaklamanos et al. are stated in absolute percentage difference in survival at 2 years. No odds ratio or hazard ration values were given

Although not designed to specifically look at esophageal cancer, the MAGIC trial provides important data on the treatment of gastric cancer and tumors of the gastroesophageal junction (GEJ) [4]. Most studies either excluded patients with predominantly gastric GEJ tumors, the so-called Siewert III GEJ adenocarcinoma or they did not clearly state if they were included. The MAGIC trial provides the most data on this group of patients. In this trial, patients were randomized to perioperative chemotherapy with CDDP, epirubicin and 5FU versus surgery only. The survival at 5 years was 36.3 % in the chemotherapy group versus 23 % in the surgery only group. The trial is criticized for the quality of surgery performed and the lack of a standard lymphadenectomy. The extent of lymphadenectomy was determined by the surgeon's discretion.

There are multiple other trials with conflicting results, some with results favoring neoadjuvant chemotherapy and some showing no difference between both approaches with regards to overall survival. There was concern that some of the negative trials were underpowered and may have been too small to identify small but important differences in overall survival, especially in the negative trials that demonstrated a difference in progression-free survival. This prompted the publication of multiple meta-analyses, which are summarized in Table 23.2 [8–10]. The most recent of those by Sjoquist et al. showed an advantage to neoadjuvant chemotherapy with a hazard ratio of mortality of 0.87 and a 2-year absolute survival benefit of 5.1 % [10]. The difference was present in a subgroup analysis looking at patients with adenocarcinoma, but was absent in patients with SCC histology.

In addition to individual criticisms for each trial, there are several weaknesses that are shared by all. First, most of the trials were started before 1994, and hence methods for diagnosis, staging, treatment delivery, perioperative care and outcome measurements indicate clinical practice during that period. For example, in most studies, endoscopic ultrasound (EUS) was rarely used and none of the studies comment on the utility of positron emission tomography (PET). Furthermore, there was no distinction between patients who had early stage cancer limited to the mucosa, and they were analyzed similarly. Without any data on the stage of patients at the time of presentation, it is difficult to determine if differences in survival are attributed to the use of neoadjuvant chemotherapy or a higher incidence of early stage cancer in one group.

Neoadjuvant Chemoradiation

Given the conflicting results yielded from trials evaluating neoadjuvant chemotherapy, an interest developed in examining the effect of adding external beam radiotherapy (XRT) to chemotherapy in the preoperative setting. A summary of the most noteworthy trials is shown in Table 23.3 [11–18]. The earliest trials did not show any advantage in overall survival between neoadjuvant chemoradiation followed by surgery in comparison to surgery alone. One exception is the trial by Walsh et al., which demonstrated a survival advantage at 3-years [12]. The overall survival in the

Table 23.3 Selected studies of surgery with or without neoadjuvant chemoradiation

Study	Histology	Treatment	No. of patients	% pCR	Treatment Related mortality (%)	Survival	Quality of evidence
Le Prise et al. [11]	SCC 100 %	CDDP+5FU +20 Gy sXRT + S	41	10	8.5	19.2 % at 3 years	Moderate
		S	45		7	13.8 % at 3 years	
Walsh et al. [12]	*ACA 100%*	*CDDP+5FU +40 Gy cXRT + S*	*58*	*25*	*8.5*	*32% at 3 years*	*Moderate*
		S	*55*		*3.6*	*6% at 3 years*	
Bosset et al. [13]	SCC 100 %	CDDP +37 Gy sXRT + S	143	26	12.3	18.6 months[a]	Moderate
		S	139		3.6	18.6 months[a]	
Urba et al. [14]	ACA 75 %	CDDP + vinblastine +5FU +45 Gy cXRT + S	50	28	2.1	30 % at 3 years	Moderate
		S	50		4	16 % at 3 years	
Burmeister et al. [15]	ACA 62 %	CDDP+5FU +35 Gy cXRT + S	128	16	4.7	22 months[a]	Moderate
		S	128		5.5	19 months[a]	
Lee et al. [16]	SCC 100 %	CDDP+5FU +45 GycXRT + S	51	43	Not stated	55 % at 2 years	Moderate
		S	50		Not stated	57 % at 2 years	
Tepper et al. [17]	*ACA 75%*	*CDDP+5FU +50.4 Gy cXRT + S*	*30*	*33*	*Not stated*	*39% at 5 years*	*Moderate*
		S	*26*		*Not stated*	*16% at 5 years*	
Van Hagen et al. (CROSS) [18]	*ACA 75%*	*Carboplatin + paclitaxel +41.4 Gy cXRT + S*	*178*	*29*	*4*	*47% at 5 years*	*Moderate*
		S	*188*		*4*	*34% at 5 years*	

Rows in italics indicate a statistically significant difference in outcomes

Abbreviations: *ACA* adenocarcinoma, *CDDP* cisplatin, *cXRT* concurrent external beam radiotherapy, *pCR* pathologic complete response, *S* surgery, *SCC* squamous cell carcinoma, *sXRT* sequential external beam radiotherapy, *5FU* 5-fluorouracil

[a]Median survival

neoadjuvant chemoradiation group was 32 % at 3-years, compared to 6 % in the surgery only group. The study is criticized for the unusually low survival in the surgery only group.

More recent trials have demonstrated a survival advantage in favor of trimodality therapy compared to surgery alone. The Cancer and Leukemia Group B (CALGB) 9,781 study was conducted recently in the United States, and it randomized patients to the trimodality arm which received 2 cycles of 5FU and CDDP with concurrent XRT at 50.4 Gy followed by surgery or a surgery only arm [17]. The study was closed prematurely due to a low accrual rate. The results that were reported showed a statistically significant improvement in overall survival in favor of trimodality therapy. Median overall survival was 4.48 years in the trimodality group versus 1.79 years in the surgery only group.

The most recent study addressing the issue is the CROSS study published in 2012 by Van Hagen et al. [18]. The study included patients with both adenocarcinoma and SCC. They excluded patients with tumors within 3 cm of the upper esophageal sphincter and tumors greater than 8 cm in length and greater than 5 cm in width. EUS was routinely performed for staging and patients had to have T1 N1 or T2-3 N0-1 disease to qualify. The study group included 178 patients who were scheduled to receive 5 cycles of paclitaxel and carboplatin with concurrent XRT at 41.4 Gy followed by surgery. The control group included 188 patients that were to undergo surgery only. The overall survival was higher the trimodality group at 1, 2, 3 and 5 years. The median survival was 49.4 months in the trimodality group versus 24 months in the surgery only group. This is a very important trial, as it most closely approximates treatment approaches of the current era in terms of preoperative staging and delivery of neoadjuvant therapy.

Similar to the data on neoadjuvant chemotherapy, there have been a number meta-analyses addressing combined chemoradiation in the neoadjuvant setting. These publications consistently yielded similar results and the data is summarized in Table 23.2 [9, 10, 19–21]. All but one of the studies demonstrated an overall survival advantage.

All these trials suffer from flaws similar to the ones discussed in the above section about neoadjuvant chemotherapy. That is to say that the older studies performed in the 90s reflected practice patterns from that era and thus may not be applicable to current therapy. This is supported by the fact that most recent trials demonstrated an improvement in survival. Also, the radiation doses in some of the earlier trials were lower than currently recommended doses. With the advent of conformal radiation techniques, current trials have used higher doses of radiation (typically 40 Gy) that are likely to result in better downstaging of overt tumors.

Neoadjuvant Chemotherapy Versus Neoadjuvant Chemoradiation

There have been two trials that directly compared preoperative chemotherapy versus preoperative chemoradiation. The first is by Stahl et al. published in 2009 [22]. This study randomized patients with adenocarcinoma of the distal esophagus and

Table 23.4 Randomized trails comparing neoadjuvant chemotherapy and chemoradiation

Study	Histology	Treatment	No. of patients	% pCR	Treatment related mortality (%)	Survival	Quality of evidence
Stahl et al. [9]	ACA 100 %	CDDP+5FU followed by + CDDP + etoposide +30 Gy cXRT + S	60	15.6	10.2	47.4 % at 3 years	Moderate
		CDDP+5FU + S	59	2	3.8	27.7 % at 3 years	
Burmeister et al. [10]	ACA 100 %	CDDP+5FU 35 Gy cXRT + S	39	13	0	45 % at 5 years	Moderate
		CDDP+5FU + S	36	0	0	36 % at 5 years	

Abbreviations: *ACA* adenocarcinoma, *CDDP* cisplatin, *cXRT* concurrent external beam radiotherapy, *pCR* pathologic complete response, *S* surgery, *sXRT* sequential external beam radiotherapy, *5FU* 5-fluorouracil

GEJ to either preoperative chemoradiation consisting of 2 cycles of CDDP and 5-FU followed by concurrent etoposide, CDDP and 30 Gy of XRT followed by surgery (n=60) versus preoperative chemotherapy only consisting of 2.5 cycles of CDDP and 5-FU followed by surgery (n=59). EUS was performed routinely and patients with T3/4 disease were eligible for the study. The rate of complete pathologic response was 15.6 % in the trimodality group versus 2 % in the chemotherapy group. The overall survival at 3 years was 47.4 % in the trimodality group versus 27.7 % in the chemotherapy group, but this fell short of statistical significance with a p-value of 0.07. The progression free survival at 3 years was better in the trimodality group at 79.5 % versus 56 % in the chemotherapy group. Of note, only 66 % of patients in the chemotherapy group completed the regime and 86 % underwent surgery, whereas in the trimodality group 75 % completed the full course and 82 % underwent surgery.

The second study by Burrmeister et al. also randomized patients with adenocarcinoma of the distal esophagus and GEJ to either preoperative chemoradiation including two cycles of CDDP and 5-FU with 35 Gy of XRT or preoperative chemotherapy only with the same chemotherapy regime. There was no difference in overall or progression free survival between the two groups. The rate of pathologic complete response was higher in the trimodality group [23].

The results of both these studies are summarized in Table 23.4. Looking strictly at survival data gained from these studies, there is no advantage to adding XRT preoperatively to chemotherapy. However, the studies suffer from similar flaws. The numbers are quite small and the studies may be underpowered to detect important differences in survival. The Stahl study showed a big difference in overall survival, but this was not statistically significant. Also, the neoadjuvant regime were much less aggressive compared to current recommendations and compared to those used in most recent trials demonstrating a survival advantage to preoperative multimodality therapy. It is also important to mention that there is a higher rate of complete pathologic response when radiation is combined with chemotherapy, and although this did not translate to an improvement in survival in these studies, it has in other studies been shown to be associated with a clinically and statistically significant improvement in overall survival [6].

The Trial of Preoperative Therapy for Gastric and Esophagogastric Junction Adenocarcinoma (TOPGEAR) is an ongoing trial that compares neoadjuvant chemotherapy versus chemoradiation in patients with adenocarcinoma of the stomach and GEJ [24]. This is being undertaken by the Australasian Gastro-Intestinal Trials Group and is a multi-institutional randomized trial that is recruiting patients with T3/4 and/or node positive biopsy-proven adenocarcinoma of the stomach or GEJ. The intervention arm in TOPGEAR consists of pre-operative chemotherapy, pre-operative chemoradiotherapy, surgery and post-operative chemotherapy. The control arm consists of pre-operative chemotherapy, surgery and post-operative chemotherapy. We hope that this trial will provide some more definitive answers on the choice of neoadjuvant regime.

Recommendations

Based on the above data, we suggest the use of induction chemoradiation in patients with resectable adenocarcinoma of the distal esophagus and Siewert I or II GEJ tumors that is at least T3 or higher or N1 and higher. We recommend use of either fluorpyrimidine/platinum or taxane/platinum regimes along with at least 40 Gy of XRT. Our preferred regimen is carboplatinum and paclitaxel with 50.2 Gy of XRT (delivered in fractions of 1.8–2 Gy per day). For patients with Siewert III adenocarcinoma of the GEJ, we suggest using preoperative chemotherapy without radiation, similar to that used in MAGIC trial [4]. Most studies either excluded these patients or did not clearly define the location of tumors of the GEJ. However, this question is currently being investigated in the TOPGEAR trial (clinicaltrials.gov Identifier: NCT01924819) and we look forward to the results of this tria [24]. For patients with resectable SCC of the esophagus that is at least staged as T3 or N1 or higher, we recommend either definitive chemoradiation or neoadjuvant chemoradiation with either a fluoropyrimidine- or taxane-based or fluorouracil based chemotherapy with concurrent external beam radiation followed by surgery in patients who demonstrate a good response on post-treatment evaluation. We strongly recommend against omitting radiotherapy in this subset of patients given the lack of improvement seen in neoadjuvant chemotherapy trails.

A Personal View of the Data

Neoadjuvant chemoradiation followed by surgery is increasingly being used to treat esophageal cancer although its benefit over neoadjuvant chemotherapy without radiation has not been unequivocally documented in prospective phase III trials to date. Although there is a slightly higher incidence of postoperative morbidity and mortality sited in some studies [11, 12], this has not been the case in most studies [11, 14, 15, 18]. The risk of postoperative complications is related, in part, to the specifics of radiation therapy. Large radiation fractions and treatment of large volumes of lung tissue are undesirable. This was observed in the trial reported by Bosset where fractions of 3 Gy were used [13]. Furthermore, when looking at trials that reported survival in relation to pathologic response, there is an undeniable survival advantage associated with a complete pathologic response [6, 14, 18]. All studies that report the rate of complete pathologic response demonstrate a considerably higher rate in the chemoradiation group. We thus believe that incorporating radiation into the regime is of utmost importance. The radiation treatment should be appropriately dosed and should be at least 40 Gy, as doses less than that are unlikely to produce sterilization of the tumor bed.

Recommendations

- We recommend the use of induction chemoradiation in patients with resectable adenocarcinoma of the distal esophagus and Siewert I or II GEJ tumors that is at least T3 or higher or N1 and higher. (Evidence quality moderate; weak recommendation)
- For patients with Siewert III adenocarcinoma of the GEJ, we recommend using preoperative chemotherapy without radiation. (Evidence quality moderate; weak recommendation)

References

1. National Comprehensive Cancer Network Clinical Practice Guidelines (NCCN Guidelines). Esophageal and esophagogastric junction cancers. Version 2. 2013. www.nccn.org.
2. Kelsen DP, Winter KA, Gunderson LL, Mortimer J, Estes NC, Haller DG, et al. Long-term results of RTOG trial 8911 (USA Intergroup 113): a random assignment trial comparison of chemotherapy followed by surgery compared with surgery alone for esophageal cancer. J Clin Oncol. 2007;25:3719–25.
3. Allum WH, Stenning SP, Bancewicz J, Clark PI, Langley RE. Long-term results of a randomized trial of surgery with or without preoperative chemotherapy in esophageal cancer. J Clin Oncol. 2009;27:5062–7.

4. Cunningham D, Allum WH, Stenning SP, Thompson JN, Van de Velde CJ, Nicolson M, et al. Perioperative chemotherapy versus surgery alone for resectable gastroesophageal cancer. N Engl J Med. 2006;355:11–20.
5. Ychou M, Boige V, Pignon JP, Conroy T, Bouché O, Lebreton G, et al. Perioperative chemotherapy compared with surgery alone for resectable gastroesophageal adenocarcinoma: an FNCLCC and FFCD multicenter phase III trial. J Clin Oncol. 2011;29:1715–21.
6. Ancona E, Ruol A, Santi S, Merigliano S, Sileni VC, Koussis H, et al. Only pathologic complete response to neoadjuvant chemotherapy improves significantly the long term survival of patients with resectable esophageal squamous cell carcinoma: final report of a randomized, controlled trial of preoperative chemotherapy versus surgery alone. Cancer. 2001;91:2165–74.
7. Boonstra JJ, Kok TC, Wijnhoven BP, van Heijl M, van Berge Henegouwen MI, Ten Kate FJ, et al. Chemotherapy followed by surgery versus surgery alone in patients with oesophageal squamous cell carcinoma: long-term results of a randomized controlled trial. BMC Cancer. 2011;11:181.
8. Urschel JD, Vasan H, Blewett CJ. A meta-analysis of randomized controlled trials that compared neoadjuvant chemotherapy and surgery to surgery alone for resectable esophageal cancer. Am J Surg. 2002;183(3):274–9.
9. Kaklamanos IG, Walker GR, Ferry K, Franceschi D, Livingstone AS. Neoadjuvant treatment for resectable cancer of the esophagus and the gastroesophageal junction: a meta-analysis of randomized clinical trials. Ann Surg Oncol. 2003;10(7):754–61.
10. Sjoquist KM, Burmeister BH, Smithers BM, Zalcberg JR, Simes RJ, Barbour A, et al. Survival after neoadjuvant chemotherapy or chemoradiotherapy for resectable oesophageal carcinoma: an updated meta-analysis. Lancet Oncol. 2011;12:681–92.
11. Le Prise E, Etienne PL, Meunier B, Maddern G, Ben Hassel M, Gedouin D, et al. A randomized study of chemotherapy, radiation therapy, and surgery versus surgery for localized squamous cell carcinoma of the esophagus. Cancer. 1994;73:1779–84.
12. Walsh TN, Noonan N, Hollywood D, Kelly A, Keeling N, Hennessy TP. A comparison of multimodal therapy and surgery for esophageal adenocarcinoma. N Engl J Med. 1996;335:462–7.
13. Bosset JF, Gignoux M, Triboulet JP, Tiret E, Mantion G, Elias D, et al. Chemoradiotherapy followed by surgery compared with surgery alone in squamous-cell cancer of the esophagus. N Engl J Med. 1997;337:161–7.
14. Urba SG, Orringer MB, Turrisi A, Iannettoni M, Forastiere A, Strawderman M, et al. Randomized trial of preoperative chemoradiation versus surgery alone in patients with locoregional esophageal carcinoma. J Clin Oncol. 2001;19:305–13.
15. Burmeister BH, Thomas JM, Burmeister EA, Walpole ET, Harvey JA, Thomson DB, et al. Is concurrent radiation therapy required in patients receiving preoperative chemotherapy for adenocarcinoma of the oesophagus? A randomised phase II trial. Eur J Cancer. 2011;47:354–60.
16. Lee JL, Park SI, Kim SB, Jung HY, Lee GH, Kim JH, et al. A single institutional phase III trial of preoperative chemotherapy with hyperfractionation radiotherapy plus surgery versus surgery alone for resectable esophageal squamous cell carcinoma. Ann Oncol. 2004;15:947–54.
17. Tepper J, Krasna MJ, Niedzwiecki D, Hollis D, Reed CE, Goldberg R, et al. Phase III trial of trimodality therapy with cisplatin, fl uorouracil, radiotherapy, and surgery compared with surgery alone for esophageal cancer: CALGB 9781. J Clin Oncol. 2008;26:1086–92.
18. van Hagen P, Hulshof MC, van Lanschot JJ, Steyerberg EW, van Berge Henegouwen MI, Wijnhoven BP, et al. Preoperative chemoradiotherapy for esophageal or junctional cancer. N Engl J Med. 2012;366(22):2074–84.
19. Urschel JD, Vasan H. A meta-analysis of randomized controlled trials that compared neoadjuvant chemoradiation and surgery to surgery alone for resectable esophageal cancer. Am J Surg. 2003;185(6):538–43.

20. Fiorica F, Di Bona D, Schepis F, Licata A, Shahied L, Venturi A, et al. Preoperative chemora-diotherapy for oesophageal cancer: a systematic review and meta-analysis. Gut. 2004;53(7): 925–30.
21. Jin HL, Zhu H, Ling TS, Zhang HJ, Shi RH. Neoadjuvant chemoradiotherapy for resectable esophageal carcinoma: a meta-analysis. World J Gastroenterol. 2009;15(47):5983–91.
22. Stahl M, Walz MK, Stuschke M, Lehmann N, Meyer HJ, Riera-Knorrenschild J, et al. Phase III comparison of preoperative chemotherapy compared with chemoradiotherapy in patients with locally advanced adenocarcinoma of the esophagogastric junction. J Clin Oncol. 2009;27:851–6.
23. Burmeister BH, Smithers BM, Gebski V, Fitzgerald L, Simes RJ, Devitt P, et al, for the Trans-Tasman Radiation Oncology Group; Australasian Gastro-Intestinal Trials Group. Surgery alone versus chemoradiotherapy followed by surgery for resectable cancer of the oesophagus: a randomized controlled phase III trial. Lancet Oncol 2005;6:659–68.
24. ClinicalTrials.gov. Identifier: NCT01924819 http://www.clinicaltrials.gov/ct2/show/NCT019 24819?term=NCT01924819&rank=1.

Chapter 24
The Role of Surgery in the Management of Regionally Advanced Esophageal Squamous Cell Cancer

Tyler R. Grenda and Andrew C. Chang

Abstract Regionally advanced squamous cell carcinoma (SCC) of the esophagus portends a poor prognosis even when esophageal resection can be accomplished. In an effort to improve patient survival, multimodal approaches to this disease have evolved that prompt re-evaluation whether esophageal resection remains a key part of treatment. In review of the available literature, multimodality approaches that include chemoradiation (CRT) may offer the best survival benefit, whereas the exact role of surgery remains unclear and continues to evolve. Further prospective studies are needed to solidify the role of surgery in regionally advanced SCC of the esophagus.

Keywords Surgery • Esophagectomy • Radiation therapy • Esophagus • Squamous cell carcinoma • Neoadjuvant treatment • Chemoradiation

Introduction

Regionally advanced squamous cell carcinoma (SCC) of the esophagus historically is associated with poor survival [1]. While surgery has been the traditional approach to treatment, chemoradiation (CRT) has developed as an effective modality that is associated with survival benefits [2–4]. Complete tumor response has been observed following chemotherapy with definitive dose radiation.

T.R. Grenda, MD • A.C. Chang, MD (✉)
Section of Thoracic Surgery, University of Michigan Health System,
Taubman Center 2120/5344, 1500 E. Medical Center Drive, Ann Arbor, MI 48109, USA
e-mail: andrwchg@umich.edu

M.K. Ferguson (ed.), *Difficult Decisions in Thoracic Surgery*,
Difficult Decisions in Surgery: An Evidence-Based Approach 1,
DOI 10.1007/978-1-4471-6404-3_24, © Springer-Verlag London 2014

As cancer staging, multimodal therapy, and surgical care have continued to improve, the optimal approach for treatment remains controversial. In patients with regionally advanced disease (T1-4N0-2), surgery alone provides poor survival results, prompting evaluation of CRT as standard treatment. It is clear that careful patient selection for consideration of esophageal resection is necessary. As survival data following chemotherapy with definitive dose radiation has become available, the role of additional surgery remains a point of controversy. This chapter will evaluate the available evidence to define the current best recommendations for the role of surgical intervention in patients with regionally advanced SCC of the esophagus.

Search Strategy

A systematic literature search was performed by the authors. We used the following medical search terms to identify relevant literature: esophageal cancer; advanced squamous cell carcinoma of the esophagus; regionally advanced esophageal cancer; surgery; neoadjuvant therapy; esophagectomy; chemoradiation. MEDLINE and Cochrane Reviews were searched to find abstracts pertinent to the topic. The literature (Table 24.1) was restricted to the most comprehensive and recent articles in order to provide up-to-date evidence. Articles included randomized controlled trials (RCTs), meta-analyses, observational studies, literature reviews, and retrospective studies in circumstances where other data was not available. All articles were restricted to those available in English. The reference lists of retrieved articles were also searched to identify additional literature. All publications were reviewed to ensure that they included the specific pathologic diagnosis, staging information, and outcome measures.

All literature was reviewed and the quality of data was classified according to the GRADE system (as outlined in Chap. 2). Specific clinical practice recommendations, based on the available evidence, were made according to the GRADE system.

Overview

While esophageal resection has been considered the standard treatment approach for patients with regionally advanced esophageal (SCC), survival following resection alone has been poor [9]. As chemotherapy with definitive dose radiation has been shown to be an effective treatment modality, it has become more difficult to determine which patients remain appropriate for surgical intervention. The initial approach to treatment strategy should be determined by the location of the primary tumor, distinguishing disease of the cervical (<5 cm from the cricopharyngeus), middle and distal esophagus. While there are no RCTs comparing resection and

Table 24.1 Quality of evidence

Authors, reference	Year of publication	Histology (no. of AC/SCC)/stage	Study design	Treatment	Effect	Hazard ratio (95 % CI)	Quality of evidence
Bedenne et al. [5]	2007	SCC(n=239); AC(n=29)/T3N0-1	RCT	Neoadjuvant CRT + surgery vs. dCRT	No benefit to additional surgery vs. continued CRT	0.90	High
Gebski et al. [3]	2007	SCC; AC/T0-3 N0-1	Meta-analysis	Neoadjuvant CRT-or-C + surgery vs. surgery	Survival benefit with neoadjuvant CRT	Neoadjuvant CRT: 0.84 (0.71–0.99; p=0.04); Neoadjuvant C: 0.88 (0.75–1.03; p=0.12)	High
Kranzfelder et al. [2]	2011	SCC T1-4N0-1	Meta-analysis	Neoadjuvant CRT-or-C + surgery vs. surgery; dCRT vs. neoadjuvant + surgery-or- surgery	Survival benefit for neoadjuvant CRT	Neoadjuvant CRT: 0.81 (0.70–0.95; p=0.008) Neoadjuvant C: 0.93 (0.81–1.08; p=0.368)	High
Sjoquist et al. [4]	2011	SCC; AC T0-3N0-1	Meta-analysis	Neoadjuvant CRT-or-C + surgery vs. surgery	Survival benefit of neoadjuvant CRT or C vs. surgery alone	CRT: 0.80 (0.68–0.93; p=0.004) C: 0.92 (0.81–1.04; p=0.18)	High
Stahl et al. [6]	2005	SCC (n=172) T3-4 N0-1	RCT	CRT + surgery vs. definitive CRT	Improved PFS in surgery arm; No difference in 2-year survival	2.1 (1.3–3.5; p=0.003)	Moderate
Teoh et al. [7]	2013	SCC (n=81)/ T1-4N0-1	RCT	Surgery vs. dCRT	Comparable long-term survival	–	Moderate
Vallböhmer et al. [8]	2010	SCC (n=118) AC (n=181)/T2N1M0, T3-4N0-1M0	Observational study	Neoadjuvant CRT-or-C + surgery	–	–	Moderate

Abbreviations: *AC* adenocarcinoma, *C* chemotherapy, *CI* confidence interval, *CRT* chemoradiation, *dCRT* definitive chemoradiation, *PFS* progression-free survival, *RCT* randomized controlled trial, *SCC* squamous cell carcinoma

definitive CRT in patients with SCC of the cervical esophagus, current recommendations state that such patients should be treated with definitive CRT [10].

In patients who have regionally advanced SCC of the middle or distal esophagus, the role of surgery is more controversial. The debate regarding the role of surgery in these patients addresses whether to provide definitive dose radiation or neoadjuvant radiation therapy in anticipation of esophageal resection. Neoadjuvant radiation therapy with concurrent chemotherapy is felt to improve local control, with better rates of complete (R0) resection as well as subsequent improvement of long-term survival. It is presumed that increased rates of complete clinical response can translate to higher rates of complete pathologic response [1, 11].

Results

A multicenter observational study evaluated the outcomes of patients with complete histopathologic response, as determined at esophagectomy, following multimodal therapy for locally advanced esophageal cancer. In this multi-center cohort study, 299 patients were identified as having a complete pathologic response out of 1,673 patients who had received neoadjuvant therapy at the six participating centers. Of the 299, 118 had been diagnosed with esophageal squamous cell carcinoma. Within the cohort of "complete responders" overall 5-year survival was 68 % (95 % CI: 62–76) and disease-specific 5-year survival was 55 % (95 % CI: 48–62). Even in this population, 70 (23 %) subjects had recurrent disease, including 10 (3 %) with local recurrence and 60 (20 %) with distant recurrence [8]. Thus, as advances in CRT potentially lead to improved complete pathologic response, resection still may carry a benefit in terms of minimizing local recurrence although patients remain at risk of recurrent systemic disease. Current non-surgical staging modalities (i.e. endoscopic ultrasound (EUS), [18F]-fluorodeoxyglucose (FDG) positron emission tomography (PET), computed tomography (CT) following induction therapy are not reliable in identifying patients with complete pathologic response, leading to continued focus on evaluating the potential benefits of CRT combined with surgery compared to CRT alone [12–14].

As the role of CRT as part of a multimodal approach has evolved, a comparison of neoadjuvant therapy and resection has been explored to help define the role of surgery. A meta-analysis of randomized trial data performed by Gebski and colleagues [3] evaluated randomized trials comparing neoadjuvant CRT followed by resection vs. surgery alone and neoadjuvant chemotherapy followed by resection vs. surgery alone. An update to this meta-analysis performed by Sjoquist and colleagues [4] revealed a survival benefit for patients undergoing neoadjuvant chemoradiotherapy (HR 0.80, 95 % CI 0.68–0.93; p=0.004) or chemotherapy (HR 0.92, 95 % CI 0.81–1.04; p=0.18) when compared to esophageal resection alone. Although these meta-analyses provide support for the benefit obtained from neoadjuvant CRT, the evaluated cohorts represented patients with heterogeneous disease stages (T0–3, N0–1), not necessarily specific for regionally advanced disease.

A randomized trial performed by Stahl and colleagues [6] compared the results of esophagectomy to definitive chemoradiation for patients with locally advanced (T3-4, N0-1) SCC. In the surgical cohort, patients underwent chemotherapy, followed by concurrent CRT prior to Ivor Lewis esophagectomy (ILE). In the definitive CRT arm, patients underwent the same induction chemotherapy, followed by CRT with an increased radiation dose (65 Gy vs. 40 Gy in the surgical cohort). Patients undergoing esophagectomy experienced improved progression-free survival (PFS) at 2 years (64.3 % vs. 40.7 %; P=0.003), although, overall 2-year survival was found to be equivalent between both arms (CRT: 35.4 %, surgery: 39.9 %). The treatment-related mortality in the surgery group was found to be significantly higher compared to the CRT arm (12.8 % vs. 3.5 %; P=0.03). This study suggests that esophageal resection and chemoradiation may improve local control compared to definitive CRT, but does not increase survival in those with regionally advanced disease.

Similarly, Bedenne and colleagues [5] reported their findings from a randomized trial that included 259 patients with predominantly SCC (88 %) and regionally advanced disease (T3-4, N0-1). Patients were treated with either CRT followed by surgery or definitive CRT. While no statistically significant difference was found in median survival (resection vs. continuation of CRT; 17.7 vs. 19.3 months) or 2-year survival (34 % vs. 40 %; P=0.44), the surgical cohort had a significantly higher mortality rate (9.3 vs. 0.8 %; P=0.002). This suggests that treatment strategies involving CRT with and without esophagectomy can result in similar survival rates.

While previous randomized trials have shown no significant difference in 2-year survival in patients undergoing treatment with CRT alone versus CRT with surgery, suggesting that the addition of surgery conferred no added survival benefit [4, 6], a more recent prospective multicenter RCT has reported comparable 5-year survival and disease-free survival in patients randomized to definitive CRT versus esophagectomy alone [7]. While there was no significant survival difference, a trend toward significance was observed in 5-year survival and disease-free survival, particularly for patients with node-positive disease, favoring the CRT group.

In patients specifically with T4 disease, overall survival historically has been very poor. Furthermore, the available literature suggests that, when compared to non-surgical therapy, esophagectomy alone, including resection of involved organs, does not improve outcomes [1, 15]. While the role of surgery is limited in these patients, definitive CRT or CRT followed by surgery offers the best survival advantage [1, 16]. Overall, the evidence in T4 disease is limited and current recommendations reflect different strategies based on T4a vs. T4b disease [10]. Current guidelines state that T4a tumors with involvement of the pericardium, pleura, or diaphragm may be appropriate for resection. While there are studies that provide some evidence addressing which patients might benefit from resection, a clearly defined role is not yet apparent [9, 17]. There are multiple factors that can confound clinical decision-making. As previously stated, currently available diagnostic modalities remain inaccurate, limiting the ability to determine the true extent of disease, particularly for patients who have undergone induction therapy, where distinguishing inflammation from residual tumor is challenging.

While neoadjuvant treatment may lead to downstaging and the possibility of R0 resection, the role of esophageal resection as part of the multimodal approach for treatment of mid and distal esophageal squamous cell carcinoma continues to evolve. Assessment of treatment response following induction therapy and elucidation of specific organ involvement may be helpful in the determining the overall prognosis and in guiding additional therapy, but the role of surgery remains controversial [1, 17].

Recommendations

Review of current literature provides important information regarding the multimodality approach that should be taken for the management of esophageal squamous cell carcinoma. CRT in the neoadjuvant setting offers an important survival benefit. Patients with regionally advanced SCC of the cervical esophagus should undergo definitive CRT. The role of surgery in disease of the non-cervical esophagus still cannot be clearly defined based on the evidence available. Current recommendations, in patients who can tolerate surgery, include neoadjuvant CRT followed by esophagectomy. Patients need to be evaluated on an individual basis for esophagectomy following CRT.

Although the surgical options for patients with evidence of local tumor invasion into adjacent organs remains limited, a multimodality approach may offer the best survival advantage [1]. In treatment of these patients, the role of neoadjuvant therapy and tumor downstaging followed by surgery continues to evolve. Specific organ involvement and the relative response to induction therapy may help to identify which patients are likely to benefit from operative intervention.

Summary

In review of the available evidence, regionally advanced SCC of the esophagus carries a poor prognosis. The approach to treatment is determined primarily by tumor location, i.e., cervical, middle or lower esophagus. Patients with disease of the cervical esophagus should undergo concurrent chemotherapy with definitive radiation therapy. Evidence to-date suggests that patients with disease of the non-cervical esophagus can benefit from neoadjuvant CRT followed by possible esophageal resection. These patients may exhibit a response from neoadjuvant CRT, which can potentially downstage disease and optimize a future attempt at an R0 resection, ultimately improving local control. While the exact role of surgery still remains to be defined, a multimodality approach to patients with regionally advanced SCC of the esophagus offers the best chance of survival.

In patients specifically with T4 tumors, the role of surgery also remains unclear. Evidence is limited and current recommendations are stratified based on T4a vs.

T4b disease. These patients should undergo CRT; however, additional studies to identify which patients may benefit from resection are needed.

Given the limited data on the role of surgery in patients with regionally advanced disease, further large prospective multicenter studies are needed to evaluate whether esophageal resection, with its attendant risks and sequelae, provides a significant survival benefit. Other considerations include assessing quality of life following treatment, as chemotherapy with definitive radiation alone carries side effects such as development of tracheo-esophageal fistula or esophageal stricture. Thus, each patient must be evaluated to determine the best approach for therapy, considering not only the ability of the patient to tolerate treatment, but also the associated risks and potential implications on quality of life.

A Personal View of the Data

In our practice, patients with cervical esophageal squamous cell carcinoma with proximal tumor involvement that would require resection of the upper esophageal sphincter with or without laryngopharyngoesophagectomy typically are referred for chemotherapy and concurrent definitive dose radiation therapy. Patients with loco-regionally advanced squamous cell carcinoma of the mid-to-distal esophagus are evaluated by a multidisciplinary team, including medical and radiation oncology, gastroenterology and thoracic surgical oncology, for combined modality treatment including preoperative concurrent chemotherapy and radiation followed by esophagectomy. If a patient has severe esophageal obstruction, enteral nutrition is maintained during neoadjuvant therapy using a naso-enteric feeding tube or surgical feeding jejunostomy, with care taken to avoid any trauma to the stomach, such as placement of a percutaneous gastrostomy, which might compromise the greater curvature vascular supply for a proposed gastric esophageal substitute. For patients with a mid-esophageal carcinoma, airway examination is imperative to assure that there is no evidence for airway invasion (thus T4b).

Recommendations

- Patients with locally advanced squamous cell carcinoma of the esophagus (T1-4aN+) should receive chemoradiation with or without resection (evidence quality moderate; strong recommendation).
- Patients with T4b SCC of the esophagus should undergo definitive CRT (evidence quality low; weak recommendation). (In patients with invasion of the trachea, great vessels, or heart, chemotherapy alone should be considered.)
- Patients with regionally advanced SCC of the cervical esophagus should undergo definitive radiation therapy (evidence quality moderate; weak recommendation).

References

1. Bharat A, Crabtree T. Management of advanced-stage operable esophageal cancer. Surg Clin North Am. 2012;92(5):1179–97.
2. Kranzfelder M, Schuster T, Geinitz H, Friess H, Buchler P. Meta-analysis of neoadjuvant treatment modalities and definitive non-surgical therapy for oesophageal squamous cell cancer. Br J Surg. 2011;98(6):768–83.
3. Gebski V, Burmeister B, Smithers BM, Foo K, Zalcberg J, Simes J. Survival benefits from neoadjuvant chemoradiotherapy or chemotherapy in oesophageal carcinoma: a meta-analysis. Lancet Oncol. 2007;8(3):226–34.
4. Sjoquist KM, Burmeister BH, Smithers BM, Zalcberg JR, Simes RJ, Barbour A, et al. Survival after neoadjuvant chemotherapy or chemoradiotherapy for resectable oesophageal carcinoma: an updated meta-analysis. Lancet Oncol. 2011;12(7):681–92.
5. Bedenne L, Michel P, Bouché O, Milan C, Mariette C, Conroy T, et al. Chemoradiation followed by surgery compared with chemoradiation alone in squamous cancer of the esophagus: FFCD 9102. J Clin Oncol. 2007;25(10):1160–8.
6. Stahl M, Stuschke M, Lehmann N, Meyer HJ, Walz MK, Seeber S, et al. Chemoradiation with and without surgery in patients with locally advanced squamous cell carcinoma of the esophagus. J Clin Oncol. 2005;23(10):2310–7.
7. Teoh AYB, Chiu PWY, Yeung WK, Liu SYW, Wong SKH, Ng EKW. Long-term survival outcomes after definitive chemoradiation versus surgery in patients with resectable squamous carcinoma of the esophagus: results from a randomized controlled trial. Ann Oncol. 2013;24(1):165–71.
8. Vallbohmer D, Holscher AH, DeMeester S, DeMeester T, Salo J, Peters J, et al. A multicenter study of survival after neoadjuvant radiotherapy/chemotherapy and esophagectomy for ypT-0N0M0R0 esophageal cancer. Ann Surg. 2010;252(5):744–9.
9. Fujita H, Sueyoshi S, Tanaka T, Tanaka Y, Matono S, Mori N, et al. Esophagectomy: is it necessary after chemoradiotherapy for a locally advanced T4 esophageal cancer? Prospective non-randomized trial comparing chemoradiotherapy with surgery versus without surgery. World J Surg. 2005;29(1):25–30.
10. Ajani JA, Barthel JS, Bekaii-Saab T, Bentrem DJ, D'Amico TA, Fuchs CS, Gerdes H, Hayman JA, Hazard L, Ilson DH, Kleinberg LR, McAleer MF, Meropol NJ, Mulcahy MF, Orringer MB, Osarogiagbon RU, Posey JA, Sasson AR, Scott WJ, Shibata S, Strong VE, Swisher SG, Washington MK, Willett C, Wood DE, Wright CD, Yang G, NCCN Esophageal Cancer Panel. Esophageal cancer. J Natl Comp Canc Netw. 2008;6(9):818.
11. Di Fiore F, Lecleire S, Rigal O, Galais MP, Ben Soussan E, David I, et al. Predictive factors of survival in patients treated with definitive chemoradiotherapy for squamous cell esophageal carcinoma. World J Gastroenterol. 2006;12(26):4185–90.
12. Vallbohmer D, Holscher AH, Dietlein M, Bollschweiler E, Baldus SE, Monig SP, et al. [18F]-Fluorodeoxyglucose-positron emission tomography for the assessment of histopathologic response and prognosis after completion of neoadjuvant chemoradiation in esophageal cancer. Ann Surg. 2009;250(6):88–94.
13. Sloof GW. Response monitoring of neoadjuvant therapy using CT, EUS, and FDG-PET. Best Pract Res Clin Gastroenterol. 2006;20(5):941–57.
14. Rebollo Aguirre AC, Ramos-Font C, Villegas Portero R, Cook GJ, Llamas Elvira JM, Tabares AR. 18 F-fluorodeoxiglucose positron emission tomography for the evaluation of neoadjuvant therapy response in esophageal cancer: systematic review of the literature. Ann Surg. 2009;250(2):247–54.
15. Shimada H, Okazumi S, Matsubara H, Nabeya Y, Shiratori T, Shimizu T, et al. Impact of the number and extent of positive lymph nodes in 200 patients with thoracic esophageal squamous cell carcinoma after three-field lymph node dissection. World J Surg. 2006;30(8):1441–9.

16. Ancona E, Ruol A, Castoro C, Chiarion-Sileni V, Merigliano S, Santi S, et al. First-line chemotherapy improves the resection rate and long-term survival of locally advanced (T4, any N,
M0) squamous cell carcinoma of the thoracic esophagus: final report on 163 consecutive
patients with 5-year follow-up. Ann Surg. 1997;226(6):714–23.
17. de Manzoni G, Pedrazzani C, Pasini F, Bernini M, Minicozzi AM, Giacopuzzi S, et al.
Chemoradiotherapy followed by surgery for squamous cell carcinoma of the thoracic esophagus with clinical evidence of adjacent organ invasion. J Surg Oncol. 2007;95(3):261–6.

Chapter 25
Optimal Surgical Approach to Esophagectomy for Distal Esophageal Adenocarcinoma

Sabha Ganai

Abstract Esophagectomy can be performed using transthoracic, transhiatal, and minimally-invasive approaches, with reconstruction via intrathoracic or cervical anastomoses. The optimal surgical approach to esophagectomy for cancer has been a subject of debate for decades, with assumed trade-offs between lymph node retrieval and perioperative morbidity. This chapter reviews the literature comparing esophageal procedures, examining studies investigating how technical considerations influence perioperative morbidity, mortality, functional outcomes, and survival for distal esophageal cancer.

Keywords Esophageal cancer • Esophagectomy • Outcomes • Complications • Transhiatal • Minimally-invasive • Transthoracic

Introduction

The past century has been distinguished by progress in the surgical management of esophageal diseases, a consequence of important developments in positive-pressure anesthesia, fluid management, nutritional support, surgical technique, and reconstructive options. A discussion on the optimal surgical approach for esophagectomy cannot proceed without an understanding of the history of esophageal resection. Esophagectomy for cancer was first successfully performed in 1913 by Franz Torek in New York City, with his patient surviving for 12 years with a cervical esophagostomy and gastrostomy [1, 2]. While others had later developed esophageal reconstructions via a subcutaneous route using transverse colon or stomach, Professor

S. Ganai, MD, PhD
Department of Surgery, Simmons Cancer Institute, Southern Illinois
University School of Medicine, 315 West Carpenter Street, Springfield, IL 62702, USA
e-mail: sganai@siumed.edu

M.K. Ferguson (ed.), *Difficult Decisions in Thoracic Surgery*,
Difficult Decisions in Surgery: An Evidence-Based Approach 1,
DOI 10.1007/978-1-4471-6404-3_25, © Springer-Verlag London 2014

Osawa at the University of Kyoto performed the first successful one-stage esopha-gectomy using an intrathoracic esophagogastrostomy in 1933, followed contempo-raneously by Dallas Phemister and William Adams at the University of Chicago in 1938 [2]. In 1945, Richard Sweet from Massachusetts General Hospital further popularized the left thoracoabdominal approach after advocating resection for can-cer with a high esophagogastric anastomosis over the Torek Procedure, which he described as both inadequate at addressing important lymph nodes and unsatisfac-tory at palliation [3].

Also in 1945, the Welsh surgeon, Ivor Lewis, was first to present an approach to the intrathoracic esophagus from the right side, dividing the esophagectomy and reconstruction into two stages [4, 5]. The first stage involved an abdominal incision, where, after excluding metastatic disease, the stomach was mobilized, leaving it dependent on the right gastric and gastroepiploic vessels, followed by a feeding jejunostomy. Approximately 2 weeks later, the second stage involved access via a right thoracotomy, where the azygous vein was divided and the esophagus dissected free, drawing the stomach into the chest where the esophagogastrostomy was com-pleted. While facing criticism from his contemporaries, Ivor Lewis favored the right thoracic approach over the then standard left thoracoabdominal incision because of improved access to the entirety of the esophagus, requiring only division of the azygous vein to allow for exposure. He implored that from the right chest, "the aortic arch… instead of being an obstacle, becomes a safety barrier between the surgeon and the other pleural cavity… Instead of separating the growth bluntly and blindly from behind the arch, it can be dissected under full vision" [4, 5].

The concept of esophagectomy without thoracotomy was explored in both ani-mals and humans by the German surgeon Alwin von Ach and the Austrian surgeon Wolfgang Denk in 1912–13 [6]. In the 1930s, the British surgeon George Gray Turner detailed the maneuvers of the transhiatal approach, with blunt mobilization of the esophagus from the abdomen followed by cervical anastomosis [7]. In the 1960–70s, the British surgeon McKeown, a junior of Grey Turner at Hammersmith, popularized a transthoracic approach that added a third cervical phase to the Ivor Lewis procedure, moving the anastomosis from the chest into the neck [8]. While transhiatal esophagectomy was largely abandoned due to concerns about mediasti-nal hemorrhage as well as increased familiarity with the transthoracic approaches, it was later revived by Hiroshi Akiyama from Tokyo in 1971 who demonstrated no operative mortality in his initial series [6, 7]. Mark Orringer from the University of Michigan further popularized this technique, developing a substantial series of over 2,000 cases of transhiatal resection with low perioperative morbidity and mortality [9, 10]. Controversy currently exists regarding the optimal approach to esophagec-tomy in light of both perioperative and oncologic outcomes.

Briefly, esophagectomy for cancer is now generally performed in one stage either by transthoracic (TTE) or transhiatal (THE) means with reconstruction using mobi-lized stomach (occasionally colon or jejunum) and creation of an anastomosis in the chest or neck. Minimally-invasive, robotic, and hybrid approaches use a combina-tion of laparoscopy and/or thoracoscopy to perform esophagectomy by any of the above methods. In a year 2000 report from the American College of Surgeons'

National Cancer Database, distal esophageal tumors that were treated surgically were resected most frequently via thoracotomy with laparotomy (45 %), followed by transhiatal approaches (25 %), thoracotomy alone (14 %), and by other techniques (16 %) [11].

Search Strategy

The methodology for this chapter comprises an English-language literature review of PubMed and OVID/Medline databases from 1993 to 2013, focusing on meta-analyses and randomized clinical trials comparing surgical techniques for esophagectomy. Multimodality trials were excluded from analysis. Results from large population-based cohorts and/or case series were also included. If patient populations were not limited to distal esophageal tumors, this was noted, with an effort to focus on surgical interventions for esophageal cancer with curative intent. Outcome measures evaluated included perioperative mortality, complications, functional outcomes, and survival.

Results

Transhiatal vs Transthoracic Resection

Table 25.1 summarizes the prospective randomized trials comparing TTE and THE for esophageal adenocarcinoma. In 1993, Goldminc and colleagues [12] randomized 67 patients from 1988 to 1991 presenting to a single French institution to either THE or TTE using an intrathoracic anastomosis via right thoracotomy. Investigators excluded patients with cervical esophageal cancers, those receiving neoadjuvant therapy, patients with preoperative evidence of extraesophageal spread, and a history of other cancers. No significant differences were seen in perioperative morbidity, mortality, postoperative dilatations, and overall survival.

In 1997, Chu and colleagues from Hong Kong reported a randomized clinical trial including patients with lower-third adenocarcinomas that accrued from 1990 to 1994 [13]. Patients were similarly excluded based on use of neoadjuvant therapy, advanced malignancy, concomitant malignancy, pulmonary function, and poor general condition. Investigators demonstrated no significant differences in postoperative complications, although anastomotic leak and chyle leak were not specified. No significant differences in mortality and tumor recurrence were seen during follow-up, although time-to-event analysis was not performed.

Jacobi and colleagues from two German institutions [14] focused on the effects of the type of esophageal resection on perioperative cardiopulmonary function. They randomized 32 patients with resectable esophageal cancer presenting between

Table 25.1 Prospective randomized trials comparing transthoracic and transhiatal esophagectomy for esophageal adenocarcinoma

Study	Patients	Outcome	TTE	THE	Relative risk for THE	Quality of evidence
Goldminc et al. (1993) [12]	TTE, n=35 THE, n=32	Anastomotic leak	9 %	6 %	0.66 (p=NS)	Level 1B
		Recurrent laryngeal nerve paralysis	3 %	3 %	1.00 (p=NS)	
		OR time (hours)	6	4	p=NR	
		Median overall survival	NR	NR	p=NS	
Chu et al. (1997) [13]	TTE, n=19 THE, n=20	Blood loss (L)	0.7	0.7	p<0.001	Level 2B
		OR time (hours)	3.5	2.9	p<0.001	
		Hospital stay (days)	27	18	p=NS	
		In-hospital mortality	0	15 %	p=NS	
		Recurrence	32 %	20 %	0.62 (p=NS)	
		Median overall survival (years)	1.1	1.3	p=NS	
Jacobi et al. (1997) [14]	TTE, n=16 THE, n=16	OR time (hours)	5.5	3.2	p=0.005	Level 1B
		Blood loss (L)	2.3	1.0	p=0.003	
		Pulmonary complications	50 %	25 %	0.5 (p)	
		Anastomotic leak	13 %	13 %	1.0 (p=NS)	
		Thirty-day mortality	6 %	6 %	1.0 (p=NS)	
		1-year overall survival	77 %	70 %	p=NS	

Hulscher et al. (2002) [15]	TTE, n=114 THE, n=106; 80 % distal esophageal, 20 % cardia; 96 % adenocarcinoma				Level 1B
	Pulmonary complications	57 %	27 %	0.47 (p<0.001)	
	Anastomotic leak	16 %	14 %	0.88 (p=NS)	
	Vocal cord paralysis	21 %	13 %	0.62 (p=NS)	
	Chyle leak	10 %	2 %	0.20 (p=0.02)	
	OR time (hours)	6.0	3.5	p<0.001	
	Blood loss (L)	1.9	1.0	p<0.001	
	Ventilator time (days)	2	1	p<0.001	
	Hospital stay (days)	19	15	p<0.001	
	In-hospital mortality	4 %	2 %	0.50 (p=NS)	
	R0 resection	71 %	72 %	1.01 (p=NS)	
	Number lymph nodes	31	16	p<0.001	
	Recurrence	50 %	58 %	p=NS	
	Median disease-free survival (years)	1.7	1.4	p=NS	
	Median overall survival (years)	2.0	1.8	p=NS	
	Median QALY (years)	1.8	1.5	p=NS	

L liter, NR not reported, NS not significant, OR operating room, R0 microscopically-negative resection, THE transhiatal esophagectomy, TTE transthoracic esophagectomy, QALA quality-adjusted life-years

1992 and 1995 to either THE or *en bloc* TTE with cervical anastomosis. Outcome measures included pulmonary arterial catheter measurements, perioperative complications, and survival. There were fewer pulmonary complications after THE, although intraoperative cardiopulmonary parameters did not correlate with complications. Similar rates of leak and postoperative mortality were noted in both groups, with no survival difference seen at a mean follow-up of 1 year.

In 2002, Hulscher and colleagues [15] reported a randomized trial that accrued from two high-volume academic centers in the Netherlands between 1994 and 2000, comparing THE (n = 106) with TTE with extended en bloc lymphadenectomy and cervical esophagogastrostomy (n = 114). Patients had histologically-confirmed adenocarcinoma of the mid to distal esophagus, or gastric cardia adenocarcinoma involving the distal esophagus, and had no distant metastases, celiac or cervical lymph node metastases, with resectable, local disease. Exclusion criteria included neoadjuvant therapy, prior cancer, and involvement of the stomach that would preclude reconstruction with a gastric conduit. Endpoints included morbidity, mortality, survival, and incremental costs per quality-adjusted life-years. Investigators found a significantly higher morbidity associated with transthoracic resection, with longer hospital length of stay, longer ICU stays, and higher costs. There was no significant difference between groups in terms of in-hospital mortality. Although disease-free and overall survival curves trended toward better outcomes with extended transthoracic resection, there were no significant differences between the groups. Further follow-up confirmed no significant overall survival difference between THE and TTE, with 5-year survival rates of 34 and 36 %, respectively [16].

Boshier and colleagues performed a meta-analysis of English-language studies up to 2010 comparing THE with TTE, including the prior randomized controlled trials [17]. A total of 52 studies comprising nearly six thousand patients were included. Lymph node yield was greater during TTE versus THE, although heterogeneity was significant. Operative time and postoperative length of stay were less for THE versus TTE. There were no significant differences in the overall incidence of cardiac complications, although respiratory complications were significantly higher in the TTE group. Early mortality was significantly greater after TTE compared to THE, without significant heterogeneity. Lower rates of anastomotic leak and vocal cord paralysis were noted after TTE compared to THE. Overall analysis of 5-year survival showed no significant differences between procedures.

Chang and colleagues [18] published the largest population-based study examining esophagectomy using the Surveillance, Epidemiology, and End Results (SEER)–Medicare linked database from 1992 to 2002, identifying 225 patients who underwent THE and 643 patients who underwent TTE. Mortality was lower after THE compared to TTE, at 7 % versus 13 % (p = 0.009). Five-year survival was similar for patients after adjusting for stage, patient, and provider factors. Overall, THE may confer an early survival advantage, but long-term survival does not appear to differ by approach. Indeed, the largest reported series of transhiatal esophagectomies (n = 2,007) described an in-hospital mortality of 1 %, a recurrent laryngeal nerve injury rate of 2 %, chylothorax rate of 1, and a 9 % leak rate across the most recent 944 patients, suggesting exceptional results in expert hands [10].

Technique of Anastomosis

Hand-sewn versus stapled esophagogastric anastomosis has been examined in 12 randomized trials and 2 meta-analyses, demonstrating similar anastomotic leak rates between techniques [19–23]. Subgroup analysis has suggested that the use of circular staplers leads to greater stricture rates compared to hand-sewn anastomoses [20]. Walther and colleagues from Sweden confirmed no differences in morbidity, mortality, hospital stay, anastomotic diameter, postoperative weight, or overall survival when comparing cervical hand-sewn versus stapled intrathoracic anastomoses, demonstrating that site of anastomosis does not adversely affect outcome [21].

Conduit Route

Seven randomized controlled trials studied the route of conduit transposition after transhiatal esophagectomy, randomizing between the anterior and posterior mediastinum [24–26]. Bartels and colleagues randomized patients presenting between 1986 and 1989 preoperatively to THE with anterior and posterior reconstruction, studying 96 patients after excluding those with colonic interpositions or who had not achieved an R0 resection [24]. Patients with anteriorly placed conduits had a significantly longer ICU stay, greater reduction in stroke volume index, and greater cardiac complications, with a non-significant increase in hospital mortality compared to those patients who received reconstruction in an orthotopic position. However, further data including a meta-analysis suggests that, while there are trends to improved outcomes with posterior gastric reconstructions, there are no significant differences in complications, mortality, and functional outcomes based on route.

The Role of Minimally Invasive Esophagectomy

To answer the question if minimally-invasive esophagectomy (MIE) confers benefit, Biere and European colleagues performed a multicenter randomized trial comparing TTE with MIE for resectable esophageal cancer [27]. Patient accrual occurred between 2009 and 2011, with exclusion of patients with cervical esophageal cancers, metastatic disease, cT4 disease, or other malignancies. Only hospitals who had performed more than 30 esophagectomies per year could participate, with a requirement that surgeons had experience performing at least 10 MIE and could also perform the procedure open. Open TTE was performed using right thoracotomy and laparotomy with a cervical or intrathoracic anastomosis. MIE was performed using a right thoracoscopy in a prone position, with laparoscopy and a cervical or intrathoracic anastomosis. Reconstruction was using a gastric conduit, with 65 % of randomized patients undergoing cervical esophagogastrostomy. The investigators studied primary outcomes focusing on pulmonary infections, with secondary outcomes including length of stay, quality of life, lymph node retrieval, intraoperative data, and postoperative complications. A total of 56 patients were randomized to open TTE and 59 to MIE, with all patients having completed neoadjuvant chemoradiation (92 %) or chemotherapy (8 %). Tumors were of distal or gastroesophageal junction in 55 % of patients. Among MIE patients, 14 % were converted to open technique in either the abdomen or chest.

Examining their primary study outcome, MIE patients had significantly less in-hospital pulmonary infections compared to open TTE (12 % vs. 34 %, $p = 0.005$) [27]. Median hospital stay was slightly shorter (11 vs. 14 days; $p = 0.04$), with greater operative time (5.5 vs. 5.0 h; $p = 0.002$) and less blood loss (0.2 vs. 0.5 L, $p < 0.001$) after MIE. Lymph node retrieval was similar in both groups (20 vs. 21, $p = 0.85$), with a trend toward higher rates of R0 resections (92 % vs. 84 %, $p = 0.08$) after MIE. There were no significant differences in in-hospital mortality, anastomotic leaks, pulmonary embolisms, or reoperations. Of note, vocal cord paralysis was less after MIE compared to TTE (2 % vs. 14 %; $p = 0.01$) Quality of life outcomes including the physical component of the SF-36 survey, the EORTC C-30 global health score, and questionnaires focusing on talking and pain scores at 6 weeks were all significantly better in patients receiving MIE compared to TTE.

James Luketich and colleagues at the University of Pittsburgh recently published their retrospective outcomes of over 1,000 MIEs [28]. After excluding planned hybrid procedures, they evaluated 481 patients who underwent MIE with cervical anastomosis (MIE-neck) and 530 patients who underwent MIE with intrathoracic anastomosis (MIE-chest), which became their preferred approach over the latter part of their series. A majority of patients had distal esophageal or gastroesophageal junction tumors (93 %), with equal rates of R0 resections (98 %). The number of lymph nodes examined were greater in patients undergoing MIE-chest compared to MIE-neck (24 vs. 19; $p < 0.001$). Postoperative length of stay (7 vs. 8 days, $p = 0.06$) and 30-day mortality were similar (1 % vs. 3 %, $p = 0.08$), with less vocal cord paralysis (1 % vs. 8 %, $p < 0.001$) after MIE-chest compared to MIE-neck. Combining both approaches, their series demonstrates a remarkable mortality rate of 1.7 and a 5 % rate of anastomotic leak requiring surgery. Prior to publication of both of these studies, two systematic reviews comprised of case-control studies also suggested improved perioperative outcomes with MIE, including reduction in hospital length of stay, ICU stay, blood loss, and pulmonary complications [29, 30]. Oncologic outcomes reviewed demonstrated higher lymph node retrieval but no evidence of survival advantage at 5 years [30]. Overall, data support several short-term benefits of MIE over TTE (Level 1B), although further follow-up is warranted to properly evaluate oncologic and functional outcomes (Level 3A).

Conclusions

There continues to be a lack of consensus on the ideal approach to esophagectomy, with similar survival benefit noted for THE and TTE, and evidence of decreased respiratory complications and perioperative mortality with THE. Hand-sewn and stapled anastomoses appear to have similar leak rates, with circular stapled anastomoses associated with a greater stricture rate, and no significant differences in outcomes between intrathoracic and cervical anastomoses. There are no important differences in complications, mortality, and functional outcomes associated with orthotopic versus heterotopic location for gastric conduit. MIE has many short-term advantages over TTE including pulmonary infections, operative time, blood loss, hospital stay, and quality of life, although significant advantages in oncologic outcomes of MIE over open esophagectomy have not yet been demonstrated.

More importantly, hospital-based quality measures and centralization are essential considerations in respect to perioperative outcomes after esophagectomy. In 1979, Luft and colleagues first suggested that regionalization of complex surgical procedures should occur based on volume-outcome relationships [31]. John Birkmeyer and the Veterans Affairs Outcomes group demonstrated that among surgical procedures performed on Medicare recipients, esophagectomy had the highest 30-day mortality rate and strongest observed relationship with hospital volume, with a significant correlation between mortality and surgeon volume when adjusted for hospital volume [32, 33]. Recent trends have shown a decrease in risk-adjusted mortality associated with esophagectomy, [34] which may reflect a redistribution of patients from low-volume to high-volume centers, [35] but also better training and perioperative care. Some debate exists on an approach to further regionalization, as low-volume hospitals with certain systems characteristics have been demonstrated to have outcomes similar to high-volume hospitals [36]. While procedure volume has become a quality measure adopted by the Leapfrog Group and the Agency for Healthcare Research and Quality, more recent analyses with large databases have suggested that patient characteristics may better predict mortality risk than hospital volume [37, 38]. Despite differences in definitions of high and low surgical volume thresholds and heterogeneity in studies, as well as changing practice patterns, there is reasonable evidence of benefit in centralization of esophagectomy to high-volume institutions with respect to mortality [39].

Recommendations

While there are similar long-term survival benefits noted for transhiatal and transthoracic esophagectomy, there is evidence of decreased respiratory complications and perioperative mortality with the transhiatal approach. Hand-sewn and stapled anastomoses have similar leak rates. Circular-stapled anastomoses are associated with greater stricture rates compared to hand-sewn anastomoses. There are no significant differences in outcomes between intrathoracic and cervical anastomoses. There are no important differences in complications, mortality, and functional outcomes associated with orthotopic versus heterotopic location for gastric conduit. Minimally-invasive esophagectomy has many short-term advantages over open transthoracic esophagectomy including pulmonary infections, operative time, blood loss, hospital stay, and quality of life, although significant advantages in oncologic outcomes have not yet been demonstrated. There is reasonable evidence of benefit in centralization of esophagectomy to high-volume institutions with respect to mortality.

Summary

In deciding the optimal surgical approach for distal esophageal cancers, it may be prudent to tailor an approach based on both the patient and the surgeon, accounting for their training, learning curve, skill set, and system of practice. Data suggest that morbidity is associated with surgical technique, and a patient at high risk for pulmonary complications may be better served by a THE or MIE in comparison to TTE. Most important is to have a surgeon with focused training in esophagectomy doing the procedure that they are comfortable with a system that can identify and address complications effectively. Access to surgeons with expertise in esophageal surgery is certainly an issue. While each technique may have some trade-offs related to lymph node retrieval rates and perioperative morbidity, there may be no important differences in longer-term oncologic outcomes like survival. While the question of optimal surgical approach in the setting of esophageal cancer has historically been a subject of heated debate, and continues to be a focus for future study, it may ultimately become less important in the setting of multimodality therapy and improved systems-based practices.

A Personal View of the Data

My approach to a typical patient with a distal or gastroesophageal junction tumor begins with preoperative staging including endoscopic ultrasound and/or PET, followed by consideration for induction chemoradiation therapy. With recognition that there is no preferred surgical technique toward esophagectomy, I would plan to perform a transhiatal approach with a side-to-side cervical esophagogastrostomy fashioned using a linear stapler. I typically place a feeding jejunostomy tube as it can be a method to intervene with existing malnutrition, possible complications, and a slow transition to oral intake by providing enteral support when needed. However, there is not sufficient evidence to suggest that routine postoperative enteral feeding is always necessary.

Recommendations

- Transhiatal and transthoracic approaches have similar overall outcomes and there is no overall advantage of one over the other. (Evidence quality high; no recommendation)
- The transhiatal approach is associated with decreased respiratory complications and perioperative mortality compared to open transthoracic resection and is recommended for higher risk patients. (Evidence quality moderate; weak recommendation)
- Hand-sewn and stapled anastomoses have similar leak rates and one technique is not recommended over the other. (Evidence quality moderate; no recommendation)
- Hand-sewn anastomoses are preferred over circular-stapled anastomoses because of their lower stricture rates. (Evidence quality moderate; weak recommendation)
- Intrathoracic and cervical anastomoses have similar outcomes and one technique is not recommended over the other. (Evidence quality moderate; no recommendation)
- Orthotopic and heterotopic locations for the gastric conduit have similar outcomes, and one technique is not recommended over the other. (Evidence quality low; no recommendation)
- Minimally-invasive esophagectomy has short-term advantages over open transthoracic esophagectomy, and should be considered for higher risk patients in specialized centers. (Evidence quality moderate; weak recommendation)
- Centralization of esophagectomy to high-volume institutions is recommended to reduce operative mortality. (Evidence quality moderate; weak recommendation)

References

1. Torek F. The first successful resection of the thoracic portion of the esophagus for carcinoma: preliminary report. JAMA. 1913;60:1533.
2. Kakegawa T, Fujita H. A history of esophageal surgery in the twentieth century. Gen Thorac Cardiovasc Surg. 2009;57:55–63.
3. Sweet RH. Surgical management of carcinoma of the midthoracic esophagus: preliminary report. N Engl J Med. 1945;233:1–7.
4. Lewis I. The surgical treatment of carcinoma of the oesophagus with special reference to a new operation for growths of the middle third. Br J Surg. 1946;34:18–31.
5. Morris-Stiff G, Hughes LE. Ivor-Lewis (1895–1982) – Welsh pioneer of the right-sided approach to the oesophagus. Dig Surg. 2003;20:546–53.
6. Dubecz A, Kun L, Stadlhuber RJ, Peters JH, Schwartz SI. The origins of an operation: a brief history of transhiatal esophagectomy. Ann Surg. 2009;249:535.

322   S. Ganai

7. Akiyama H, Hiyama M, Miyazono H. Total esophageal reconstruction after extraction of the esophagus. Ann Surg. 1975;182:547–52.
8. McKeown KC. Total three-stage oesophagectomy for cancer of the oesophagus. Br J Surg. 1976;63:259–62.
9. Orringer MB, Sloan H. Esophagectomy without thoracotomy. J Thorac Cardiovasc Surg. 1978;76:643–54.
10. Orringer MB, Marshall B, Chang AC, Lee J, Pickens A, Lau CL. Two thousand transhiatal esophagectomies: changing trends, lessons learned. Ann Surg. 2007;246:363–74.
11. Daly JM, Fry WA, Little AG, Winchester DP, McKee RF, Stewart AK, Fremgen AM. Esophageal cancer: results of an American College of Surgeons Patient Care Evaluation Study. J Am Coll Surg. 2000;190:562–73.
12. Goldminc M, Maddern G, Le Prise E, Meunier B, Campion JP, Launois B. Oesophagectomy by a transhiatal approach or thoracotomy: a prospective randomized trial. Br J Surg. 1993;80: 367–70.
13. Chu KM, Law SY, Fok M, Wong J. A prospective randomized comparison of transhiatal and transthoracic resection for lower-third esophageal carcinoma. Am J Surg. 1997;174:320–4.
14. Jacobi CA, Zieren HU, Muller JM, Pichlmaier H. Surgical therapy of esophageal carcinoma: the influence of surgical approach and esophageal resection on cardiopulmonary function. Eur J Cardiothorac Surg. 1997;11:32–7.
15. Hulscher JB, van Sandick JW, de Boer AG, Wijnhoven BP, Tijssen JG, Fockens P, Stalmeier PF, ten Kate FJ, van Dekken H, Obertop H, Tilanus HW, van Lanschot JJ. Extended transthoracic resection compared with limited transhiatal resection for adenocarcinoma of the esophagus. N Engl J Med. 2002;347:1662–9.
16. Omloo JM, Lagarde SM, Hulscher JB, Reitsma JB, Fockens P, van Dekken H, ten Kate FJ, Obertop H, Tilanus HW, van Lanschot JJ. Extended transthoracic resection compared with limited transhiatal resection for adenocarcinoma of the mid/distal esophagus: five-year survival of a randomized clinical trial. Ann Surg. 2007;246:992–1001.
17. Boshier PR, Anderson O, Hanna GB. Transthoracic versus transhiatal esophagectomy for the treatment of esophagogastric cancer: a meta-analysis. Ann Surg. 2011;254:894–906.
18. Chang AC, Ji H, Birkmeyer NJ, Orringer MB, Birkmeyer JD. Outcomes after transhiatal and transthoracic esophagectomy for cancer. Ann Thorac Surg. 2008;85:424–9.
19. Beitler AL, Urschel JD. Comparison of stapled and hand-sewn esophagogastric anastomoses. Am J Surg. 1998;175:337–40.
20. Honda M, Kuriyama A, Noma H, Nunobe S, Furukawa TA. Hand-sewn versus mechanical esophagogastric anastomosis after esophagectomy: a systematic review and meta-analysis. Ann Surg. 2013;257:238–48.
21. Walther B, Johansson J, Johnsson F, von Holstein CS, Zilling T. Cervical of thoracic anastomosis after esophageal resection and gastric tube reconstruction: a prospective randomized trial comparing sutured neck anastomosis with stapled intrathoracic anastomosis. Ann Surg. 2003;238:803–12.
22. Hsu HH, Chen JS, Huang PM, Lee JM, Lee YC. Comparison of manual and mechanical cervical esophagogastric anastomosis after esophageal resection for squamous cell carcinoma: a prospective randomized controlled trial. Eur J Cardiothorac Surg. 2004;25:1097–101.
23. Okuyama M, Motoyama S, Suzuki H, Saito R, Maruyama K, Ogawa J. Hand-sewn cervical anastomosis versus stapled intrathoracic anastomosis after esophagectomy for middle or lower thoracic esophageal cancer: a prospective randomized controlled study. Surg Today. 2007;37: 947–52.
24. Bartels H, Thorban S, Siewert JR. Anterior versus posterior reconstruction after transhiatal oesophagectomy: a randomized controlled trial. Br J Surg. 1993;80:1141–4.
25. Khiria LS, Pal S, Peush S, Chattopadhyay TK, Deval M. Impact on outcome of the route of conduit transposition after transhiatal oesophagectomy: a randomized controlled trial. Dig Liver Dis. 2009;41:711–6.
26. Urschel JD, Urschel DM, Miller JD, Bennett WF, Young JE. A meta-analysis of randomized controlled trials of route of reconstruction after esophagectomy for cancer. Am J Surg. 2001;182:470–5.

27. Biere SS, van Berge Henegouwen MI, Maas KW, Bonavina L, Rosman C, Garcia JR, Gisbertz SS, Klinkenbikl JH, Hollmann MW, de Lange ES, Jaap Bonjer H, van der Peet DL, Cuesa MA. Minimally invasive versus open oesophagectomy for patients with oesophageal cancer: a multicentre, open-label randomised controlled trial. Lancet. 2012;379:1887–92.
28. Luketich JD, Pennathur A, Awais O, Levy RM, Keeley S, Shende M, Christie NA, Weksler B, Landreneau RJ, Abbas G, Schuchert MJ, Nason KS. Outcomes after minimally invasive esophagectomy: review of over 1000 patients. Ann Surg. 2012;256:95–103.
29. Verhage RJ, Hazebroek EJ, Boone J, Van Hillegersberg R. Minimally invasive surgery compared to open procedures in esophagectomy for cancer: a systematic review of the literature. Minerva Chir. 2009;64:135–46.
30. Dantoc MM, Cox MR, Esllick GD. Does minimally invasive esophagectomy (MIE) provide for comparable oncologic outcomes to open techniques? A systematic review. J Gastrointest Surg. 2012;16:486–94.
31. Luft HS, Bunker JP, Enthoven AC. Should operations be regionalized? The empirical relation between surgical volume and mortality. N Engl J Med. 1979;301:1364–9.
32. Birkmeyer JD, Siewers AE, Finlayson EV, Stukel TA, Lucas FL, Batista I, Welch HG, Wennberg DE. Hospital volume and surgical mortality in the United States. N Engl J Med. 2002;346:1128–37.
33. Birkmeyer JD, Stukel TA, Siewers AE, Goodney PP, Wennberg DE, Lucas FL. Surgeon volume and operative mortality in the United States. N Engl J Med. 2003;349:2117–27.
34. Finks JF, Osborne NH, Birkmeyer JD. Trends in hospital volume and operative mortality for high-risk surgery. N Engl J Med. 2011;364:2128–37.
35. Stitzenberg KB, Meropol NJ. Trends in centralization of cancer surgery. Ann Surg Oncol. 2010;17:2824–31.
36. Funk LM, Gawande AA, Semel ME, Lipsitz SR, Berry WR, Zinner MJ, Jha AK. Esophagectomy outcomes at low-volume hospitals: the association between systems characteristics and mortality. Ann Surg. 2011;253:912–7.
37. Wright CD, Kucharczuk JC, O'Brien SM, Grab JD, Allen MS. Predictors of major morbidity and mortality after esophagectomy for esophageal cancer: a Society of Thoracic Surgeons General Thoracic Surgery Database risk adjustment model. J Thorac Cardiovasc Surg. 2009;137:587–96.
38. LaPar DJ, Kron IL, Jones DR, Stukenborg GJ, Kozower BD. Hospital procedure volume should not be used as a measure of quality. Ann Surg. 2012;256:606–15.
39. Markar SR, Karthikesalingam A, Thrumurthy S, Low DE. Volume-outcome relationship in surgery for esophageal malignancy: systematic review and meta-analysis 2000–2011. J Gastrointest Surg. 2012;16:1055–63.

Chapter 26
Regional Extent of Lymphadenectomy for Esophageal Cancer

Hirofumi Kawakubo, Hiryoya Takeuchi, and Yuko Kitagawa

Abstract Surgery has been most frequently used to obtain locoregional control and has played a major role in esophageal cancer treatment. Thoracic esophageal carcinoma is commonly accompanied by extensive lymph node metastasis in the cervical, thoracic, and abdominal regions. However, the distribution and incidence of lymph node metastasis both may vary according to the location, size, and depth of tumor invasion. The cervical lymph nodes are at risk of cancer metastasis from either upper or middle thoracic esophageal cancers. Therefore, three-field lymphadenectomy is recommended. In patients with lower thoracic esophageal cancers, the appropriate extent of regional lymphadenectomy is defined by mediastinal and abdominal lymphadenectomy.

Keywords Esophageal cancer • Minimally invasive esophagectomy • VATS • Sentinel node navigation surgery • Three-field lymph node dissection • Esophagectomy • Lymphadenectomy • Extended lymphadenectomy and three-field lymph node dissection

Introduction

The global incidence of esophageal cancer has increased in the past few decades [1, 2]. Many therapeutic options are used to treat esophageal cancer, and multimodality treatment including surgery, radiotherapy, and chemotherapy is necessary for advanced esophageal carcinoma. However, traditionally, surgery has been

H. Kawakubo, MD, PhD • H. Takeuchi, MD • Y. Kitagawa, MD, PhD (✉)
Department of Surgery, Keio University School of Medicine,
35 Shinanomachi, Shinjuku-ku, 160-8582 Tokyo, Japan
e-mail: kitagawa@sc.itc.keio.ac.jp

most frequently used to obtain locoregional control and has played a major role in esophageal cancer treatment. The main controversy surrounding the surgical treatment of esophageal cancer surrounds the extent of lymph node dissection required during esophagectomy. The concept of extensive three-field lymph node dissection including the dissection of cervical, mediastinal, and abdominal lymph nodes for surgically curable esophageal cancer located in the middle or upper thoracic esophagus was developed in Japan in the 1980s. Although the effectiveness of extended lymphadenectomy for esophageal cancer has not yet be proven by randomized prospective studies, better survival can be obtained with three-field lymph node dissection than with two-field lymph node dissection in Japan [3–6]. There have been disagreements about the strategy for surgical management of esophageal cancer between the majority of Western surgical groups and Japanese groups. Many investigators in Europe and the United States have reported that the results of concurrent chemoradiotherapy are comparable with those of surgery [7, 8] however, many Japanese and some Western surgeons have reported the importance of radical lymph node dissection for locoregional control of esophageal cancer [9, 10].

Search Strategy

We searched Pub Med for the period 1994 and 2013 using the search terms: esophagectomy, lymphadenectomy, extended lymphadenectomy and three-field lymph node dissection.

Defining the Extent of Lymphadenectomy

The naming and numbers of lymph nodes are defined according to the location of lymph nodes [11].

The Cervical Field

This field includes the superficial lymph nodes, cervical paraesophageal lymph nodes, deep cervical lymph nodes, peripharyngeal lymph nodes, and supraclavicular lymph nodes. These lymph nodes also include the lymphatic chain along both recurrent nerves throughout their mediastinal and cervical course and the deep cervical nodes posterior and lateral to the jugular vein and supraclavicular nodes.

The Mediastinal Field

This field includes the upper, middle, and lower mediastinal lymph nodes. The upper mediastinal lymph nodes include the upper thoracic paraesophageal lymph nodes, both recurrent nerve lymph nodes, pretracheal lymph nodes, and left tracheo-bronchial lymph nodes. The middle mediastinal lymph nodes also include middle thoracic paraesophageal, subcarinal, and both main bronchial lymph nodes. The lower mediastinal lymph nodes include lower thoracic paraesophageal lymph nodes, supradiapharagmatic lymph nodes and posterior mediastinal lymph nodes.

The Abdominal Field

This field includes both cardiac lymph nodes, lymph nodes along the lesser curvatures, lymph nodes along the left gastric artery, lymph nodes along the common hepatic artery, lymph nodes along the celiac artery, and lymph nodes along the splenic artery.

Regional Extent of Lymphadenectomy

Lymphadenectomy for Thoracic Esophageal Carcinoma

Thoracic esophageal carcinoma is commonly accompanied by extensive lymph node metastasis in the cervical, thoracic, and abdominal regions. However, the distribution and incidence of lymph node metastasis both may vary according to the location, size, and depth of tumor invasion. Therefore, preoperative evaluation using computed tomography, ultrasonography, magnetic resonance imaging, or positron emission tomography for each patient is important for determining the extent of the lymph node dissection. The concept of three-field dissection was developed in Japan in the 1980s. In Japan, three-field lymph node dissection, including dissection of the cervical, mediastinal, and abdominal lymph nodes, is the standard procedure for surgically curable esophageal cancer located in the middle or upper thoracic esophagus. The effectiveness of extended lymphadenectomy for esophageal cancer has not yet been proven by randomized prospective studies; better survival can be obtained with three-field lymph node dissection than with two-field lymph node dissection in Japan.

Since a nation-wide retrospective study by Isono et al. in 1991 showed the potential benefits of esophagectomy with three-field dissection, many reports have been published [3]. The largest study demonstrating the benefits of the three-field lymph node dissection from a single institution was reported by Akiyama et al. in 1994 [4]. The authors performed 393 cases of esophagectomy with a two-field lymph node dissection between 1973 and 1984 and 324 cases of esophagectomy with a three-field lymph node dissection between 1984 and 1993. The 5-year survival rate of node-negative patients was 83.9 % after three-field lymph node dissection and 55.0 % after two-field lymph node dissection. The 5-year survival rate of node-positive patients was 43.1 % after three-field lymph node dissection and 27.9 % after two-field lymph node dissection. In both groups, the node-negative and node-positive groups, the survival of patients after extensive three-field dissection was significantly better than that after the less extensive two-field dissection. The authors speculated that the differences may be because of occult cancer-positive nodes in the cervical region and other areas, which may have been present and omitted from dissection and analysis in the group with less extensive dissections, were removed by extensive dissection. The 5-year survival rate of patients with all depth of cancer invasion after extensive three-field and the less extensive two-field dissection were 53.3 % and 37.5 %, respectively. Although this study was a non-randomized, historical control study, the 5-year survival rate of 53.3 % in the patient after three-field dissection in those days remained very high. Turumaru et al. studied the state of lymph node metastasis in cases with only a single node metastasis [12]. A single node metastasis in patients with thoracic esophageal cancer may be located in the cervical (14.1 %), mediastinal (upper, 31.0 %; middle, 11.3 %; and lower, 8.5 %) and abdominal areas (35.2 %). They also studied the state of lymph node metastasis in 5-year survivors of these cases and showed that 14.2 % had a single node metastasis in the cervical area, 49.3 % had a single node in the mediastinum (upper, 19.4 %; middle, 22.4 %; and lower 7.5 %), and 37.3 % had a single node in the abdomen. These results showed that even if there were lymph node metastases in either the cervical or abdominal areas, many patients could be cured by extended lymphadenectomy. These results also suggested that lymph nodes in the cervical and abdominal areas were regional lymph nodes of the thoracic esophagus.

Only two prospective studies have been published from Japan. One was a prospective randomized trial comparing three-field with two-field lymph node dissection published by Nishihara et al. [13]. They showed a survival benefit for three-field over two-field lymph node dissection (65 % vs. 48 %); however, the study was a low volume study at a single institution and the difference was not statistically significant. Another prospective study was published from the National Cancer Center in Tokyo [14]. It was a non-randomized, case-matched trial and showed that the 5-year survival rate was significantly better after three-field dissection (48 % vs. 33 %; p=0.03). The 5-year survival rate in the group of patients with a cervical lymph node was as high as 30 %. These results suggested that there was a survival advantage in the three-field lymph node dissection and that lymph nodes in the cervical and abdominal areas were regional lymph nodes for thoracic esophageal squamous cell carcinoma. Although the incidence of esophageal cancer is increasing, the number of candidates for potentially curative resection is limited. For this reason, a prospective randomized study will be difficult to complete within a reasonable timeframe. It can also be very difficult to set up high-volume multi-institutional prospective randomized studies.

There have been two reports that have supported the three-field dissection in Western countries. Altorki et al. from New York performed esophagectomy with three-field dissection on 80 patients (adenocarcinoma, 48; squamous cell cancer (SCC), 32) during the period from 1994 to 2001 [9]. Hospital mortality was 5 % and morbidity was 47 %, and 69 % presented with nodal metastases. Metastases to the recurrent laryngeal and/or deep cervical nodes occurred in 36 % patients regardless of the cell type or location of the tumor within the esophagus. Overall, the 5-year and disease-free survival rates were 51 and 46 %, respectively. The 5-year survival rate in patients with positive cervical nodes was 25 % (SCC, 40 %; adenocarcinoma, 15 %). The authors concluded that esophagectomy with three-field lymph node dissection could be performed with low mortality and reasonable morbidity and that the data suggested a true survival benefit. Lerut et al. reported on their experience with esophagectomy with three-field dissection in Belgium [10]. They performed an esophagectomy with the three-field dissection in 174 patients (adenocarcinoma, 96; SCC, 78) during the period from 1991 to 1999. Hospital mortality was 1.4 % and morbidity was 57 %. Overall, the 5-year and disease-free survival rates were 41.9 and 46.3 %, respectively. In addition, the overall 5-year survival rate with positive cervical nodes was 27.7 % for squamous cell carcinoma located in the middle third of the esophagus, 11.9 % for adenocarcinoma in the distal third of the esophagus (the 4-year survival rate was 35.7 %), and 0 % for gastroesophageal junction (GEJ) adenocarcinoma. They concluded that esophagectomy by the three-field lymph node dissection can be performed with low mortality and acceptable morbidity and that data may indicate a real survival benefit. Role of the three-field dissection for adenocarcinoma of the distal third of the esophagus remains unclear.

In cases of lower thoracic esophageal carcinoma, lymph node metastasis occurs primarily in the mediastinal and abdominal regions, but metastasis to cervical lymph nodes can also occur at a lower frequency. The prognosis of a patient with cervical lymph node metastases from a lower thoracic esophageal carcinoma is very unfavorable [15]. Thus, mediastinal and abdominal lymphadenectomy may be adequate for lower thoracic esophageal carcinoma.

In summary, the cervical lymph nodes are at a risk of being involved by cancer metastasis from either upper or middle thoracic esophageal cancers. Therefore, three-field lymphadenectomy, bilateral cervical lymphadenectomy, mediastinal lymphadenectomy, and abdominal lymphadenectomy are recommended. In contrast, in patients with lower thoracic esophageal cancer, the appropriate extent of regional lymphadenectomy is mediastinal and abdominal lymphadenectomy.

Lymphadenectomy for Gastroesophageal Junction Arcinoma

The incidence of adenocarcinoma of the esophagus and gastroesophageal junction is rapidly increasing. Surgery is still considered the best curative treatment. However considerable debate exists as to the most appropriate surgical approach, transhiatal, or transthoracic esophagectomy. A transhiatal esophagectomy limits the extent of surgical trauma without an extended lymphadenectomy. However, a transthoracic esophagectomy with an en bloc extended lymphadenectomy in the posterior mediastinum and upper abdomen is intended to improve long-term survival. Several retrospective studies have shown little difference in the perioperative and survival outcomes between transhiatal and transthoracic esophagectomy. Rindani et al. reviewed the results from 44 series published between 1986 and 1996 [16]. The 30-day mortality rate was 6.3 % after transhiatal and 9.5 % after transthoracic esophagectomy. Overall, the 5-year survival rate was 24 % after transhiatal esophagectomy and 26 % following transthoracic resection. The Hulscher et al. analysis included data abstracted from 50 articles published between 1990 and 1999 with a total of 7,500 patients [17]. There was no statistically significant difference in the overall 3-year and 5-year survival rates between the two procedures. Recently, Boshier et al. reviewed the results from 52 studies, including 5,905 patients, which compared transthoracic with transhiatal esophagectomy (transthoracic, 3,389; transhiatal, 2,516) until 2010 [18]. The results showed that transhiatal esophagectomy was associated with significantly reduced operative time, length of hospital stay, postoperative respiratory complications, and early mortality. In comparison, transthoracic esophagectomy was associated with significantly fewer anastomotic leaks, anastomotic strictures, and vocal cord palsies. Overall, the 5-year survival rate was found to not significantly differ. These findings were comparable with the results of two previous meta-analyses. Although the survival was shown to be equivalent, transhiatal esophagectomy was chosen significantly more frequently for early-stage tumors and transthoracic esophagectomy chosen for more advanced tumors. The authors concluded that the findings of equivalent survival should be viewed with caution.

Some randomized studies have been performed to compare these two approaches. Hulscher et al. randomly assigned 220 patients with adenocarcinoma of the mid-to-distal esophagus or adenocarcinoma of the gastric cardia involving the distal esophagus either to transhiatal esophagectomy or transthoracic esophagectomy with extended en bloc lymphadenectomy [19]. The mean number of resected lymph nodes was 31 nodes after the transthoracic esophagectomy and 16 after transhiatal esophagectomy. Perioperative morbidity was higher after transthoracic esophagectomy, but there was no significant difference in the in-hospital mortality. Although the difference in survival was not statistically significant, there was a trend toward a survival benefit with the extended approach at 5 years. The 5-year disease-free survival rate was 27 % in the transhiatal esophagectomy group compared with 39 % in the transthoracic esophagectomy group, whereas the overall survival rate was 29 % in the transhiatal esophagectomy group compared with 39 % in the transthoracic esophagectomy group. The authors concluded that there was a trend toward improved long-term survival rate at 5 years with the extended transthoracic approach.

The most recent randomized clinical trial was performed by Omloo et al. [20]. A total of 220 patients with adenocarcinoma of the distal esophagus (type I) or gastric cardia involving the distal esophagus (type II) were randomly assigned to limited transhiatal esophagectomy or to extended transthoracic esophagectomy with en bloc lymphadenectomy. Overall, the 5-year survival rate was 34 % after transhiatal resection and 36 % after transthoracic resection. In a subgroup analysis that was based on the location of the primary tumor, no overall survival benefit was seen in

115 patients with type II tumor (p=0.81). In 90 patients with a type I tumor, the survival benefit of 14 % was observed with the transthoracic approach (51 % vs. 37 %, p=0.33). There was no significant difference in the survival rate between transhiatal and transthoracic esophagectomy for patients with type II tumors. However, compared with limited transhiatal resection, extended transthoracic esophagectomy for type 1 esophageal adenocarcinoma showed an ongoing trend toward better 5-year survival rate.

Sasako et al. reported the results of a phase III trial comparing transhiatal to left thoracoabdominal approaches in patients with gastric adenocarcinoma of the cardia or subcardia with esophageal invasion of 3 cm or less (types II and III) [21]. The 5-year overall survival rate was 52.3 % in the transhiatal approach group and 37.9 % in the left thoracoabdominal approach group. Morbidity was worse after a left thoracoabdominal approach than in the transhiatal approach. They concluded that the left thoracoabdominal approach did not improve survival after transhiatal approach and led to increased morbidity in patients with this type of gastric adenocarcinoma. The authors also concluded that a left thoracoabdominal approach could not be justified to treat these tumors.

In summary, there were no significant differences in the survival between transhiatal and transthoracic esophagectomy for patients with type II tumors. However, better survival may be obtained after an extended transthoracic esophagectomy compared with a limited transhiatal resection for type 1 esophageal adenocarcinomas.

Future Perspectives

The concepts of the sentinel lymph node (SLN), intraoperative lymphatic mapping, and sentinel lymphadenectomy appear attractive. We have performed radio-guided SLN mapping for cT1aN0 or cT2N0 esophageal cancer to verify the feasibility of SLN mapping. SLN is defined as the lymph node that is first to receive lymphatic drainage from a tumor site [22]. The SLN is believed to be the first probable micrometastasis site along the lymphatic drainage route from the primary lesion. If the SLN is recognized and is negative for metastasis, there may be no metastasis in other lymph nodes. The pathological status of SLN may predict the status of all the regional lymph nodes and may thus prevent unnecessary radical lymph node dissection.

SLN mapping and biopsy were first applied to melanoma and subsequently extended to breast cancer and many other solid tumors [23–26]. These techniques can benefit patients by avoiding the various complications that may result from unnecessary radical lymph node dissections in cases wherein SLN was negative for metastasis. We developed a radio-guided method to detect SLN in esophageal cancer [27] rather than the conventional blue-dye method. One day (within 16 h) before surgery, 2.0-mL of technetium-99 m tin colloid solution (150 MBq) is injected into the submucosal layer at four quadrants around the primary tumor using an endoscopic puncture needle. Preoperative lymphoscintigraphy is usually obtained 3–4 h after injection. The distribution of SLNs in esophageal cancers is widely spread from the cervical to abdominal areas. Takeuchi reported our results of the validation of radio-guided SLN navigation study of esophageal cancer [28]; 75 consecutive patients who were diagnosed before surgery with T1N0M0 or T2N0M0 primary esophageal cancer were enrolled. SLNs were identified in 71 (95 %) of 75 patients. The mean number of identified SLNs per case was 4.7; furthermore, 29 (88 %) of the 33 patients with LN metastasis revealed positive SLNs, and on the basis of SLN status, the diagnostic accuracy was 94 %.

Intraoperative SLN (i.e., radio-labeled lymph nodes) sampling is performed using a handheld gamma probe (GPS Navigator, Covidien, Tokyo, Japan). In addition, gamma probing may be feasible for thoracoscopic or laparoscopic sampling of SLN using a special gamma detector, which is introducible from trocar ports. SLNs located in the cervical area can be identified using percutaneous gamma probing. All SLNs were sent for an intraoperative pathological examination. SLN mapping was successful during thoracoscopic esophagectomy as well as during a conventional surgical procedure.

In the future, SLN mapping may play a significant role by eliminating the necessity of uniform application of a highly invasive surgery by obtaining individual information to allow adjustments and modifications to the surgical procedure for patients. If an SLN is recognized and is negative for metastasis, unnecessary extended lymph node dissection can be avoided. For instance, if the SLN was identified only in the mediastinum or abdominal area and all SNL were pathologically negative in patients with middle or lower thoracic esophageal cancer, the cervical lymph node dissection could be avoided. If the SLN was identified along the recurrent laryngeal nerves in the upper mediastinum and positive for metastasis or the SLN is identified in cervical lymph nodes, extended three-field lymph node dissection may be considered. The SLN mapping and biopsy may be useful for adenocarcinoma of the distal esophagus or gastroesophageal junction. If the SLN was identified only in the abdominal area and was pathologically negative, the patient would be treated with limited transhiatal resection. In contrast, if the SLN was positive for metastasis in the lower mediastinum, the patients should be treated with transthoracic esophagectomy with an extended en bloc lymphadenectomy. SLN mapping and navigation may become a promising strategy for less invasive, individualized surgery for esophageal carcinoma.

Recommendations

The cervical lymph nodes are at risk of cancer metastasis from either upper or middle thoracic esophageal cancers. Therefore, three-field lymphadenectomy is recommended. In patients with lower thoracic esophageal cancers, the appropriate extent of regional lymphadenectomy is mediastinal and abdominal lymphadenectomy. There was no significant difference in the survival rate between transhiatal and transthoracic esophagectomy for patients with type II (GEJ) tumors. However, better survival can be obtained after extended transthoracic esophagectomy compared with limited transhiatal resection for type I (distal esophageal) adenocarcinoma.

A Personal View of the Data

We typically perform three-field nodal dissection for cancers of the middle and upper thoracic esophagus. Our technical approach is outlined below.

Upper Mediastinal Procedure

After the azygous arch is divided, the posterior portion of the right upper mediastinal pleura is incised along the posterior edge of the esophagus up to right subclavian artery. The right bronchial artery is carefully isolated and preserved for open esophagectomy. The dorsal and left sides of the upper esophagus are dissected from the left pleura. The right upper mediastinal pleura is incised along the right vagal nerve up to right subclavian artery. The right recurrent laryngeal nerve is identified at the caudal end of the right sublavian artery, and lymph nodes around right recurrent laryngeal nerve are dissected carefully to prevent nerve injury. The anterior part of the upper esophagus is circumferentially dissected along with the surrounding nodes. By shifting the taped esophagus posteriorly and retracting the trachea anteriorly, it is possible to approach the left anterior side of trachea. The nodes around the left recurrence laryngeal nerve are dissected from the aortic arch to the cervical level. The left subclavian artery is exposed to dissect the left recurrence laryngeal lymph nodes. During dissection of the left tracheobronchial lymph nodes, the left recurrence laryngeal nerve and left bronchial artery are preserved on the face of the trunk of the left pulmonary artery between the aortic arch and the left main bronchus.

Middle and Lower Mediastinal Procedure

The mediastinal pleura is incised along the anterior edge of the vertebrae to the hiatus. The posterior side of the middle to lower esophagus is dissected to expose the aortic arch and descending aorta. The thoracic duct is ligated and divided behind the lower esophagus and resected together with the esophagus. The mediastinal pleura of the anterior side of the esophagus is then incised. The esophagus is divided using a linear stapler above the primary tumor, and the caudal stump of the esophagus and surrounding tissue are dissected up to the hiatus. The subcarinal nodes are separately resected. Esophageal mobilization and mediastinal lymphadenectomy are thus completed.

Abdominal Procedure

The greater omentum is divided 4–5 cm from the arcade of the gastroepiploic vessels. The left gastroepiploic and short gastric vessels are divided along the splenic hilum. The lesser omentum is opened, and the right gastric vessels are preserved. The distal esophagus is dissected and mobilized. The distal stump of the esophagus and the dissected mediastinal tissue are then extracted from the thorax to the abdomen. Lymph node around the left gastric artery, common hepatic artery and splenic artery are dissected, and the left gastric artery is ligated and divided. Lymph nodes around the celiac artery are dissected up to the hiatus. The stomach is divided from the lesser curvature to the fornix using linear staplers. Thus, gastric conduit formation and abdominal lymphadenectomy are completed.

Recommendations

- Because the cervical lymph nodes are at risk of cancer metastasis from either upper or middle thoracic esophageal cancers, a three-field lymphadenectomy is recommended. (Evidence quality low; weak recommendation)
- In patients with lower thoracic esophageal cancers, the appropriate extent of regional lymphadenectomy is mediastinal and abdominal lymphadenectomy. (Evidence quality low; weak recommendation)
- There is no advantage for transhiatal vs transthoracic esophagectomy for patients with type II (GEJ) tumors. (Evidence quality low; no recommendation)
- Better survival can be obtained after extended transthoracic esophagectomy compared with limited transhiatal resection for type I (distal esophageal) adenocarcinoma. (Evidence quality low; weak recommendation)

References

1. Parkin DM, Pisani P, Ferlay J. Global cancer statistics. CA Cancer J Clin. 1999;49:33–64.
2. Jamal A, Bray F, Center MM, et al. Global cancer statistics. CA Cancer J Clin. 2011;61: 69–90.
3. Isono K, Sato H, Nakayama K. Results of nationwide study of the tree-field lymph node dissection of esophageal cancer. Oncology. 1991;48:411–20.
4. Akiyama H, Tsurumaru M, Udagawa H, et al. Radical lymph node dissection for cancer of the thoracic esophagus. Ann Surg. 1994;220:364–73.
5. Fujita H, Kakegawa T, Yamana H, et al. Mortality and morbidity rates, postoperative course, quality of life, and prognosis after extended radical lymphadenectomy for oesophageal cancer. Comparison of three-field lymphadenctomy with two- field lymphadenctomy. Ann Surg. 1995;222:654–62.
6. Ando N, Ozawa S, Kitagawa Y, et al. Improvement in the results of surgical treatment of advanced squamous esophageal carcinoma during 15 consecutive years. Ann Surg. 2000;232:225–32.
7. Bedenne L, Michel P, Bouche O, et al. Chemoradiation followed by surgery compared with chemoradiation alone in squamous cancer of the esophagus: FFCD 9102. J Clin Oncol. 2007;25:1160–8.
8. Suntharalingam M. Definitive chemoradiation in the management of locally advanced esophageal cancer. Semin Radiat Oncol. 2007;17:22–8.
9. Altorki N, Kent M, Ferrara RN, et al. Three-field lymph node dissection for squamous cell and adenocarcinoma of the esophagus. Ann Surg. 2002;236:177–83.
10. Lerut T, Nafteux P, Moons J, et al. Three-field lymphadenectomy for carcinoma of the esophagus and gastroesophageal junction in 174 R0 resections: impact on staging, disease-free survival, and outcome: a plea for adaptation of TNM classification in upper-half esophageal carcinoma. Ann Surg. 2004;240:962–72.
11. Japanese Society for Esophageal Diseases. Japanese classification of esophageal cancer, tenth edition: part I. Esophagus. 2009;6:1–25.
12. Tsurumaru M, Kajiyama Y, Udagawa H, et al. Outcomes of extended lymph node dissection for squamous cell carcinoma of the thoracic esophagus. Ann Thorac Cardiovasc Surg. 2001;7:325–9.

13. Nishihira T, Hirayama K, Mori S. A prospective randomized control trial of extended cervical and superior mediastinal lymphadenectomy for carcinoma of the thoracic esophagus. Am J Surg. 1998;175:47–51.
14. Kato H, Watanabe H, Tachimori Y, et al. Evaluation of the neck lymph node dissection for thoracic esophageal carcinoma. Ann Thorac Surg. 1991;51:931–5.
15. Nishimaki T, Suzuki T, Tnanaka Y, et al. Evalutating the rational extent of dissection in radical esophagectomy for invasive carcinoma of the thoracic esophagus. Surg Today. 1997;27:3–8.
16. Rindani R, Martin CJ, Cox MR. Transhiatal versus Lvor-Lewis esophagectomy: is there a difference? Aust N Z J Surg. 1999;69:187–94.
17. Hulscher JB, Tijssen JG, Oberop H, et al. Transthoracic versus transhiatal resection for carcinoma of the esophagus: a meta-analysis. Ann Thorac Surg. 2001;72:306–13.
18. Boshier PR, Anderson O, Hanna GB. Transthoracic versus transhiatal esophagectomy for the treatment of esophagogastric cancer. Ann Surg. 2011;254:894–906.
19. Hulscher JB, van Sandick JW, de Boer AG, et al. Extended transthoracic resection compared with limited transhiatal resection for adenocarcinoma of the esophagus. N Engl J Med. 2002;347:1662–9.
20. Omloo JM, Lagarde SM, Hulsche JB, et al. Extended transthoracic resection compared with limited transhiatal resection for adenocarcinoma of the mid/distal esophagus. Ann Surg. 2007;246:992–1000.
21. Sasako M, Sano T, Yamamoto S, et al. Left thoracoabdominal approach versus abdominal-transhiatal approach for gastric cancer of the cardia or subcardia: a randomized controlled trial. Lancet Oncol. 2006;7(8):644–51.
22. Morton DL, Wen DR, Wong JH, et al. Technical details of intraoperative lymphatic mapping for early stage melanoma. Arch Surg. 1992;127:392–9.
23. Morton DL, Thompson JF, Essner R, et al. Multicenter Selective Lymphadenectomy Trial Group. Validation of accuracy of intraoperative lymphatic mapping and sentinel lymphadenectomy for early-stage melanoma: a multicenter trial. Ann Surg. 1999;230:453–63.
24. Krag D, Weaver D, Ashikage T, et al. The sentinel node in breast cancer – a multicenter validation study. N Engl J Med. 1998;339:941–6.
25. Blichik AJ, Saha S, Wiese D, et al. Molecular staging of early colon cancer on the basis of sentinel node analysis: a multicenter phase II trial. J Clin Oncol. 2001;19:1128–36.
26. Kitagawa Y, Fujii H, Mukai M, et al. The role of the sentinel lymph node in gastrointestinal cancer. Surg Clin North Am. 2000;80:1799–809.
27. Kitagawa Y, Fujii H, Mukai M, et al. Intraoperative lymphatic mapping and sentinel lymph node sampling in esophageal and gastric cancer. Surg Oncol Clin N Am. 2002;11:293–304.
28. Takeuchi H, Fujii H, Ando N, et al. Validation study of radio-guided sentinel lymph node navigation in Esophageal cancer. Ann Surg. 2009;249:757–63.

Chapter 27
Optimal Lymph Node Dissection in Esophageal Cancer

Nasser K. Altorki and Brendon M. Stiles

Abstract Surgical resection remains the cornerstone of treatment protocols for both early stage and locally advanced esophageal cancer (EC). However, considerable controversy exists as to the best surgical approach to esophagectomy and to the extent of lymph node dissection (LND) necessary during the course of the operation. Some hold that the disease is systemic at the time of diagnosis and that extensive operative procedures and nodal dissection lead to increased operative morbidity and mortality without appreciable improvements in survival. The countervailing opinion is that an aggressive en bloc dissection with extensive LND eliminates locoregional disease and contributes to improved overall survival. This chapter describes the rationale for lymphadenectomy in esophageal cancer.

Keywords Esophageal cancer • Lymphadenectomy • Extended lymphadenectomy • Lymph node dissection • Esophagectomy

Introduction

Surgical resection remains the cornerstone of treatment protocols for both early stage and locally advanced esophageal cancer (EC). However, considerable controversy exists as to the best surgical approach to esophagectomy and to the extent of lymph node dissection (LND) necessary during the course of the operation. Some hold that the disease is systemic at the time of diagnosis and that extensive operative procedures and nodal dissection lead to increased operative morbidity and mortality

N.K. Altorki, MB, BCh (✉) • B.M. Stiles, MD
Department of Surgery, Division of Cardiothoracic Surgery,
Weill Cornell Medical College-New York Presbyterian Hospital,
525 East 68th Street, Suite M404/110, New York, NY 10065, USA
e-mail: nkaltork@med.cornell.edu; brs9035@med.cornell.edu

M.K. Ferguson (ed.), *Difficult Decisions in Thoracic Surgery*,
Difficult Decisions in Surgery: An Evidence-Based Approach 1,
DOI 10.1007/978-1-4471-6404-3_27, © Springer-Verlag London 2014

without appreciable improvements in survival. The countervailing opinion is that an aggressive en bloc dissection with extensive LND eliminates locoregional disease and contributes to improved overall survival. This chapter describes the rationale for lymphadenectomy in esophageal cancer.

Search Strategy

For this systematic review, search terms were identified and targeted searches were run in PubMed through November 2013. The search was limited to reports in English language and to human studies. The following Medical Subject Heading (MeSH) terms were used: "Esophageal cancer" and "Lymph node dissection". Initially, 1,635 articles and abstracts were identified through the PubMed/Medline search. Additional MeSH terms used to further stratify studies were: esophageal neoplasm, esophagectomy, en bloc esophagectomy, minimally invasive esophagectomy, lymph node excision, three-field dissection, targeted lymphadenectomy, or neoadjuvant therapy. After narrowing the search focus using MeSH headings, 32 articles served as the source for the review.

The Importance of Lymphadenectomy

The extent of lymph node dissection undertaken in patients with esophageal cancer depends upon the surgeon's preferences, upon the extent and location of the tumor, and upon the surgical approach utilized. Relatively unique to the esophagus is the pervasive submucosal and muscular networks of lymphatics, which run longitudinally in the esophageal wall with extensive intercommunication. As such, high rates of lymph node metastases are present in EC, 20–30 % in T1 cancers, 45–75 % in T2 cancers, and 80–85 % in T3 cancers [1, 2]. Importantly, although often adjacent to the primary tumor, these nodal metastases can be occult and may be present in multiple locations including the celiac axis and upper abdomen, the mediastinum, and along the recurrent laryngeal nerves up to the cervical esophagus, sometimes skipping more proximal stations. The extent of lymphadenectomy is necessarily an important component of esophagectomy with regard to optimal staging, but also for its potential impact on disease control and survival.

Lymph Node Stations and Fields

Great variability exists with regard to the extent of lymphadenectomy undertaken during the course of esophagectomy. A numbering system is used to define individual lymph node stations. However, the extent of lymphadenectomy is typically described by fields, as opposed to stations. These nodal regions or fields include:

1. The abdominal field, which encompasses the greater and lesser curvatures, left gastric, celiac, common hepatic, and splenic artery nodes. In addition, all retroperitoneal tissues between the superior border of the pancreas and the crus of the diaphragm are included within this dissection.
2. The mediastinal field, which includes the middle and lower periesophageal nodes, the subcarinal nodes, and the thoracic duct with its associated lymph nodes as it courses through the middle and lower mediastinum.
3. The "third" field, which includes the chain of lymph nodes along both recurrent nerves throughout their mediastinal and cervical course, as well as the deep cervical nodes posterior and lateral to the jugular vein and the supraclavicular nodes. Thus, the third field encompasses a group of nodal stations that span the superior posterior mediastinum and the lower neck.

Most surgeons resect nodes from at least the first and second fields, while a minority also perform nodal dissection of the third field [3].

Some discrepancies exist as to the definition of the third field. In Japan and other eastern countries where squamous cell carcinoma predominates, dissection of lymph nodes from the superior mediastinum and along both recurrent laryngeal nerves is typically included in the second thoracic field, while the third field is meant to describe cervical lymph node dissection. Conversely, in western countries in which adenocarcinomas of the gastroesophageal junction predominate, the upper mediastinal dissection is typically not included from the thoracic approach. Therefore, most western authors refer to the inclusion of the superior mediastinal and recurrent laryngeal nodal basins as the third field dissection.

Procedures can be described as either radical, referred to as "en bloc", or as nonradical, which generally indicates lymph node sampling rather than intent for complete dissection. The extent of lymphadenectomy is influenced by the surgical approach. Many different techniques for esophagectomy exist, including a transhiatal approach (TH), a transthoracic approach (TT) with anastomosis in the chest, and a TT McKeown approach with the anastomosis in the neck. Minimally invasive techniques have been utilized in all of these approaches and can be used for radical lymphadenectomy. Although the fields amenable to lymph node dissection are governed by the operative approach, the radicality of the dissection is not. Rather, it is defined by the approach to and handling of the lymphatic tissues.

Evidence for Extended Lymphadenectomy

Reliable evidence in support of extended lymphadenectomy has been obtained from large population based registries and multi-institutional observational studies [4–7]. In these studies (Table 27.1), the total number of lymph nodes removed is consistently an independent predictor of survival. Two of these studies analyzed data from

Table 27.1 Evidence in support of extended lymphadenectomy from large population based registries and multi-institutional observational studies

Author	Patients	Findings	Recommendations
Schwarz et al. (2007): SEER database 1973–2003 [4]	5,620	Higher total LN count (>30) and negative LN count (>15) associated with improved survival (p<0.001); Relative increase in OS of 4–5 % at 5 years for every 10 LN identified	Obtain ≥30 LN to optimize staging, survival, and locoregional control
Groth et al. (2010): SEER database 1988–2005 [5]	4,882 (including patients with neoadjuvant therapy)	Significant difference between stratified LN groups in all-cause (p<0.001) and cancer-specific (p=0.004) mortality. Cancer specific morality HR of 0.58 (CI 0.44–0.78) with ≥30 LN	Obtain ≥15 LN to maximize the likelihood of detecting LN metastases; obtain ≥30 LN to optimize cancer-specific mortality
Peyre et al. (2008): Patients from nine international centers prior to 2002 [8]	2,303 (surgery alone)	Best threshold of LN removed to maximize survival was 23–29; even when minimum threshold of 23 nodes was achieved, 5 year survival was better after en bloc resection than after lesser types	To maximize outcome of surgical resection, ≥23 nodes should be removed. En bloc resection is most likely to meet this threshold
Rizk et al. (2010): Worldwide esophageal cancer collaboration [7]	4,627 (surgery alone)	Optimum LN dissection is defined by T classification and histopathologic type; for pN0M0 moderately or poorly differentiated cancers and for all pN + cancers, 5 year survival improved with increasing LN dissection	Resect ≥10 LN for pT1, ≥20 LN for pT2, and ≥30 LN for pT3/T4 cancers

the SEER database for an association between the total number of lymph nodes removed and overall survival (OS) in EC. Schwarz et al. analyzed data from approximately 2,600 EC patients treated by esophagectomy, on whom full nodal staging information was available [4]. Multivariate analysis indentified that total nodal count, modeled as a continuous variable, was an independent predictor of OS regardless of nodal status (N0 or N1) or tumor histology. The best OS was observed when >30 LN were examined. Using linear regression modeling, the authors calculated a 10 and 3 % relative increase in 5 year OS for every ten extra lymph nodes examined for N0 and N1 patients, respectively. Groth et al. also analyzed the SEER database for EC to examine the association between lymph node count and all cause mortality [5]. Recursive partitioning analysis was used to stratify 4,882 patients based on the number of lymph nodes examined. The authors concluded that to maximize all cause and cancer specific survival, EC patients should have at least 30 lymph nodes examined pathologically (HR 0.58 for CSS).

In addition to these population-based studies, two large multi-institutional studies were recently reported that examined the association between the number of lymph nodes and survival in EC patients treated by esophagectomy without preoperative therapy. Peyre et al. constructed a database of over 2,300 EC patients from nine esophageal centers worldwide [6]. Cox regression analysis showed that the number of lymph nodes removed was an independent predictor of survival (p < 0.0001). The optimal threshold predicted by Cox regression for this survival benefit was removal of a minimum of 23 nodes. From the Worldwide Esophageal Cancer Collaboration (WECC) database, Rizk et al. reported on 4,627 EC patients with both adenocarcinoma and SCC treated at 13 different institutions worldwide. Risk adjusted survival was estimated using random survival forests and was averaged for each number of lymph nodes resected [7]. The optimum number of lymph nodes resected was dependent on T-classification, N-classification, and cell type. Optimum lymphadenectomy for pN0M0 patient was 10–12, 15–22, and 31–42 for pT1, pT2 and pT3/4 tumors, respectively. For pN + M0 cancers with up to six positive nodes, optimum lymphadenectomy was 10, 15, and 29–50 for pT1, T2 and T3/4 tumors respectively.

Comparison of Surgical Techniques for Lymphadenectomy

Transhiatal Versus Transthoracic Esophagectomy

Comparison of transhiatal (THE) to transthoracic (TTE) esophagectomy perhaps more accurately evaluates surgical access rather than extent of lymphadenectomy. However, as the extent of lymph node removal is clearly different between the two approaches, data from randomized trials may be used to infer the importance of lymphadenectomy. In 2002, Hulscher reported the largest randomized trial comparing THE to TTE [9]. Two hundred and twenty treatment naive patients, were randomly assigned to either THE with single field upper abdominal lymph node dissection (D2 lymphadenectomy) or TTE with two-field (D2 lymphadenectomy and middle and lower mediastinal node dissection) performed by an en-bloc technique. The total lymph nodes removed were significantly higher in the TTE approach, 31 ± 14 versus 16 ± 9 with the TTE approach ($p = 0.001$). Although THE was associated with lower morbidity, there was a non-significant trend for improved survival favoring the transthoracic en-bloc procedure (TTE 39 % vs. THE 29 %). A subsequent per-protocol subgroup analysis showed that patients most likely to benefit from the extended resection were those with adenocarcinoma of the distal tubular esophagus (51 % vs. 37 %; p=0.33) and those with limited nodal involvement (1–8 positive nodes) (TTE: 64 %, THE: 25 %; p=0.02) [10]. Patients with tumors of the gastroesophageal junction and those with either no or extensive nodal metastases (>8 nodes) had similar survival with either type of resection.

The most recent meta-analysis of TTE versus THE reviewed 5,905 patients from 52 articles, including recent literature from the 2000s [11]. Patients undergoing TTE had an average of eight more lymph nodes removed than those undergoing THE (p=0.02, CI 1–14). However, lymph node yield was adequately reported in only four studies. There was no significant difference in 5-year overall survival between patients undergoing TTE versus THE, although significant heterogeneity existed among studies.

The Role of En Bloc Esophagectomy

Logan introduced the en bloc concept in 1963, which was later re-introduced by Skinner in 1979 [12, 13]. The basic premise of the en bloc operation is to maximize local tumor control by resection of the tumor bearing esophagus within a wide envelope of adjoining tissues that includes both pleural surfaces laterally and the pericardium anteriorly where these structures are intimately related to the esophagus. In addition to providing for a greater circumferential margin, en bloc esophagectomy leads to enhanced lymphadenectomy. Posteriorly, the lymphatics wedged dorsally between the esophagus and the aorta, including the thoracic duct throughout its mediastinal course, are resected en bloc with the specimen. This posterior mediastinectomy necessarily results in a complete mediastinal node dissection from the tracheal bifurcation to the esophageal hiatus. Additionally, as part of the en bloc operation, an upper abdominal lymphadenectomy is performed including the common hepatic, celiac, left gastric, lesser curvature, parahiatal, and the retroperitoneal nodes. Local recurrence rates reported by proponents of this approach have been in the 2–10 % range, much lower than those reported following either transhiatal esophagectomy or standard transthoracic resections [1, 14].

The only randomized trial reported to date comparing transthoracic en-bloc resection with non en bloc resection (transhiatal) esophagectomy is the Hulscher trial, previously discussed [9]. Again, as differences exist in the surgical access, approach, and fields of lymph node dissection this trial should not be taken as only a direct comparison of en-bloc versus non en-bloc strategies. However, as mentioned, en bloc esophagectomy enhanced lymphadenectomy and appeared to improve survival in patients with limited nodal involvement (one to eight positive nodes) (TTE: 64 %, THE: 25 %; p=0.02).

Several retrospective case series also exist describing enhanced lymphadenectomy and patient survival with en bloc techniques. Lee et al. have recently updated their institution's series of resections for esophageal cancer patients, from which they had previously reported the superiority of en bloc resection to non-en bloc approaches [15]. This included 465 patients who had an R0 resection, 179 patients resected following induction therapy and 286 patients treated with surgery alone. Three hundred twenty-eight patients (71 %) had an en bloc resection. The remaining 137 patients (29 %) had a non-en bloc resection (88 transhiatal, 49 transthoracic). The number of resected lymph nodes was significantly higher for the en bloc group (median 31 vs. 17, p < 0.001). For patients with pathologic stage 0/I disease, there was no significant difference in disease free survival (DFS) between the en bloc group and the standard resection group (5 year-DFS 75.7 % (95 % CI: 62.2–90.4) vs. 76.3 % (95 % CI: 65.3–86.1). However, for patients with pathologic stage II/III/IV disease, DFS was significantly improved following en bloc resection compared to standard resection [HR: 0.66, (0.50–0.88), p = 0.004]. Median DFS was 19.0 months (95 % CI: 14.0–24.0) after en bloc and 12.2 months (95 % CI: 7.7–16.7) following standard resection. An important criticism of most of this and other retrospective studies is the failure to clearly define the criteria for patient selection for one procedure versus another. For example, in the studies by Lee et al and by Hagen et al, the patients receiving a transhiatal resection were either significantly older than the en-bloc group or had a worse performance status with respect to cardiopulmonary function [15, 16].

The Role of Three-Field Lymphadenectomy

The concept of 3-field lymph node dissection for esophageal cancer was developed by Japanese surgeons in the 1980s in response to the observation that as many as 40 % of patients with resected squamous cell esophageal cancer developed isolated cervical lymph node metastases [17]. A nationwide retrospective study was subsequently reported describing the findings and potential benefits of esophagectomy with 3-field dissection [18]. The additional third field of dissection included excision of the nodes along both recurrent nerves as they course through the mediastinum and neck, as well as a modified cervical node dissection. Previously, unsuspected cervical nodal metastases, primarily in the recurrent nodes, were seen in approximately one third of patients. Furthermore, the authors reported a significantly higher overall 5-year survival after 3-field dissection in comparison to 2-field dissection.

The largest Japanese study from a single institution was reported by Akiyama in 1994 [19]. The authors reported their experience with 717 patients in whom a complete (R0) resection was performed using either a two-field (n = 393) or a three-field technique (n = 324). Five-year survival in node-negative patients was 84 % after the three-field procedure compared to 55 % after two-field lymphadenectomy (p = 0.004). Patients with node-positive disease also fared better after three-field dissection with a 5-year survival rate of 43 % compared to a 28 % 5-year survival rate after two-field dissection (p = 0.0008).

Two prospective studies have been reported [20, 21]. The study by Nishihira was a prospective randomized trial that showed a survival advantage for three-field over two-field lymph node dissection (65 % versus 48 %); however the difference was not statistically significant [20]. The study from the National Cancer Hospital in Tokyo was a prospective non-randomized case- matched study that showed that 5-year survival was significantly better after three-field dissection (48 % versus 33 %; p=0.03) [21].

A recent meta-analysis of the eastern literature was published by Ye et al. including 13 studies for analysis, of which two were randomized trials [22]. Total number of lymph nodes removed with each technique was not analyzed. Among 2,379 patients, a better 5-year survival rate was demonstrated in patients undergoing three-field versus two-field lymphadenectomy (HR for three-field 0.64, CI: 0.56–0.73, p<0.001). Patients undergoing three-field lymphadenectomy had similar rates of perioperative mortality (RR 0.64, CI: 0.38–1.10, p=0.110) and pulmonary complications (RR 1.00, CI: 0.89–1.12, p=0.760), but higher rates of anastomotic leakage (RR 1.46, CI 1.19–1.79, p<0.001).

The relevance of these findings to a western population afflicted primarily by esophageal adenocarcinoma remains unknown. The early experience in North America with this technique was reported by Altorki et al, in 2002 [23]. The procedure was performed in 80 patients, 60 % of which had adenocarcinoma of the esophagus. Recurrent nerve injury occurred in 6 % of patients. An average of 60 nodes were resected per patient. The prevalence of cervical nodal metastases was 37 % in patients regardless of cell type or location of the tumor within the esophagus. Overall and disease-free survival was 50 and 46 %, respectively, and was not influenced by cell types. Patients with adenocarcinoma who had metastases to the recurrent laryngeal lymph nodes had a 3- and 5-year survival of 30 and 15 %, respectively. In contrast patients with squamous cell carcinoma and positive recurrent laryngeal nodes had a 5-year survival of 40 %.

Lerut reported the most significant European experience with esophagectomy and three-field lymph node dissection [24]. One hundred and seventy four patients had an R0 three-field esophagectomy with a hospital mortality of 1.4 % and morbidity of 57 %. Fifty five percent of patients had adenocarcinoma of the esophagus or cardia. Overall and disease-free survival at 5 years was 42 and 46 %, respectively. The incidence of positive cervical nodes in patients with adenocarcinoma was 23 % and was slightly higher for those with esophageal versus cardial tumors (26 % vs. 18 %). Four- and 5-year survival for patients with adenocarcinoma and positive cervical nodes were 35 and 11 %, respectively.

Targeted Lymphadenectomy

A number of investigations regarding selection of patients for dissection of the third field have been reported. Preoperative ultrasonography has been reported to have a sensitivity, specificity, and accuracy of 75–82 %, 94 %, and 85–95 % respectively [25, 26]. However it is not clear what role ultrasonography plays with the addition of PET scans to the preoperative workup. Other groups have suggested the use of intraoperative pathological examination of superior mediastinal nodes as a predictor of cervical node metastases [27]. The rate of cervical node positivity was 41 % in patients with positive intrathoracic recurrent laryngeal nerve nodes, compared to 10 % in patients without positive recurrent laryngeal nodes ($p=0.007$). More recently, Stiles et al. have described predictors of positive cervical and recurrent laryngeal nerve (CRL) nodal metastases [28]. Among 470 patients undergoing three-field lymph node dissection, 47 (25 %) had positive CRL node metastases. On multivariate analysis, advanced (cT3-4 or cN1-3 or both) clinical stage predicted positive CRL nodes (HR 2.56, CI 0.91–7.2, $p=0.07$), as did histology (HR 6.0 for squamous vs. adenocarcinoma, CI 2.2–16.6, $p<0.0001$), and pathologic nodal status (HR 16.3 for pN2-3 vs. pN0-1, CI 5.4–48.9, $p<0.0001$).

Lymphadenectomy Following Neoadjuvant Therapy

Recommendations regarding optimum lymphadenectomy for esophageal cancer have been based only upon series of patients undergoing surgery alone and do not include an analysis of patients receiving multimodality therapy. Unfortunately, most patients with EC present with locally advanced disease. As such, neoadjuvant chemotherapy or chemoradiotherapy is commonly used in the treatment of these patients. Limited studies exist to define the importance of lymphadenectomy during esophagectomy following neoadjuvant chemotherapy and/or radiation therapy. Some groups have suggested that the extent of resection and lymphadenectomy affect outcome of EC patients, even following neoadjuvant therapy [8, 29]. Rizzetto et al described outcomes of 58 patients undergoing either en bloc TTE (n=40) or THE (n=18) following neoadjuvant therapy [8]. Locoregional failures were higher in the THE group (16.6 % vs. 0 %, p=0.02). Overall 5-year survival was significantly better in the TTE group, 51 % vs. 22 %, p=0.04). However, the groups weren't well matched, as patients undergoing THE were older and had more comorbidities, factors which potentially affected long term survival.

More recently, Stiles et al. evaluated the WECC recommendations for lymphadenectomy with respect to esophageal cancer patients undergoing neoadjuvant therapy, predominantly chemotherapy alone [29]. For analysis, adequacy of lymph node dissection (optimal lymphadenectomy) was defined as removing a minimum of 10 lymph nodes for ypTis/T0/T1 cancers, 20 lymph nodes for ypT2 cancers, and 30 lymph nodes for ypT3 /T4 cancers. Optimal lymphadenectomy predicted OS (0.50, CI 0.29–0.85, p=0.011), although it was collinear with ypT-classification, which was also predictive. Patients not downstaged from clinical to pathologic T classification (n=66, 49 %) experienced a trend toward improved 3-year survival with optimal lymphadenectomy (51 % vs. 29 %, p=0.144). Similarly, of patients with persistent nodal disease (n=79, 59 %), those who had optimal lymphadenectomy (n=51) experienced improved 3-year overall survival compared to those with suboptimal lymphadenectomy (n=28), (55 % versus 36 %, p=0.087). The retrospective nature of these studies makes drawing overarching conclusions difficult.

Minimally Invasive Surgery and Lymphadenectomy

There has been a steady increase in the use of minimally invasive techniques to facilitate esophagectomy, either thoracoscopic, laparoscopic, or both. Additionally, robot-assisted minimally invasive techniques have been utilized by several centers. These approaches are often grouped together under the broad category of minimally invasive esophagectomy (MIE). Until recently, limited randomized trial information was available for evaluation. Decker et al. performed a comprehensive review of the literature on MIE in through 2007 [30]. The extent of lymph nodes removed was reported in 29 papers, in which the median of all series was 14 nodes [5–31]. More recently, a meta-analysis of MIE versus open esophagectomy was performed in 2010 by Sgourakis et al, analyzing 1,008 patients in eight comparative studies [32]. The authors reported no difference in the number of lymph nodes removed between the two approaches, however they didn't report the numbers. Additionally, data from only 79 patients in two studies were available for this analysis.

The most compelling evidence in support of the equivalency of MIE to open esophagectomy was recently published as part of the TIME trial [31]. Patients were randomly assigned to either open esophagectomy (n=56) or MIE (n=59). All patients underwent neoadjuvant chemoradiotherapy or chemotherapy alone. There was no difference in total lymph nodes retrieved in the open (median = 21) or MIE (median = 20) groups (p=0.85). A similar randomized trial (ROBOT) is planned to evaluate robotic-assisted MIE versus open esophagectomy.

Conclusions and Recommendations

Lymph node dissection is a recommended key component of esophageal resection of invasive cancer as it provides important staging information and may lead to a survival. To optimize staging in treatment naive T1, T2, and T3 tumors, at least ten lymph nodes for T1 and 20–30 lymph nodes for T2 and above should be resected. There is limited data regarding the optimal number of lymph nodes to be resected after neoadjuvant chemoradiation. Transthoracic esophageal resection, particularly using en bloc resection techniques, enhances lymphadenectomy compared to transhiatal and non en-bloc surgical techniques. Three-field lymph node dissection may be considered in either squamous cell or adenocarcinoma. Three-field dissection leads to enhanced lymphadenectomy, however its survival benefit remains uncertain. Minimally invasive esophagectomy can be expected to yield numbers of lymph nodes resected equivalent to open esophagectomy.

A Personal View of the Data

The personal view of the authors is a two field lymphadenectomy that includes the middle and lower mediastinal as well as the upper abdominal retroperitoneal nodes has been convincingly shown to improve staging and survival of patients with esophageal cancer. We thus advocate an en bloc, transthoracic resection for all patients except those with appropriately staged clinical T1aN0 disease. The en bloc dissection can be performed by either open or minimally invasive approaches. For all patients with squamous cell cancer and for adenocarcinoma patients with locally advanced disease of the thoracic esophagus, dissection of the recurrent laryngeal and cervical lymph node basins should be strongly considered.

Recommendations

- Lymph node dissection is recommended as part of esophagectomy for invasive cancer. (Evidence quality low; weak recommendation)
- To optimize staging in treatment naive tumors, at least ten lymph nodes for T1 and 20–30 lymph nodes for T2 and above should be resected. (Evidence quality low; weak recommendation)
- No recommendation can be made regarding the optimal number of lymph nodes that should be resected after neoadjuvant chemoradiation. (Evidence quality very low; no recommendation)
- Three-field lymph node dissection may be considered in either squamous cell or adenocarcinoma. (Evidence quality low; weak recommendation)
- Minimally invasive esophagectomy can be expected to yield numbers of lymph nodes resected equivalent to open esophagectomy. (Evidence quality low; weak recommendation)

References

1. Nigro JJ, DeMeester SR, Hagen JA, DeMeester TR, Peters JH, Kiyabu M, et al. Node status in transmural esophageal adenocarcinoma and outcome after en bloc esophagectomy. J Thorac Cardiovasc Surg. 1999;117:960–8.
2. Rice TW, Zuccaro Jr G, Adelstein DJ, Rybicki LA, Blackstone EH, Goldblum JR. Esophageal carcinoma: depth of tumor invasion is predictive of regional lymph node status. Ann Thorac Surg. 1998;65:787–92.
3. Enestvedt CK, Perry KA, Kim C, McConnell PW, Diggs BS, Vernon A, et al. Trends in the management of esophageal carcinoma based on provider volume: treatment practices of 618 esophageal surgeons. Dis Esophagus. 2010;23(2):136–44.
4. Schwarz RE, Smith DD. Clinical impact of lymphadenectomy extent in resectable esophageal cancer. J Gastrointest Surg. 2007;11(11):1384–94.

5. Groth SS, Virnig BA, Whitson BA, DeFor TE, Li ZZ, Tuttle TM, et al. Determination of the minimum number of lymph nodes to examine to maximize survival in patients with esophageal carcinoma: data from the Surveillance Epidemiology and End Results database. J Thorac Cardiovasc Surg. 2010;139(3):612–20.

6. Peyre CG, Hagen JA, DeMeester SR, Altorki NK, Ancona E, Griffin SM, et al. The number of lymph nodes removed predicts survival in esophageal cancer: an international study on the impact of extent of surgical resection. Ann Surg. 2008;248(4):549–56.

7. Rizk NP, Ishwaran H, Rice TW, Chen LQ, Schipper PH, Kesler KA. Optimum lymphadencectomy for esophageal cancer. Ann Surg. 2010;251:46–50.

8. Rizzetto C, DeMeester SR, Hagen JA, Peyre CG, Lipham JC, DeMeester TR. En bloc esophagectomy reduces local recurrence and improves survival compared with transhiatal resection after neoadjuvant therapy for esophageal adenocarcinoma. J Thorac Cardiovasc Surg. 2008;135(6):1228–36.

9. Hulscher JB, van Sandick JW, de Boer AG, Wijnhoven BP, Tijssen JG, Fockens P. Extended transthoracic resection compared with limited transhiatal resection for adenocarcinoma of the esophagus. N Engl J Med. 2002;347(21):1662–9.

10. Omloo JM, Lagarde SM, Hulscher JB, Reitsma JB, Fockens P, van Dekken H, et al. Extended transthoracic resection compared with limited transhiatal resection for adenocarcinoma of the mid/distal esophagus: five-year survival of a randomized clinical trial. Ann Surg. 2007;246(6):992,1001.

11. Boshier PR, Anderson O, Hanna GB. Transthoracic versus transhiatal esophagectomy for the treatment of esophagogastric cancer: a meta-analysis. Ann Surg. 2011;254:894–906.

12. Logan A. The surgical treatment of carcinoma of the esophagus and cardia. J Thorac Cardiovasc Surg. 1963;46:150–61.

13. Skinner DB. En-bloc resection for neoplasms of the esophagus and cardia. J Thorac Cardiovasc Surg. 1983;85:59–69.

14. Altorki NK, Girardi L, Skinner DB. En-bloc esophagectomy improves survival for stage III esophageal cancer. J Thorac Cardiovasc Surg. 1997;114(6):948–55.

15. Lee PC, Mirza FM, Port JL, Stiles BM, Paul S, Christos P, et al. Predictors of recurrence and disease-free survival in patients with completely resected esophageal carcinoma. J Thorac Cardiovasc Surg. 2011;141(5):1196–206.

16. Hagen JA, Peters JH, De Meester TR. Superiority of extended en bloc esophagogastrectomy for carcinoma of the lower esophagus and cardia. J Thorac Cardiovasc Surg. 1993;106(5): 850–8.

17. Isono K, Onoda S, Okuyama K, Sato H. Recurrence of intrathoracic esophageal cancer. Jpn J Clin Oncol. 1985;15:49–60.

18. Isono K, Sato H, Nakayama K. Results of nationwide study of the three-field lymph node dissection of esophageal cancer. Oncology. 1991;48:411–20.

19. Akiyama H, Tsurumaru M, Udagawa H, Kajiyama Y. Radical lymph node dissection for cancer of the thoracic esophagus. Ann Surg. 1994;220:364–72.

20. Nishihira T, Hirayama K, Mori S. A prospective randomized trial of extended cervical and superior mediastinal lymphadenectomy for carcinoma of the thoracic esophagus. Am J Surg. 1998;175:47–51.

21. Kato H, Watanabe H, Tachimori Y, Iizuka T. Evaluation of the neck lymph node dissection for thoracic esophageal carcinoma. Ann Thorac Surg. 1991;51:931–5.

22. Ye T, Sun Y, Zhang Y, Zhang Y, Chen H. Three-field or two-field resection for thoracic esophageal cancer: a meta-analysis. Ann Thorac Surg. 2013. doi:10.1016/j.athoracsur.2013.06.050 [pii: S0003-4975(13)01378-7], [Epub ahead of print].

23. Altorki N, Kent M, Ferrara C, Port J. Three-field lymph node dissection for squamous cell and adenocarcinoma of the esophagus. Ann Surg. 2002;236(2):177–83.

24. Lerut T, Nafteux P, Moons J, Coosemans W, Decker G, De Leyn P. Three-field lymphadenectomy for carcinoma of the esophagus and gastroesophageal junction in 174 R0 resections: impact on staging, disease-free survival, and outcome: a plea for adaptation of TNM classification in upper-half esophageal carcinoma. Ann Surg. 2004;240(6):962–72.

25. Natsugoe S, Yoshinaka H, Shimada M, Shirao K, Nakano S, Kusano C. Assessment of cervical lymph node metastasis in esophageal carcinoma using ultrasonography. Ann Surg. 1999;229:62–6.
26. Tachimori Y, Kato H, Watanabe H, Yamaguchi H. Neck ultrasonography for thoracic esophageal carcinoma. Ann Thorac Surg. 1994;57:1180–3.
27. Ueda Y, Shiozaki A, Itoi H, Okamoto K, Fujiwara H, Ichikawa D. Intraoperative pathological investigation of recurrent nerve nodal metastasis can guide the decision whether to perform cervical lymph node dissection in thoracic esophageal cancer. Oncol Rep. 2006;16:1061–6.
28. Stiles BM, Mirza F, Port JL, Lee PC, Paul S, Christos P. Predictors of cervical and recurrent laryngeal lymph node metastases from esophageal cancer. Ann Thorac Surg. 2010;90(6): 1805–11.
29. Stiles BM, Nasar A, Mirza FA, Lee PC, Paul S, Port JL, et al. Worldwide Oesophageal Cancer Collaboration guidelines for lymphadenectomy predict survival following neoadjuvant therapy. Eur J Cardiothorac Surg. 2012;42(4):659–64.
30. Decker G, Coosemans W, De Leyn P, Decaluwé H, Nafteux P, Van Raemdonck D, et al. Minimally invasive esophagectomy for cancer. Eur J Cardiothorac Surg. 2009;35(1):13–21.
31. Biere SS, van Berge Henegouwen MI, Maas KW, Bonavina L, Rosman C, Garcia JR, et al. Minimally invasive versus open oesophagectomy for patients with oesophageal cancer: a multicentre, open-label, randomised controlled trial. Lancet. 2012;379(9829):1887–92.
32. Sgourakis G, Gockel I, Radtke A, Musholt TJ, Timm S, Rink A, et al. Minimally invasive versus open esophagectomy: meta-analysis of outcomes. Dig Dis Sci. 2010;55(11):3031–40.

Chapter 28
Salvage Esophagectomy for Persistent or Recurrent Disease After Definitive Chemoradiotherapy

David Rice and Clara S. Fowler

Abstract It is not uncommon for patients to either undergo definitive chemoradiotherapy with the expectation that locally recurrent tumor may possibly be treated by 'salvage' esophagectomy, or that patients be treated with chemoradiothearpy followed by selective use of surgery in cases of persistent disease. The literature supporting use of salvage esophagectomy is sparse. Nevertheless, esophagectomy has been shown to result in better survival than what can be achieved by either supportive care or non-operative strategies. Consideration should be given to performing salvage esophagectomy in carefully selected patients with persistent or recurrent cancer who are physiologically fit and who have a high likelihood of being able to undergo complete resection of their tumor.

Keywords Esophageal cancer • Esophagectomy • Recurrent cancer • Salvage esophagectomy • Neoadjuvant therapy • Chemoradiotherapy

Introduction

The treatment of locally advanced esophageal cancer remains controversial. Several randomized controlled trials and meta-analyses have demonstrated survival benefit for induction chemoradiation (CRT) and surgery over surgery alone for patients

D. Rice, MB, BCh (✉)
Department of Thoracic and Cardiovascular Surgery, University of Texas MD Anderson Cancer Center, 1515 Holcombe Blvd, Unit 1499, Houston, TX 77030, USA
e-mail: drice@mdanderson.org

C.S. Fowler, MSLS
Research Medical Library, The University of Texas MD Anderson Cancer Center, 1515 Holcombe Blvd., Unit 1499, Houston, TX 77030, USA
e-mail: cfowler@mdanderson.org

M.K. Ferguson (ed.), *Difficult Decisions in Thoracic Surgery*,
Difficult Decisions in Surgery: An Evidence-Based Approach 1,
DOI 10.1007/978-1-4471-6404-3_28, © Springer-Verlag London 2014

with esophageal and gastroesophageal junction (GEJ) tumors (mainly adenocarcinomas). However, two other recent phase III studies have failed to show a benefit to
the addition of surgery in patients with predominantly squamous cell cancers who
responded to CRT [1–4]. Proponents of the trimodality approach (chemotherapy +
radiotherapy + surgery) argue that local failure following definitive CRT is high,
ranging between 40 and 60 %, and that residual cancer is found in the resected
specimen in up to 70 % in patients who undergo surgery after induction CRT.
Conversely, approximately 30 % of patients undergoing trimodality therapy will
have a complete pathologic response and it is questionable whether such patients
needlessly endure the operative morbidity and long-term functional deficits associated with esophagectomy. For this reason, it is not uncommon for patients to either
undergo definitive CRT (dCRT) with the expectation that locally recurrent tumor
may possibly be treated by 'salvage' esophagectomy, or that patients be treated with
CRT followed by selective use of surgery in cases of persistent disease. This chapter
reviews the available literature regarding the short and long-term outcomes of
patients undergoing salvage esophagectomy following definitive CRT.

Search Strategy

A MEDLINE (Ovid) search was performed using the terms "esophageal neoplasms", "esophagectomy", "oesophageal cancer", "esophageal cancer" "esophageal adenocarcinoma", "combined modality therapy/ or chemoradiotherapy/ or
chemotherapy, adjuvant/ or neoadjuvant therapy/ or radiotherapy, adjuvant", "salvage oesophagectomy", "salvage esophagectomy" and "salvage resection". Details
of the search process is provided in Appendix 28.1. After removing duplicate studies, 115 citations were identified. Studies that reported soley on outcomes of planned
esophagectomy following neoadjuvant CRT (nCRT) were excluded. Selection of
studies for review required that they include more than ten patients in the salvage
group and have been published in English in peer-reviewed journals from Jan 2000
until Dec 2013. A total of 16 studies were identified that specifically addressed
perioperative outcomes and survival of patients who had undergone salvage esophagectomy (Table 28.1) [5–16, 18–20]. All of these were retrospective studies and
thus constitute a low or very low grade of evidence. Ten studies were identified that
retrospectively compared outcomes of patients undergoing salvage esophagectomy
with a control group that included either patients undergoing planned esophagectomy following nCRT (n=8), esophagectomy without CRT (n=2) or patients who
had failed CRT but did not undergo surgery (n=1). One study compared salvage
resections to patients undergoing either surgery only or surgery after nCRT. Only
one of these studies used matched controls. A single phase II study was identified
that prospectively examined the feasibility of performing selective esophagectomy
following after dCRT to 50.4 Gy, however perioperative outcomes of patients who
underwent salvage surgery were not described [21]. Several literature review articles were identified but no formal systematic reviews or meta-analyses were found.

Table 28.1 Study design and quality of evidence according to the GRADE system. nCRT, neoadjuvant chemoradiation

Author, year	n	Study design	Quality of evidence
Wilson et al. (2002) [5]	16	Comparative (appropriate statistical methodology not used)	Very low
Swisher et al. (2002) [6]	13	Comparative (nCR + planned surgery, non-matched)	Very low
Nakamura et al. (2004) [7]	27	Comparative (nCRT + planned surgery, non-matched)	Very low
Tomimaru et al. (2006) [8]	24	Comparative (nCRT + planned surgery, non-matched)	Very low
Oki et al. (2007) [9]	14	Case series	Very low
Nishimura et al. (2007) [10]	46	Case series	Very low
Smithers et al. (2007) [11]	14	Comparative (nCRT + planned surgery, non-matched)	Very low
D'Journo et al. (2008) [12]	24	Case series	Very low
Pinto et al. (2009) [13]	15	Case series	Very low
Miyata et al. (2009) [14]	33	Comparative (nCRT + planned surgery, non-matched)	Very low
Chao et al. (2009) [15]	27	Comparative (nCRT + planned surgery, non-matched)	Very low
Tachimori et al. (2009) [16]	59	Comparative (surgery only, non-matched)	Very low
Morita et al. (2011) [17]	27	Comparative (nCR + planned surgery, surgery alone, non-matched)	Very low
Marks et al. (2012) [18]	65	Comparative (nCRT + planned surgery, matched)	Low
Yoo et al. (2012) [19]	12	Comparative (dCRT with recurrence, no surgery, non-matched)	Very low
Schieman et al. (2013) [20]	12	Case series	Very low

Results

Patients

Salvage esophagectomy was performed infrequently. The average study reported on only 27 patients (range 12–65). Ten articles reported a denominator that included the total number of esophagectomies performed during the study period (mean 558, range 268–780) and of all esophagectomies, salvage cases accounted for on average only 5.3 %. Only three articles reported the total number of patients undergoing dCRT during the study period [11, 14, 15]. Chao et al. reported salvage esophagectomy having been performed in 27 of 47 (57 %) patients with locally recurrent tumor out of a group of 84 patients who had undergone dCRT. Smithers et al. reported salvage esophagectomy in 11 of 235 (4 %) patients undergoing dCRT at their institution and Miyata and colleagues performed salvage surgery in 33 of 219 (15 %) patients treated with dCRT. Eight studies, all from Asia, reported exclusively on patients with recurrent or persistent squamous cell cancer (SCC) [7–10, 14–16, 19]. A single study from North America reported outcomes of patients undergoing salvage esophagectomy for adenocarcinoma (ACA) only [18]. Radiation doses used for dCRT were generally between 50 and 60 Gy, with two exceptions; Schieman et al. reported a dosage range between 30 and 72 Gy in patients with recurrent SCC of the proximal esophagus (defined as tumor arising less than 20 cm from the incisors), and in the study by Chao and colleagues the total dosage of radiation was 30 Gy in 25 fractions [15, 20]. All 16 studies reviewed described salvage esophagectomy for persistent or recurrent tumor, however, D'Journo et al. included in their analysis six patients who underwent esophagectomy for benign etiologies (intractable stenosis in three, perforation in two and radiation induced esophagitis in one) [12]. Eleven studies provided details regarding whether salvage esophagectomy was performed for persistent or recurrent disease.

Combined analysis of 251 patients included in these studies shows even distribution between persistent (50.2 %) and recurrent tumors (49.8 %), however studies by Swisher et al and Yoo et al consisted of a very high proportion of recurrent tumors (100 and 92 %, respectively), whereas the study by Nakamura et al had a predominance of persistent tumors following dCRT (89 %) [6, 19, 22]. This may be relevant with respect to perioperative outcomes because the deleterious fibrotic effects of radiation are more likely to be encountered when performing esophagectomy for recurrent tumors which typically occur many months or even years after the completion of dCRT. The mean time from completion of dCRT until esophagectomy ranged from 1.7 to 18 months, and averaged 7.1 months among 11 studies where data were available (Table 28.2).

Surgical Approaches

Surgical approaches usually included either a transthoracic or a three-hole technique. Reports from Asia tended to include a higher utilization of three-hole (McKeown) esophagectomy and cervical anastomoses compared to North American, Australian and European series. Three-field lymphadenectomy was reported exclusively in reports from Asian centers. The transhiatal approach was used infrequently (mean 5.5 %, range 0–15 % of cases, 11 studies). Complete resection with negative margins averaged 79 % (range 50–100 %, 15 studies) and the mean complete pathologic response rate (ypT0N0M0) was 4.1 % (range 0–13 %, 12 studies, benign cases excluded). Regarding perioperative morbidity, complications were reported in 35–79 % cases (mean 53 %, 8 studies). The most common postoperative events were respiratory complications, which were reported in 9–62 % of cases (mean 28 %, 15 studies [6–16, 18, 20]).

Complications

Seven comparative studies evaluated incidence of postoperative complications and all showed higher rates in patients undergoing salvage procedures compared to controls undergoing surgery alone or planned surgery after nCRT (Table 28.3). In only

Table 28.2 Demographic, morbidity and survival outcomes for patients undergoing salvage esophagectomy

	n	Gy (mean)	Months from dCRT (mean)	Persistent disease (%)	R0 (%)	Morbidity Respiratory (%)	Leak (%)	Overall (%)	Mortality 30-day (%)	90-day (%)	Survival
Wilson et al. (2002) [5]	16	60	na	63	na	na	na	na	3	na	5-years 37 %
Swisher et al. (2002) [6]	13	57	18 (4–56)	0	77	62	38	77	15	na	5-years 25 %
Nakamura et al. (2004) [7]	27	60	4 (1–15)	89	67	11	22	na	4	na	~5-years 30 %
Tomimaru et al. (2006) [8]	24	62	6 (1–25)	54	67	21	21	na	4	12	na
Oki et al. (2007) [9]	14	65	9 (1–34)	36	50	21	29	na	0	14	5-years 32 %
Nishimura et al. (2007) [10]	46	50–60	2 (1–7)	na	100	9	22	60	9	11	3-years 17 %
Smithers et al. (2007) [11]	14	60	7 (3–14)	57	86	57	14	79	7	7	3-years 24 %
D'Journo et al. (2008) [12]	24	56	2 (1–8)	na	88	41	13	50	21	25	5-years 35 %
Pinto et al. (2009) [13]	15	50	7 (2–35)	na	93	33	20	71	0	na	na
Miyata et al. (2009) [14]	33	60	8 (1–46)	39	88	30	39	na	3	12	5-years 35 %
Chao et al. (2009) [15]	27	30	na	na	63	33	15	na	na	22 (in hospital)	5-years 25 %
Tachimori et al. (2009) [16]	59	>60 Gy	na	61	85	32	31	na	na	8 (in hospital)	3-year 38 %
Morita et al. (2011) [17]	27	>60 Gy	na	33	70	30	38	59		7	5-years 51 %
Marks et al. (2012) [18]	65	50	7	na	91	23	19	35	3	5	5-years 32 %
Yoo et al. (2012) [19]	12	54	8 (2–33)	8	67	42	8	na	0	0	3-years 58 %
Schieman et al. (2013) [20]	12	30–72	31, recurrent; 7, persistent	58	83	17	17	42	8	8	5-years 17 %

R0 resection with negative margins, *nCRT* neoadjuvant chemotherapy, *na* not available, ~ survival estimated by author from Kaplan Meier survival curve

two studies was the difference significant, however. In 27 patients undergoing salvage surgery, Chao et al. reported respiratory complications in 33 % compared to 12 % in non-matched patients undergoing planned surgery after nCRT (p=0.006) [15]. Similarly, Smithers et al reported higher rates of respiratory events in 14 patients undergoing salvage surgery (57 % vs. 30 %, p<0.05) [11]. However analysis of a larger group of patients (n=65) undergoing salvage esophagectomy by Marks and colleagues showed no significant differences in rates postoperative respiratory events between salvage patients and propensity score matched controls (23 % vs. 19 %, p=0.664) [18]. Anastomotic leak was reported to occur in between 8 and 38 % of cases (mean 23 %, 15 studies). The highest leak rate (38 %) was reported by Swisher and colleagues, however, this small series of 13 patients consisted exclusively of patients who had recurrent tumors that presented at an average of 18 months after dCRT (mean dose 56 Gy) which is the longest disease free interval reported in any of the studies reviewed [6].

Nine comparative studies reported data on leak rates, all showing a higher incidence in patients undergoing salvage procedures compared to control groups and in five (all with non-matched controls) this difference reached significance. However in the matched analysis by Marks and colleagues which accounted for factors such as age, body mass index, smoking status, diabetes mellitus, clinical stage, tumor location, radiation dose, and type of esophagectomy, the difference in leak rate between salvage patients and matched controls that underwent esophagectomy after nCRT was small and not significant (19 % vs. 17 %, p=1.0) [18].

Other serious complications that were reported include gastric tube necrosis (seven cases, four studies [6, 13, 16, 18]), tracheal necrosis/fistulization (seven cases, six studies [8, 10, 13, 14, 16, 20]) and major hemorrhage (nine cases, six studies [8–10, 14, 16, 19]). The latter two complications are rarely encountered with esophagectomy performed after nCRT and it has been speculated that extensive lymphadenectomy performed in an already heavily radiated region may contribute to their occurrence. Of the bleeding complications that were reported, three were manifest by hemoptysis (all fatal), three involved the common carotid artery (fatal in two cases), and one case each involved the innominate artery (fatal), an unspecified artery (fatal) and an omental artery.

Only one of sixteen studies did not report on operative mortality [5]. Thirty-day mortality ranged between 0 and 15 % (mean 6.2 %, 12 studies) and 90 day or in-hospital mortality ranged between 0 and 25 % (mean 10.6 %, 13 studies). Eight comparative studies reported higher perioperative mortality in patients undergoing salvage esophagectomy compared to esophagectomy alone or after nCRT, however this difference was significant in only two series. Chao et al. reported 22 % in-hospital mortality in 27 salvage cases compared to 8 % in 191 patients undergoing planned esophagectomy after nCRT (p=0.03) [15], and in the series by Tachimori et al. in-hospital mortality was 8 % in the salvage group (n=59) but only 2 % in 553 patients undergoing esophagectomy without any preoperative treatment (p=0.01) [16]. In contrast, in the propensity-matched analysis by Marks and colleagues, 90-day mortality was actually higher in the neoadjuvant control group (5 %) than in the salvage group (3 %), though this difference was not significant [18].

Table 28.3 Comparative studies showing demographic, perioperative and survival outcomes

Author, year	Groups	n	Age	Upper or cervical (%)	R0 (%)	Morbidity Respiratory (%)	Leak (%)	Mortality (%)	Survival	Survival predictors
Swisher et al. (2002) [6]	Salvage	13	65	31	73	62	38	15	5-years 25 %	UVA: cT1/2 N0, R0 DFI > 12 months
	nCRT + surgery	99	61	1	na	na	7	6	~5-years 30 %	
Nakamura et al. (2004) [7]	Salvage	27	63	15	67	11	22	7	~5-years 30 %	UVA: R0
	nCRT + surgery	28	62	18	61	11	11	4	~5-years 37 %	
Tomimaru et al. (2006) [8]	Salvage	24	63	21	16	21	21	4	na	UVA: R0, cT1/2, CR; MVA: R0
	nCRT + surgery	26	65	35	23	12	8	0	na	
Smithers et al. (2007) [11]	Salvage	14	66	7	86	57	14	7	3-years 24 %	No analysis performed
	nCRT + surgery	53	60	0	91	30	8	0	3-years 53 %	
Chao et al. (2009) [15]	Salvage	27	62	29	63	33	15	29	~5-years 33 %	MVA: R0 HR 4.92 (1.08–22.4) p=.039
	nCRT + surgery	191	55	20	84	12	1	8	~5-years 22 %	
Tachimori et al. (2009) [16]	Salvage	59	63	22	85	32	31	8	3-years 38 %	UVA: R0 , cT1; MVA: cT1, M1
	Surgery only	553	62	16	91	20	25	2	3-years 61 %	
Miyata et al. (2009) [14]	Salvage	33	63	30	88	30	39	3	5-years 35 %	UVA cT1/2, cN0, R0
	nCRT + surgery	112	60	2	88	22	22	0	5-years 31 %	
Morita et al. (2011) [17]	Salvage	27	63	33	70	30	37	7	5-years 50.6 %	UVA: R0, recurrent vs. persistent tumor; MVA: R0
	nCRT + surgery	197	62	27	77	15	23	2	5-years 41 %	
	Surgery only	253	64	13	87	10	13	2	5-years 58 %	
Yoo et al. (2012) [19]	Salvage	12	63	25	67	25	8	0	3-years 58 %	UVA: cT1/T2, R0
	dCRT + recurrence	21	69	4	na	na	na	na	3-years 0 %	
Marks et al. (2012) [18]	Salvage	65	63	5	91	23	19	3	3-years 48 %	UVA: R0, early stage, DFI; MVA: None significant
	nCRT + surgery (matched)	65	63	6	99	19	17	5	3-years 57 %	

R0 resection with negative margins, *nCRT* neoadjuvant chemotherapy, *na* not available, ~ survival estimated by author from Kaplan Meier survival curve. *UVA* univariate analysis, *MVA*, multivariate analysis

Completeness of Resection

Data regarding resectability was available from 14 studies and complete resection (R0) was achieved in 50–100 % of cases (mean 79 %). Five series reported lower R0 rates for salvage cases compared to patients undergoing surgery alone or after nCRT, but in only two series was the difference significant. Chao reported R0 resection in 63 % of 27 patients undergoing salvage esophagectomy compared to 84 % in patients undergoing planned surgery (p = 0.001) and complete resection was achieved in 91 % of 65 salvage cases compared to 99 % in matched controls in the study by Marks et al. (p < 0.005) [15, 18]. Miyata et al. reported identical resectability rates among salvage and control groups and Nakamura et al. found a higher (non-significant) R0 rate in the salvage group compared to non-matched patients undergoing planned surgery after nCRT [7, 14].

Survival

Survival following salvage esophagectomy varies considerably among studies. Reported survival rates at 3 and 5 years range from 17 to 58 % and 17 to 51 %, respectively. Median survival ranging between 16 and 32 months has been reported. In a comparison of salvage esophagectomy to patients undergoing surgery alone, Tachimori reported 3-year survival rates of 38 and 61 %, respectively (p value not reported) [16]. On univariate analysis R0 resection and early T c-stage predicted improved survival, but only earlier T c-stage was predictive in multivariate analysis. Similarly, Morita and colleagues reported 3-year survival of 51 and 63 % for patients undergoing salvage esophagectomy and esophagectomy without preoperative treatment, respectively [23]. On multivariate analysis incomplete resection was an independent predictor of poor survival (5-year survival 15 % if R1/2 vs. 70 % if R0, p = 0.0118). Eight studies reported survival of patients undergoing salvage esophagectomy and those undergoing planned surgery after nCRT. With the exception of the series of 14 patients reported by Smithers et al., survival in both groups at 5 years is similar in all [11]. In five studies where survival differences were compared statistically, there were no significant differences. Seven studies reported R0 resection to be predictive of improved survival (by univariate analysis in six and multivariate in two). Earlier clinical T-stage was associated with improved survival by univariate analysis in four studies. Three reports provided information regarding outcomes of patients with residual or recurrent tumors following dCRT who did not receive salvage esophagectomy. Nakamura et al reported a 3-year survival of 17 % in patients who had salvage esophagectomy but fewer than <10 % of patients who had a partial response following dCRT survived 2 years or longer (p = 0.004) [7]. Chao et al reported 20 patients who had failed dCRT and who did not undergo salvage surgery [15]. All patients had died within 18 months, however, 5-year survival in the salvage resection group was 25 % (p = 0.003). Lastly, Yoo et al.

examined outcomes of 21 patients with recurrent or persistent disease after dCRT and showed median survival of 2.1 months for patients receiving only supportive care and 7.5 months for those who received additional chemotherapy or radiotherapy without any 3-year survivors [19]. In comparison, 58 % of patients who had salvage esophagectomy survived 3 years or more and the median survival had yet to be reached.

A single prospective phase II study evaluated the strategy of definitive chemoradiation using selective surgery as a salvage strategy for isolated local recurrence or persistent disease [21]. Forty-one patients with potentially resectable esophageal cancer (76 % T3/4) received 2 cycles of induction chemotherapy and 37 completed induction chemotherapy followed by concurrent nCRT (50.4 Gy). Twenty-one patients (57 %) underwent surgery for residual (17 patients) or recurrent (3 patients) tumor, and 1 patient because of choice. Of the 23 patients who did not receive surgery immediately following nCRT 14 had a complete clinical response, 3 had developed distant metastases, 1 was medically inoperable and 5 had died (2 from tumor progression and 3 from treatment-related causes). The 1-year survival was 71 %, longer than the 60 % 1-year survival estimated from the RTOG database and comparable to 1-year survival rates reported in other phase II trials of planned surgery after nCRT (1-year, 59–72 %) [24–26].

Recommendations

Though the majority of studies reviewed were retrospective series and contained small numbers of patients, together constituting a low level of evidence, certain recommendations regarding salvage esophagectomy can be made. First, the overall outcome of patients with residual or recurrent tumor following dCRT is poor, and the available literature points to very limited survival with either supportive care or salvage strategies using chemotherapy or radiation. In highly selected patients, salvage esophagectomy has resulted in 5-year survival rates between17 and 51 % and should therefore be considered for patients with localized recurrent or residual disease following definitive CRT. Second, the majority of studies have shown survival benefit only in patients who can achieve complete resection (R0) at salvage surgery. R0 resection can be achieved in the majority of cases, particularly when preoperative assessment does not suggest T4 status. Thus, all patients undergoing consideration for salvage surgery should undergo thorough axial, metabolic and endoscopic imaging to ensure likelihood of resectability. Third, the majority of studies reveal a trend toward higher postoperative morbidity and mortality in patients undergoing salvage esophagectomy compared to patients undergoing planned esophagectomy with or without nCRT. Patients should be counseled regarding the probability of higher surgical risk and care should be taken to perform a careful physiologic assessment of patients who are potential candidates for salvage esophagectomy.

A Personal View of the Data

Salvage esophagectomy is feasible following definitive chemoradiation, however it is often a more complex and more risky operation compared to planned esophagectomy, which typically follows within a couple of months of the completion of induction treatment. This is particularly true when recurrence occurs many months or even years after treatment when tissue planes are often obscured by post-radiation fibrosis, and the deleterious effect of radiation on microvascular structures and tissue perfusion may complicate the healing process. What the data clearly demonstrate is that complete surgical resection is so far the only treatment modality that can offer a reasonable hope of cure to patients with locally recurrent tumors. The main determinant of unresectability is invasion of esophageal tumors into non-resectable organs, chiefly the airway and the aorta. Unfortunately our current imaging modalities and endoscopic ultrasound (EUS) are much less accurate for predicting T and N stage following neoadjuvant therapy than they are for initial staging [27, 28]. Nonetheless all three should be performed prior to salvage esophagectomy. The overall accuracy of EUS for T staging ranges from 27 to 82 % compared to histopathology because of its inability to distinguish inflammation and fibrosis from tumor [29]. Nonetheless it may reveal absence of tissue plane between the esophagus and aorta, which may alert the surgeon of the possibility of T4 disease. CT imaging is important not only because of the anatomic information that it provides that help determine resectability but also because it may disclose late pulmonary effects of radiation such as pleural effusion and pulmonary fibrosis, which may influence perioperative morbidity. A recent study indicated that abutment of tumor against more than 90° of the circumference of the descending aorta correlated highly with T4 status and unresectability [30]. Integrated PET/CT imaging is vital to ensure absence of metastatic disease, and though it may offer more accurate information regarding nodal metastases, residual FDG activity in the esophagus does not usually help in the determination of tumor extent [31]. For recurrent tumors that involve the mid or upper esophagus and where airway involvement is in question, bronchoscopy is mandatory to rule out endobronchial invasion, and radial endobronchial ultrasound may occasionally be helpful in establishing tracheobronchial invasion that is not visually apparent [32].

The literature review revealed a higher than expected incidence of often fatal large vessel hemorrhage and tracheobronchial fistulization or necrosis. Apart from one case of invasion by locally recurrent tumor causes of hemorrhage were not clarified in the reports, however one might postulate that the combination of fragile irradiated vessels, vascular skeletonization, possibly subadventitial dissection during three-field nodal dissection, and possibly localized infection/abscess following anastomotic leak may have had some role to play. Similarly, aggressive lymphadenectomy with devascularization of the trachea, anastomotic leakage and iatrogenic injury during dissection in obliterated tissue planes may have resulted in many of the airway events. Careful judgment is required, especially in the setting of tumors that recur long after the completion of dCRT where the effect of radiation induced fibrosis is usually greater, balancing the benefits of an extensive lymphadenectomy with the attendant risks. At least two groups modified their techniques of lymphadenectomy over the course of their respective study periods in response to the increased risk of morbidity in salvage patients. The use of soft tissue interposition between the conduit and vascular and airway structures should always be considered. A pedicled omental flap based on branches off the right gastroepiploic artery is a simple and effective option as it will easily reach to the neck if needed. Sepesi et al. showed a reduction in leak rate from 15 to 4.6 % when omentum was used in patients undergoing salvage esophagectomy [33]. Additionally, patients requiring salvage esophagectomy are often in frail condition, either because of age and comorbidities or because of malnourishment or the side effects of concurrent chemoradiation. In compromised patients who are expected to undergo an extensive resection, staged esophagectomy and reconstruction is sometimes a useful option to lessen perioperative morbidity [17].

Conclusion

The literature supporting use of salvage esophagectomy is sparse and constitutes a low level of evidence. Nevertheless, esophagectomy has been shown to result in better survival than what can be achieved by either supportive care or non-operative strategies. Consideration should therefore be given to performing salvage esophagectomy in carefully selected patients with persistent or recurrent cancer who are physiologically fit and who have a high likelihood of being able to undergo complete resection of their tumor.

Recommendations

- Patients with persistent or locally recurrent esophageal cancer after definitive chemotherapy and radiation should be considered for salvage esophagectomy (Evidence quality low; weak recommendation).
- Potential candidates for salvage esophagectomy should undergo thorough preoperative axial, metabolic and endoscopic imaging to ensure likelihood of achieving R0 resection (Evidence quality low; weak recommendation).
- Potential candidates for salvage esophagectomy should undergo thorough physiologic and nutritional assessment and optimization prior to salvage surgery (Evidence quality low; weak recommendation).

Appendix 28.1

Database: Ovid MEDLINE(R) In-Process & Other Non-Indexed Citations and Ovid
    MEDLINE(R) <1946 to Present>

Search strategy:

1. Esophageal neoplasms/ (38568)
2. Esophagectomy/ (6211)
3. Oesophageal cancer.mp. (2178)
4. Esophageal cancer.mp. (11718)
5. Esophagectomy.mp. (8452)
6. Oesophagus.mp. (10955)
7. Esophagus.mp. (65778)
8. Esophageal adenocarcinoma.mp. (2502)
9. 1 or 2 or 3 or 4 or 5 or 6 or 7 or 8 (95127)
10. Combined modality therapy/ or chemoradiotherapy/ or chemotherapy, adjuvant/ or neoadjuvant therapy/ or radiotherapy, adjuvant/ (185157)
11. Antineoplastic combined chemotherapy protocols/ (115868)
12. Radiochemotherapy.mp. (2641)
13. Chemoradiotherapy.mp. (10841)
14. Chemotherapy.mp. (318941)
15. Radiotherapy.mp. (181917)
16. Radiation therapy.mp. (51814)
17. 10 or 11 or 12 or 13 or 14 or 15 or 16 (552048)
18. 9 and 17 (10173)
19. Salvage esophagectomy.mp. (49)
20. Salvage oesophagectomy.mp. (5)
21. Salvage surgery.mp. (1942)
22. Surgical salvage.mp. (424)
23. Salvage resection.mp. (64)
24. 19 or 20 or 21 or 22 or 23 (2374)
25. 18 and 24 (121)

After removing duplicate results, there were 115 articles published since 1987 that matched the search criteria.

References

1. Tepper J, et al. Phase III trial of trimodality therapy with cisplatin, fluorouracil, radiotherapy, and surgery compared with surgery alone for esophageal cancer: CALGB 9781. J Clin Oncol. 2008;26(7):1086–92.
2. Stahl M, et al. Chemoradiation with and without surgery in patients with locally advanced squamous cell carcinoma of the esophagus. J Clin Oncol. 2005;23(10):2310–7.
3. Bedenne L, et al. Chemoradiation followed by surgery compared with chemoradiation alone in squamous cancer of the esophagus: FFCD 9102. J Clin Oncol. 2007;25(10):1160–8.
4. van Hagen P, et al. Preoperative chemoradiotherapy for esophageal or junctional cancer. N Engl J Med. 2012;366(22):2074–84.
5. Wilson KS, Wilson AG, Dewar GJ. Curative treatment for esophageal cancer: Vancouver Island Cancer Centre experience from 1993 to 1998. Can J Gastroenterol. 2002;16(6):361–8.

6. Swisher SG, et al. Salvage esophagectomy for recurrent tumors after definitive chemotherapy and radiotherapy. J Thorac Cardiovasc Surg. 2002;123(1):175–83.

7. Nakamura T, et al. Salvage esophagectomy after definitive chemotherapy and radiotherapy for advanced esophageal cancer. Am J Surg. 2004;188(3):261–6.

8. Tomimaru Y, et al. Factors affecting the prognosis of patients with esophageal cancer undergoing salvage surgery after definitive chemoradiotherapy. J Surg Oncol. 2006;93(5):422–8.

9. Oki E, et al. Salvage esophagectomy after definitive chemoradiotherapy for esophageal cancer. Dis Esophagus. 2007;20(4):301–4.

10. Nishimura M, et al. Salvage esophagectomy following definitive chemoradiotherapy. Gen Thorac Cardiovasc Surg. 2007;55(11):461–4; discussion 464–5.

11. Smithers BM, et al. Outcomes from salvage esophagectomy post definitive chemoradiotherapy compared with resection following preoperative neoadjuvant chemoradiotherapy. Dis Esophagus. 2007;20(6):471–7.

12. D'Journo XB, et al. Indications and outcome of salvage surgery for oesophageal cancer. Eur J Cardiothorac Surg. 2008;33(6):1117–23.

13. Pinto CE, et al. Salvage esophagectomy after exclusive chemoradiotherapy: results at the Brazilian National Cancer Institute (INCA). Dis Esophagus. 2009;22(8):682–6.

14. Miyata H, et al. Salvage esophagectomy after definitive chemoradiotherapy for thoracic esophageal cancer. J Surg Oncol. 2009;100(6):442–6.

15. Chao YK, et al. Salvage surgery after failed chemoradiotherapy in squamous cell carcinoma of the esophagus. Eur J Surg Oncol. 2009;35(3):289–94.

16. Tachimori Y, et al. Salvage esophagectomy after high-dose chemoradiotherapy for esophageal squamous cell carcinoma. J Thorac Cardiovasc Surg. 2009;137(1):49–54.

17. Morita M, et al. Clinical significance of salvage esophagectomy for remnant or recurrent cancer following definitive chemoradiotherapy. J Gastroenterol. 2011;46(11):1284–91.

18. Marks JL, et al. Salvage esophagectomy after failed definitive chemoradiation for esophageal adenocarcinoma. Ann Thorac Surg. 2012;94(4):1126–32; discussion 1132–3.

19. Yoo C, et al. Salvage esophagectomy for locoregional failure after chemoradiotherapy in patients with advanced esophageal cancer. Ann Thorac Surg. 2012;94(6):1862–8.

20. Schieman C, et al. Salvage resections for recurrent or persistent cancer of the proximal esophagus after chemoradiotherapy. Ann Thorac Surg. 2013;95(2):459–63.

21. Swisher SG, et al. A Phase II study of a paclitaxel-based chemoradiation regimen with selective surgical salvage for resectable locoregionally advanced esophageal cancer: initial reporting of RTOG 0246. Int J Radiat Oncol Biol Phys. 2012;82(5):1967–72.

22. Nakamura T, et al. Multimodal treatment for lymph node recurrence of esophageal carcinoma after curative resection. Ann Surg Oncol. 2008;15(9):2451–7.

23. Morita M, et al. Two-stage operation for high-risk patients with thoracic esophageal cancer: an old operation revisited. Ann Surg Oncol. 2011;18(9):2613–21.

24. Kelsen DP, et al. Long-term results of RTOG trial 8911 (USA Intergroup 113): a random assignment trial comparison of chemotherapy followed by surgery compared with surgery alone for esophageal cancer. J Clin Oncol. 2007;25(24):3719–25.

25. Urba SG, et al. Randomized trial of preoperative chemoradiation versus surgery alone in patients with locoregional esophageal carcinoma. J Clin Oncol. 2001;19(2):305–13.

26. Minsky BD, et al. INT 0123 (Radiation Therapy Oncology Group 94-05) phase III trial of combined-modality therapy for esophageal cancer: high-dose versus standard-dose radiation therapy. J Clin Oncol. 2002;20(5):1167–74.

27. Ajani JA, et al. Clinical parameters model for predicting pathologic complete response following preoperative chemoradiation in patients with esophageal cancer. Ann Oncol. 2012;23(10):2638–42.

28. Hayashi Y, et al. A nomogram associated with high probability of malignant nodes in the surgical specimen after trimodality therapy of patients with oesophageal cancer. Eur J Cancer. 2012;48(18):3396–404.

29. Lightdale CJ, Kulkarni KG. Role of endoscopic ultrasonography in the staging and follow-up of esophageal cancer. J Clin Oncol. 2005;23(20):4483–9.

30. Piessen G, et al. Patients with locally advanced esophageal carcinoma nonresponder to radio-chemotherapy: who will benefit from surgery? Ann Surg Oncol. 2007;14(7):2036–44.
31. Monjazeb AM, et al. Outcomes of patients with esophageal cancer staged with [(1)(8)F]fluo-rodeoxyglucose positron emission tomography (FDG-PET): can postchemoradiotherapy FDG-PET predict the utility of resection? J Clin Oncol. 2010;28(31):4714–21.
32. Garrido T, et al. Endobronchial ultrasound application for diagnosis of tracheobronchial tree invasion by esophageal cancer. Clinics (Sao Paulo). 2009;64(6):499–504.
33. Sepesi B, et al. Omental reinforcement of the thoracic esophagogastric anastomosis: an analysis of leak and reintervention rates in patients undergoing planned and salvage esophagectomy. J Thorac Cardiovasc Surg. 2012;144(5):1146–50.

Chapter 29
Gastric Emptying Procedure After Esophagectomy

Puja Gaur and Scott James Swanson

Abstract A systematic review of the literature was performed to assess the necessity of a pyloric drainage procedure during an esophagectomy. Fourteen individual studies were identified from the past decade that published patient outcome after undergoing an esophagectomy either with or without a pyloric drainage procedure. Careful analysis demonstrated that pyloric drainage procedure was associated with a non-significant trend for delayed gastric emptying and biliary reflux, while not affecting the incidence of dumping. No correlation was identified between a pyloric drainage procedure and anastomotic leaks, postoperative pulmonary complications, length of hospital stay, and overall perioperative morbidity.

Keywords Esophagectomy • Pyloric drainage • Botox • Delayed gastric emptying • Dumping • Biliary reflux

Introduction

One of the most controversial debates that still exists in the field of thoracic surgery is the necessity of performing a pyloric drainage procedure for patients undergoing an esophagectomy with gastric conduit reconstruction for benign or malignant pathology. Advocates of a concomitant pyloric drainage procedure argue that it avoids delayed gastric emptying (DGE), gastric outlet obstruction (GOO), and anastomotic leak that results from bilateral truncal vagotomy and a dysfunctional pylorus. On the contrary, surgeons who do not routinely perform a pyloric drainage procedure debate

P. Gaur, MD • S.J. Swanson, MD (✉)
Division of Thoracic Surgery, Brigham and Women's Hospital,
15 Francis Street, Boston, MA 02115, USA
e-mail: pujakhaitan@hotmail.com; sjswanson@partners.org

M.K. Ferguson (ed.), *Difficult Decisions in Thoracic Surgery*,
Difficult Decisions in Surgery: An Evidence-Based Approach 1,
DOI 10.1007/978-1-4471-6404-3_29, © Springer-Verlag London 2014

that it only leads to increased biliary reflux due to negative intra-thoracic pressure and worsened dumping symptoms [1]. Studies have shown that post-esophagectomy foregut function improves with time regardless of the level of the anastomosis or pyloric drainage procedure [1, 2]. Despite conflicting views, there are a few selective surgeons who individualize the pyloric drainage procedure to patients depending on how their pylorus looks on the preoperative endoscopy. In this chapter, we will attempt to review some of the more recent studies on this controversial subject.

Search Strategy

Search Terms

Only articles published in English and in peer-reviewed journals were selected for our study. Search engines such as Embase, Cochrane Review, PubMed, and Medline (OVID) databases were explored for a span of 12 years, starting from January 1, 2001 to September 1, 2013. Keywords explored in the title or abstract were: {(o)esophagectomy} and/or {pyloroplasty, pyloromyotomy, pyloric drainage procedure, and botulinum toxin/botox}. Considering that several studies over the last decade have demonstrated comparable results between the minimally invasive and the three open surgical techniques (Ivor Lewis, transhiatal, and three-hole McKeown), we disregarded the specific technique used in each study to answer our question [3–5]. We limited our search to the last decade due to many of the technical changes that surgeons have adapted in their practice more recently such as use of staplers, minimally invasive techniques, and employing a tubularized gastric conduit as opposed to the whole stomach.

Selection of Articles

In order to have a large cohort of patients to compare, we were reasonably liberal in our selection criteria. We investigated all published studies that reported results of patients undergoing an esophagectomy with gastric interposition with or without a concomitant pyloric drainage procedure. Despite a rigorous search, we only found 14 such studies and three meta-analyses/reviews of previously published studies. Studies were limited to those involving human subjects, and, as stated before, they were not excluded because of the technique employed; i.e. open and minimally invasive approaches were deemed equally suitable for the purposes of our question. Likewise, all patients undergoing either a pyloroplasty, pyloromyotomy, pyloric digital fracture, pyloric balloon dilatation, or botulinum toxin injections or a combination thereof were defined as the 'treatment group' and the 'control group' only included those patients who did not undergo any pyloric drainage procedure. The results from these studies were tabulated and data was contrasted with the other two meta-analyses and one review published during the same time-frame.

Outcomes of Interest

The primary outcomes we reviewed were DGE/GOO, dumping symptoms, and reflux as reported in each study related to patient's clinical recovery. Secondary outcomes included anastomotic leaks, pulmonary morbidity, length of hospital stay, and perioperative mortality. DGE, dumping, and reflux were reported according to each study author's definitions. While some studies reported DGE and reflux symptoms based on radiographic and endoscopic criteria [6–8], others based their results solely on patient symptomatology and questionnaire [3, 6]. Similarly, while some studies reported anastomotic leaks as clinical leaks and others as radiographic leaks [7, 8], other studies lumped both types of leaks into one category or did not even define an anastomotic leak [3, 6], thus making data interpretation difficult among studies. Pulmonary complications and symptoms of dumping were also specific to study authors' definitions.

Data Extraction

During our initial search, a total of 63 abstracts and papers were reviewed. After elimination of duplicate studies, case reports, case series, and review articles, 17 full studies were selected meeting our selection criteria [3, 6–21]. Other studies were removed for the following reasons: lack of substantial data and measurable outcome, mere description of a particular technique, unavailability of study, multiple publications of single patient group, and lack of gastric conduit use (such as colon or jejunal interposition). Finally, we excluded the three meta-analyses from our analysis to avoid bias and duplication of data from already selected studies [9, 10, 20]. This resulted in a final total of 14 studies for our review.

Results

The 2002 meta-analysis review by Urschel et al. reviewed nine randomized controlled trials (RCTs) published between the years 1984–1996 and the 2007 meta-analysis by Khan et al. concluded results from 6 RCTs between 1986 and 1996 and Urschel et al.'s 2002 meta-analysis [9, 10]. Both of these meta-analyses favored pyloric drainage. They both concluded that a pyloric drainage procedure reduces the incidence of GOO and speeds up gastric emptying. All other complications including esophagogastric anastomotic leak, pulmonary morbidity, and operative mortality were comparable between the two groups in both meta-analyses.

On the contrary, the 14 studies included in our study (summarized in Table 29.1) were published between the years 2001 and 2011. The majority of these studies were retrospective in nature and four of them were prospective. None of the studies were randomized, although one study from MD Anderson Cancer Center did

Table 29.1 Patient demographics as reported in the 14 studies and methods of measuring outcomes

Study	Design	Patient group	Primary outcomes	Secondary outcomes	Level of evidence
Ludwig et al. [11]	Prospective	48 patients No pyloric drainage	No DGE 25 % reflux 8.3 % dumping	38 % anastomotic stricture	Moderate
Maier et al. [12]	Prospective	18 patients No pyloric drainage	12 reflux	12 esophagitis	Low
Lee et al. [19]	Retrospective	50 patients 46 finger disruption 4 pyloroplasty	37.5 % DGE		Moderate
Kent et al. [15]	Retrospective	12 patients All botox injections	No DGE	No aspiration pneumonia	Low
Lanuti et al. [8]	Retrospective	242 patients 83 no drainage 159 pyloromyotomy	DGE/GOO 9.6 % vs. 18.2 % P: 0.078	Anastomotic leak No difference Pulmonary complications 27.7 % vs. 19.5 % P: 0.15 Respiratory failure 8.4 % vs. 4.4 % P: 0.20 Length of stay 10 vs. 11 days P: 0.18 Perioperative mortality 2.4 % vs. 2.5 % P: 0.96	Moderate

Maffetone et al. [17]	Retrospective	35 patients Whole stomach and no pyloric drainage	No DGE		Low
Palmes et al. [7]	Retrospective	198 patients 46 no drainage 152 pyloromyotomy or pyloroplasty	Reflux 0 % vs. 14.9 % P: 0.069	Esophagitis 10.3 vs. 34.5 % $P < 0.05$ Anastomotic leak 17.4 % vs. 14.5 % $P > 0.05$ Aspiration 13 % vs. 15.8 % $P > 0.05$ Length of stay 21.7 vs. 23.2, 16 days $P > 0.05$ Perioperative mortality 2.2 % vs. 2.6 % $P > 0.05$	Moderate
Kim et al. [16]	Retrospective	257 patients All finger fracture	8 % GOO	21 % anastomotic stricture	Moderate

(continued)

Table 29.1 (continued)

Study	Design	Patient group	Primary outcomes	Secondary outcomes	Level of evidence
Cerfolio et al. [13]	Retrospective	221 patients	DGE on POD#4	Stricture-dilated	Moderate
		54 no drainage	96 %	7.4 %	
		71 pyloromyotomy	93 %	8.4 %	
		28 pyloroplasty	96 %	14 %	
		68 botox	59 %	7.3 %	
			Bile reflux	Anastomotic leak	
			9 %	1	
			20 %	0	
			38 %	0	
			6 %	0	
				Aspiration/ pneumonia	
				22 %	
				14 %	
				32 %	
				13 %	
				Mortality	
				4 %	
				6 %	
				4 %	
				4.4 %	
				Length of stay	
				8.2 days	
				9.5 days	
				8.7 days	
				7.3 days	
Martin et al. [18]	Prospective	45 patients	4.4 % early DGE		Moderate
		All botox injections	6.7 % late DGE		

Deng et al. [14]	Prospective	78 patients 30 no drainage 48 digital fracture	Early DGE 13.3 % vs. 0 %	Anastomotic leaks 23.3 % vs. 16.7 % Cardiopulmonary complication 10 % vs. 4.2 %	Moderate
Nguyen et al. [6]	Retrospective	140 patients 109 no drainage 31 pyloroplasty	DGE/GOO 5.5 % vs. 3.2 % P: NR	Leak rate 9.6 % vs. 9.7 % P: NS	Moderate
Lanuti et al. [21]	Retrospective	436 patients 257 no drainage 179 pyloromyotomy	GOO 18 % vs. 28 % P: 0.01		Moderate
Mehran et al. [3]	Retrospective	88 patients 44 no drainage 44 pyloric drainage	DGE/GOO 11.3 % vs. 2.2 % P: 0.219 Dumping No difference Reflux score 5.5 vs. 3.5 P: 0.021	Anastomotic leaks 25 % vs. 13.6 % P: 0.267 Pulmonary complication 31.8 % vs. 34 % P: 1.00	Moderate

Abbreviations: *DGE* delayed gastric emptying, *GOO* gastric outlet obstruction, *POD* postoperative day

perform a propensity score-matched analysis [3]. Indeed, over the last decade, no prospective randomized controlled study has been performed to compare the advantage of pyloric drainage procedure versus no drainage procedure. The three primary outcomes that we focused on for the purposes of our study were: DGE/GOO, dumping, and reflux. While 12 of the 14 studies evaluated how a pyloric drainage procedure did or did not negatively impact gastric emptying, only one of them was significant with a p-value of 0.01 [21]. Overall, there was no clear trend regarding whether a pyloric drainage procedure alleviated GOO or not. Only two studies evaluated dumping and while one study found that a pyloric drainage procedure did not impact dumping based on a questionnaire [3], another study highlighted how 8.3 % of its 48 patients reported symptoms of dumping after no pyloric drainage procedure [11]. Lastly, we reviewed each study for reflux with or without a pyloric drainage procedure. Overall, 5 of the 14 studies had evaluated reflux in their patient cohort; while three studies reported a significantly high association of reflux with patients not undergoing a pyloric drainage procedure [3, 11, 12], two of the comparative studies that directly compared a control and a treatment group strongly associated reflux with patients who had undergone a pyloric drainage procedure [7, 13].

We also analyzed the studies for secondary outcomes including development of stricture requiring dilatation, anastomotic leaks, pulmonary morbidity, length of hospital stay, and perioperative mortality. While the treatment arm favored lesser incidence of anastomotic leak and lower risk of post-operative pulmonary complications, it was associated with longer length of hospital stay and higher overall perioperative mortality.

Summary and Recommendations

Despite the fact that pyloric drainage was once routinely performed during an esophagectomy and gastric conduit reconstruction, its role has been questioned over the last decade. In this chapter, we sought to determine the advantages and disadvantages of performing a pyloric drainage procedure during an esophagectomy in the present era using more recent studies.

Because the two meta-analyses by Urschel et al. (2002) and Khan et al. (2007) reviewed data from the 1980s and 1990s and both of them used a majority of the same studies with inherent limitations [9, 10], we recently published a review of the more recent literature on this issue of performing a concomitant pyloric drainage procedure or not during an esophagectomy [20]. We had looked into the literature and only selected those individual studies that compared two groups of patients undergoing an esophagectomy with or without a pyloric drainage procedure. We concluded that a pyloric drainage procedure is unwarranted and can be safely omitted. We explained our discrepant results from the four studies that we used in our paper from the two meta-analyses published in 2002 and 2007 by stating that some of the studies [22–24] used for the two meta-analysis utilized a whole stomach as the gastric conduit, which is now known to result in gastric stasis and DGE due to gastric denervation [25]. In the more recent four individual studies performed, a tubularized gastric conduit was utilized that eliminates the 'baggy' reservoir.

In this chapter, we extended our search and included all cohort studies, and when we carefully analyzed the data from the 14 studies in Table 29.1, we found that pyloric drainage procedure was once again associated with DGE/GOO; although that is counter-intuitive, no explanation was given in any of the studies. Possible explanations could include early postoperative edema and long-term stricture or scar formation resulting in delayed emptying from the gastric conduit. Similarly, the biliary reflux associated with a pyloric drainage procedure could be explained by lack of sphincter control and negative intrathoracic pressure predisposing a patient to aspiration. Although these are merely conjectures to explain real-life phenomenon, they certainly need to be studied and proven and they serve to explain the data.

A Personal View of the Data

Advocates of a pyloric drainage procedure emphasize how not performing the drainage procedure merely negates the ultimate goal of an esophagectomy in ridding the patient of obstructive symptoms. However opponents, and likewise we, claim that the esophagectomy itself has palliated the patient of his symptoms. We feel that a pyloric drainage procedure puts patients at risk for potential complications of DGE/GOO and biliary reflux in addition to all the risks and complications associated with the esophagectomy itself. Therefore, at our institution, we favor not performing a pyloric drainage procedure unless clinically indicated, such as in patients with a severely fibrotic or radiated pylorus. Given that we only see a fraction of patients ever developing gastric emptying problems after an esophagectomy and that most of these patients either regain foregut function with time [26] or are managed with prokinetic agents, botox injections, and/or endoscopic dilations [6, 27, 28], a pyloric drainage procedure seems to be less warranted. On the contrary, an alternative approach is to perform preoperative endoscopic pyloric balloon dilatation 1–2 weeks prior to an esophagectomy to reduce the risk of subsequent pyloric stenosis as suggested in a recent publication by Swanson et al. [29].

In our opinion, there is no conclusive evidence that routine addition of a pyloric drainage procedure leads to equivalent or better outcomes following esophagectomy. Prospectively designed, randomized studies would be needed to justify its omission with established criteria for defining gastric emptying, biliary reflux, anastomotic leak, and pulmonary complications where patients are propensity score-matched for smoking history, diabetic gastroparesis, functional status, neoadjuvant chemoradiation therapy, gastric conduit width, surgical technique (open vs MIE and stapled vs hand-sewn anastomosis), and level of anastomosis (chest vs neck). Additionally, a standardized method of measuring and documenting use of promotility agents, vocal cord injury resulting in aspiration, reflux, DGE/GOO, and dumping should be used, whether that involves a questionnaire of patient symptoms, time to nutritional independence, routine follow-up endoscopies and/or need for dilations, radioisotope nuclear, or fluoroscopic/pH probe studies so that justified conclusions are drawn.

Recommendation

• A pyloric drainage procedure during an esophagectomy with gastric interposition is not routinely indicated. (Evidence quality low; weak recommendation)

References

1. Velanovich V. Esophagogastrectomy without pyloroplasty. Dis Esophagus. 2003;16(3):243–5.
2. Berger AC, Bloomenthal A, Weksler B, Evans N, Chojnacki KA, Yeo CJ, et al. Oncologic efficacy is not compromised, and may be improved with minimally invasive esophagectomy. J Am Coll Surg. 2011;212(4):560–6; discussion 566–8. Epub 2011/04/06.
3. Mehran R, Rice D, El-Zein R, Huang JL, Vaporciyan A, Goodyear A, et al. Minimally invasive esophagectomy versus open esophagectomy, a symptom assessment study. Dis Esophagus. 2011;24(3):147–52.
4. Luketich JD, Alvelo-Rivera M, Buenaventura PO, Christie NA, McCaughan JS, Litle VR, et al. Minimally invasive esophagectomy: outcomes in 222 patients. Ann Surg. 2003; 238(4):486–94; discussion 494–5.
5. Verhage RJ, Hazebroek EJ, Boone J, Van Hillegersberg R. Minimally invasive surgery compared to open procedures in esophagectomy for cancer: a systematic review of the literature. Minerva Chir. 2009;64(2):135–46.
6. Nguyen NT, Dholakia C, Nguyen XM, Reavis K. Outcomes of minimally invasive esophagectomy without pyloroplasty: analysis of 109 cases. Am Surg. 2010;76(10):1135–8.
7. Palmes D, Weilinghoff M, Colombo-Benkmann M, Senninger N, Bruewer M. Effect of pyloric drainage procedures on gastric passage and bile reflux after esophagectomy with gastric conduit reconstruction. Langenbecks Arch Surg. 2007;392(2):135–41.
8. Lanuti M, de Delva PE, Wright CD, Gaissert HA, Wain JC, Donahue DM, et al. Post-esophagectomy gastric outlet obstruction: role of pyloromyotomy and management with endoscopic pyloric dilatation. Eur J Cardiothorac Surg. 2007;31(2):149–53.
9. Urschel JD, Blewett CJ, Young JE, Miller JD, Bennett WF. Pyloric drainage (pyloroplasty) or no drainage in gastric reconstruction after esophagectomy: a meta-analysis of randomized controlled trials. Dig Surg. 2002;19(3):160–4.
10. Khan OA, Manners J, Rengarajan A, Dunning J. Does pyloroplasty following esophagectomy improve early clinical outcomes? Interact Cardiovasc Thorac Surg. 2007;6(2):247–50.
11. Ludwig DJ, Thirlby RC, Low DE. A prospective evaluation of dietary status and symptoms after near-total esophagectomy without gastric emptying procedure. Am J Surg. 2001; 181(5):454–8.
12. Maier A, Tomaselli F, Sankin O, Anegg U, Fell B, Renner H, et al. Acid-related diseases following retrosternal stomach interposition. Hepato-Gastroenterol. 2001;48(39):899–902.
13. Cerfolio RJ, Bryant AS, Canon CL, Dhawan R, Eloubeidi MA. Is botulinum toxin injection of the pylorus during Ivor-Lewis esophagogastrectomy the optimal drainage strategy? J Thorac Cardiovasc Surg. 2009;137(3):565–72.
14. Deng B, Tan QY, Jiang YG, Zhao YP, Zhou JH, Chen GC, et al. Prevention of early delayed gastric emptying after high-level esophagogastrostomy by "pyloric digital fracture". World J Surg. 2010;34(12):2837–43.
15. Kent MS, Pennathur A, Fabian T, McKelvey A, Schuchert MJ, Luketich JD, et al. A pilot study of botulinum toxin injection for the treatment of delayed gastric emptying following esophagectomy. Surg Endosc. 2007;21(5):754–7.
16. Kim JH, Lee HS, Kim MS, Lee JM, Kim SK, Zo JI. Balloon dilatation of the pylorus for delayed gastric emptying after esophagectomy. Eur J Cardiothorac Surg. 2008;33(6):1105–11.

17. Maffettone V, Rossetti G, Rambaldi P, Russo F, Cuccurullo V, Brusciano L, et al. Whole stomach transposition without gastric drainage procedure: a good surgical option to restore digestive continuity after esophagectomy. Int Surg. 2007;92(2):73–7.

18. Martin JT, Federico JA, McKelvey AA, Kent MS, Fabian T. Prevention of delayed gastric emptying after esophagectomy: a single center's experience with botulinum toxin. Ann Thorac Surg. 2009;87(6):1708–13; discussion 1713–4.

19. Lee HS, Kim MS, Lee JM, Kim SK, Kang KW, Zo JI. Intrathoracic gastric emptying of solid food after esophagectomy for esophageal cancer. Ann Thorac Surg. 2005;80(2):443–7. Epub 2005/07/26.

20. Gaur P, Swanson SJ. Should we continue to drain the pylorus in patients undergoing an esophagectomy? Dis Esophagus; 2013. Epub 2013/02/28.

21. Lanuti M, DeDelva P, Morse CR, Wright CD, Wain JC, Gaissert HA, et al. Management of delayed gastric emptying after esophagectomy with endoscopic balloon dilatation of the pylorus. Ann Thorac Surg. 2011;91(4):1019–24.

22. Cheung HC, Siu KF, Wong J. Is pyloroplasty necessary in esophageal replacement by stomach? A prospective, randomized controlled trial. Surgery. 1987;102(1):19–24.

23. Mannell A, McKnight A, Esser JD. Role of pyloroplasty in the retrosternal stomach: results of a prospective, randomized, controlled trial. Br J Surg. 1990;77(1):57–9.

24. Fok M, Cheng SW, Wong J. Pyloroplasty versus no drainage in gastric replacement of the esophagus. Am J Surg. 1991;162(5):447–52.

25. Bemelman WA, Taat CW, Slors JF, van Lanschot JJ, Obertop H. Delayed postoperative emptying after esophageal resection is dependent on the size of the gastric substitute. J Am Coll Surg. 1995;180(4):461–4.

26. Collard JM, Romagnoli R, Otte JB, Kestens PJ. The denervated stomach as an esophageal substitute is a contractile organ. Ann Surg. 1998;227(1):33–9.

27. Hill AD, Walsh TN, Hamilton D, Freyne P, O'Hare N, Byrne PJ, et al. Erythromycin improves emptying of the denervated stomach after oesophagectomy. Br J Surg. 1993;80(7):879–81.

28. Bemelman WA, Brummelkamp WH, Bartelsman JF. Endoscopic balloon dilation of the pylorus after esophagogastrostomy without a drainage procedure. Surg Gynecol Obstet. 1990; 170(5):424–6.

29. Swanson EW, Swanson SJ, Swanson RS. Endoscopic pyloric balloon dilatation obviates the need for pyloroplasty at esophagectomy. Surg Endosc. 2012;26(7):2023–8.

Chapter 30
Postoperative Adjuvant Therapy After Resection of Regionally Advanced Esophageal Cancer

Elizabeth Won and David H. Ilson

Abstract For regionally advanced esophageal cancer, surgical resection alone has been shown to be inadequate due to the systemic nature of the disease. Effective local radiotherapy and systemic chemotherapy, directed at micrometastases and added to surgical resection, may lead to increased survival. Studies have evaluated preoperative, perioperative, and postoperative treatment approaches in combination with surgery. This chapter will discuss the evidence for postoperative radiotherapy, chemotherapy, and chemoradiotherapy and discuss areas of controversy as well as of ongoing research.

Keywords Postoperative therapy • Adjuvant therapy • Regionally advanced • Locally advanced • Esophageal cancer

Introduction

Esophagectomy remains the cornerstone treatment of clinically localized esophageal cancer. While huge progress has been made in refining preoperative staging, patient selection, operative technique, and postoperative care, the overall survival for patients undergoing surgical resection alone remains poor. The failure of surgery alone is attributed to the systemic nature of disease. Effective local radiotherapy and systemic chemotherapy – directed at micrometastases and added to surgical resection – may lead to increased survival.

Multiple clinical trials have addressed the preferred treatment sequence in managing locally advanced esophageal cancer. In Western countries, combined

E. Won, MD • D.H. Ilson, MD, PhD (✉)
Gastrointestinal Oncology Service, Department of Medicine,
Memorial Sloan Kettering Cancer Center,
300 East 66th Street, New York, NY 10065, USA
e-mail: ilsond@mskcc.org

M.K. Ferguson (ed.), *Difficult Decisions in Thoracic Surgery*,
Difficult Decisions in Surgery: An Evidence-Based Approach 1,
DOI 10.1007/978-1-4471-6404-3_30, © Springer-Verlag London 2014

preoperative chemoradiotherapy has become a preferred preoperative strategy for locally advanced esophageal cancer in the United States for both squamous cell and adenocarcinoma. However, upfront surgical resection followed by postoperative adjuvant therapy remains a standard approach in East Asian countries, in particular for adenocarcinomas of the gastric cardia or more distal stomach. This upfront surgical approach allows for the surgeon to avoid the potential increased operative morbidity after neoadjuvant therapy and for more pathologic staging of disease permitting more accurate selection of appropriate high risk patients for postoperative therapy. The role of postoperative therapy, in particular for esophageal squamous cell and adenocarcinoma, however, remains less clear.

This chapter will discuss the evidence for postoperative radiotherapy, chemotherapy, and chemoradiotherapy after for locally advanced cancer (tumors higher than T1 or node positive) and discuss areas of controversy as well as of ongoing research.

Search Strategy

A PubMed search was conducted with the search terms Chemotherapy, Adjuvant "[Mesh] OR "Radiotherapy" AND "Esophageal Neoplasms" [Mesh] AND postoperative. A Scopus database search was conducted with the search terms [Postoperative OR adjuvant] AND ("regionally advanced" OR "locally advanced") AND esophageal. All titles and abstracts from 1990 to 2013 were scanned and appropriate citations reviewed for meta-analyses, systemic reviews, and eligible clinical trials. Only English-language literature was included in the search. A manual search was made to identify relevant articles published in the New England Journal of Medicine and Journal of Clinical Oncology. Recommendations given are graded according to the GRADE system.

Postoperative Radiotherapy

There are five randomized clinical trials that have evaluated postoperative radiotherapy and surgery compared to surgery alone in esophagus cancer [1–5]. All studies included only squamous cell histology. The studies included a heterogenous patient population, with one study including patients with celiac lymph nodes [4, 5] and R1 resections [2]. Varying radiation doses with differing fractionation were utilized in the studies, administered 6–12 weeks following surgery. Three showed no survival benefit for adjuvant radiation compared to surgery alone [1, 3, 5], regardless of lymph node status. In the study by Fok et al. [2], worse survival outcomes in the postoperative radiotherapy group were seen compared to surgery alone (median survival 15.2 months versus 8.7 months). The shorter survival in the radiation group was attributed to radiation-related toxicity deaths. Another trial showed improved quality of life in the surgery-only arm compared with the adjuvant radiation arm due to postradiation complications [4]. The rate of local recurrence with radiotherapy was lower in three of the trials [1, 2, 5] but in two of these trials [1, 2], this benefit was achieved at the expense of increased morbidity.

There is one meta-analysis published in 2004 which looked at adjuvant therapy for resectable esophageal cancer authored by Malthaner et al. on behalf of the Gastrointestinal Cancer Disease Site Group [6]. In the pooled analysis of five trials that reported 1-year mortality data, there was no significant difference in the risk of mortality with postoperative radiotherapy and surgery compared to surgery alone (RR 1.23; 95 % CT, 0.95–1.59, p=0.11).

Postoperative Chemotherapy

There are only a few randomized studies comparing postoperative chemotherapy and surgery to surgery alone. All studies used cisplatin-based regimens. Pouliquen et al. found no improvement in survival with adjuvant cisplatin and 5-Fluorauracil (5-FU) compared to surgery alone in patients with squamous cell carcinoma [7]. Patients with node negative disease at time of resection were excluded from the study. Quality of life parameters was similar between both groups.

One recent non-randomized study suggests an overall survival benefit to adjuvant chemotherapy. The ECOG8296 trial was a multicenter phase II trial of postoperative paclitaxel and cisplatin in patients with resected T2 node positive or T3–4 any node status adenocarcinoma distal esophagus, gastroesophageal junction (GEJ) or gastric cardia with a R0 resection [8]. The primary endpoint of 2-year survival was met, with the 2-year survival rate 60 %, compared to historical control rate of 38 % (95 % CI, 46–73 %, one-sided p=0.0008). The authors concluded that adjuvant paclitaxel and cisplatin may improve survival in completely resected patients.

The Japanese Clinical Oncology Group (JCOG) has conducted a series of trials leading to two large phase III studies evaluating postoperative chemotherapy in squamous cell esophageal cancer. The JCOG8806 study showed no survival benefit of adjuvant cisplatin and vindesine compared to surgery alone, (p=0.60), even with lymph node stratification [9]. The subsequent JCOG9204 randomized 242 patients to surgery alone or surgery followed by postoperative cisplatin and 5-FU for 2 cycles [10]. The primary endpoint of disease free survival (DFS) was met, with a benefit seen in the postoperative chemotherapy group with the 5-year DFS 55 % in this arm versus 45 % with surgery alone (p=0.037). There was no difference in overall survival in the two groups (p=0.13). In the subgroup analysis, the node negative patients did not have a DFS benefit from postoperative chemotherapy and a benefit was seen only for node positive patients.

The above results led to a follow up study (JCOG 9907, Ando et al.) to evaluate the optimal timing for chemotherapy (preoperative vs postoperative) in patients with locally advanced SCC [11]. Patients were randomized to either preoperative chemotherapy or postoperative chemotherapy with 5-FU/cisplatin. Patients had CT or MRI staging; endoscopic ultrasound staging was recommended but not required for clinical staging. All patients underwent transthoracic esophagectomy with extended lymphadenectomy. In the postoperative chemotherapy arm, those with pathologic node-negative disease did not receive chemotherapy because the prior JCOG9204 study discussed above did not find a benefit of chemotherapy in the subset of node-negative patients [10]. Due to this study design, 140 patients received all the preoperative chemotherapy, while only 81 patients completed the prescribed postoperative therapy (49 % randomized to postoperative arm). The primary endpoint of progression-free survival was not met. The authors concluded that overall survival was superior with preoperative chemotherapy with a 5-year survival of 55 % in this group versus 43 % in the postoperative arm (p=0.04), despite the imbalance in treatment arms. Further confirming these results was the observation that a survival benefit for preoperative chemotherapy was limited only to patients with node negative disease, in contrast to their prior observation of a benefit for postoperative chemotherapy only in node positive disease.

Postoperative Chemoradiotherapy

The Intergroup 0116 (INT-0116) was a randomized phase III trial conducted to compare observation versus adjuvant chemoradiation following curative gastric adenocarcinoma resection [12]. The chemoradiation arm received post-operative combination of bolus 5-FU and leucovorin and 45 Gy of radiation. 20 % had gastroesophageal junction (GEJ) tumors. The results showed an improved median survival in the chemoradiation group of 36 months compared to 27 months in the surgery-only group (HR1.35, 95 % CI, 1.23–1.86; p<0.001). In the chemoradiotherapy group, grade 3 and 4 toxicity rates were high and occurred in 41 % and 32 % of patients, respectively. In addition, 1 % (3 patients) suffered toxicity-related deaths and 31 % did not complete treatment due to toxicity. A major criticism of this trial was the limited extent of surgical resection in most cases. D2 dissection was only performed in 10 % of patients; 36 % had D1 resection, and the majority of patients (54 %) had D0 surgery. The benefit of adjuvant chemoradiotherapy was limited only to reducing local disease recurrence, further calling into question the adequacy of surgical resection on this trial.

The subsequent CALBG 80101study was designed to compare the INT-0116 regimen to a regimen of epirubicin, cisplatin, and 5-FU (ECF) in combination with radiation (45 Gy) in patients with resected gastric and GEJ adenocarcinoma. In the preliminary results presented at the 2011 meeting of the American Society of Clinical Oncology (ASCO), toxicity was increased in the ECF arm with 40 % experiencing grade 4 toxicity compared to 25 % in the 5-FU arm. There was no significant improvement in median overall survival (HR 1.03. 95 % CI, 0.80–1.34, p=0.80) with the more intense ECF regimen. The study was not powered for non-inferiority. Because nearly 25 % of patients had GEJ cancers, the results from this study reinforce a survival benefit for postoperative 5-FU and radiotherapy but indicate no benefit for the use of cisplatin based combination chemotherapy over 5-FU alone when combined with radiotherapy.

Recommendations

Postoperative radiation for resected esophageal cancer does not improve overall survival compared to surgery alone. The use of postoperative radiation may be harmful with increased rates of toxicity. We strongly recommend against the use of postoperative radiation alone.

The efficacy of postoperative chemotherapy in improving overall survival has not been established in a randomized trial for patients with esophageal cancer and cannot be recommended as standard therapy. In patients who have not received any preoperative therapy, postoperative chemotherapy may lead to improvements in disease-free survival, but not overall survival, in patients with node positive, squamous cell histology. In T2 node positive or T3-T4 distal or GEJ adenocarcinoma, the phase II data of adjuvant paclitaxel and cisplatin are promising but merit further investigation. The recent positive data for preoperative combined carboplatin, paclitaxel, and radiotherapy followed by surgery in esophageal squamous cell and adenocarcinoma argue for a benefit of taxane based adjuvant therapy in esophageal cancer [13]. The data favoring use of the adjuvant chemotherapy in gastric cancer, largely from Asian trials, cannot clearly be extrapolated to the treatment of esophageal cancer.

The available evidence for the use of postoperative chemoradiation for adenocarcinoma histology comes from two U.S. phase III randomized trials involving patients with gastric cancer that included patients with distal esophageal and GEJ adenocarcinoma (quality of evidence moderate). Postoperative chemoradiation has been shown to improve overall survival in patients with T3-T4a tumors and node positive T1-T2 tumors, however is associated with significant toxicity with the published INT-0116 regimen. This approach can be carefully considered in a select high-risk patient population. In CALBG 80101, the addition of cisplatin and epirubicin to conventional postoperative 5-FU and radiotherapy did not improve outcome compared to 5-FU based chemotherapy alone.

A Personal View of the Data

The recommendations above are made on the basis of published evidence. The evidence is dependent on the quality of surgery and radiotherapy regimen at the time the studies were undertaken. Pre and perioperative therapy studies (INT 0113, OEO2 [14], MAGIC [15], and the FNCLCC/FFCD trials [16]) which have shown inconsistent benefits in survival compared to surgery were not included for discussion in this chapter. All the studies included in this review are strictly post-operative studies, in which the pathological staging was available for patients. The exception is the JCOG9907 which compared preoperative to postoperative chemotherapy. Despite its substantial problems this study led to a new standard approach of treatment in Japan, and therefore important to address in this review.

The data on postoperative adjuvant therapy for locally advanced esophageal cancer are limited and the potential benefits of postoperative therapy are less clear compared to the efficacy of treatments seen in the neoadjuvant setting. In the United States and Western Europe, the preferred approach for locally advanced esophageal and gastroesophageal junction cancers has become neoadjuvant chemotherapy or chemoradiotherapy prior to surgical resection. While pre- and peri-operative chemotherapy have been shown to improve outcomes, the very low rate of pathologic complete response rates and inconsistent impact on curative resection rates in esophageal/GEJ cancers makes us favor neoadjuvant chemoradiotherapy for this patient population. The significant benefits of the CROSS trial, employing preoperative carboplatin, paclitaxel, and radiotherapy, underpin our recommendation for neoadjuvant chemoradiotherapy for patients with locally advanced (T2 node positive, T3-T4 node any). In this study, patients with esophageal or GEJ cancer randomized to the chemoradiotherapy-surgery arm (carboplatin, paclitaxel, and concurrent radiation 41.4 Gy) had a significant survival benefit (49.4 months versus 24.0 months, HR 0.657; 95 % CI, 0.495–0871, p=0.003) compared to patients who received surgery alone. The pathological complete response rates seen in the chemoradiotherapy-surgery arm were among the highest reported in the literature, 49 % in squamous histology and 23 % in adenocarcinoma. Curative resection rates were increased from 69 % with surgery alone to 92 % with preoperative therapy.

We recognize, however, that there are geographic and institutional differences in the management of regionally advanced esophageal cancer. In Asia, the upfront surgery with extended lymphadenectomy remains the common treatment approach for both esophageal and gastric cancer. It is clear that surgery alone is not adequate in esophageal cancer due to the systemic nature of this disease. The data on adjuvant therapy after resection have not been as robust as the preoperative evidence. Postoperative chemotherapy alone has not been shown to improve survival in a randomized phase III trial.

The study design and results of the JCOG9907 phase III trial comparing preoperative to postoperative need to be analyzed critically. The study design precluded over 50 % of patients randomized to the postoperative chemotherapy arm from getting treatment because node-negative patients were felt not to benefit from treatment, based on a subset analysis from a prior study. Consequently, the analysis is comparing node positive and node negative patients who received preoperative therapy to only node positive patients treated with postoperative therapy. In addition, the primary endpoint of progression-free survival was not met, but the overall survival was in favor of the preoperative group. Due to this imbalance in treatment arms and the study design, we cannot agree with the authors' conclusion that this study establishes the superiority of preoperative chemotherapy to postoperative chemotherapy in squamous cell carcinomas of the esophagus.

The INT 0116 study did show an overall survival benefit in patients who received adjuvant chemoradiation compared to surgery alone in adenocarcinoma. The long-term followup of the study shows a persistent overall and relapse-free survival benefit in the chemoradiation group; and the data suggests the reduction of loco-regional failure (LRF) may account for the majority of relapse reduction. However, the following points need to be made about this study: (1) The majority of patients in this study had inadequate surgical resection, with 54 % having less than a D1 dissection. (2) The regimen was toxic and not well tolerated, with almost one-third of patients unable to complete the full treatment course. We would not recommend the chemotherapy as administrated in the original study, and recommend infusional 5-FU or capecitabine to be used in place of bolus 5-FU and leucovorin. Robust younger patients with high risk, node positive or T3-T4 tumors adenocarcinoma who did not undergo preoperative therapy can be considered for adjuvant chemoradiation based on this data. Adding cisplatin and epirubicin to 5-FU adjuvant therapy did not improve outcome compared to 5-FU alone.

Further randomized trials comparing chemotherapy with or without radiotherapy will shed greater light on the role of radiotherapy, and such trials are ongoing both in the pre- and postoperative setting. The ongoing TOPGEAR trial being conducted in Australia compares perioperative chemotherapy with or without preoperative radiotherapy in esophageal and gastric adenocarcinoma. The about to be completed CRITIS trial conducted in Sweden and Netherlands compares perioperative chemotherapy with or without postoperative radiotherapy in GEJ and gastric adenocarcinoma. These studies, hopefully with accurate pre-therapy clinical staging including endoscopic ultrasound, as well as hopefully uniform high quality surgical resections will help answer the clinically important questions to help further define the optimal treatment paradigm for regionally advanced esophageal cancer.

Recommendations

- We recommend against postoperative radiation therapy as it does not improve overall survival in squamous cell carcinoma and may be harmful compared to surgical resection alone. (Evidence quality high; strong recommendation)
- We recommend against the routine use of postoperative adjuvant chemotherapy as it has not been shown to improve survival compared to surgery alone. (Evidence quality moderate; weak recommendation)
- For younger, robust patients who did not get preoperative treatment with T3-T4, or node positive adenocarcinoma, postoperative chemoradiation can be considered. (Evidence quality moderate; weak recommendation)

References

1. Ténière P, Hay JM, Fingerhut A, Fagniez PL. Postoperative radiation therapy does not increase survival after curative resection for squamous cell carcinoma of the middle and lower esophagus as shown by a multicenter controlled trial. French University Association for Surgical Research. Surg Gynecol Obstet. 1991;173:123–30.
2. Fok M, Sham JS, Choy D, Cheng SW, Wong J. Postoperative radiotherapy for carcinoma of the esophagus: a prospective, randomized controlled study. Surgery. 1993;113:138–47.
3. Fok MMJ, Law SYK, Wong J. Prospective randomised study in the treatment of oesophageal carcinoma. Asian J Surg. 1994;17:223–9.
4. Zieren HU, Müller JM, Jacobi CA, Pichlmaier H, Müller RP, Staar S. Adjuvant postoperative radiation therapy after curative resection of squamous cell carcinoma of the thoracic esophagus: a prospective randomized study. World J Surg. 1995;19:444–9.
5. Xiao ZF, Yang ZY, Liang J, Miao YJ, Wang M, Yin WB, Gu XZ, Zhang DC, Zhang RG, Wang LJ. Value of radiotherapy after radical surgery for esophageal carcinoma: a report of 495 patients. Ann Thorac Surg. 2003;75:331–6.
6. Malthaner RA, Wong RK, Rumble RB, Zuraw L, Members of the Gastrointestinal Cancer Disease Site Group of Cancer Care Ontario's Program in Evidence-based Care. Neoadjuvant or adjuvant therapy for resectable esophageal cancer: a systematic review and meta-analysis. BMC Med. 2004;2:35.
7. Pouliquen X, Levard H, Hay JM, McGee K, Fingerhut A, Langlois-Zantin O. 5-fluorouracil and cisplatin therapy after palliative surgical resection of squamous cell carcinoma of the esophagus. A multicenter randomized trial. French Associations for Surgical Research. Ann Surg. 1996;223:127–33.
8. Armanios M, Xu R, Forastiere AA, Haller DG, Kugler JW, Benson 3rd AB, Eastern Cooperative Oncology Group. Adjuvant chemotherapy for resected adenocarcinoma of the esophagus, gastro-esophageal junction, and cardia: phase II trial (E8296) of the Eastern Cooperative Oncology Group. J Clin Oncol. 2004;22:4495–9.
9. Ando N, Iizuka T, Kakegawa T, Isono K, Watanabe H, Ide H, et al. A randomized trial of surgery with and without chemotherapy for localized squamous carcinoma of the thoracic esophagus: the Japan Clinical Oncology Group study. J Thorac Cardiovasc Surg. 1997;114:205–9.
10. Ando N, Iizuka T, Ide H, Ishida K, Shinoda M, Nishimaki T, et al. Surgery plus chemotherapy compared with surgery alone for localized squamous cell carcinoma of the thoracic esophagus: a Japan Clinical Oncology Group Study – JCOG9204. J Clin Oncol. 2003;21:4592–6.

11. Ando N, Kato H, Igaki H, Shinoda M, Ozawa S, Shimizu H, et al. A randomized trial comparing postoperative adjuvant chemotherapy with cisplatin and 5-Fluorouracil versus preoperative chemotherapy for localized advanced squamous cell carcinoma of the thoracic esophagus (JCOG9907). Ann Surg Oncol. 2012;19:68–74.
12. Macdonald JS, Smalley SR, Benedetti J, Hundahl SA, Estes NC, Stemmermann GN, et al. Chemoradiotherapy after surgery compared with surgery alone for adenocarcinoma of the stomach or gastroesophageal junction. N Engl J Med. 2001;345(10):725–30.
13. van Hagen P, Hulshof MC, van Lanschot JJ, Steyerberg EW, van Berge Henegouwen MI, Wijnhoven BP, et al. Preoperative chemoradiotherapy for esophageal or junctional cancer. N Engl J Med. 2012;366:2074–84.
14. Allum WH, Stenning SP, Bancewicz J, Clark PI, Langley RE. Long-term results of a randomized trial of surgery with or without preoperative chemotherapy in esophageal cancer. J Clin Oncol. 2009;28:5062–7.
15. Cunningham D, Allum WH, Stenning SP, Thompson JN, Van de Velde CJ, Nicolson M, et al. Perioperative chemotherapy versus surgery alone for resectable gastroesophageal cancer. N Engl J Med. 2006;355:11–20.
16. Ychou M, Boige V, Pignon JP, Conroy T, Bouché O, Lebreton G, et al. Perioperative chemotherapy compared with surgery alone for resectable gastroesophageal adenocarcinoma: an FNCLCC and FFCD multicenter phase III trial. J Clin Oncol. 2001;29:1715–21.

Chapter 31
Prophylactic Antireflux Surgery in Lung Transplantation

Brian C. Gulack, Matthew G. Hartwig, and R. Duane Davis

Abstract Lung transplantation has seen immense growth over the past two decades. There are, however, many remaining uncertainties with regards to patient selection and post-operative care. In this chapter we have reviewed the literature in order to answer three important questions. First, does fundoplication following lung transplant improve symptomatology, lung function, and overall survival? Second, is fundoplication safe in this patient population? Third, does the timing of fundoplication matter, early after transplant or in a delayed fashion in those who develop allograft dysfunction? Based on our findings, we have made two recommendations. We furthermore discuss our own view of the data and how it should influence clinical decision making.

Keywords Lung transplantation • Gastroesophageal reflux disease • Fundoplication • Lung function • Bronchiolitis obliterans syndrome • Survival • Safety

Introduction

Since its induction in 1963, lung transplantation has evolved significantly [1]. Steady increases in the number of bilateral lung transplants has increased yearly transplant rates to almost 3,000 a year. Despite these advancements, allograft failure

B.C. Gulack, MD • M.G. Hartwig, MD
Division of Cardiothoracic Surgery, Department of Surgery,
Duke University Medical Center, Durham, NC, USA

R.D. Davis, MD, MBA (✉)
Division of Cardiothoracic Surgery, Department of Surgery,
Duke University Medical Center, DUMC Box 3864, Durham, NC 27710, USA
e-mail: davis053@mc.duke.edu

M.K. Ferguson (ed.), *Difficult Decisions in Thoracic Surgery*,
Difficult Decisions in Surgery: An Evidence-Based Approach 1,
DOI 10.1007/978-1-4471-6404-3_31, © Springer-Verlag London 2014

(both acute and chronic) continues to produce significant morbidity and mortality [2]. Following lung transplant, Bronchiolitis Obliterans Syndrome (BOS) is the most common cause of mortality responsible for roughly 40 % of deaths [3]. Despite its prevalence, there is debate as to the etiology of this syndrome. Numerous risk factors have been reported including early acute rejection, CMV serologic status, airway ischemia, and gastro-esophageal reflux disease (GERD) [4,5]. Recent evidence has further implicated aspiration from GERD as a causative factor in BOS, complicated by the finding that GERD may be increased secondary to the transplant procedure itself [6–15]. Oropharyngeal dysphagia secondary to transplant and the attendant increased risk of aspiration may furthermore progress the development of BOS [16]. Despite the correlation of GERD with BOS, not all studies have demonstrated a direct effect of post-transplant GERD on outcomes, and some authors have pointed out that current studies demonstrate only correlation, not causation [17,18].

Due to the evidence linking lung transplant patients with an increased incidence of GERD, and GERD with the progression of BOS, clinical equipoise with regards to the management of GERD in this population persists. Data has demonstrated that management of the acidity of gastric reflux alone will not prevent the negative consequences of GERD [19]. Therefore, in order to decrease the prevalence of micro-aspiration from GERD and hopefully BOS, many centers have turned to antireflux surgical procedures consisting of various forms of gastric fundoplication [20–22]. Despite increasing use of these procedures, there remains limited evidence to support the use of early antireflux surgery to prevent BOS and increase survival. In this chapter, we review the current literature analyzing antireflux surgery in lung transplant patients, and make formal recommendations with regards to its use.

Search Strategy

A literature search was performed using PubMed. The search terms "antireflux and lung transplant," "fundoplication and lung transplant," and "GERD and lung transplant" were used. Searches were limited from 1995 to the present. References from all sources of interest were also researched for use in this review. Studies specific to subgroups or performed on the same patient population while not adding significant additional findings were excluded. A summary of our methodology is present in Table 31.1.

Table 31.1 Summary of our search methodology including PICO terms

Patient population (P)	Intervention (I)	Comparison (C)	Outcome (O)
Lung transplant recipients	Fundoplication	No fundoplication	Symptomatology, lung function, survival, operative mortality
Lung transplant patients who Received Fundoplication	Timing of fundoplication	Early vs. late intervention	Symptomatology, lung function, survival

Review of the Literature

There are three pertinent questions that we have chosen to explore. The first is whether antireflux surgery has a beneficial effect on GERD and aspiration, an effect on the development of BOS, or an effect on overall outcomes including survival. The second is whether antireflux surgery is safe in the lung transplant population. The third questions the proper timing of antireflux surgery in transplant patients. We will review the literature examining the strengths of studies, and determining areas for further exploration. We will later discuss appropriate recommendations based on the current literature.

Effect of Antireflux Surgery on GERD, the Development of BOS, and Outcomes

Unfortunately, there are no prospective, randomized controlled trials examining the effect of antireflux surgery on GERD and aspiration in lung transplant patients. Lung transplant patients differ from the traditional patient population due to differing mechanisms underlying the reflux, likely related to the procedure itself, and therefore data from the general population cannot necessarily be extrapolated to lung transplant patients [15–17,23]. Furthermore, trials investigating GERD often rely on surrogate measures of aspiration such as pH data. D'Ovidio et al. demonstrated that only 72 % of patients with bile acid detected upon bronchoalveolar lavage (BAL), which is more likely indicative of gastro-duodenal aspiration, had abnormal pH findings [11]. Studies have also demonstrated that it is likely not the acidity of the reflux but other gastro-duodenal contents which contribute to the adverse effects following lung transplantation [19]. Despite the absence of randomized controlled trial data in this patient population, there have been numerous retrospective and prospective observational and non-randomized controlled studies examining antireflux surgery after lung transplantation which will be described here. The quality of evidence associated with each study as determined based on the GRADE criteria can be found in Table 31.2.

Cantu et al. reported on a total of 381 lung transplant patients, 201 of whom had documented reflux. Of those with reflux, 76 had a fundoplication while 125 did not. They further delineated those who received surgery into two groups, one who underwent early fundoplication (range 0–87 days) and one who underwent late fundoplication (range 106–2,999 days). They measured freedom from BOS, rates of acute rejection, and overall survival among patients. They discovered that recipients undergoing early fundoplication had significantly increased freedom from BOS than patients with no documented GERD, patients with GERD who did not receive fundoplication, and patients who received delayed fundoplication. With regards to acute rejection, they found no significant differences among the four groups. With regards to survival, the early surgery group had significantly increased survival at 1

Table 31.2 Studies investigating the effect of fundoplication on lung transplant patients evaluated in our review including study characteristics and the overall quality of evidence based on the GRADE criteria

Study	Patients	Study type	Outcome recorded	Quality of evidence
Cantu et al. [21]	381 total, 201 with GERD, 76 had fundoplication	Retrospective, controlled study	Freedom from BOS, acute rejection, survival	Low
Hartwig et al. [24]	297 total, 222 with GERD, 157 had fundoplication	Prospective, non-randomized controlled study	PFTs	Low
Neujahr et al. [9]	21 total, 8 had fundoplication	Non-randomized controlled prospective study	Frequency of CD8 cells from BAL expressing granzyme B and PFTs	Low
Lau et al. [20]	18 total	Retrospective, non-controlled study	PFTs	Low
Robertson et al. [22]	16 total	Prospective, non-controlled study	PFTs, and RSI and GIQLI questionnaires	Low
Abbassi-Ghadi et al. [25]	40 total	Retrospective, non-controlled study	PFTs	Low
Davis et al. [26]	43 total	Retrospective, non-controlled study	PFTs, survival	Low
Fisichella et al. [27]	8 total	Prospective non-controlled study	Leukocyte differential and inflammatory mediators in BAL and PFTs	Low
Burton et al. [28]	21 total	Prospective, non-controlled study	Questionnaire on symptomatology, PFTs	Low
Hoppo et al. [29]	43 total, 19 pre-transplant and 24 post-transplant	Prospective, non-controlled study	PFTs, pneumonia, acute rejection	Low

GERD gastroesophageal reflux disease, *BOS* bronchiolitis obliterans syndrome, *PFTs* pulmonary function tests, *BAL* bronchioalveolar lavage, *RSI* Reflux Symptom Index, *GIQLI* Gastro-Intestinal Quality of Life Index

and 3 years than any other group [21]. An interesting finding in this study was that patients with no documented reflux fared worse than those following early fundoplication. It can be hypothesized that this may be secondary to reflux and micro-aspiration that was not discovered via evaluative studies, raising the question how should patients be chosen for fundoplication following transplant?

Another study was performed by Hartwig et al. who analyzed 297 patients from a prospective database who underwent pH probe evaluation either before or immediately following lung transplantation. Two hundred twenty-two of these patients had an abnormal pH study, 157 of whom underwent fundoplication within 1 year of transplant. They evaluated pulmonary function tests (PFTs) and found that patients who had documented GERD but no fundoplication had significantly decreased FEV_1 measurements when compared to the no-GERD and GERD with fundoplication groups. Those latter two groups had similar measurements [24].

Neujahr et al. analyzed eight patients following lung transplant who underwent gastric fundoplication, and compared them with 13 patients who were determined to have GERD but did not undergo fundoplication. GERD was diagnosed by a DeMeester score greater than or equal to 14. Patients were evaluated by BAL including flow cytometry assessing for CD8+ effector cells, and PFTs. They found a significant decrease in the frequency of CD8 cells expressing granzyme B, a cytotoxic intracellular protein, between patients before and after gastric fundoplication. Furthermore, patients who did not undergo fundoplication had increased numbers of CD8 cells expressing granzyme B. Despite these findings, the study did not find any significant difference in pulmonary function between the two groups [9].

In a retrospective review of PFTs in 18 patients who had undergone an antireflux procedure following lung transplant, Lau et al. found an improvement in 67 % of the subjects' FEV_1 following the procedure [20]. A prospective review by Robertson et al. examined 16 patients who underwent laparoscopic Nissen fundoplication following lung transplant, evaluating pre and post-operative PFTs along with Reflux Symptom Index (RSI) and Gastro-Intestinal Quality of Life Index (GIQLI) questionnaires. They discovered a significant improvement in symptoms based on the questionnaires, but no improvement in lung function [22].

Abbassi-Ghadi et al. performed a retrospective study of lung transplant patients who underwent anti-reflux surgery at their institution. They evaluated pre and post-operative PFTs. They discovered that among 40 patients, only those with a positive pre-operative impedance and declining FEV_1 had a significant PFT improvement post procedure [25].

Davis et al. performed a retrospective review of 43 patients who underwent an antireflux procedure following lung transplant. They evaluated patients with PFTs and studied overall survival. A significant improvement was seen in the fundoplication group with regards to FEV_1. Furthermore, 26 patients in the fundoplication group met the criteria for BOS prior to the procedure, whereas only 13 met the criteria post-procedure. With regards to survival, the fundoplication group had a significantly improved survival compared to the overall series [26].

Fisichella et al. performed a prospective study on eight transplant patients with known GERD. They evaluated for leukocyte differential and inflammatory mediators from BAL samples pre and post-fundoplication, and also examined PFTs. They found a significant decrease in the percentage of neutrophils and lymphocytes following the procedure as well as significant decreases in interferon-gamma and interferon-1beta. They hypothesized that this may be indicative of a protective effect against the development of BOS. Despite this, they found no significant differences in PFTs [27].

A review of a prospectively maintained database of 21 patients who underwent fundoplication following lung transplant was performed by Burton et al. They evaluated symptomatology, lung function, and type of fundoplication. They found 76 % of patients had an improvement in symptoms following fundoplication. However, they found no significant improvements in lung function. Only two were performed within 6 months of transplant. With regards to type of fundoplication, 16 patients had a Toupet while five had a Nissen. When looking at patient satisfaction, dysphagia, or gas bloating, there was no significant differences between the two [28].

Lastly, Hoppo et al. performed an analysis of a prospectively compiled database containing 43 patients with end stage lung disease and GERD, including both pre and post-transplant patients (24 were post-transplant). All 43 underwent antireflux procedures. They evaluated changes in PFTs along with episodes of pneumonia and acute rejection. They found significant improvements in the FEV_1 of both groups, as well as a significant reduction in pneumonia and acute rejection in the post-transplant group [29].

None of the studies presented here evaluated the efficacy of fundoplication with respect to decreasing the incidence or the severity of gastro-duodenal reflux and aspiration. This is particularly important in that failed or slipped fundoplication procedures are frequently associated with worsened reflux and aspiration. To date, there have been no randomized controlled trials evaluating the effect of antireflux surgery on GERD and aspiration, BOS, or survival in patients following lung transplant, significantly affecting the availability of high grade evidence. There have been numerous small prospective and retrospective studies at individual institutions, however based on the GRADE criteria, these are all ranked as low with regards to quality of evidence. Therefore, further higher grade research is still necessary in order to reach definitive conclusions with regards to these questions.

Safety of Antireflux Surgery in the Post-lung Transplant Population

Antireflux surgery has been found to be an effective and safe tool for the management of GERD in the general population [30,31]. However, lung transplant recipients have underlying issues that raise concern when contemplating even the simplest procedures. This is secondary to their immune suppression and lung physiology, which could cause an increased rate of infection or sepsis and possible ventilation issues during and following surgery [32,33]. We have therefore reviewed the current literature to investigate the safety of this procedure in lung transplant patients. As before, the GRADE criteria was used to evaluate each study presented in this section for quality of evidence. The evaluation of any study not described in Table 31.2 was compiled in Table 31.3.

Numerous studies presented previously in this chapter reported on operative mortality. Including the studies by Hoppo et al., Burton et al., Abbassi-Ghadi et al., Robertson et al., and Cantu et al., and additional studies presented by Gasper et al. and Fisichella et al., we have compiled 30-day mortality data [21–23,25,28,29,34].

Table 31.3 Studies investigating the safety of fundoplication in lung transplant patients evaluated in our review including study characteristics and the overall quality of evidence based on the GRADE criteria (does not include studies already presented in Table 31.1)

Study	Patients	Study type	Outcome used	Quality of evidence
Gasper et al. [34]	35 total (20 post-transplant)	Retrospective non-controlled study	30-day mortality	Low
Fisichella et al. [23]	29 total	Retrospective non-controlled study	30-day mortality	Low
Zheng et al. [35]	11 total	Retrospective non-controlled study	30-day mortality	Low

Studies reporting from the same data population (i.e. same institution) as another were omitted, with the attempt to use the most recent data sample from each center. There were a total of 235 operations and two 30-day mortalities (0.86 %) described, although one death was attributed to an unrelated infection. This is comparable to the overall mortality following antireflux procedures for the general population (0.34 %, p=0.20) [36].

An additional study by Zheng et al. reported on the outcomes following 12 Nissen fundoplications in 11 pediatric patients following either lung or heart-lung transplantations. There were no 30 day mortalities in this population, although one exploratory laparotomy was performed for free air following a procedure [35].

There have been no high quality studies examining the safety of antireflux procedures in the post-lung transplant population. There have, however, been numerous small observational studies that reported 30-day mortality. By combining the data from these studies, we see that 30-day mortality is not significantly different from that reported from a nationwide sampling of antireflux procedures in the general public [36]. However, this does not take into account morbidity or delayed complications and mortality beyond 30 days. As described before, Lau et al. compared fundoplication in transplanted and non-transplanted patients. They evaluated for inpatient length of stay and found a significantly increased length of stay for post-transplant patients, which could be indicative of additional morbidity or just more intensive post-operative care in this high-risk population [20]. Secondary to the lack of high quality evidence, further studies are paramount in providing sufficient evidence as to the safety of these procedures in the post-lung transplant population.

Timing of Anti-reflux Surgery in the Post-Lung Transplant Population

Although the evidence is of low quality, the aforementioned studies have demonstrated that antireflux surgery helps prevent GERD, that it may help prevent BOS, and that it may improve outcomes [9,21]. Furthermore, the 30-day mortality from antireflux procedures in this patient population is similar to that of the general public [36]. Therefore, a subsequent topic that should be discussed is the optimal timing to perform this surgery. Surgery within a short period of time may help prevent the negative effects of reflux earlier, but it may also be at a time when the patient is still recovering from the transplant. Surgery at a later time may allow sufficient recovery from transplant, but the negative effects from the reflux may have already had a significant effect. Here we will review some of the aforementioned studies that have discussed timing of surgery.

Cantu et al. has the most significant study to date with regards to timing of surgery. As stated earlier, they separated their patients into two groups based roughly on a 90 day post-transplant separation point (Range 0–87 and 106–2,999 days). They found significant differences in the presence of BOS and overall survival favoring earlier surgery. Unfortunately, their findings have to be viewed with the understanding that their groups' baseline demographics are not equivalent, as the earlier surgery group tended to contain younger patients with a diagnosis of Cystic Fibrosis, and patients with cystic fibrosis have better mean survival than most other diagnoses [2,21].

As discussed before, Burton et al. did not find an effect on lung function following fundoplication, which could be attributable to delayed operations (only two were before 6 months, and both were after 3 months) [28]. Consequently, due to the lack of high grade evidence, further research into this question including higher grade trials is necessary.

Recommendations

We have evaluated ten studies which either investigated the effect of fundoplication on GERD [2], on lung function including evolution of BOS [9], or on overall outcomes including survival and rejection [3]. However, due to the nature of each study being observational in nature without any additional strengths, the overall quality of the evidence is low based on the GRADE criteria. Furthermore, there has not been sufficient investigation as to the determination of which patients will benefit from an antireflux procedure or which type of antireflux procedure is superior. That being said, the desirable effect of prolonged survival, improved pulmonary function, and decreased symptomatology along with the safety of this procedure in this patient population leads us to make the following recommendation based on the current literature: Lung Transplant patients with abnormal levels of gastroesophageal reflux either by diagnostic testing or symptomatology should receive a fundoplication.

This recommendation should be taken in light of the aforementioned evidence that our current diagnostic studies evaluating GERD may not be sufficient. Despite the presence of only one small observational study looking at the timing of fundoplication, in light of the likely increased survival and lung function of an earlier wrap along with the lack of adverse outcomes, we make the following recommendation: Lung Transplant patients who receive a fundoplication for diagnosed or symptomatic reflux should receive a fundoplication within 3 months of transplant, or as soon as clinically appropriate.

There are many questions remaining with regards to fundoplication post-lung transplant that exist secondary to the current paucity of data. For instance, are there certain groups within the lung transplant population that may have increased benefit from fundoplication than other groups? *Gasper* et al. demonstrated that patients presenting for lung transplant with connective tissue disorders have high levels of esophageal dysmotility, perhaps indicating a higher risk for post-transplant GERD and aspiration, but also a higher risk of dysphagia or intra-esophageal reflux following fundoplication [37]. Mendez et al. also determined that patients with cystic fibrosis have a higher prevalence of GERD than the general pre-transplant population, and idiopathic pulmonary fibrosis has also been implicated as a disease with increased aspiration events [38,39]. Other questions include how to best diagnose gastro-duodenal aspiration in this population as pH studies may not be sufficiently sensitive or specific. Furthermore, the optimal fundoplication technique to prevent aspiration has not been determined [11,19].

A Personal View of the Data

We feel that all potential lung transplant recipients should be evaluated before and after transplant for GERD due to the increased prevalence in this patient population, the effects of transplantation on gastrointestinal motility, and the possibility of asymptomatic GERD leading to gastro-duodenal aspiration. Patients with abnormal studies, especially those with evidence of proximal esophageal reflux, should undergo fundoplication as soon as clinically safe after transplant. Data from the general population in terms of indications for fundoplication and techniques are not necessarily generalizable to the transplant population. The impact of esophageal motility and gastric emptying, along with the determination of the optimal type of fundoplication require additional studies in order to appropriately direct clinical practice.

Recommendations
- Lung Transplant patients with abnormal levels of gastro-esophageal reflux either by diagnostic testing or symptomatology should receive a fundoplication (evidence quality low; weak recommendation).
- Lung Transplant patients who receive a fundoplication for diagnosed or symptomatic reflux should receive a fundoplication within 3 months of transplant, or as soon as clinically appropriate (evidence quality low; weak recommendation).

References

1. Hardy JD, Webb WR, Dalton Jr ML, Walker Jr GR. Lung homotransplantation in man. JAMA. 1963;186:1065–74.
2. Christie JD, Edwards LB, Kucheryavaya AY, Aurora P, Dobbels F, Kirk R, et al. The Registry of the International Society for Heart and Lung Transplantation: twenty-seventh official adult lung and heart-lung transplant report–2010. J Heart Lung Transplant. 2010;29(10):1104–18.
3. Meyers BF, de la Morena M, Sweet SC, Trulock EP, Guthrie TJ, Mendeloff EN, et al. Primary graft dysfunction and other selected complications of lung transplantation: a single-center experience of 983 patients. J Thorac Cardiovasc Surg. 2005;129(6):1421–9.
4. Heng D, Sharples LD, McNeil K, Stewart S, Wreghitt T, Wallwork J. Bronchiolitis obliterans syndrome: incidence, natural history, prognosis, and risk factors. J Heart Lung Transplant. 1998;17(12):1255–63.
5. Bando K, Paradis IL, Similo S, Konishi H, Komatsu K, Zullo TG, et al. Obliterative bronchiolitis after lung and heart-lung transplantation. An analysis of risk factors and management. J Thorac Cardiovasc Surg. 1995;110(1):4–13. discussion -4.
6. Davis CS, Shankaran V, Kovacs EJ, Gagermeier J, Dilling D, Alex CG, et al. Gastroesophageal reflux disease after lung transplantation: pathophysiology and implications for treatment. Surgery. 2010;148(4):737–44; discussion 744–5.
7. Shah N, Force SD, Mitchell PO, Lin E, Lawrence EC, Easley K, et al. Gastroesophageal reflux disease is associated with an increased rate of acute rejection in lung transplant allografts. Transplant Proc. 2010;42(7):2702–6.
8. Meltzer AJ, Weiss MJ, Veillette GR, Sahara H, Ng CY, Cochrane ME, et al. Repetitive gastric aspiration leads to augmented indirect allorecognition after lung transplantation in miniature swine. Transplantation. 2008;86(12):1824–9.
9. Neujahr DC. Surgical correction of gastroesophageal reflux in lung transplant patients is associated with decreased effector CD8 cells in lung lavages. A case series. CHEST J. 2010;138(4):937.
10. Ward C, Forrest IA, Brownlee IA, Johnson GE, Murphy DM, Pearson JP, et al. Pepsin like activity in bronchoalveolar lavage fluid is suggestive of gastric aspiration in lung allografts. Thorax. 2005;60(10):872–4.
11. D'Ovidio F, Mura M, Ridsdale R, Takahashi H, Waddell TK, Hutcheon M, et al. The effect of reflux and bile acid aspiration on the lung allograft and its surfactant and innate immunity molecules SP-A and SP-D. Am J Transplant. 2006;6(8):1930–8.
12. Blondeau K, Mertens V, Vanaudenaerde BA, Verleden GM, Van Raemdonck DE, Sifrim D, et al. Gastro-oesophageal reflux and gastric aspiration in lung transplant patients with or without chronic rejection. Eur Respir J. 2008;31(4):707–13.
13. Stovold R, Forrest IA, Corris PA, Murphy DM, Smith JA, Decalmer S, et al. Pepsin, a biomarker of gastric aspiration in lung allografts: a putative association with rejection. Am J Respir Crit Care Med. 2007;175(12):1298–303.
14. Hartwig MG, Appel JZ, Li B, Hsieh C-C, Yoon YH, Lin SS, et al. Chronic aspiration of gastric fluid accelerates pulmonary allograft dysfunction in a rat model of lung transplantation. J Thorac Cardiovasc Surg. 2006;131(1):209–17.
15. Fisichella PM, Davis CS, Shankaran V, Gagermeier J, Dilling D, Alex CG, et al. The prevalence and extent of gastroesophageal reflux disease correlates to the type of lung transplantation. Surg Laparosc Endosc Percutan Tech. 2012;22(1):46–51.
16. Atkins BZ, Trachtenberg MS, Prince-Petersen R, Vess G, Bush EL, Balsara KR, et al. Assessing oropharyngeal dysphagia after lung transplantation: altered swallowing mechanisms and increased morbidity. J Heart Lung Transplant. 2007;26(11):1144–8.
17. Molina EJ, Short S, Monteiro G, Gaughan JP, Macha M. Symptomatic gastroesophageal reflux disease after lung transplantation. Gen Thorac Cardiovasc Surg. 2009;57(12):647–53.
18. Fisichella PM, Davis CS, Kovacs EJ. A review of the role of GERD-induced aspiration after lung transplantation. Surg Endosc. 2011;26(5):1201–4.
19. Tang T, Chang JC, Xie A, Davis RD, Parker W, Lin SS. Aspiration of gastric fluid in pulmonary allografts: effect of pH. J Surg Res. 2013;181(1):e31–8.

20. Lau CL, Palmer SM, Howell DN, McMahon R, Hadjiliadis D, Gaca J, et al. Laparoscopic antireflux surgery in the lung transplant population. Surg Endosc. 2002;16(12):1674–8.
21. Cantu E, Appel JZ, Hartwig MG, Woreta H, Green C, Messier R, et al. Early fundoplication prevents chronic allograft dysfunction in patients with gastroesophageal reflux disease. Ann Thorac Surg. 2004;78(4):1142–51.
22. Robertson AGN, Krishnan A, Ward C, Pearson JP, Small T, Corris PA, et al. Anti-reflux surgery in lung transplant recipients: outcomes and effects on quality of life. Eur Respir J. 2011;39(3):691–7.
23. Fisichella PM, Davis CS, Gagermeier J, Dilling D, Alex CG, Dorfmeister JA, et al. Laparoscopic antireflux surgery for gastroesophageal reflux disease after lung transplantation. J Surg Res. 2011;170(2):e279–86.
24. Hartwig MG, Anderson DJ, Onaitis MW, Reddy S, Snyder LD, Lin SS, et al. Fundoplication after lung transplantation prevents the allograft dysfunction associated with reflux. Ann Thorac Surg. 2011;92(2):462–8; discussion; 468–9.
25. Abbassi-Ghadi N, Kumar S, Cheung B, McDermott A, Knaggs A, Zacharakis E, et al. Anti-reflux surgery for lung transplant recipients in the presence of impedance-detected duodeno-gastroesophageal reflux and bronchiolitis obliterans syndrome: a study of efficacy and safety. J Heart Lung Transplant. 2013;32(6):588–95.
26. Davis Jr RD, Lau CL, Eubanks S, Messier RH, Hadjiliadis D, Steele MP, et al. Improved lung allograft function after fundoplication in patients with gastroesophageal reflux disease under-going lung transplantation. J Thorac Cardiovasc Surg. 2003;125(3):533–42.
27. Fisichella PM, Davis CS, Lowery E, Pittman M, Gagermeier J, Love RB, et al. Pulmonary immune changes early after laparoscopic antireflux surgery in lung transplant patients with gastroesophageal reflux disease. J Surg Res. 2012;177(2):e65–73.
28. Burton PR, Button B, Brown W, Lee M, Roberts S, Hassen S, et al. Medium-term outcome of fundoplication after lung transplantation. Dis Esophagus. 2009;22(8):642–8.
29. Hoppo T, Jarido V, Pennathur A, Morrell M, Crespo M, Shigemura N, et al. Antireflux surgery preserves lung function in patients with gastroesophageal reflux disease and end-stage lung disease before and after lung transplantation. Arch Surg. 2011;146(9):1041–7.
30. Bammer T, Hinder RA, Klaus A, Libbey JS, Napoliello DA, Rodriquez JA. Safety and long-term outcome of laparoscopic antireflux surgery in patients in their eighties and older. Surg Endosc. 2002;16(1):40–2.
31. Dassinger MS, Torquati A, Houston HL, Holzman MD, Sharp KW, Richards WO. Laparoscopic fundoplication: 5-year follow-up. Am Surg. 2004;70(8):691–4; discussion 694–5.
32. Santacruz JF, Mehta AC. Airway complications and management after lung transplantation: ischemia, dehiscence, and stenosis. Proc Am Thorac Soc. 2009;6(1):79–93.
33. Sims KD, Blumberg EA. Common infections in the lung transplant recipient. Clin Chest Med. 2011;32(2):327–41.
34. Gasper WJ, Sweet MP, Hoopes C, Leard LE, Kleinhenz ME, Hays SR, et al. Antireflux surgery for patients with end-stage lung disease before and after lung transplantation. Surg Endosc. 2007;22(2):495–500.
35. Zheng C, Kane TD, Kurland G, Irlano K, Spahr J, Potoka DA, et al. Feasibility of laparoscopic Nissen fundoplication after pediatric lung or heart-lung transplantation: should this be the standard? Surg Endosc. 2011;25(1):249–54.
36. Colavita PD, Belyansky I, Walters AL, Tsirline VB, Zemlyak AY, Lincourt AE, et al. Nationwide inpatient sample: have antireflux procedures undergone regionalization? J Gastrointest Surg. 2013;17(1):6–13; discussion p 13.
37. Gasper WJ, Sweet MP, Golden JA, Hoopes C, Leard LE, Kleinhenz ME, et al. Lung transplantation in patients with connective tissue disorders and esophageal dysmotility. Dis Esophagus. 2008;21(7):650–5.
38. Davis CS, Mendez BM, Flint DV, Pelletiere K, Lowery E, Ramirez L, et al. Pepsin concentrations are elevated in the bronchoalveolar lavage fluid of patients with idiopathic pulmonary fibrosis after lung transplantation. J Surg Res. 2013;185:e101.
39. Mendez BM, Davis CS, Weber C, Joehl RJ, Fisichella PM. Gastroesophageal reflux disease in lung transplant patients with cystic fibrosis. Am J Surg. 2012;204(5):e21–6.

Chapter 32
Surgical Versus Endoscopic Management for Esophageal Perforations

Henner M. Schmidt and Donald E. Low

Abstract Esophageal perforations remains a challenging clinical problem and is associated with a high mortality rate. Since the introduction of conservative and endoscopic therapies treatment has been increasingly diversified. In this chapter the currently available surgical and endoscopic treatment strategies are introduced and discussed against the background of the most recent literature. The published experiences of esophageal perforations are limited and typically reported from single centers. Timely initial assessment and diagnosis as well as providing a tailored approach for each patient are critically importance to achieve best outcomes. Best evidence currently suggests that this is best provided in high-volume centers where a multidisciplinary team with expertise in esophageal surgery, interventional radiology and endoscopy is available.

Keywords Esophageal perforation • Treatment • Outcome • Surgery • Endoscopy • Stent • Clip • Vacuum • Hybrid • Procedures

Introduction

Esophageal perforations remains a challenging clinical problem and has historically been associated with a high mortality rate. Esophageal perforation remains a relatively uncommon clinical problem and treatment approaches continue to evolve. An incidence rate from 3 to 6/1,000,000 and a mean rate of 3.9 cases per year for major referral centers has been reported [1, 2]. Historically the mainstay of therapy was early initiation of surgical therapy [3] but as the treatment approach to esophageal

H.M. Schmidt, MD • D.E. Low, MD, FACS, FRCS(c) (✉)
Digestive Disease Institute, Esophageal Center of Excellence, Virginia Mason Medical Center, Mail Stop C6-GS 1100 Ninth Ave, Buck Pavilion 6th Floor, Seattle, WA 98111, USA
e-mail: donald.low@vmmc.org

M.K. Ferguson (ed.), *Difficult Decisions in Thoracic Surgery*,
Difficult Decisions in Surgery: An Evidence-Based Approach 1,
DOI 10.1007/978-1-4471-6404-3_32, © Springer-Verlag London 2014

perforation has become increasingly diversified management controversies have increased [4]. Mortality rates have progressively decreased likely secondary to a combination of factors including improvements in diagnosis, diversification in treatment approaches and evolution of resuscitation and critical care protocols in these patients.

In the heterogeneous group of patients presenting with iatrogenic, spontaneous and other esophageal perforations we believe that treatment outcomes are affected not only by early detection but also by the experience of the managing team [3, 4]. Tailored approaches for each patient are optimum and most efficiently applied in specialized centers, with expertise in surgery, endoscopy and radiology.

In this review we will summarize the current options for diagnosis and treatment for esophageal perforations described in the most recent literature as well as providing a management algorithm for patients presenting with esophageal perforation.

Search Strategy

The literature search in PubMed© includes publications from January 2009 till July 2013. A total of one Meta-Analysis and 29 observational studies were analyzed. The published data is divide in those studies focusing on comparing treatment modalities and outcomes and in those for endoscopic treatment options. The available data for endoscopic therapy is mostly derived from reports of case reports or small heterogeneous patient groups from single centers.

Etiology and Diagnosis

Iatrogenic perforation is currently the most common etiology accounting for approximately 60 % of presentations predominately related to the endoscopic treatment of stricture or achalasia. Spontaneous perforation, including Boerhaave Syndrome, which had been the leading cause historically, currently accounts for 30 % [5, 6]. The incidence of iatrogenic perforations associated with a variety of endoscopic procedures include: diagnostic procedures 0.03 % [7], transesophageal ultrasound 0.18 %, sclerotherapy for varices 2 % [8] and pneumatic dilation for achalasia at 4 % [9].

Other causes are traumatic or operative injury, foreign body ingestions, chronic diseases or esophageal cancer accounting for the remaining cases. The symptoms can be diverse such as fever, nausea, vomiting, dyspnea, dysphagia, thoracic, epigastric or back pain may occur as well as severe presentations such as hypotension or sepsis [6]. The triad of vomiting, chest pain and subcutaneous emphysema is known as the Mackler triad [10]. Presentation is often inconclusive as symptoms mimics other causes, such as myocardial infarction, peptic ulcer perforation, pancreatitis, aortic aneurysm dissection, spontaneous pneumothorax or pneumonia.

Tachycardia is common with later onset of fever [11]. Moreover hemodynamic instability and sepsis can be present at initial referral or can evolve in an uncontained, thoracic or abdominal perforation within 24–48 h [6]. Therefore a high index of suspicion is often a prerequisite to make a timely diagnosis and the treatment and resuscitation of pain, hypotension or sepsis is critical before proceeding to the diagnostic work-up.

In stable patients an initial upper gastrointestinal contrast study with water-soluble contrast as first line screening is recommended. Water-soluble agents have been associated with an approximately 20 % false-negative rate [12]. If water-soluble survey is negative but clinical suspicious remains high the survey should be repeated with thin barium contrast agent, because this has shown a 22 % higher accuracy in detecting perforations compared to water-soluble agents [12]. Historical concerns that barium extravasation into the mediastinum will increase inflammation is inaccurate. However extravasated barium in the chest or abdomen will remain longer and may impair the accuracy of subsequent ct-scans. The accuracy of this initial assessment will be significantly increased by first having a member of the surgical team present at the time of the study and second irrespective of the outcome of the swallow study carrying out a chest and abdominal ct scan immediately following the swallow study to provide additional information on the presence and extent of extravasation or to identify undrained fluid collections or other chest or abdominal abnormalities [13, 14]. Computed tomography scans are utilized as an initial assessment where patient instability precludes contrast studies [5].

We now routinely do upper endoscopy on all patients with esophageal perforation. This can be done in the endoscopy suite for stable patients who may be appropriate for endoscopic management. Alternatively for patients requiring surgery for large free perforations with extensive undrained fluids collections or mediastinal contamination it should be done in the operating room to provide specific information of the location and extent of the perforation which can help guide decisions on operative approach. The accuracy of endoscopic assessment in esophageal injury was described as 99 % in a case series in trauma patients, with a sensitivity and specificity of more than 90 % [15, 16]. Historically concerns that air insufflation amplifies the contamination in mediastinal or pleural cavities has not been validated.

Operative Therapy

Operative therapy is more commonly required in free perforation with extensive mediastinal and pleural contamination which is most often associated with Boerhaave Syndrome. Current operative approaches include surgical drainage alone, decortication, primary repair (done either transabdominal or transthoracic) with or without buttress (with pleural, pericardial, omental or muscle flaps and stomach), repair over T-Tube to establish a controlled fistula, esophageal resection with immediate reconstruction or esophageal exclusion with cervical

Table 32.1 Summary of recent publication comparing surgical and endoscopic treatment

				Management		Mortality		
Author	Date	Study period	Pat. n	Operative (%)	Non-operative (%)	Operative (%)	Non-operative (%)	Overall (%)
Vallboehmer et al. [21]	2009	1996–2008	44	55	45	8	5	6.8
Abbas et al. [3]	2009	1998–2008	119	76	24	15	4	14.2
Schmidt et al. [20]	2010	1998–2006	62	51	49	16	13	14.5
Keeling et al. [22]	2010	1997–2008	97	74	26	8	8	8.3
Shaker et al. [17]	2010	2002–2008	27	83	17	12	25	18.5
Hermansson et al. [23]	2011	1970–2006	125	79	21	20	15	19
Bhatia et al. [24]	2011	1981–2007	119	67	33	16	35	18.4.
Kuppusamy et al. [25]	2011	1989–2009	84	59.	41.	2.	6.	4.
Minnich et al. [26]	2011	1998–2009	81	64	36	12	10	11
Søreide et al. [11]	2012	2000–2010	47	45	55	–	–	23.4
Lindenmann et al. [18]	2013	2002–2012	120	55	45	16.7	5.6	11.7
Schweigert et al. [27]	2013	2002–2012	33	61	39	5	15	9.1

esophagostomy. A feeding jejunostomy or gastrostomy are often simultaneously placed particularly when recovery is expected to be prolonged. The approach selected depends on patients' stability, extent of the perforation and condition of the esophagus as well as the presence of other esophageal pathology. Many series have documented the outcome advantages of initiation of surgical treatment within 24 h [17–20]. In the most recent studies (Table 32.1) mortality rates for surgical treated patients varies from 4 to 24 % [3, 11, 17, 18, 20–26]. A Meta-Analysis from Biancari highlights that non-randomized mortality rates for stenting versus primary repair versus esophagectomy are 7.3, 9.5 and 13.8 % respectively [2]. The results of this meta-analysis are shown in Table 32.2.

Drainage alone is typically used when the patient is unstable and more demanding procedures are not feasible or in late presenting patients, after failed or inadequate previous treatment. Decortication is required in patients with extensive pleural contamination and trapped lung.

Primary repair represents the main approach in esophageal perforation and should be applied to large perforations with healthy esophageal tissue. The approach is determined by the site and size of the perforation and can be performed via a cervical, thoracic or abdominal approach. Typically the perforation is reapproximated and sutured in one to two layers. Buttressing of primary repairs, using pleura, pericardial fat, intercostal, chest wall or diaphragmatic muscle flaps, stomach or omentum, have also been described.

In large esophageal defects, in which primary repair would lead to stricture of the esophagus or in very unstable patients a T-Tube can be placed in order to establish a controlled fistula.

Esophagectomy should be reserved for malignant perforations in non-disseminated cancers. Esophageal exclusion have been applied in the past in extensive perforations in unstable patients. The use of exclusions procedures in

Table 32.2 Meta-analysis, Biancari et al. [2]	Studies included	75
	Study period	2000–2012
	N pat.	2,971
	Mortality	
	Overall	11.9 %
	Location	
	Cervical	5.9 %
	Thoracic	10.9 %
	Abdominal	13.2 %
	Cause	
	Foreign body	2.1 %
	Iatrogenic	13.2 %
	Spontaneous	14.8 %
	Treatment	
	<24 h	7.4 %
	>24 h	20.3 %
	Primary repair	9.5 %
	Esophagectomy	13.8 %
	T-tube, any other repair	20 %
	Stent	7.3 %

experienced centers is decreasing. Esophageal resection with esophagostomy and gastrostomy should only be performed in a non-viable esophagus which cannot be primarily repaired.

Open surgery historically had been strongly advocated for patients with Boerhaave Syndrome, with mortality rates ranging from 2 to 36 %. In a recent meta-analysis spontaneous perforations had an average mortality of 14.8 % [2]. Schweigert recently reported a morbidity rate in patients with Boerhaave Syndrome treated with either surgery or endoscopic stents of 30 % and 84 % respectively [27]. However, recent studies reported successful conservative and endoscopic management for spontaneous perforations and Boerhaave Syndrome [28–30].

Minimally Invasive Surgery

Minimally invasive approaches are being increasingly applied in both iatrogenic and spontaneous perforations especially in stable patients with limited contamination [31]. Cho and colleagues compared thoracotomy versus thoracoscopy with decortication and repair in 15 patients with Boerhaave Syndrome. The seven patients with the thoracoscopic approach were hemodynamically more stable, had shorter operation time, less prolonged ventilation time and reduced mortality [32]. Laparoscopic primary repair of pneumatic perforations in patients with achalasia with subsequent fundoplication has also been reported [33].

Endoscopic Therapy

Recent published data shows a substantial increase in the use of endoscopic techniques in managing esophageal perforations and its current application in the literature ranges from 17 to 55 %. With the etiological shift from spontaneous to iatrogenic perforations endoscopic treatment is increasingly appropriate in selected patients. Kuppusamy and colleagues highlighted the increased fraction of non-operative treatment from nearly 0 % in the early nineties to 75 % of cases treated in 2009 [4]. Furthermore the ability to combine diagnostic and therapeutic goals at the time of endoscopy increases efficiency. Endoscopy is currently utilized in up to 70 % of cases as a component of the initial assessment [4].

Endoluminal Stenting

Stent deployment is typically performed under endoscopic visualization with or without fluoroscopic guidance to position the stent correctly and maximize the opportunity to exclude the perforation. Full stent deployment can take up to 24 h, therefore follow-up contrast esophagography can be performed either shortly after stent placement or the following day to confirm exclusion of the perforation. Pleural and mediastinal fluid collections and contaminated spaces must be radiologically drained subsequently. Ideally an experienced surgeon should be involved when non-operative therapy is being contemplated [5].

A variety of removable stents are currently available. The majority of current reports utilizing stents in patients with esophageal perforation have used the self-expandable plastic PolyFlex Stent (SEPS) or the self-expandable metallic stent (SEMS), an example being the UltraFlex (Boston Scientific, Natick, MA, USA). Both of these stents have versions with complete or partial silicone cover. Other SEMS-options include the WallFlex (Boston Scientific, Natick, MA, USA), the ALIMAXX (Merit Medical System, Inc, South Jordan, UT, USA), the Evolution (Cook Medical, Bloomington, IN, USA) and the Niti-S (Taewoong Medical, Geyonggi-Do, South Korea). Van Boeckel and colleagues compared in their study fully covered SEMS, SEPS and partially covered SEMS with no significant difference in efficacy with success rates of 73, 83 and 83 % respectively [34]. SEMS have been introduced for the palliative treatment for patients with esophageal cancer whereas SEPS have seen application in both malignant and benign diseases. The PolyFlex-Stent is the only stent currently approved by the FDA for removal in benign disease.

The reported success rates of treating acute perforations with stents vary from 60 to 94 %. Virtually all current reports were conducted in single centers. The most commonly reported complication is stent migration. Migration occurs in approximately 25 % of cases with reported ranges varying from 3 to 38 % [28, 30, 35–42]. Table 32.3 provides a summary of recent studies reporting stent treatment in esophageal perforations. Van Boeckel and colleagues reported associated migration rates of 20, 14 and 12 % for fully covered SEMS, SEPS and partially covered SEMS respectively [34]. However, no current comparison of the efficacy of individual stents is available. Typically fully covered stents are associated with a higher migration rate [35]. In contrast partially covered stents allows granulation into the uncovered portions which can decrease migration but potentially make removal more challenging. Using the appropriate size and whenever possible avoiding placing the stent across the lower esophageal sphincter can minimize the incidence of migration. Diverse options for stent fixation are described in the literature [43, 44]. Endoscopical clipping of the stent edges and transcervical or transnasal fixation are options but efficacy of these techniques are currently poorly defined [45].

Endoscopic Clips

Currently two different types of endoscopic clips are available which are both FDA approved for closure of perforations. The Resolution Clip (Boston Scientific, Natick, MA, USA) which is used through the working channel of the scope and previously has been applied for hemostasis in gastrointestinal bleeding. These clips have rather limited opening diameter of 11 mm and therefore are most appropriate for mucosal tears or very small esophageal perforations which are recognized at the time of occurrence [46, 47]. There is an evolving experience in routinely closing the mucosal layer after the peroral endoscopic myotomy (POEM) procedure with the application of several clips to close the mucosal tunnel. In selected cases clips and stents can be used in combination. Swallow studies to verify closure of the perforation must be done and selected drainage of mediastinal or pleural fluid must be performed separately.

The second type of endoscopic clips is the newer OTSC (Over-The-Scope-Clip, Ovesco Endoscopy AG, Tübingen, Germany) which is attached as a cap over the end of the endoscope. These nitinol-clips are 11–14 mm wide and 3–6 mm depth forming a crescent clip with atraumatic or penetrating teeth. This clip may provide the opportunity to seal larger defects. The current literature assessing the efficacy of the OTSC device (Table 32.4) is limited [48–51]. Kirschniak and colleagues described their experience of seven esophageal perforations (out of 50) treated with the OTSC with a healing rate of 100 %. However follow-up endoscopy after an average of 9 days showed a 10 % rate of displaced clips, without any complications identified [49].

Endoscopic Vacuum Device

Endoscopic vacuum therapy (EVT) has been described for anastomotic leakage of colorectal anastomosis [52, 53]. As shown in Table 32.5 there are limited reports where these Polyurethane sponges (EndoSponge by B.BRAUN®, Melsungen, Germany) were applied in esophageal perforations [54–56]. The sponge is either placed in the esophageal lumen or in the extraluminal cavity created by the perforation. The vacuum

Table 32.3 Endoscopic stents

Author	Date	Pat. n	Perforation I/S	Treatment	Mean LOS	Success (%)	Migration (%)	Morbidity (%)	Mortality (%)
Leers et al. [35]	2009	9	9/0	SEMS	6	94	3	13	6
Salminen et al. [37]	2009	8	4/4	SEMS	–	75	10	20	25
Van Heel et al. [38]	2010	29	19/10	SEMS/SEPS	–	74	33	33	21
Freeman et al. [36]	2011	36	17/19	SEPS	9	92	19	24	0
Dai et al. [39]	2011	7	–	SEPS	32	85	35	35	2
David et al. [40]	2011	12	6/6	SEMS	–	73	7	40	10
D'Cunha et al. [41]	2011	15	13/2	SEMS/SEPS	33	60	16	24	13.5
van Boeckel et al. [42]	2012	17	13/4	SEMS/SEPS	39	76	30	46	2
Koivukangas et al. [30]	2012	14	0/14	SEMS	34	86	–	14	14

I/S iatrogenic/spontaneous, *LOS* length of stay in days, *SEMS* self-expanding metal stent, *SEPS* self-expanding plastic stent

Table 32.4 Endoscopic clips

Author	Date	Pat. n	Perforation I/ S	Treatment	Success (%)	LOS
Qadeer et al. [46]	2007	7	5/2	EndoClip	100	9.6 days
Pohl et al. [48]	2010	2	1/1	OTSC	50	–
Kirschniak et al. [49]	2011	7	–	OTSC	100	–
Rokszin et al. [47]	2011	1	0/1	EndoClip	100	14
Hagel et al. [50]	2012	2	2/0	OTSC	0	–
Bona et al. [51]	2013	1	0/1	OTSC	100	28

I/S iatrogenic/spontaneous, *OTSC* Over the Scope Clip, OVESCO, *EndoClip Resolution Clip, Boston Scientific, LOS* length of stay in days

Table 32.5 Endoscopic vacuum therapy

Author	Date	Pat. n	Perforation I/S	Mean LOS	Mean scope	Success (%)	Morbidity (%)	Mortality (%)
Loske et al. [54]	2010	1	0/1	18	2	100	0	0
Kuehn et al. [55]	2012	4	3/1	22	6.75	89	44	11
Schorsch et al. [56]	2013	7	7/0	5	1.7	100	0	0

I/S iatrogenic/spontaneous, *LOS* length of stay in days

device is then connected through a nasal drainage tube to an external pump. EVT induces secondary wound healing but does not achieve it primarily, therefore complete healing needs to be monitored with repetitive endoscopies. Nutritional support is achieved by endoscopic placement of an additional enteric feeding tube.

Kuehn and colleagues describes four Patients (three iatrogenic, one spontaneous) who were treated with this approach for esophageal perforation and showed healing of the perforation in all four patients [55]. The single patient presenting with Boerhaave Syndrome had the sponge placed in the extraluminal cavity and needed 13 sponge changes over 44 days for successful healing. Schorsch and colleagues published 7patients (out of a series of 24) with iatrogenic esophageal perforations which all had been successfully treated with EVT. The median perforation size was 13 mm, with only one patient having an endoscopically visible extraluminal cavity, all patients had been diagnosed within 1 h after perforation and all patients had been in a stable condition. Mean duration of therapy in that group was 5 days and with a mean change interval of 3 days only one to two sponges has been needed for complete healing [56]. This approach provides an additional option in patients with contained cavities associated with esophageal perforations.

Hybrid Procedures

A combination of radiologic, endoscopic and open or minimally invasive surgical techniques demonstrates that multidisciplinary approaches can provide the possibility of tailoring approaches for each patient with esophageal perforation. Radiologic guided drainage in patients with undrained mediastinal abscesses or pleural fluid collections after endoscopic or surgical treatment is a frequently applied example of combination therapy, as is the subsequent endoscopic placement of nasogastric or external feeding tubes in conjunction with transthoracic primary repair. Intraoperative endoscopy can facilitate operative repair by helping confirm the location and extent of the perforation to decide whether a transthoracic or transabdominal approach is recommended, guide the dissection of the esophagus and placement of sutures and test the repair by insufflating air [5].

In addition hybrid procedures at the time of surgical drainage or decortication can involve the placement of external surgical sutures to stabilize endoscopically placed stents to decrease migration and increase the chances of an uncomplicated recovery [57]. We have treated five patients in whom the esophageal perforation has been simultaneously approached surgically and endoscopically. After surgical decortication, drainage or primary repair an endoscopically deployed stent was fixated by a chromic suture placed during surgery to stabilize the stent. This technique ensures correct stent deployment and decreases the incidence of stent migration. Complete occlusion of the perforation was achieved in four out of five cases. All stents remained in position during the post-operative period and were removed uneventfully 2–4 weeks later.

Summary

The diagnostic and therapeutic technologies available to treat esophageal perforations continues to evolve. Timely diagnosis and initiation of treatment remains an important factor to achieve good outcomes but as treatment options diversify, treatment is best administered in high-volume centers which can potentially apply all surgical, radiological and endoscopic options. The treatment approach will vary according to the physiological stability of the patient, site and size of the perforation and underlying esophageal disease. Ideally the treatment should be supervised by an experienced surgical team which can match the treatment to the individual circumstances of the patients' physiology, the extent and nature of the perforation and the presence of a secondary esophageal pathology.

Recommendations

Timely diagnosis and treatment optimizes outcomes. Management by an experienced multidisciplinary team optimizes outcomes. Initial contrast esophagography immediately followed by a chest and abdominal CT-scan is the best approach to assess the extent of the esophageal perforation and mediastinal or pleural fluid collections. Early utilization of endoscopy is appropriate for assessing esophageal perforations. Endoscopic assessment can guide treatment decision making and provide additional information on the site and size of the perforation, the viability of the esophagus and underlying pathologies. Endoscopic treatment is appropriate in selected cases of esophageal perforation, especially iatrogenic and contained spontaneous perforations. The diversified treatment approaches are most commonly available in high-volume centers with expertise in esophageal surgery, interventional radiology and endoscopy. In stable patients with small contained perforations and no significant contamination conservative management may be appropriate. In contained spontaneous perforations with limited contamination endoscopic therapy can be considered. Perforations associated with extensive mediastinal, pleural or abdominal contamination are most suitable for surgical or hybrid (combined approach) therapy. Esophagectomy should be considered in patients with acute perforations in non-disseminated cancer. Endoscopy during surgery (hybrid procedure) can improve treatment decision-making.

A Personal View of the Data

Acute esophageal perforation is best managed in high volume esophageal units where multidisciplinary teams including interventional radiology and gastroenterology are routinely available. Initial assessment is best accomplished with a member of the surgical team present at the time of contrast study and endoscopic assessment, preferably done by the surgeon, should be a component of initial work-up whenever feasible. Surgical management remains an essential component of therapy for large uncontained perforations. However endoscopic treatment, particularly the placement of removable stents, will be appropriate in selected patients but typically must be accompanied by external drainage of contained perforations. Nutritional support should be a component of the management of all major perforations. Future clinical assessment should include the development and testing of new methodologies for stent fixation to decrease the incidence of migration in patients with benign esophageal perforations.

Recommendations

- Endoscopic treatment is appropriate in selected cases of esophageal perforation (Evidence quality moderate; weak recommendation).
- In stable patients with small contained perforations and no significant contamination conservative management may be appropriate (Evidence quality low; weak recommendation).
- Perforations associated with extensive mediastinal, pleural or abdominal contamination are most suitable for surgical or hybrid (combined approach) therapy (Evidence grade moderate; weak recommendation).
- Esophagectomy should be considered in patients with acute perforations in non-disseminated cancer (Evidence level low; weak recommendation).

References

1. Vidarsdottir H, Blondal S, Alfredsson H, Geirsson A, Gudbjartsson T. Oesophageal perforations in Iceland: a whole population study on incidence, aetiology and surgical outcome. Thorac Cardiovasc Surg. 2010;58(8):476–80.
2. Biancari F, D'Andrea V, Paone R, Di MC, Savino G, Koivukangas V, et al. Current treatment and outcome of esophageal perforations in adults: systematic review and meta-analysis of 75 studies. World J Surg. 2013;37(5):1051–9.
3. Abbas G, Schuchert MJ, Pettiford BL, Pennathur A, Landreneau J, Landreneau J, et al. Contemporaneous management of esophageal perforation. Surgery. 2009;146(4):749–55.
4. Kuppusamy MK, Felisky C, Kozarek RA, Schembre D, Ross A, Gan I, et al. Impact of endoscopic assessment and treatment on operative and non-operative management of acute oesophageal perforation. Br J Surg. 2011;98(6):818–24.
5. Carrott Jr PW, Low DE. Advances in the management of esophageal perforation. Thorac Surg Clin. 2011;21(4):541–55.
6. Brinster CJ, Singhal S, Lee L, Marshall MB, Kaiser LR, Kucharczuk JC. Evolving options in the management of esophageal perforation. Ann Thorac Surg. 2004;77(4):1475–83.
7. Merchea A, Cullinane DC, Sawyer MD, Iqbal CW, Baron TH, Wigle D, et al. Esophagogastroduodenoscopy-associated gastrointestinal perforations: a single-center experience. Surgery. 2010;148(4):876–80.
8. Terblanche J, Krige JE, Bornman PC. The treatment of esophageal varices. Annu Rev Med. 1992;43:69–82.
9. Vaezi MF. Should surgery replace pneumatic dilation in achalasia? Gastroenterology. 2008;135(5):1794–6.
10. Nia AM, Abel J, Semmo N, Gassanov N, Er F. 86-year-old patient with vomiting and loss of consciousness: the Mackler triad. Dtsch Med Wochenschr. 2011;1779(36).
11. Soreide JA, Konradsson A, Sandvik OM, Ovrebo K, Viste A. Esophageal perforation: clinical patterns and outcomes from a patient cohort of Western Norway. Dig Surg. 2012;29(6):494–502.
12. Buecker A, Wein BB, Neuerburg JM, Guenther RW. Esophageal perforation: comparison of use of aqueous and barium-containing contrast media. Radiology. 1997;202(3):683–6.
13. Strauss C, Mal F, Perniceni T, Bouzar N, Lenoir S, Gayet B, et al. Computed tomography versus water-soluble contrast swallow in the detection of intrathoracic anastomotic leak complicating esophagogastrectomy (Ivor Lewis): a prospective study in 97 patients. Ann Surg. 2010;251(4):647–51.
14. Hogan BA, Winter DC, Broe D, Broe P, Lee MJ. Prospective trial comparing contrast swallow, computed tomography and endoscopy to identify anastomotic leak following oesophagogastric surgery. Surg Endosc. 2008;22(3):767–71.
15. Arantes V, Campolina C, Valerio SH, de Sa RN, Toledo C, Ferrari TA, et al. Flexible esophagoscopy as a diagnostic tool for traumatic esophageal injuries. J Trauma. 2009;66(6):1677–82.
16. Wu JT, Mattox KL, Wall Jr MJ. Esophageal perforations: new perspectives and treatment paradigms. J Trauma. 2007;63(5):1173–84.
17. Shaker H, Elsayed H, Whittle I, Hussein S, Shackcloth M. The influence of the 'golden 24-h rule' on the prognosis of oesophageal perforation in the modern era. Eur J Cardiothorac Surg. 2010;38(2):216–22.
18. Lindenmann J, Matzi V, Neuboeck N, Anegg U, Maier A, Smolle J, et al. Management of esophageal perforation in 120 consecutive patients: clinical impact of a structured treatment algorithm. J Gastrointest Surg. 2013;17(6):1036–43.
19. Soreide JA, Viste A. Esophageal perforation: diagnostic work-up and clinical decision-making in the first 24 hours. Scand J Trauma Resusc Emerg Med. 2011;19:66.
20. Schmidt SC, Strauch S, Rosch T, Veltzke-Schlieker W, Jonas S, Pratschke J, et al. Management of esophageal perforations. Surg Endosc. 2010;24(11):2809–13.

21. Vallbohmer D, Holscher AH, Holscher M, Bludau M, Gutschow C, Stippel D, et al. Options in the management of esophageal perforation: analysis over a 12-year period. Dis Esophagus. 2010;23(3):185–90.
22. Keeling WB, Miller DL, Lam GT, Kilgo P, Miller JI, Mansour KA, et al. Low mortality after treatment for esophageal perforation: a single-center experience. Ann Thorac Surg. 2010;90(5):1669–73.
23. Hermansson M, Johansson J, Gudbjartsson T, Hambreus G, Jonsson P, Lillo-Gil R, et al. Esophageal perforation in South of Sweden: results of surgical treatment in 125 consecutive patients. BMC Surg. 2010;10:31.
24. Bhatia P, Fortin D, Inculet RI, Malthaner RA. Current concepts in the management of esophageal perforations: a twenty-seven year Canadian experience. Ann Thorac Surg. 2011;92(1):209–15.
25. Kuppusamy MK, Hubka M, Felisky CD, Carrott P, Kline EM, Koehler RP, et al. Evolving management strategies in esophageal perforation: surgeons using nonoperative techniques to improve outcomes. J Am Coll Surg. 2011;213(1):164–71.
26. Minnich DJ, Yu P, Bryant AS, Jarrar D, Cerfolio RJ. Management of thoracic esophageal perforations. Eur J Cardiothorac Surg. 2011;40(4):931–7.
27. Schweigert M, Beattie R, Solymosi N, Booth K, Dubecz A, Muir A, et al. Endoscopic stent insertion versus primary operative management for spontaneous rupture of the esophagus (Boerhaave syndrome): an international study comparing the outcome. Am Surg. 2013;79(6):634–40.
28. Freeman RK, Van Woerkom JM, Vyverberg A, Ascioti AJ. Esophageal stent placement for the treatment of spontaneous esophageal perforations. Ann Thorac Surg. 2009;88(1):194–8.
29. Vogel SB, Rout WR, Martin TD, Abbitt PL. Esophageal perforation in adults: aggressive, conservative treatment lowers morbidity and mortality. Ann Surg. 2005;241(6):1016–21.
30. Koivukangas V, Biancari F, Merilainen S, Ala-Kokko T, Saarnio J. Esophageal stenting for spontaneous esophageal perforation. J Trauma Acute Care Surg. 2012;73(4):1011–3.
31. Kimberley KL, Ganesh R, Anton CK. Laparoscopic repair of esophageal perforation due to Boerhaave syndrome. Surg Laparosc Endosc Percutan Tech. 2011;21(4):e203–5.
32. Cho JS, Kim YD, Kim JW, I HS, Kim MS. Thoracoscopic primary esophageal repair in patients with Boerhaave's syndrome. Ann Thorac Surg. 2011;91(5):1552–5.
33. Hunt DR, Wills VL, Weis B, Jorgensen JO, DeCarle DJ, Coo IJ. Management of esophageal perforation after pneumatic dilation for achalasia. J Gastrointest Surg. 2000;4(4):411–5.
34. van Boeckel PG, Dua KS, Weusten BL, Schmits RJ, Surapaneni N, Timmer R, et al. Fully covered self-expandable metal stents (SEMS), partially covered SEMS and self-expandable plastic stents for the treatment of benign esophageal ruptures and anastomotic leaks. BMC Gastroenterol. 2012;12:19.
35. Leers JM, Vivaldi C, Schafer H, Bludau M, Brabender J, Lurje G, et al. Endoscopic therapy for esophageal perforation or anastomotic leak with a self-expandable metallic stent. Surg Endosc. 2009;23(10):2258–62.
36. Freeman RK, Ascioti AJ. Esophageal stent placement for the treatment of perforation, fistula, or anastomotic leak. Semin Thorac Cardiovasc Surg. 2011;23(2):154–8.
37. Salminen P, Gullichsen R, Laine S. Use of self-expandable metal stents for the treatment of esophageal perforations and anastomotic leaks. Surg Endosc. 2009;23(7):1526–30.
38. van Heel NC, Haringsma J, Spaander MC, Bruno MJ, Kuipers EJ. Short-term esophageal stenting in the management of benign perforations. Am J Gastroenterol. 2010;105(7):1515–20.
39. Dai Y, Chopra SS, Kneif S, Hunerbein M. Management of esophageal anastomotic leaks, perforations, and fistulae with self-expanding plastic stents. J Thorac Cardiovasc Surg. 2011;141(5):1213–7.
40. David EA, Kim MP, Blackmon SH. Esophageal salvage with removable covered self-expanding metal stents in the setting of intrathoracic esophageal leakage. Am J Surg. 2011;202(6):796–801.
41. D'Cunha J, Rueth NM, Groth SS, Maddaus MA, Andrade RS. Esophageal stents for anastomotic leaks and perforations. J Thorac Cardiovasc Surg. 2011;142(1):39–46.
42. van Boeckel PG, Sijbring A, Vleggaar FP, Siersema PD. Systematic review: temporary stent placement for benign rupture or anastomotic leak of the oesophagus. Aliment Pharmacol Ther. 2011;33(12):1292–301.

43. Endo M, Kaminou T, Ohuchi Y, Sugiura K, Yata S, Adachi A, et al. Development of a new hanging-type esophageal stent for preventing migration: a preliminary study in an animal model of esophagotracheal fistula. Cardiovasc Intervent Radiol. 2012;35(5):1188–94.

44. Manes G, Corsi F, Pallotta S, Massari A, Foschi D, Trabucchi E. Fixation of a covered self-expandable metal stent by means of a polypectomy snare: an easy method to prevent stent migration. Dig Liver Dis. 2008;40(9):791–3.

45. Vanbiervliet G, Filippi J, Karimdjee BS, Venissac N, Iannelli A, Rahili A, et al. The role of clips in preventing migration of fully covered metallic esophageal stents: a pilot comparative study. Surg Endosc. 2012;26(1):53–9.

46. Qadeer MA, Dumot JA, Vargo JJ, Lopez AR, Rice TW. Endoscopic clips for closing esophageal perforations: case report and pooled analysis. Gastrointest Endosc. 2007;66(3):605–11.

47. Rokszin R, Simonka Z, Paszt A, Szepes A, Kucsa K, Lazar G. Successful endoscopic clipping in the early treatment of spontaneous esophageal perforation. Surg Laparosc Endosc Percutan Tech. 2011;21(6):e311–2.

48. Pohl J, Borgulya M, Lorenz D, Ell C. Endoscopic closure of postoperative esophageal leaks with a novel over-the-scope clip system. Endoscopy. 2010;42(9):757–9.

49. Kirschniak A, Subotova N, Zieker D, Konigsrainer A, Kratt T. The Over-The-Scope Clip (OTSC) for the treatment of gastrointestinal bleeding, perforations, and fistulas. Surg Endosc. 2011;25(9):2901–5.

50. Hagel AF, Naegel A, Lindner AS, Kessler H, Matzel K, Dauth W, et al. Over-the-scope clip application yields a high rate of closure in gastrointestinal perforations and may reduce emergency surgery. J Gastrointest Surg. 2012;16(11):2132–8.

51. Bona D, Aiolfi A, Rausa E, Bonavina L. Management of Boerhaave's syndrome with an over-the-scope clip. Eur J Cardiothorac Surg. 2014;45(4):752–4.

52. Chopra SS, Mrak K, Hunerbein M. The effect of endoscopic treatment on healing of anastomotic leaks after anterior resection of rectal cancer. Surgery. 2009;145(2):182–8.

53. Weidenhagen R, Gruetzner KU, Wiecken T, Spelsberg F, Jauch KW. Endoluminal vacuum therapy for the treatment of anastomotic leakage after anterior rectal resection. Rozhl Chir. 2008;87(8):397–402.

54. Loske G, Schorsch T, Muller C. Endoscopic vacuum sponge therapy for esophageal defects. Surg Endosc. 2010;24(10):2531–5.

55. Kuehn F, Schiffmann L, Rau BM, Klar E. Surgical endoscopic vacuum therapy for anastomotic leakage and perforation of the upper gastrointestinal tract. J Gastrointest Surg. 2012;16(11):2145–50.

56. Schorsch T, Muller C, Loske G. Endoscopic vacuum therapy of anastomotic leakage and iatrogenic perforation in the esophagus. Surg Endosc. 2013;27(6):2040–5.

57. Ben-David K, Lopes J, Hochwald S, Draganov P, Forsmark C, Collins D, et al. Minimally invasive treatment of esophageal perforation using a multidisciplinary treatment algorithm: a case series. Endoscopy. 2011;43(2):160–2.

Chapter 33
Stents for Esophageal Anastomotic Leak

Shanda H. Blackmon and Laurissa Gann

Abstract The appropriate therapy for managing esophageal anastomotic leaks is not clearly established. For uncontained leaks, no trials exist demonstrating superiority of esophageal stenting over what is considered to be the gold standard of surgical intervention (surgical repair with a vascularized, pedicled muscle flap and drainage). Esophageal stenting should be reserved to clinical trials, as it remains investigative in nature. Patients who are offered this intervention should be warned of its off-label application and the potential complications associated with it.

Keywords Anastomotic leak • Esophagus • Stent • Esophagectomy • Complications

Introduction

The current practice among most thoracic surgeons who discover a patient has an uncontained esophageal anastomotic leak is surgical debridement to healthy tissue and primary repair (whenever possible) reinforced with a vascularized, pedicled muscle flap and drainage. Determining the optimal therapy for such patients requires examining all available options, including surgery alone, surgery plus a muscle flap, stenting, hybrid procedures such as stenting with surgical drainage and a muscle flap, clipping or suturing with stenting, and other means. Unfortunately, there are too few retrospective and no prospective studies comparing these techniques against

S.H. Blackmon, MD, MPH (✉)
Division of Thoracic Surgery, Departments of Thoracic Surgery and General Surgery,
Houston Methodist Hospital, Texas, Weill Cornell Medical College,
6550 Fannin Street, Smith Tower, Suite 1661, Houston, TX 77030, USA
e-mail: shblackmon@houstonmethodist.org

L. Gann, MSLS
Research Medical Library, The University of Texas MD Anderson Cancer Center,
Houston, TX USA

M.K. Ferguson (ed.), *Difficult Decisions in Thoracic Surgery*,
Difficult Decisions in Surgery: An Evidence-Based Approach 1,
DOI 10.1007/978-1-4471-6404-3_33, © Springer-Verlag London 2014

each other. The objective of this chapter is to determine the efficacy and safety of the use of stents of various types when used to treat anastomotic leakage after esophagectomy.

Search Strategy

To obtain data to determine the efficacy and safety of stenting for esophageal anasto- motic leaks, published outcomes from a variety of studies were reviewed. Electronic databases searched were MEDLINE (Ovid SP), EMBASE (Ovid SP), and the Cochrane Library from January 2000 to September 2013. The search strategies were developed using keywords, adjacency searching, and medical subject headings under existing database organizational schemes. We restricted our search to English-language articles only. Terms used for the search included anastomotic leak or leakage, esopha- geal neoplasms/surgery, esophagus/surgery, esophagectomy, and stent. The search was limited to humans. British spelling variations were also included. Additionally, PubMed was keyword searched for newly published articles. One hundred eleven abstracts were reviewed and an article search was performed on selected abstracts. Additional references from article bibliographies were included as appropriate.

Search Results

Twenty-eight articles were excluded because the English version and/or PDF version was not available for review. Twenty additional articles were excluded because they did not actually include esophageal stents for anastomotic leakage or were from a bariatric series. In articles in which the authors appeared to re-publish data from the same series, the largest series was used and the smaller, earlier series from the same patient popula- tion were excluded. Articles reporting the use of a stent to treat anastomotic leaks but not including success rate or mortality rate were excluded. Three review articles were also excluded. Because of a size limitation for the reference list and because it is unlikely an author would report a single case that was unsuccessful, ten additional individual case reports or single cases reported of anastomotic leak stenting from a larger series were excluded to limit owing to bias in reporting. Careful review revealed no randomized controlled trials, meta-analyses, or systematic reviews comparing surgi- cal therapy vs stenting for anastomotic leak management. Of the 36 remaining selected articles included in this review of literature, there were only 2 prospective studies.

Results

The success rate of stenting for anastomotic leaks from the aggregated selected series was calculated to be 72.77 % (326/448 cases), Table 33.1 [1–36]. The mortality rate of stenting for anastomotic leak was 15 % (67/448 cases) compared to a mortality rate of 3.3–11.6 % for surgical repair, Table 33.1 [1–36]. Analyzing each series by type of stent used, cSEMS-only (covered self-expanding metal stent) reports included 236 patients with a 72.9 % (172/236) success rate and a 13.6 % (32/236) mortality rate while self-expanding plastic stents (SEPS)-only reports included 96 patients with an 81.3 % (78/96) success rate and a 9.4 % (9/96) mortality rate.

Many stenting patients had hybrid procedures performed (surgical repair with or without muscle flap and drainage plus stenting), a variety of stents used, a variety of locations for the stents, and disparate time intervals between leak and stenting, which limited our interpretation of outcomes. Several stent-related complications were also reported in these studies. We found at least nine cases of large vessel erosion resulting in hemorrhage and death and seven cases in which the stent had made the leak worse (Table 33.1). Because so many studies reported adjunctive surgical procedures in addition to stenting (hybrid procedures), it appeared that stenting alone was inadequate treatment.

Comparison against surgical repair is difficult, but Kassis et al. recently analyzed the Society of Thoracic Surgeons (STS) database in 2013 and reviewed 7,595 esophagectomies, with 804 (10.6 %) leaks. They reported an 11.6 % mortality rate (38 of 327) for patients requiring "surgical management" of an anastomotic leak [37] compared to our reported 15 % mortality rate [1–36] on the basis of our study results. While mortality from leakage is high in both groups, it appears to be slightly worse in the stenting cohort. In another study, mortality from anastomotic leakage was reported to be as low as 3.3 %, with aggressive use of intra-thoracic muscle flaps, early debridement, evacuation of all contaminated spaces, and the use of enteral nutrition [38].

Evidence Quality

The data discussed above come from multiple disparate sources of varying quality, mostly in a retrospective manner and with small numbers. The retrospective studies (as well as two prospective series) summarizing stent treatment for a variety of indications are case series, include small numbers, and have few comparisons against what is considered to be current standard of care. The overall evidence quality is low.

Discussion

Because there is no standardized reporting system for esophageal stenting and no clinical trials exist, and because stenting is often used as an adjunct to surgical therapy, interpreting the efficacy of stenting for anastomotic leakage is difficult. Many studies report the ability of a stent to seal but not heal the leak [31]. Many other studies are unclear about the role of adjunctive surgical intervention such as a concomitant operative decortication and muscle flap with stenting versus percutaneous drainage and stenting, stenting over a sponge, stenting with clipping, or stenting

Table 33.1 Outcomes of stenting for anastomotic leak

Author, year (ref)	Stent for anastomotic leak n = patients	Type of stent	Notes	Heal success n = patients (%)	Mortality n = patients (%)
Babor et al. (2009) [1]	4	cSEMS		4 (100)	0
Blackmon et al. (2009) [2]	3	cSEMS		2 (67)	1 (33)
Bona et al. (2010) [3]	3	cSEMS		2 (67)	0
Brangewitz et al. (2013) [4]	39	cSEMS or SEPS		21 (54)	11 (28)
Cerna et al. (2011) [5]	4	BD		4 (100)	0
Dai et al. (2011) [6]	33	fcSEPS		30 (91)	3 (9)
David et al. (2011) [7]	5	cSEMS		4 (80)	1 (20)
D'Cuhna et al. (2011) [8]	22	cSEMS or SEPS	1 LVEH	13 (59)	4 (18)
Eloubeidi et al. (2009) [9]	2	fcSEMS		2 (100)	0
Evrard et al. (2004) [10]	4	SEPS		4 (100)	0
Feith et al. (2011) [11]	115	fcSEMS		81 (70)	10 (9)
Fernandez et al. (2010) [12]	4	SEPS		3 (75)	1 (25)
Freeman et al. (2011) [13]	17	SEPS and cSEMS		16 (94)	0
Gelbmann et al. (2004) [14]	5	SEPS	1 MLW	3 (60)	2 (40)
Gubler et al. (2013) [15]	2	SEMS		2 (100)	0
Han et al. (2006) [16]	8	cSEMS	1 LVEH	6 (75)	2 (25)
Hirdes et al. (2011) [17]	2	pcSEMS	2 MLW	1 (50)	0
Hunerbein et al. (2004) [18]	9	SEPS		9 (100)	0
Jiang et al. (2011) [19]	2	cSEMS	2 LVEH, 2 MLW	0 (0)	2 (100)
Johnsson et al. (2005) [20]	2	cSEMS		1 (50)	1 (50)
Kauer et al. (2008) [21]	10	cSEMS		7 (70)	2 (20)
Keeling et al. (2010) [22]	3	cSEMS		3 (100)	0
Kim et al. (20080 [23]	4	MSBT	1 LVEH	4 (100)	0
Kotzampassakis et al. (2009) [24]	3	Not reported		3 (100)	0
Langeret al. (2005) [25]	24	SEPS	2 MLW	16 (67)	3 (13)
Lee et al. (2010) [26]	7	pcSEMS		4 (57)	0
Leenders et al. (2013) [27]	15	SEMS- mix		11 (73)	5 (33)
Leers et al. (2009) [28]	15	cSEMS		13 (87)	1 (7)
Lindenmann et al. (2008) [29]	6	cSEMS		6 (100)	0

Pennathur et al. (2008) [30]	5	SEPS	1 LVEH	2 (40)	nr
Salminen et al. (2009) [31]	2	SEMS		2 (100)	1 (50)
Schniewind et al. (2013) [32]	12	SEMS and SEPS		2 (17)	10 (83)
Schubert et al. (2005) [33]	12	SEPS		11 (92)	0
Schweigert et al. (2011) [34]	17	cSEMS	3 LVEH	13 (76)	4 (24)
Tuebergen et al. (2008) [35]	19	cSEMS		14 (74)	1 (5)
Zsis et al. (2008) [36]	9	cSEMS		7 (78)	2 (22)
Total	448		9 LVEH, 7 MLW	326 (73 %)	67 (15 %)

Abbreviations: *cSEMS* covered self-expanding metal stent, *pcSEMS* partially covered self-expanding metal stent, *fcSEMS* fully covered self-expanding metal stent, *bd* biodegradable stent, *SEPS* self-expanding plastic stent, *MSBT* Montgomery salivary bypass tub⁺, *LVEH* large vessel erosion hemorrhage, *MLW* made the leak worseHeal success means that the stent is reported to heal the leak and not just seal with radiograph. The seal rate will always be higher than the actual heal rate with drainage. What is clear is that in order for stenting to work, all contaminated spaces have to be drained completely.

There are reports of surgical drains preventing the sealing and healing of a leak because of the drain being in direct contact with the stent. In those cases, the drain would need to be pulled back to allow tissue ingrowth and healing. Additionally, there are complications associated with stents that are left in place for several weeks. There are studies reporting the stent enlarging a leak or eroding into large adjacent vascular structures when left in place for more than 3–4 weeks. Comparing the values of surgical repair and stenting for leak mortality in patients may not be fair, since most patients relegated to stenting may have been considered too ill for surgical intervention, resulting in selection bias. Stenting appears to be a complex treatment, and repeat endoscopic intervention is reported in most series. Leak classification and techniques used to achieve a complete seal require complex decision-making. Because of this, we recommend that stent management be only at the direction of a surgical team and not a non-surgical team. Since stenting for leak and fistula is not approved by the Federal Drug Administration in many cases, we are unsure how internal review boards are approving the investigational use of stents without an investigational device exemption.

Recommendations Based on the Data

Early experience with stenting for esophageal anastomotic leaks suggests potential benefit, but also potentially compromises in safety, when stents are used off-label. Surgical drainage and adjunctive treatment still appears to play a major role in the management of esophageal leaks in situations in which stenting alone would not be adequate. And although mortality is high when the leak is not controlled by either method (stenting or surgery), stenting is still a useful tool in a surgeon's armamentarium to help patients who are poor surgical candidates. Since the management of esophageal anastomotic leaks with stents is considered an off-label use of a device, patients should be warned of potential risks. Esophageal stenting for the management of esophageal anastomotic continues to remain experimental.

A Personal View of the Data

My approach to esophageal leaks and fistulas is individualized. When a patient presents with a leak from the esophagus, management depends on several factors: the condition of the patient, the duration of leakage, the etiology of the leak, the condition of the esophagus distal to the leak, and available options for treatment. In general, stenting is only one of the tools a surgeon may choose to treat such patients.

Our service is careful to make the patient aware of the off-label nature of this new technology and has enrolled some of them onto a prospective trial in conjunction with the FDA (Federal Drug Administration) as part of an IDE (Investigational device Exemption). Frequently, the stent requires adjunctive procedures such as thoracostomy tubes to ensure good drainage of all infected spaces, occasional muscle flaps to cover a leak that is close to vascular or airway structures, endoluminal suturing or bridling the stent to empirically prevent migration, enteral nutrition through the stent or downstream to the stent through a feeding tube, or drainage gastrostomy tubes to drain leaks located at the esophago-gastric junction. Every patient requires a leak evaluation within 24 h of stenting. Persistent leaks require re-intervention if undrained. Undrained contamination around the outside of the stent may make a leak worse. Stents should never be left in place for more than 3 weeks to prevent erosion into major vascular structures. When a patient exhibits signs or symptoms of sepsis and stenting does not seal the leak, operative repair or diversion is performed.

Recommendation

- Stents are potentially useful in treating anastomotic leaks in patients who are poor surgical candidates, although surgical drainage and adjunctive treatments are often necessary (evidence level low; weak recommendation).

References

1. Babor R, Talbot M, Tyndal A. Treatment of upper gastrointestinal leaks with a removable, covered, self-expanding metallic stent. Surg Laparosc Endosc Percut Tech. 2009;19(1):e1–4.
2. Blackmon SH, Santora R, Schwarz P, Barroso A, Dunkin BJ. Utility of removable esophageal covered self-expanding metal stents for leak and fistula management. Ann Thorac Surg. 2010;89(3):931–6; discussion 936–7.
3. Bona D, Laface L, Bonavina L, Abate E, Schaffer M, Ugenti I, et al. Covered nitinol stents for the treatment of esophageal strictures and leaks. World J Gastroenterol. 2010;16(18):2260–4.
4. Brangewitz M, Voigtlander T, Helfritz FA, Lankisch TO, Winkler M, Klempnauer J, et al. Endoscopic closure of esophageal intrathoracic leaks: stent versus endoscopic vacuum-assisted closure, a retrospective analysis. Endoscopy. 2013;45(6):433–8.
5. Cerna M, Kocher M, Valek V, Aujesky R, Neoral C, Andrasina T, et al. Covered biodegradable stent: new therapeutic option for the management of esophageal perforation or anastomotic leak. Cardiovasc Intervent Radiol. 2011;34(6):1267–71.
6. Dai Y, Chopra SS, Kneif S, Hunerbein M. Management of esophageal anastomotic leaks, perforations, and fistulae with self-expanding plastic stents. J Thorac Cardiovasc Surg. 2011;141(5):1213–7.
7. David EA, Kim MP, Blackmon SH. Esophageal salvage with removable covered self-expanding metal stents in the setting of intrathoracic esophageal leakage. Am J Surg. 2011;202(6):796–801; discussion 801.

8. D'Cuhna J, Rueth NM, Groth SS, Maddaus MA, Andrade RS. Esophageal stents for anastomotic leaks and perforations. J Thorac Cardiovasc Surg. 2011;142(1):39–46.
9. Eloubeidi MA, Lopes TL. Novel removable internally fully covered self-expanding metal esophageal stent: feasibility, technique of removal, and tissue response in humans. Am J Gastroenterol. 2009;104(6):1374–81.
10. Evrard S, Le Moine O, Lazaraki G, Dormann A, El Nakadi I, Deviere J. Self-expanding plastic stents for benign esophageal lesions. Gastrointest Endosc. 2004;60(6):894–900.
11. Feith M, Gillen S, Schuster T, Theisen J, Friess H, Gertler R. Healing occurs in most patients that receive endoscopic stents for anastomotic leakage; dislocation remains a problem. Clin Gastroenterol Hepatol. 2011;9(3):202–10.
12. Fernandez A, Vila JJ, Vasquez C, Gonzalez-Portela C, de la Iglesia M, Lozano M, et al. Self-expanding plastic stents for the treatment of post-operative esophago-jejuno anastomosis leak. A case series study. Rev Esp Enferm Dig. 2010;102(12):704–10.
13. Freeman RK, Vyverberg A, Ascioti AJ. Esophageal stent placement for the treatment of acute intrathoracic anastomotic leak after esophagectomy. Ann Thorac Surg. 2011;92(1):204–8; discussion 208.
14. Gelbmann C, Ratiu NL, Rath HC, Rogler G, Lock G, Scholmerich J, et al. Use of self-expandable plastic stents for the treatment of esophageal perforations and symptomatic anastomotic leaks. Endoscopy. 2004;36(8):695–9.
15. Gubler C, Schneider PM, Bauerfeind P. Complex anastomotic leaks following esophageal resections: the new stent over sponge approach. Dis Esophagus. 2013;26(6):598–602.
16. Han XW, Li YD, Wu G, Li MH, Ma XX. New covered mushroom-shaped metallic stent for managing anastomotic leak after esophagogastrostomy with a wide gastric tube. Ann Thorac Surg. 2006;82(2):702–6.
17. Hirdes MMC, Vleggaar FP, Van der Linde K, Willems M, Totte ER, Siersema PD. Esophageal perforation due to removal of partially covered self-expanding metal stents placed for a benign perforation or leak. Endoscopy. 2011;43(2):156–9.
18. Hunerbein M, Stroszczynski C, Moesta KT, Schlag PM. Treatment of thoracic anastomotic leaks after esophagectomy with self-expanding plastic stents. Ann Surg. 2004;240(5):801–7.
19. Jiang F, Yu MF, Ren BH, Yin GW, Zhang Q, Xu L. Nasogastric placement of sump tube through the leak for the treatment of esophagogastric anastomotic leak after esophagectomy for esophageal carcinoma. J Surg Res. 2011;171(2):448–51.
20. Johnsson E, Lundell L, Liedman B. Sealing of esophageal perforation or ruptures with expandable metallic stents: a prospective controlled study on treatment efficacy and limitations. Dis Esophagus. 2005;18(4):262–6.
21. Kauer WK, Stein HJ, Dittler HJ, Siewert JR. Stent implantation as a treatment option in patients with thoracic anastomotic leaks after esophagectomy. Surg Endosc. 2008;22(1):50–3.
22. Keeling WB, Miller DL, Lam GT, Kilgo P, Miller JI, Mansour KA, et al. Low mortality after treatment for esophageal perforation: a single-center experience. Ann Thorac Surg. 2010;90:1669–73.
23. Kim AW, Liptay MJ, Snow N, Donahue P, Warren WH. Utility of silicone esophageal bypass stents in the management of delayed complex esophageal disruptions. Ann Thorac Surg. 2008;85(6):1962–7; discussion 1967.
24. Kotzampassakis N, Christodoulou M, Krueger T, Demartines N, Vuillemeier H, Cheng C, et al. Esophageal leaks repaired by a muscle onlay approach in the presence of mediastinal sepsis. Ann Thorac Surg. 2009;88(3):966–72.
25. Langer FB, Schoppmann SF, Prager G, Riegler FM, Zacherl J. Solving the problem of difficult stent removal due to tissue ingrowth in partially uncovered esophageal self-expanding metal stents. Ann Thorac Surg. 2010;89(5):1691–2.
26. Lee KM, Shin SJ, Hwang JC, Yoo BM, Cheong JY, Lim SG, et al. Proximal-releasing stent insertion under transnasal endoscopic guidance in patients with postoperative esophageal leakage. Gastrointest Endosc. 2010;72(1):180–5.
27. Leenders BJ, Stronkhorst A, Smulders FJ, Nieuwenhuijzen GA, Gilissen LP. Removable and repositionable covered metal self-expandable stents for leaks after upper gastrointestinal surgery: experiences in a tertiary referral hospital. Surg Endosc. 2013;27(8):2751–9.

28. Leers JM, Vivaldi C, Schafer H, Bludau M, Brabender J, Lurje G, et al. Endoscopic therapy for esophageal perforation or anastomotic leak with a self-expandable metallic stent. Surg Endosc. 2009;23(10):2258–62.
29. Lindenmann J, Matzi V, Porubsky C, Anegg U, Sankin O, Gabor S, et al. Self-expandable covered metal tracheal type stent for sealing cervical anastomotic leak after esophagectomy and gastric pull-up: pitfalls and possibilities. Ann Thorac Surg. 2008;85(1):354–6.
30. Pennathur A, Chang AC, McGrath KM, Steiner G, Alvelo-Rivera M, Awais O, et al. Polyflex expandable stents in the treatment of esophageal disease: initial experience. Ann Thorac Surg. 2008;85(6):1968–72; discussion 1973.
31. Salminen P, Gullichsen R, Laine S. Use of self-expandable metal stents for the treatment of esophageal perforations and anastomotic leaks. Surg Endosc. 2009;23(7):1526–30.
32. Schniewind B, Schafmayer C, Voehrs G, Egberts J, von Schoenfels W, Rose T, et al. Endoscopic endoluminal vacuum therapy is superior to other regimens in managing anastomotic leakage after esophagectomy: a comparative retrospective study. Surg Endosc. 2013;27(10):3883–90.
33. Schubert D, Scheibach H, Kuhn R, Wex C, Weiss G, Eder F, et al. Endoscopic treatment of thoracic esophageal anastomotic leaks by using silicone-covered, self-expanding polyester stents. Gastrointest Endosc. 2005;61(7):891–6.
34. Schweigert M, Dubecz A, Stadlhuber RJ, Muschweck H, Stein HJ. Risk of stent-related aortic erosion after endoscopic stent insertion for intrathoracic anastomotic leaks after esophagectomy. Ann Thorac Surg. 2011;92(2):513–8.
35. Tuebergen D, Rijcken E, Mennigen R, Hopkins AM, Senninger N, Bruewer M. Treatment of thoracic esophageal anastomotic leaks and esophageal perforations with endoluminal stents: efficacy and current limitations. J Gastrointest Surg. 2008;12(7):1168–76.
36. Zisis C, Guillin A, Heyries L, Lienne P, D'Journo XB, Doddoli C, et al. Stent placement in the management of oesophageal leaks. Eur J Cardiothorac Surg. 2008;33(3):451–6.
37. Kassis ES, Kosinski AS, Ross P, Koppes KE, Donahue JM, Daniel VC. Predictors of anastomotic leak after esophagectomy: an analysis of the Society of Thoracic Surgeons general thoracic database. Ann Thorac Surg. 2013;96(6):1919–26.
38. Martin LW, Swisher SG, Hofstetter W, Correa AM, Mehran RJ, Rice DC, et al. Intrathoracic leaks following esophagectomy are no longer associated with increased mortality. Ann Surg. 2005;242(3):392–9; discussion 399–402.

Chapter 34
Management of Small Esophageal GIST Tumors

Richard G. Berrisford and Samuel J. Ford

Abstract Esophageal gastrointestinal stromal tumors (GIST) are very rare. There is a very small literature reporting on lesions larger than 3 cm in diameter. Management of small (<2 cm) submucosal esophageal lesion is limited by difficulty in obtaining a histological diagnosis. Submucosal lesions <2 cm in diameter have, at most, a 10 % chance of being an esophageal GIST, and the likely malignant potential of such a GIST is low. However, there is insufficient data on esophageal GISTs to extrapolate malignant behavior of GISTs from elsewhere in the gastrointestinal tract. Endoscopic ultrasound (EUS) may help to identify rare malignant behavior and allows precise measurement for surveillance. Consensus opinion supports conservative treatment and regular surveillance of esophageal submucosal lesions <2 cm in diameter.

Keywords Esophageal tumor • Esophagus • Gastrointestinal stromal tumor • Esophageal GIST

Introduction

Small submucosal lesions (less than 2 cm in diameter) are a relatively common incidental finding in the esophagus during upper GI endoscopy. These lesions are difficult to biopsy in their submucosal location, and uncommonly turn out to be esophageal Gastrointestinal Stromal Tumors (GISTs). The issue for the surgeon is that of balancing the low likelihood of such lesions being GISTs and the low

R.G. Berrisford, MD (✉) • S.J. Ford, MB, ChB, PhD, FRCS
Peninsula Oesophagogastric Unit, Derriford Hospital,
Level 7, Derriford Road, Plymouth, Devon PL6 8DH, UK
e-mail: richard.berrisford@nhs.net; samuelford1@nhs.net

M.K. Ferguson (ed.), *Difficult Decisions in Thoracic Surgery*,
Difficult Decisions in Surgery: An Evidence-Based Approach 1,
DOI 10.1007/978-1-4471-6404-3_34, © Springer-Verlag London 2014

likelihood of small GISTs having poor prognostic features, against the rare but high malignant potential of larger esophageal GISTs. We have very little reported data with which to plan our approach.

Among the main questions to be answered include how likely it is that an esophageal submucosal mass <2 cm diameter is a GIST. Identifying esophageal GIST may be possible with Endoscopic Ultrasound (EUS) or EUS guided Fine Needle Aspiration (FNA. If it is established that a small esophageal lesion is a GIST, it is uncertain whether it will behave in a malignant manner. It is unclear whether the behavior of GISTs elsewhere in the GI tract can be used to make assumptions about the behavior of esophageal GISTs. Whether surveillance or resection of small esophageal GISTs is unclear.

Search Strategy

The PICO question for this chapter was whether enucleation or esophagectomy was more appropriate for patients with small GIST tumors that were without evident adenopathy on clinical staging. The search terms for this chapter were "gastrointestinal stromal tumor" or "GIST" and "esophageal" or "esophageal". These terms were applied to a PubMed search of the English literature from 2000 to 2013. The reference lists of identified papers were also searched along with National Consensus Guidelines from the US, Europe and Britain.

Epidemiology

Esophageal GISTs are very rare. There are few solitary case reports and very few small retrospective series in the literature shown in Table 34.1 [1–12]. The smallest esophageal GIST in this literature had a diameter of 2.6 cm, although Abraham [3] identified coincidental microscopic GISTs in esophageal resection specimens. Esophageal GISTs are three times less common than leiomyomas [2], GISTs being variably reported to comprise from 12 % [3] to 25 % [2] of all esophageal mesenchymal tumors. Given that lesions other than mesenchymal tumors have a similar appearance, the chance of such a lesion being a GIST is likely to be much less than 10 %.

Diagnosis

EUS should be considered to distinguish a small GIST from extrinsic impression from normal or pathological adjacent structures as well as providing an accurate diameter which can be used to monitor the lesion. Esophageal GISTs appear hypoechoic on EUS and are seen to lie within the muscularis propria [2]. For this reason, endoscopic

Table 34.1 Summary of case reports and small retrospective series for small esophageal GISTs

Study	Patients	Size	Treatment	Outcome
Jiang et al. [1]	8	3–16 cm	Local resection/ oesophagectomy largest surgical series	4 recurred despite R0 resection
Miettinen et al. [2]	17	2.6–25 cm	Local and radical resection/ transmural	9 recurred despite R0 resection and 1 was a palliative resection
Abraham et al. [3]	18	0.2–3 mm	Incidental lesions found in esophageal resection specimens	No data
Manu et al. [4]	1	14 cm		
Padula et al. [5]	1	12 cm		
Feakins et al. [6]	1	7 cm		
Basoglu et al. [7]	1	27 cm		
Huang et al. [8]	1	4 cm		
Masuda et al. [9]	1	8 cm		
Portale et al. [10]	2	13 cm, 5 cm		
Iannicelli et al. [11]	2	9 cm, 5 cm		
Dan et al. [12]	1	15 cm		

GIST gastrointestinal stromal tumors

mucosal resection or endoscopic submucosal dissection are not diagnostic or therapeutic options. However, the authors could not identify any references to EUS appearances being able to reliably differentiate between GIST and leiomyoma or other mesenchymal tumor. EUS can, however, suggest higher malignant potential in some GIST tumors which display irregular extraluminal margins or cystic spaces [13].

Some authors suggest that EUS FNA may be used to differentiate esophageal GIST from leiomyoma [14, 15]. This is dependent on lesion size and on local endoscopic and pathology expertise and can often be inconclusive [3, 16]. The National Comprehensive Cancer Network guidelines do not suggest biopsy if a lesion is to be resected due to concern around tumor dissemination and bleeding, and if local resection of a potential leiomyoma is undertaken, mucosal injury is more likely [16]. This may not hold for larger lesions requiring extensive resection for which histological confirmation may be appropriate. Where EUS appearance suggests malignant behavior, EUS FNA or core biopsy may be indicated. For small submucosal tumors of the esophagus without EUS features of concern, therefore, EUS FNA is probably not indicated, and this is in accord with European guidelines [17].

Clinical Behavior of GISTs

Most small (<2 cm) GISTs elsewhere in the GI tract have negligible mitotic activity and have a very low malignant potential. There is some uncertainty in extrapolating this data for GISTs in the combined anatomical sites of esophagus, mesentery, omentum, colon or rectum which together make up only 10 % of all GISTs [18, 19]. Esophageal GISTs may have a higher malignant potential and further data on small esophageal GISTs is not likely to be forthcoming. For this reason, Rubinet al. [20] omits esophageal GIST from the table of likely malignant behavior for GISTs elsewhere.

Management of GISTs

Non-operative management mandates repeat assessment with EUS in 6 months with consideration given to further repeat imaging after another 12 months and potentially indefinitely. It seems reasonable to extend the period between observations if the lesion remains <2 cm and does not change in size.

Consensus opinion loosely supports the non-operative management of small asymptomatic GISTs, however this recommendation is not founded on an evidence base. Consensus opinion suggests that all symptomatic as well as asymptomatic GISTs >2 cm should be resected if possible. This recommendation is derived from guidelines for managing GISTs elsewhere in the GI tract; with a possible higher malignant potential, this advice would certainly seem appropriate for esophageal GISTs. Such a resection would ideally be radical, *en bloc*, with a 2 cm margin [19]. Rupture of the tumor must be avoided [21]. While GISTs do not tend to spread to lymph nodes, such spread has been reported and the few larger resected esophageal GISTs reported in the literature had a high recurrence rate despite R0 resection.

A case series of surgical resections for esophageal GISTs recommends that local resection is limited to small (<2 cm) GISTs and only then with the proviso that clear surgical resections can be achieved [15]. In patients with lesions larger than this, EUS guided biopsy should be undertaken to guide more extensive surgical resection [22].

Summary

GIST are very rare, and management recommendations are limited by the small amount of published information on these tumors. Submucosal lesions <2 cm in diameter have a <10 % chance of being an esophageal GIST with a low malignant potential. However, there is insufficient data on esophageal GISTs to extrapolate malignant behavior of GISTs from elsewhere in the gastrointestinal tract. Endoscopic ultrasound (EUS) may help to identify rare malignant behavior and allows precise measurement for surveillance. Consensus opinion supports nonoperative treatment and regular surveillance of esophageal submucosal lesions <2 cm in diameter.

A Personal View of the Data

The author manages submucosal oesophageal lesions less than 1 cm diameter as incidental findings and does not investigate further unless the patient is symptomatic. In patients with dysphagia, a marshmallow contrast swallow is performed to identify symptom correlation with a bolus passing the lesion (this often shows no correlation). Patients with lesions 1–2 cm in diameter, whether symptomatic or not, are investigated with EUS, with a follow-up EUS at 6 months undertaken (sooner if symptoms dictate). Patients in this group whose contrast swallow correlates with dysphagia may have the lesion excised locally (without oesophageal resection). EUS FNA is only undertaken if there are concerns about malignant potential on initial EUS. Alternative diagnoses discussed above are always considered, and we have a low threshold to request CT scan.

Recommendations for Small (<2 cm) Suspected GIST Tumors

- Co-incidental submucosal esophageal lesions identified at endoscopy should be evaluated by EUS (evidence quality low; weak recommendation)
- Small esophageal GISTs (≤2 cm) can be managed with surveillance alone (evidence quality low; weak recommendation)
- Symptomatic small esophageal GISTs (≤2 cm) can potentially be resected by minimally invasive enucleation (evidence quality low; weak recommendation)
- Larger GISTs (>2 cm) or those encroaching on the gastro-esophageal junction should be considered for more invasive surgery (evidence quality low; weak recommendation)

References

1. Jiang P, Jiao Z, Han B, Zhang X, Sun X, Su J, et al. Clinical characteristics and surgical treatment of esophageal gastrointestinal stromal tumors. Eur J Cardiothorac Surg. 2010;38:223–7.
2. Miettinen M, Sarlomo-Rikala M, Sobin LH, Lasota J. Esophageal stromal tumors: a clinicopathologic, immunohistochemical, and molecular genetic study of 17 cases and comparison with esophageal leiomyomas and leiomyosarcomas. Am J Surg Pathol. 2000;24:211–22.
3. Abraham SC, Krasinskas AM, Hofstetter WL, Swisher SG, Wu TT. "Seedling" mesenchymal tumors (gastrointestinal stromal tumors and leiomyomas) are common incidental tumors of the esophagogastric junction. Am J Surg Pathol. 2007;31:1629–35.
4. Manu N, Richard P, Howard S. Bleeding esophageal GIST. Dis Esophagus. 2005;18:281–2.
5. Padula A, Chin NW, Azeez S, Resetkova E, Andriko JA, Miettinen M. Primary gastrointestinal stromal tumor of the esophagus in an HIV-positive patient. Ann Diagn Pathol. 2005;9:49–53.
6. Feakins RM, Mears L, Atkinson P, Hughes F. Esophageal gastrointestinal stromal tumor masquerading as neuroendocrine carcinoma. Histopathology. 2005;47:327–9.

7. Basoglu A, Kaya E, Celik B, Yildiz L. Giant gastrointestinal stromal tumor of the esophagus presenting with dyspnea. J Thorac Cardiovasc Surg. 2006;131:1198–9.
8. Huang CS, Hsu WH, Wu YC, Chau GY, Tsay SH, Huang MH. Enucleation of an advanced esophageal gastrointestinal stromal tumor with liver metastasis. J Gastroenterol Hepatol. 2006;21:482–3.
9. Masuda T, Toh Y, Kabashima A, Aoki Y, Harimoto N, Ito S, et al. Overt lymph node metastases from a gastrointestinal stromal tumor of the esophagus. J Thorac Cardiovasc Surg. 2007; 134:810–1.
10. Portale G, Zaninotto G, Costantini M, Rugge M, Pennelli GM, Rampado S, et al. Esophageal GIST: case report of surgical enucleation and update on current diagnostic and therapeutic options. Int J Surg Pathol. 2007;15:393–6.
11. Iannicelli E, Sapori A, Panzuto F, Pilozzi E, Delle FG, David V. Esophageal GIST: MDCT findings of two cases and review of the literature. J Gastrointest Cancer. 2012;43:481–5.
12. Dan D, Seetahal S, Persad R. Gastrointestinal stromal tumor of the esophagus. J Natl Med Assoc. 2009;101:462–5.
13. Palazzo L, Landi B, Cellier C, Cuillerier E, Roseau G, Barbier JP. Endosonographic features predictive of benign and malignant gastrointestinal stromal cell tumors. Gut. 2000;46:88–92.
14. Stelow EB, Jones DR, Shami VM. Esophageal leiomyosarcoma diagnosed by endoscopic ultrasound-guided fine-needle aspiration. Diagn Cytopathol. 2007;35:167–70.
15. Blum MG, Bilimoria KY, Wayne JD, de Hoyos AL, Talamonti MS, Adley B. Surgical considerations for the management and resection of esophageal gastrointestinal stromal tumors. Ann Thorac Surg. 2007;84:1717–23.
16. Demetri GD, Benjamin RS, Blanke CD, Blay JY, Casali P, Choi H, et al. NCCN Task Force report: management of patients with gastrointestinal stromal tumor (GIST) – update of the NCCN clinical practice guidelines. J Natl Compr Canc Netw. 2007;5 Suppl 2:S1–29.
17. Gastrointestinal stromal tumors. (ESMO) European Sarcoma Network Working Group clinical practice guidelines for diagnosis, treatment and follow-up. Ann Oncol. 2012; 23(Suppl 7):vii49–55.
18. Emory TS, Sobin LH, Lukes L, Lee DH, O'Leary TJ. Prognosis of gastrointestinal smooth-muscle (stromal) tumors: dependence on anatomic site. Am J Surg Pathol. 1999;23:82–7.
19. Connolly EM, Gaffney E, Reynolds JV. Gastrointestinal stromal tumors. Br J Surg. 2003;90: 1178–86.
20. Rubin BP, Heinrich MC, Corless CL. Gastrointestinal stromal tumor. Lancet. 2007;369: 1731–41.
21. Ng EH, Pollock RE, Munsell MF, Atkinson EN, Romsdahl MM. Prognostic factors influencing survival in gastrointestinal leiomyosarcomas. Implications for surgical management and staging. Ann Surg. 1992;215:68–77.
22. Gervaz P, Huber O, Morel P. Surgical management of gastrointestinal stromal tumors. Br J Surg. 2009;96:567–78.

Chapter 35
Surgery for Minimally Symptomatic Pulsion Diverticula of the Thoracic Esophagus

Parise Paolo and Zaninotto Giovanni

Abstract Diverticula of the thoracic esophagus (ED) are rare. The main symptoms are regurgitation and dysphagia, and sometimes respiratory symptoms too. The literature is unable to provide a high level of evidence because it consists mainly of case series or case reports. Although a linear correlation between symptoms and the size of ED has not been firmly demonstrated, it is clinically common to find that larger diverticula are more symptomatic. Some studies have found that ED patients with mild or no symptoms do not experience any worsening of their symptoms with time, whereas moderately or severely symptomatic patients tend to progress. Surgery (completed via a minimally invasive access nowadays) has achieved high success rates with extremely low rates of recurrence, but it is burdened by a far from negligible incidence of complications, particularly relating to suture line leakage. Surgery is consequently only justified in symptomatic patients, reserving a conservative approach to asymptomatic or minimally-symptomatic cases, which involves a clinical follow-up and the prescription of proton pump inhibitors or endoscopic pneumatic dilation.

Keywords Esophageal diverticulum • Surgery • Diverticulectomy • Natural history • Symptoms • Complications • Conservative treatment

Introduction

Historically, diverticula of the thoracic esophagus were considered "traction diverticula" when they arose in the middle third, and "pulsion diverticula" when in the distal third. The former originate from a chronic inflammatory process, such as tuberculosis, and involve a mediastinal lymph node attaching to and retracting the

P. Paolo, MD • Z. Giovanni, MD, FACS (✉)
General Surgery Unit, "SS. Giovanni e Paolo" Hospital,
University of Padova, Castello 6777, Venice, Italy
e-mail: paolo.parise@ulss12.ve.it; giovanni.zaninotto@unipd.it

M.K. Ferguson (ed.), *Difficult Decisions in Thoracic Surgery*,
Difficult Decisions in Surgery: An Evidence-Based Approach 1,
DOI 10.1007/978-1-4471-6404-3_35, © Springer-Verlag London 2014

esophageal wall; the latter derive from an esophageal motor disorder that leads to a high intraluminal pressure. Jordan recently wrote that small diverticula may originate anywhere in the distal half of the esophagus and, when they are larger and come closer to the diaphragm, they take the name of "epiphrenic diverticula" [1].

Esophageal diverticula (ED) are rare and their real prevalence remains uncertain. Radiological studies have reported quite different prevalence rates in different countries, ranging from about 0.015 % in the USA to 0.77 % in Japan, or 2 % in Europe [2–4]. The prevalence of the main symptoms, such as dysphagia, regurgitation or aspiration-related respiratory symptoms, is extremely variable in the literature, ranging from 0 to 40 % [5–8], and no linear correlation has emerged with the size of the ED, which cannot be considered as a reliable guide to treatment.

Since the natural history of ED is extremely difficult to predict, and the presence of a diverticulum is not per se an indication for surgery, the question is which ED need surgery? Nowadays, the treatment of choice accepted by most of surgeons is diverticulectomy associated with a myotomy and an antireflux procedure via a minimally-invasive laparoscopic access. The alternative is conservative treatment, consisting of proton pump inhibitors (PPI) in cases with associated gastroesophageal reflux disease (GERD) symptoms, endoscopic pneumatic dilation of the gastro-esophageal junction for patients with mild obstructive symptoms, or clinical follow-up alone.

Search Strategy

A PubMed search was performed of the literature published in the English language over the last 10 years. Given the rarity of ED, no randomized controlled trials were identified, only cohort studies or case series, and numerous case reports with a low level of evidence. Case series with less than ten patients were ruled out. Case reports were only considered in the event of rare complications of the disease's natural history. Cricopharyngeal (Zenker's) diverticula were also excluded.

Results

The main issue when it comes to managing patients with ED is whether or not they all warrant surgical treatment. The need for surgery is still being debated and this will probably continue for some time to come because the natural history of ED is still not completely clear. Surgeons should balance the potential benefits of surgery and the risk of ED-related complications against the risks related to surgery. Although an ED's size should not be considered a reliable guide because no linear correlation with symptoms has been demonstrated, it is common in clinical practice to find small ED mildly symptomatic or not at all symptomatic, while large ones are associated with food retention, regurgitation and aspiration symptoms. This empirical observation was confirmed by an interesting radiological study conducted in 2003 by Fasano at the University of Pennsylvania [9], reviewing 27 patients presenting with ED from 1990 to 2000: 100 % of the patients with an ED at least 5 cm in size were symptomatic, as opposed to 41 % of cases with a smaller ED (p=0.0031). A significant correlation was also found between preferential filling of the ED with barium and symptoms: 91 % of patients with preferential filling of their diverticulum were symptomatic, as opposed to 44 % of cases without preferential filling (p=0.0031). No correlation emerged between radiographically-identified motility disorders (e.g. spastic or abnormal contractions) and symptoms. Although Fasano's findings do not entitle us to consider ED size as an indication for or against surgery, they do provide evidence of larger diverticula being more likely to cause symptoms and consequently to warrant surgery for their treatment.

The natural history of ED is extremely difficult to predict. Some severe outcomes have been described in the literature, such as diverticular perforation, rupture and malignant degeneration, but these reports remain mainly anecdotal [10–12]. On the whole, it was estimated in two interesting reviews from Australia and Italy that less than 10 % of asymptomatic or mildly symptomatic patients will progress or experience a complication of their disease and that patients with moderately or severely symptomatic disease will tend to have progressively worsening symptoms in about 90 % of cases, sometimes even to the point of making surgery unfeasible [13, 14].

An important factor to consider when offering surgery for ED is the surgical risk. In fact the mortality and the overall morbidity rates, and the risk of leakage are high, especially for a benign disease. The mortality rate ranges from 0 to 7.7 %, the overall morbidity from 6.7 to 45 %, and suture leakage occurs in 3.3–23.1 % of cases. These data are summarized in Table 35.1 [15–21]. Although the level of evidence is

Table 35.1 Morbidity and mortality after surgery

Author	Pts n.	Type of surgery	Overall morbidity	Leaks	Mortality	Quality of evidence
Nehra et al. [15]	17	17 thorac	2(11.7)	1(5.8)	1(5.8)	Moderate
Klaus et al. [16]	11	10 lps 1 thorac	2(18)	1(9)	0	Moderate
Del Genio et al. [17]	13	13 D + M + A	–	3(23.1)	1(7.7)	Moderate
Fernando et al. [18]	20	10 D + M + A lps 7 D + M + A VATS 3 D + M + A lps + VATS	9(45)	4(20)	0	Moderate
Melman et al. [19]	13	12D + M + A lps 1 D + M lps	2(15.4)	1(7.7)	0	Moderate
Zaninotto et al. [20]	24	17 D + M + A lps 7 D + M + A lps + thorac	6(25)	4(16.6)	0	Moderate
Fumagalli et al. [21]	30	30 D + M + A lps	2(6.7)	1(3.3)	0	Moderate

Values in parentheses are percentages

Thorac thoracotomy, *Lps* laparoscopy, *D* diverticulectomy, *M* myotomy, *A* antireflux procedure, *VATS* video-assisted thoracic surgery

Table 35.2 Results of surgery

Author	Pts n.	Type of surgery	F.U. (months)	Asymptomatic patients	Diverticular recurrence	Quality of evidence
Nehra et al. [15]	17	17 thorac	24	15(88)	–	Moderate
Klaus et al. [16]	11	10 lps 1 thorac	26.4	11(100)	–	Moderate
Del Genio et al. [17]	13	13 D + M + A	58	13(100)	0	Moderate
Fernando et al. [18]	20	10 D + M + A lps 7 D + M + A VATS 3 D + M + A lps + ATS	15	15(75)	2(10)	Moderate
Melman et al. [19]	13	12D + M + A lps 1 D + M lps	13.6	11(84.6)	0	Moderate
Zaninotto et al. [20]	24	17 D + M + A lps 7 D + M + A lps + thorac	96	17(70.8)	0	Moderate
Fumagalli et al. [21]	30	30 D + M + A lps	52	30(100)	0	Moderate

Values in parentheses are percentages
Thorac thoracotomy, *Lps* laparoscopy, *D* diverticulectomy, *M* myotomy, *A* antireflux procedure, *VATS* video-assisted thoracic surgery

only moderate for these data (because the studies were case series with limited numbers of patients), it is worth noting that all these studies produced similar results. The picture they paint was also recently confirmed in an interesting review from Japan that calculated, for a total sample of 133 patients, a mortality rate of 2 %, a morbidity rate of 21 % and a suture leakage rate of 15 % [22]. Surgery seems to be extremely effective, however, putting a stop to symptoms in 70–100 % of cases, with a recurrence rate no higher than 10 %. These data are summarized in Table 35.2 [15–21].

Few studies have drawn a direct comparison between the results obtained in surgically-treated versus conservatively-managed patients. The main reason for adopting a conservative treatment in these reports was that patients had minimal or no symptoms, or general contraindications to surgery. PPI or H2-blockers were administered to patients who had symptoms of GERD. If esophageal motor disorders or lower esophageal sphincter relaxation alterations were detected with esophageal manometry, patients underwent endoscopic pneumatic dilation. Patients referred for surgery were treated with a diverticulectomy + myotomy + antireflux procedure through a minimally-invasive approach. The outcome in surgically-treated patients was comparable with those previously described: the overall morbidity rate ranged from 18 to 22.7 %, the suture leakage rate from 9 to 18 % and mortality was nil. The vast majority of conservatively-managed patients (85–90 %) experienced no change or an improvement in their symptoms during the follow-up [16, 23].

Recommendations

Given that most patients with minimally symptomatic or asymptomatic ED experience no exacerbation of their symptoms with time, that complications such as rupture or malignant degeneration are extremely rare, and that surgery is burdened with a high rate of severe complications, only patients with moderately or severely symptomatic ED should undergo surgery. Patients with asymptomatic or minimally symptomatic ED can be safely managed with conservative treatments. A clinical and endoscopic follow-up, administering PPI or H2-blockers in the event of GERD symptoms, and performing endoscopic pneumatic dilations for mild dysphagia, suffices for most minimally symptomatic patients.

A Personal View of the Data

Because ED are so rare, data in the literature are often obtained from case series with low or moderate levels of evidence, but most reports and the few meta-analyses available tend to converge toward the same conclusions, thus combining to reinforce our recommendations more than the single papers could do alone. We agree wholeheartedly with something Orringer said some years ago: '*A masterful inactivity in asymptomatic or mildly disturbing diverticula is a good practice even if, in this time of minimally-invasive surgery and stapling devices, an esophageal diverticulectomy may represent a tempting trophy for a hyperactive surgeon*' [24]. An exception could be represented by patients presenting with a large asymptomatic ED. In our opinion, respiratory symptoms should be particularly carefully investigated in such patients, and surgery may be justified if they are at high risk of aspiration. The final decision should nonetheless be made with the patient, after clearly explaining the risks and benefits of surgery and of conservative treatments.

Finally, we are firmly convinced that surgery should be completed using a minimally invasive approach. Laparoscopy enables us to better expose the gastroesophageal junction and esophagus, facilitating the myotomy and antireflux procedure. It also makes it easier to transect the diverticular neck because the laparoscopic stapler jaws lie parallel to the esophagus. For an ED with a massive neck, or located high in the mediastinum, transection may involve firing twice or more, thus increasing the risk of suture leakage, so we prefer to add a left or right thoracotomy in such cases, and we resect the ED with a TA stapler because its longer jaws mean that a single firing is enough [20].

Recommendations

- Only patients with moderately or severely symptomatic esophageal pulsion diverticula should undergo surgery. (Evidence quality low; weak recommendation)
- A minimally invasive approach should be used for surgical treatment of esophageal pulsion diverticula. (Evidence quality low; weak recommendation)

References

1. Jordan PH, Kinner BM. New look at epiphrenic diverticula. World J Surg. 1999;23(2): 147–52.
2. Wheeler D. Diverticula of the foregut. Radiology. 1947;49:476–81.
3. Dobashi Y, Goseki N, Inutake Y, Kawano T, Endou M, Nemoto T. Giant epiphrenic diverticulum with achalasia occurring 20 years after Heller's operation. J Gastroenterol. 1996;31:844–7.
4. Schima W, Schober E, Stacher G, Franz P, Uranitsch K, Pokieser P, et al. Association of mido-esophageal diverticula with oesophageal motor disorders. Videofluoroscopy and manometry. Acta Radiol. 1997;38:108–14.
5. Altorki NK, Sunagawa M, Skinner DB. Thoracic esophageal diverticula. Why is operation necessary? J Thorac Cardiovasc Surg. 1993;105:260–5.
6. Benacci JC, Deschamps C, Trastek VF, Allen MS, Daly RC, Pairolero PC. Epiphrenic diverticulum: results of surgical treatment. Ann Thorac Surg. 1993;55:1109–014.
7. Castrucci G, Porziella V, Granone PL, Picciocchi A. Tailored surgery for esophageal body diverticula. Eur J Cardiothorac Surg. 1998;14:380–7.
8. Streitz Jr JM, Glick ME, Ellis Jr FH. Selective use of myotomy for treatment of epiphrenic diverticula. Manometric and clinical analysis. Arch Surg. 1992;127:585–7.
9. Fasano NC, Levine MS, Rubesin SE, Redfern RO, Laufer I. Epiphrenic diverticulum: clinical and radiographic findings in 27 patients. Dysphagia. 2003;18:9–15.
10. Hung JJ, Hsieh CC, Lin SC, Wang LS. Squamous cell carcinoma in a large epiphrenic esophageal diverticulum. Dig Dis Sci. 2009;54:1365–8.
11. Herbella FAM, Del Grande JC. Benign esophagopulmonary fistula through an epiphrenic diverticulum and asymptomatic achalasia. Dig Dis Sci. 2010;55:1177–8.
12. Lee JH, Chae HS, Kim KH, Kim JW, Wang YP, Lee SH, et al. Delayed primary repair of perforated epiphrenic diverticulum. J Korean Med Sci. 2004;19:887–90.
13. Thomas ML, Anthony AA, Fosh BG, Finch JG, Maddern GJ. Oesophageal diverticula. Br J Surg. 2001;88:629–42.
14. Zaninotto G, Portale G, Costantini M, Zanatta L, Salvador R, Ruol A. Therapeutic strategies for epiphrenic diverticula: systematic review. World J Surg. 2011;35(7):1447–53.
15. Nehra D, Lord RV, DeMeester TR, Theisen J, Peters JH, Crookes PF, et al. Physiologic basis for the treatment of epiphrenic diverticulum. Ann Surg. 2002;235(3):346–54.
16. Klaus A, Hinder RA, Swain J, Achem SR. Management of epiphrenic diverticula. J Gastrointest Surg. 2003;7(7):906–11.
17. Del Genio A, Rossetti G, Maffetton V, Renzi A, Brusciano L, Limongelli P, et al. Laparoscopic approach in the treatment of epiphrenic diverticula: long-term results. Surg Endosc. 2004;18:741–5.
18. Fernando HC, Luketich JD, Samphire J, Alvelo-Rivera M, Christie NA, Buenaventura PO, et al. Minimally invasive operation for esophageal diverticula. Ann Thorac Surg. 2005;80:2076–81.
19. Melman L, Quinlan J, Robertson B, Brunt LM, Halpin VJ, Eagon JC, et al. Esophageal manometric characteristics and outcome for laparoscopic esophageal diverticulectomy, myotomy and partial fundoplication for epiphrenic diverticula. Surg Endosc. 2009;23:1337–41.
20. Zaninotto G, Parise P, Salvador R, Costantini M, Zanatta L, Rella A, et al. Laparoscopic repair of epiphrenic diverticulum. Semin Thorac Cardiovasc Surg. 2012;24(3):218–22.
21. Fumagalli Romario U, Ceolin M, Porta M, Rosati R. Laparoscopic repair of epiphrenic diverticulum. Semin Thorac Cardiovasc Surg. 2012;24(3):213–7.
22. Hirano Y, Takeuchi H, Oyama T, Saikawa Y, Niihara M, Sako H, et al. Minimally invasive surgery for esophageal epiphrenic diverticulum: the results of 133 patients in 25 published series and our experience. Surg Today. 2013;43(1):1–7.
23. Zaninotto G, Rizzetto C, Zambon P, Guzzinati S, Finotti E, Costantini M, et al. Long-term outcome of operated and unoperated epiphrenic diverticula. J Gastrointest Surg. 2008;12:1485–90.
24. Orringer MB. Epiphrenic diverticula: fact and fable. Ann Thorac Surg. 1993;55:1067–8.

Chapter 36
Partial Versus Total Fundoplication for GERD in Patients with Normal Esophageal Motility

Marco E. Allaix and Marco G. Patti

Abstract A laparoscopic total fundoplication is considered today the gold standard for the surgical treatment of gastroesophageal reflux disease (GERD). Short-term outcome is excellent, with low perioperative morbidity and fast recovery; symptom relief and reflux control are achieved in about 80–90 % of patients 10 years after surgery. However, a small but clinically relevant incidence of postoperative dysphagia and gas-related symptoms is reported. Debate still exists about the best antireflux operation and during the last two decades the surgical outcomes of laparoscopic partial fundoplication (anterior or posterior) have been compared to those achieved after a laparoscopic total fundoplication. This chapter reviews the results of partial and total fundoplication for the treatment of GERD in patients with normal esophageal motility.

Keywords Gastroesophageal reflux disease • Total fundoplication • Partial anterior fundoplication • Partial posterior fundoplication • Dysphagia • Gas bloating

Introduction

A laparoscopic total fundoplication (LTF) is considered today the procedure of choice for the surgical treatment of gastroesophageal reflux disease (GERD): it increases the resting pressure and length of the lower esophageal sphincter (LES), decreases the number of transient LES relaxations, and improves quality of

Conflict of Interest The authors have no conflicts of interest to declare.

M.E. Allaix, MD • M.G. Patti, MD (✉)
Department of Surgery, Center for Esophageal Diseases, University of Chicago
Pritzker School of Medicine,
5841 S. Maryland Ave, MC 5031, Room G-207, Chicago, IL 60637, USA
e-mail: mpatti@surgery.bsd.uchicago.edu

M.K. Ferguson (ed.), *Difficult Decisions in Thoracic Surgery*,
Difficult Decisions in Surgery: An Evidence-Based Approach 1,
DOI 10.1007/978-1-4471-6404-3_36, © Springer-Verlag London 2014

esophageal peristalsis [1, 2]. A LTF is associated with less morbidity and similar long-term outcomes compared with open fundoplication [3]. Long follow-up studies have shown that control of symptoms is achieved in about 80–90 % of patients 10 years after surgery [4, 5], with similar safety and efficacy in young and elderly patients [6].

Several randomized clinical trials (RCTs), mostly from Australia, have found that a LTF is as effective in controlling reflux as a laparoscopic partial fundoplication (LPF), but it is associated with a higher incidence of postoperative dysphagia and gas-related symptoms. [7] On the other hand, many studies from the United States have reported similar rates of postoperative dysphagia after LTF and LPF, with a LPF being less effective in controlling reflux than a LTF. [1, 8, 9] The following chapter reviews the surgical outcomes of LTF and LPF in the treatment of GERD in patients with normal esophageal motility.

Search Strategy

Full text articles in English were selected from searches of the Pub-Med database (from 1991 to present) using the following search terms, either alone or in combination: "gastroesophageal reflux disease", "laparoscopic", "total fundoplication", "partial anterior fundoplication", "partial posterior fundoplication", "dysphagia", "recurrent reflux", "gas-bloat syndrome". The reference list of all the identified papers was checked for additional articles for inclusion in this review.

Results

Laparoscopic Fundoplication: Total or Partial?

LTF is a very effective surgical procedure for the treatment of GERD with excellent results in most patients; however it is associated with a small but significant incidence of postoperative dysphagia and gas-related symptoms. Several strategies have been proposed to minimize or prevent these adverse effects, such as division of short gastric vessels during LTF, and use of several variants of LPF (posterior, anterior 90°, anterior 180°) (Table 36.1).

Short gastric vessels division has been suggested as possible factor that might improve postoperative outcomes. Long-term results of several RCTs failed to demonstrate any reduction of postoperative dysphagia in patients undergoing total fundoplication with short gastric division compared with those who underwent total fundoplication without short gastric vessel division [20–22]. Two of these RCTs have shown an association between short gastric vessel division and wind-related effects [20, 22]. However, the studies were characterized by heterogeneity and

Table 36.1 Surgical outcomes after laparoscopic anterior partial fundoplication and laparoscopic total fundoplication (LTF)

Reference	Fundoplication	N	Follow-up	Heartburn	Acid exposure	Dysphagia	Quality of evidence
Watson et al. [10]	Anterior 180°	54	6 months	Partial =	Partial =	Partial < LTF	Moderate
	LTF	53		LTF	LTF		
Ludemann et al. [11]	Anterior 180°	50	5 years	Partial =	NP	Partial < LTF	Moderate
	LTF	51		LTF			
Cai et al. [12]	Anterior 180°	41	10 years	Partial =	NP	Partial = LTF	Moderate
	LTF	48		LTF			
Broeders et al. [13]	Anterior 180°	36	14 years	Partial >	Partial >	Partial < LTF	Moderate
	LTF	41		LTF	LTF[a]		
Baigrie et al. [14]	Anterior 180°	79	2 years	Partial =	NP	Partial < LTF	Moderate
	LTF	84		LTF			
Watson et al. [15]	Anterior 90°	60	6 months	Partial >	Partial =	Partial < LTF	Moderate
	LTF	52		LTF	LTF		
Watson et al. [16]	Anterior 90°	53	5 years	Partial >	NP	Partial = LTF	Moderate
	LTF	44		LTF			
Spence et al. [17]	Anterior 90°	40	1 year	Partial =	Partial >	Partial < LTF	Moderate
	LTF	39		LTF	LTF		
Watson et al. [18]	Anterior 90°	37	5 years	Partial =	NP	Partial < LTF	Moderate
	LTF	37		LTF			
Broeders et al. [19][b]	Anterior 90°	90	5 years	Partial >	NP	Partial < LTF	Moderate
	LTF	81		LTF			

NP not performed

[a]Performed in 8 LPF and 10 LTF

[b]Combined analysis of Refs [16]. and [18]

inherent poor methodological quality, and experts in North America advocate routine division of the short gastric vessels [23]. In the open era, small RCTs with short follow-up periods did not show significant differences in the incidence of dysphagia between a total and a posterior partial fundoplication [24–26]. In the laparoscopic era, several RCTs aimed to find the ideal antireflux technique, comparing LTF to posterior LPF, 180° anterior LPF, and 90° anterior LPF.

Anterior 180° vs. LTF

Watson et al. [10] reported in 1999 the short-term results of a prospective double-blind RCT that compared 53 GERD patients treated with LTF and 54 GERD patients undergoing an anterior 180° LPF. Patients with a severe esophageal motility disorder were excluded. Postoperative dysphagia, heartburn and patients satisfaction were assessed using standardized clinical grading systems. At 6 months, LPF patients experienced significantly less dysphagia for solid food (15 % vs. 40 %, p=0.008), were more likely to belch normally, reported less flatulence, and their level of satisfaction was higher than in patients treated with LTF. No differences were observed in terms of heartburn (9 % in both groups), and mean acid exposure at 24-h pH monitoring. The authors concluded that anterior 180° LPF achieves equivalent control of reflux and is associated with improved clinical outcomes at 6 months.

The 5-year follow-up results of this RCT based on standardized questionnaires confirmed in 101 patients (51 LTF, 50 LPF) similar heartburn control in the two groups (10 % LTF vs. 20 % LPF, p=0.172), lower incidence of dysphagia, abdominal bloating and inability to belch among LPF patients, with high patients satisfaction scores in both groups, proving the durability of anterior 180° LPF. [11]

Finally, 10-year follow-up data obtained in 89 patients (48 LTF and 41 LPF) using a standard clinical questionnaire showed that both LTF and anterior 180° LPF are durable, safe and effective, with no significant differences in terms of heartburn control, use of Proton Pump Inhibitors (PPIs), incidence of dysphagia, and overall satisfaction [12]. However, when patients were tested with manometry and ambulatory 24-h impedance- pH monitoring at 14 years follow-up, mean LES resting and relaxation pressures were lower and acid, weakly acidic, liquid and mixed reflux episodes were more common after LPF. LPF patients experienced more frequent heartburn than LTF patients, while dysphagia was less common. [13]

Similar results were obtained by Baigrie et al. [14] They randomized 163 GERD patients, regardless of motility findings, to a LTF (84 patients) or an anterior 180° LPF (79 patients), with no division of the short gastric vessels. There were no significant differences in heartburn according to the assessment by visual analogue scale between the two groups at 3, 12, and 24 months. Patients after LPF had significantly less dysphagia at each follow-up interval. No differences were reported in patient satisfaction scores.

Anterior 90° vs. LTF

Although postoperative dysphagia and gas-related problems are reduced after anterior 180° LPF compared to LTF, they are still reported in some patients. This led in the late 1990s to the development of a 90° anterior LPF, that was compared to LTF in several RCTs.

Watson et al. [15] published in 2004 the short-term outcomes of a multicenter, prospective, double-blind RCT: 112 GERD patients were randomized to anterior 90° LPF (60 patients) or LTF with division of the short gastric vessels (52 patients). Patients with esophageal motility disorders were excluded from the study. Clinical outcomes in terms of dysphagia, heartburn and overall satisfaction were measured using multiple clinical grading systems at 1, 3, and 6 months postoperatively. Esophageal manometry, 24-h pH monitoring, and upper endoscopy were performed 3–4 months after surgery. No significant differences were observed in terms of early postoperative morbidity and length of postoperative stay. At 6 months, dysphagia and flatulence were more frequently experienced by patients undergoing LTF. LES pressure, acid exposure and endoscopic findings were similar at 3–4 months after both procedures. The incidence of heartburn assessed by yes/no questions was similar in the two groups at 1 and 3 months, while it was significantly higher after LPF at 6 months (19 % vs. 4 %, p=0.03). Overall satisfaction was higher after LPF. Based on these data, the authors concluded that anterior 90° LPF provides effective reflux control, and it is followed by less dysphagia and gas-related symptoms than LTF. The 12-month follow-up of clinical outcome based on analog scales showed that patients after LPF were less likely to experience dysphagia than patients treated with LTF, while no differences were observed at 5 years. A reduced incidence of heartburn was reported after LTF compared to LPF at 12 months and 5 years. Overall satisfaction was similar in both groups of patients over time. [16]

Spencer et al. [17] published in 2006 the short-term results of a RCT that compared 40 patients undergoing anterior 90° LPF and 39 patients treated with LTF without division of the short gastric vessels. Patients with severe esophageal motility that contraindicated a LTF were excluded from the study. At 1-year follow-up, LTF was associated with higher rates of dysphagia, while no differences were reported for the assessment of heartburn by the visual analogue scale. However, 24-h pH monitoring showed a significantly lower percentage time with pH less than four in the LTF group. At manometry, postoperative LES resting pressure was similar in the two groups, while LES residual relaxation pressure was significantly higher after LTF. Seventy-four patients were available for analysis of clinical outcome using standardized questionnaires at 5 years [18]. The authors found that the incidence of dysphagia and bloating was higher after LTF when measured by an analogue score. There were no significant differences in terms of heartburn control and overall satisfaction, although PPIs were more frequently used after LPF (29.7 % vs. 8.1 %). However, manometry and pH monitoring were not performed.

Broeders et al. [19] combined raw data sets from these 2 RCTs, and used the original data to determine the clinical outcomes at 5 years follow-up. Data were available from a subset of 90 patients undergoing LPF and 82 patients treated with LTF. Heartburn scores were significantly higher after LPF, and the use of PPIs was more common. In this group of patients, however, dysphagia and gas-related symptoms were less frequent. Overall satisfaction with the surgical outcomes was similar. No differences were observed in terms of endoscopic dilatations performed for dysphagia (2 % vs. 6 %, p=0.202), and the number of reoperations (10 % vs. 4.9 %, p=0.212). In particular, the most frequent indication for reoperation was recurrent reflux in the LPF group, and dysphagia in the LTF group.

Summary

Both 180° and 90° anterior LPF are associated with less postoperative dysphagia than LTF at 5 year follow-up. However, at 10 years after surgery, the outcome following anterior 180° LPF and LTF are not significantly different [12]. At 5 years, the incidence of reflux symptoms (i.e. heartburn) and use of PPIs after anterior 180° LPF and LTF were similar, but higher after 90° anterior LPF than LTF. Recurrent reflux is the most common indication for surgical revision of an anterior LPF, while persistent dysphagia is the leading cause for reoperation after LTF. However, the overall number of surgical revisions is not significantly different comparing LPF and LTF. Overall patient satisfaction rating is similar after both subtypes of anterior LPF and LTF.

However, these results should be interpreted with caution. Indeed, most RCTs included small number of patients, did not perform 24-h pH monitoring to evaluate the incidence of reflux at long-term follow-up, and used symptom control and use of PPIs as a marker of surgical outcome. Many studies have in fact shown that when ambulatory 24-h pH monitoring is performed to test patients with recurrent heartburn, pathological reflux is present in less than 40 % of cases [27–30]. On the other hand, long-term studies have shown a less effective control of gastroesophageal reflux with a LPF rather than a LTF. [1, 8, 9] Recurrence of gastroesophageal reflux confirmed by pH monitoring at 5 years is reported in more than 50 % of patients after LPF. [1, 8, 9] Based on these data, we feel that a LTF is the procedure of choice for the treatment of GERD in patients with normal esophageal motility.

Posterior vs. LTF

Laparoscopic posterior fundoplication has been proposed as an alternative to LTF to reduce the incidence of postoperative dysphagia and gas-related symptoms in GERD patients with normal esophageal peristalsis. Several large RCTs have been published, but the results of these studies did not show significant differences and did not permit definitive conclusion (Table 36.2). Broeders et al. [7] recently published a systematic review and meta-analysis of RCTs that compared LTF to Toupet

Table 36.2 Surgical outcomes after laparoscopic posterior partial fundoplication (Toupet) and laparoscopic total fundoplication (LTF)

Reference	Fundoplication	N	Follow-up (months)	Heartburn	Acid exposure	Dysphagia	Quality of evidence
Booth et al. [31]	Toupet	63	12	Toupet = LTF	Toupet = LTF	Toupet = LTF	Low
	LTF	64					
Chrysos et al. [32]	Toupet	19	12	NA	NA	Toupet = LTF	Low
	LTF	14					
Guérin et al. [33]	Toupet	63	12	Toupet = LTF	NA	Toupet = LTF	Low
	LTF	77					
Laws et al. [34]	Toupet	16	27	Toupet = LTF	NA	Toupet = LTF	Low
	LTF	23					
Mickevicius et al. [35]	Toupet	77	12	Toupet = LTF	NA	Toupet = LTF	Low
	LTF	76					
Shaw et al. [36]	Toupet	50	60	Toupet = LTF	Toupet = LTF	Toupet = LTF	High
	LTF	50					
Strate et al. [37]	Toupet	100	24	Toupet = LTF	Toupet > LTF	Toupet < LTF	Low
	LTF	100					
Broeders et al. [7][a]	Toupet	388		Toupet = LTF	Toupet = LTF	Toupet < LTF	Low
	LTF	404					

NA not available

[a]Metanalysis of the RCTs included in the table

(posterior partial) for GERD, aiming to establish the best surgical procedure of choice according to the highest level of evidence. They identified 7 RCTs comparing 404 LTF patients and 388 Toupet patients [31–37]. The methodological quality of the included RCTs ranged from poor to excellent, with a median Jadad score of 2 (range, 1–5). Follow-up ranged between 12 (4 RCTs) and 60 months (1 RCT). LTF was associated with a significantly higher prevalence of dysphagia, inability to belch and gas bloating after surgery, more endoscopic dilatations and more surgical reoperations. No differences were observed for recurrent pathological acid exposure, esophagitis, reflux symptoms, and overall patient satisfaction.

Summary

Toupet fundoplication and LTF achieve similar reflux control. Toupet fundoplication is associated with reduced postoperative dysphagia, need for endoscopic dilatation, reoperation rates and prevalence of gas-related symptoms compared with LTF. These initial mechanical advantages however seem to disappear over time, as recently demonstrated by Mardani et al.. [38]

However, this metanalysis presents some major limitations. There was heterogenous methodological quality of the RCTs included in the study. The studies included different indications for surgery (GERD proven on 24-h pH monitoring, GERD proven on upper endoscopy, GERD requiring daily PPI therapy). The follow-up was short-term. Only a small number of patients was enrolled in each RCT. There was no objective evaluation of heartburn by 24-h pH monitoring after antireflux surgery.

Longer follow-up data are necessary to confirm similar long-term outcomes after Toupet and LTF beyond 5 years, since several large prospective and retrospective studies suggested poorer long-term reflux control after Toupet fundoplication. For instance, Jobe et al. [39] found in 100 consecutive GERD patients that 24-h ph monitoring was abnormal in 51 % of all patients and in 39 % of asymptomatic patients after laparoscopic Toupet fundoplication. Similarly, Patti et al. [1] found that at 70 months after surgery, 56 % of patients after laparoscopic posterior fundoplication but only 28 % after LTF had persistent reflux confirmed by 24-h pH monitoring. After posterior fundoplication, more patients took PPIs (25 % vs. 8 %) or required a second operation (9 % vs. 3 %). The incidence of postoperative dysphagia was similar in the two groups, showing that the type of fundoplication (total vs. partial) is not a risk factor for dysphagia. Based on these data, we feel that a LTF is today the procedure of choice for the treatment of GERD in patients with normal esophageal motility.

Laparoscopic Partial Fundoplication: Anterior or Posterior?

Based on the similar reflux control and reduced postoperative dysphagia after LPF reported in several RCTs, a few studies investigated the surgical outcomes of different partial fundoplications. Hagedorn et al. [40] looked at the efficacy and mechanical consequences in 95 GERD patients who were randomized to have an anterior 120° LPF (47 patients) or a posterior (Toupet) LPF (48 patients). At 12-months, both procedures were effective in reducing reflux symptoms. However, significantly fewer patients experienced postoperative heartburn and regurgitation after a posterior LPF. Similarly, significant differences were observed in 24-h pH monitoring in favor of posterior LPF: even if acid exposure was reduced after both operations, normal levels were achieved only after a posterior LPF. No significant differences between the two groups were recorded in terms of postoperative dysphagia and ability to belch. At 5 years, the long-term results of this RCT showed that a posterior LPF provided significantly better heartburn and regurgitation control, with lower number of reoperations and use of PPIs. [41]

In summary, posterior LPF achieves better reflux control, with no increase in postoperative dysphagia at short- and long-term follow-up. However, further large RCTs with long-term follow-up are needed to confirm these results. Based on these limited data, we feel that a posterior LPF is superior to an anterior LPF.

Conclusions

A LTF is the procedure of choice for the treatment of GERD patients. A LPF, either anterior (180°) or posterior, should be performed only in patients with GERD secondary to scleroderma and in patients with achalasia, since a LTF would impair esophageal emptying and cause dysphagia.

A Personal View of the Data

In patients with GERD and normal esophageal peristalsis I perform a total fundoplication. In my experience, long term follow up has shown that a total fundoplication is superior to a partial fundoplication in terms of reflux control, and it is associated to a similar incidence of post-operative dysphagia.

Recommendation

- A total laparoscopic fundoplication is recommended for patients in whom surgical therapy of gastroesophageal reflux disease is indicated. (Evidence quality moderate; weak recommendation)

References

1. Patti MG, Robinson T, Galvani C, Gorodner MV, Fisichella PM, Way LW. Total fundoplication is superior to partial fundoplication even when esophageal peristalsis is weak. J Am Coll Surg. 2004;198:863–9.

 2. Herbella FA, Tedesco P, Nipomnick I, Fisichella PM, Patti MG. Effect of partial and total laparoscopic fundoplication on esophageal body motility. Surg Endosc. 2007;21:285–8.
 3. Broeders JA, Rijnhart-de Jong HG, Draaisma WA, Bredenoord AJ, Smout AJ, Gooszen HG. Ten-year outcome of laparoscopic and conventional Nissen fundoplication: randomized clinical trial. Ann Surg. 2009;250(5):698–706.
 4. Dallemagne B, Weerts J, Markiewicz S, Dewandre JM, Wahlen C, Monami B, Jehaes C. Clinical results of laparoscopic fundoplication at ten years after surgery. Surg Endosc. 2006;20:159–65.
 5. Morgenthal CB, Shane MD, Stival A, Gletsu N, Milam G, Swafford V, Hunter JG, Smith CD. The durability of laparoscopic Nissen fundoplication: 11-year outcomes. J Gastrointest Surg. 2007;11:693–700.
 6. Tedesco P, Lobo E, Fisichella PM, Way LW, Patti MG. Laparoscopic fundoplication in elderly patients with gastroesophageal reflux disease. Arch Surg. 2006;141:289–92.
 7. Broeders JAJL, Mauritz FA, Ahmed Ali U, Draaisma WA, Ruurda JP, Gooszen HG, Smout AJ, Broeders IA, Hazebroek EJ. Systematic review and meta-analysis of laparoscopic Nissen (posterior total) versus Toupet (posterior partial) fundoplication for gastro-oesophageal reflux disease. Br J Surg. 2010;97:1318–30.
 8. Horvath KD, Jobe BA, Herron DM, Swanstrom LL. Laparoscopic Toupet fundoplication is an inadequate procedure for patients with severe reflux disease. J Gastrointest Surg. 1999;3:583–91.
 9. Oleynikov D, Eubanks TR, Oelschlager BK, Pellegrini CA. Total fundoplication is the operation of choice for patients with gastroesophageal reflux and defective peristalsis. Surg Endosc. 2002;16:909–13.
10. Watson DI, Jamieson GG, Pike GK, Davies N, Richardson M, Devitt PG. Prospective randomized double-blind trial between laparoscopic Nissen fundoplication and anterior partial fundoplication. Br J Surg. 1999;86:123–30.
11. Ludemann R, Watson DI, Jamieson GG, Game PA, Devitt PG. Five-year follow-up of a randomized clinical trial of laparoscopic total versus anterior 180° fundoplication. Br J Surg. 2005;92:240–3.
12. Cai W, Watson DI, Lally CJ, Devitt PG, Game PA, Jamieson GG. Ten-year clinical outcomes of a prospective randomized clinical trial of laparoscopic Nissen versus anterior 180° partial fundoplication. Br J Surg. 2008;95:1501–5.
13. Broeders JA, Broeders EA, Watson DI, Devitt PG, Holloway RH, Jamieson GG. Objective outcomes 14 years after laparoscopic anterior 180-degree partial versus Nissen fundoplication: results from a randomized trial. Ann Surg. 2013;258(2):233–9.
14. Baigrie RJ, Cullis SNR, Ndhluni AJ, Cariem A. Randomized double-blind trial of laparoscopic Nissen fundoplication versus anterior partial fundoplication. Br J Surg. 2005;92:819–23.
15. Watson DI, Jamieson GG, Lally C, Archer S, Bessell JR, Booth M, Cade R, Cullingford G, Devitt PG, Fletcher DR, Hurley J, Kiroff G, Martin CJ, Martin IJ, Nathanson LK, Windsor JA, International Society for Diseases of the Esophagus–Australasian Section. Multicenter, prospective, double-blind, randomized trial of laparoscopic Nissen vs. anterior 90 degrees partial fundoplication. Arch Surg. 2004;139(11):1160–7.
16. Nijjar RS, Watson DI, Jamieson GG, Archer S, Bessell JR, Booth M, Cade R, Cullingford GL, Devitt PG, Fletcher DR, Hurley J, Kiroff G, Martin IJ, Nathanson LK, Windsor JA, International Society for the Diseases of the Esophagus-Australasian Section. Five-year follow-up of a multicenter, double-blind randomized clinical trial of laparoscopic Nissen vs anterior 90 degrees partial fundoplication. Arch Surg. 2010;145(6):552–7.
17. Spence GM, Watson DI, Jamiesion GG, Lally CJ, Devitt PG. Single center prospective randomized trial of laparoscopic Nissen versus anterior 90 degrees fundoplication. J Gastrointest Surg. 2006;10(5):698–705.
18. Watson DI, Devitt PG, Smith L, Jamieson GG. Anterior 90° partial vs Nissen fundoplication–5 year follow-up of a single-centre randomised trial. J Gastrointest Surg. 2012;16(9):1653–8.
19. Broeders JA, Roks DJ, Jamieson GG, Devitt PG, Baigrie RJ, Watson DI. Five-year outcome after laparoscopic anterior partial versus Nissen fundoplication: four randomized trials. Ann Surg. 2012;255(4):637–42.

20. Luostarinen ME, Isolauri JO. Randomized trial to study the effect of fundic mobilization on long-term results of Nissen fundoplication. Br J Surg. 1999;86(5):614–8.
21. Blomqvist A, Dalenbäck J, Hagedorn C, Lönroth H, Hyltander A, Lundell L. Impact of complete gastric fundus mobilization on outcome after laparoscopic total fundoplication. J Gastrointest Surg. 2000;4(5):493–500.
22. O'Boyle CJ, Watson DI, Jamieson GG, Myers JC, Game PA, Devitt PG. Division of short gastric vessels at laparoscopic Nissen fundoplication: a prospective double-blind randomized trial with 5-year follow-up. Ann Surg. 2002;235(2):165–70.
23. Patti MG, Arcerito M, Feo CV, De Pinto M, Tong J, Gantert W, Tyrrell D, Way LW. An analysis of operations for gastroesophageal reflux disease. Identifying the important technical elements. Arch Surg. 1998;133:600–6.
24. Thor KB, Silander T. A long-term randomized prospective trial of the Nissen procedure versus a modified Toupet technique. Ann Surg. 1989;210(6):719–24.
25. Walker SJ, Holt S, Sanderson CJ, Stoddard CJ. Comparison of Nissen total and Lind partial transabdominal fundoplication in the treatment of gastro-oesophageal reflux. Br J Surg. 1992;79(5):410–4.
26. Lundell L, Abrahamsson H, Ruth M, Rydberg L, Lönroth H, Olbe L. Long-term results of a prospective randomized comparison of total fundic wrap (Nissen-Rossetti) or semifundoplication (Toupet) for gastro-oesophageal reflux. Br J Surg. 1996;83(6):830–5.
27. Khajanchee YS, O'Rourke RW, Lockhart B, Patterson EJ, Hansen PD, Swanstrom LL. Postoperative symptoms and failure after antireflux surgery. Arch Surg. 2002;137:1008–14.
28. Lord RV, Kaminski A, Oberg S, Bowrey DJ, Hagen JA, DeMeester SR, Sillin LF, Peters JH, Crookes PF, DeMeester TR. Absence of gastroesophageal reflux disease in a majority of patients taking acid suppression medications after Nissen fundoplication. J Gastrointest Surg. 2002;6(1):3–9.
29. Galvani C, Fisichella PM, Gorodner MV, Perretta S, Patti MG. Symptoms are a poor indicator of reflux status after fundoplication for gastroesophageal reflux disease: role of esophageal functions tests. Arch Surg. 2003;138:514–8.
30. Thompson SK, Jamieson GG, Myers JC, Chin KF, Watson DI, Devitt PG. Recurrent heartburn after laparoscopic fundoplication is not always recurrent reflux. J Gastrointest Surg. 2007;11:642–7.
31. Booth MI, Stratford J, Jones L, Dehn TC. Randomized clinical trial of laparoscopic total (Nissen) versus posterior partial (Toupet) fundoplication for gastro-oesophageal reflux disease based on preoperative oesophageal manometry. Br J Surg. 2008;95(1):57–63.
32. Chrysos E, Tsiaoussis J, Zoras OJ, Athanasakis E, Mantides A, Katsamouris A, Xynos E. Laparoscopic surgery for gastroesophageal reflux disease patients with impaired esophageal peristalsis: total or partial fundoplication? J Am Coll Surg. 2003;197(1):8–15.
33. Guérin E, Bétroune K, Closset J, Mehdi A, Lefèbvre JC, Houben JJ, Gelin M, Vaneukem P, El Nakadi I. Nissen versus Toupet fundoplication: results of a randomized and multicenter trial. Surg Endosc. 2007;21(11):1985–90.
34. Laws HL, Clements RH, Swillie CM. A randomized, prospective comparison of the Nissen fundoplication versus the Toupet fundoplication for gastroesophageal reflux disease. Ann Surg. 1997;225(6):647–53.
35. Mickevicius A, Endzinas Z, Kiudelis M, Jonaitis L, Kupcinskas L, Maleckas A, Pundzius J. Influence of wrap length on the effectiveness of Nissen and Toupet fundoplication: a prospective randomized study. Surg Endosc. 2008;22(10):2269–76.
36. Shaw JM, Bornman PC, Callanan MD, Beckingham IJ, Metz DC. Long-term outcome of laparoscopic Nissen and laparoscopic Toupet fundoplication for gastroesophageal reflux disease: a prospective, randomized trial. Surg Endosc. 2010;24(4):924–32.
37. Strate U, Emmermann A, Fibbe C, Layer P, Zornig C. Laparoscopic fundoplication: Nissen versus Toupet two-year outcome of a prospective randomized study of 200 patients regarding preoperative esophageal motility. Surg Endosc. 2008;22(1):21–30.

38. Mardani J, Lundell L, Engström C. Total or posterior partial fundoplication in the treatment of GERD: results of a randomized trial after 2 decades of follow-up. Ann Surg. 2011;253(5):875–8.
39. Jobe BA, Wallace J, Hansen PD, Swanstrom LL. Evaluation of laparoscopic Toupet fundoplication as a primary repair for all patients with medically resistant gastroesophageal reflux. Surg Endosc. 1997;11(11):1080–3.
40. Hagedorn C, Jönson C, Lönroth H, Ruth M, Thune A, Lundell L. Efficacy of an anterior as compared with a posterior laparoscopic partial fundoplication: results of a randomized, controlled clinical trial. Ann Surg. 2003;238(2):189–96.
41. Engström C, Lönroth H, Mardani J, Lundell L. An anterior or posterior approach to partial fundoplication? Long-term results of a randomized trial. World J Surg. 2007;31y:1221–5.

Part IV
Diaphragm

Chapter 37
Diaphragm Pacing

Françoise Le Pimpec-Barthes

Abstract Diaphragm Pacing (DP) is a rare surgical procedure restoring breathing by an active contraction of the diaphragm independently from the central command. The main goal of DP is to wean chronically dependent patients from mechanical ventilation. The two validated and most studied indications are high cervical spinal cord injury (CSCI) above C3 and central alveolar hypoventilation in strictly selected patients with damaged central command but with functional phrenic nerves and diaphragm. The only available device has long been a radiofrequency system, introduced by cervical or thoracic approach giving success rate of around 90 % for ventilator weaning with a persistent improvement of quality of life. Eleven years ago, an intramuscular device introduced laparoscopically was evaluated in patients with CSCI or hypoventilation such as Amyotrophy Lateral Sclerosis in order to delay the necessity for mechanical ventilation. Recently the feasibility of a transvenous procedure has also been evaluated in Central Sleep Apnoea. Moreover, current research on an animal model makes us think that this technique could be used as a temporary training tool for the diaphragm in intensive care.

Keywords Diaphragm pacing • Phrenic nerve pacing • Tetraplegia • Amyotrophic lateral Sclerosis • Respiratory weaning • Quality of life • Prognosis • Intensive care

F. Le Pimpec-Barthes, MD
Department of Thoracic Surgery and Lung Transplantation,
Pompidou European Hospital, Paris-Descartes University,
HEGP 20 rue Leblanc, Paris, 75908 Cedex 15, France
e-mail: francoise.lepimpec-barthes@egp.aphp.fr

M.K. Ferguson (ed.), *Difficult Decisions in Thoracic Surgery*,
Difficult Decisions in Surgery: An Evidence-Based Approach 1,
DOI 10.1007/978-1-4471-6404-3_37, © Springer-Verlag London 2014

Introduction

Diaphragm pacing (DP) is a tool and a technique restoring active contractions of the diaphragm independently from the central command. Today there are two available techniques: an intrathoracic approach with implanted electrodes around the two phrenic nerves with radiofrequency (RF) technology and a laparoscopic (LDP) approach with direct intradiaphragmatic implantation. DP through cervical (CDP) or thoracic (TDP) approach is an old concept with the first human applications in the 1970s by Glenn, to wean selected patients from a ventilator [1]. The two techniques, CDP/TDP and LDP, require integrity of the phrenic nerves and effective diaphragm muscular function. The most studied indications are high cervical spinal cord injuries (CSCI) above C3 and Congenital Central Hypoventilation Syndrome (CCHS). More recently implantations have been proposed to patients with amyotrophic lateral sclerosis (ALS) in order to delay irreversible respiratory failure. The feasibility of intramuscular DP has also been evaluated in special situations like Central Sleep Apnoea (CSA). The goal of recent research is to determine the place of DP in a more common practice in intensive care.

In this chapter we give an update concerning each available technique, in each indication with a focus on results concerning ventilator weaning and its impact on patients' quality of life.

Search Strategy

We performed a PubMed search covering a long period of time (late 60s until today) because of the scarcity of cases concerned by DP all over the world. The search terms, according to PICO heading, are detailed in Table 37.1. We included the largest series to get the widest possible clinical experience. Only the articles published in English language were collected.

Results

The exact number of DP implanted all over the world is not well known but is probably less than 5,000 procedures having been performed since the first implanted tetraplegic patient [1].

Cervical or Thoracic Approach for DP

The first available device was an RF system including an implanted internal component—Platinum electrodes surrounding the phrenic nerve connected to the subcutaneous receiver—and an external component—an antenna stitched on the skin facing

Table 37.1 PICO used for search

Concerned population	Tetraplegia or cervical cord injury	CCHS		Intensive care unit
	Adults/children	Adults/children	ALS	
Intervention being studied	Diaphragm pacing	Phrenic nerve pacing	Diaphragm stimulation	//
Control population of patients	Patients under mechanical ventilation	Spontaneous evolution in ALS	Ventilated tetraplegic patients	//
Analyzed criteria in outcomes	Mortality	Number of patients weaned from ventilator	Quality of life	Time for mechanical ventilation in ALS
	Morbidity Phrenic nerve injury	Early and long-term survival	(Mobility, speech, smell, taste)	

Abbreviations: *ALS* amyotrophic lateral sclerosis, *CCHS* Congenital Central Hypoventilation Syndrome.

the receiver connected to the battery-powered transmitter. The initial concept was alternate-side pacing because bilateral high-frequency pacing was not well tolerated, resulting in diaphragm fatigue. The introduction of low-frequency pacing after a reconditioning period allowed continuous bilateral stimulation [2]. The first and largest international study was reported by Glenn in 1988 [3]. It included 477 implanted patients with detailed data and complete follow-up reported for 165 patients. The indication for DP was primarily medullar injury (Table 37.2). The goal of ventilator weaning (full or part time) was achieved in 84.24 % of patients. In summary, some ventilator-dependent patients following central respiratory paralysis can be weaned from their ventilator after the implantation of a Diaphragm Pacing. Standardized neuromuscular tests are recommended to select patients for diaphragm pacing.

Failure to pace, in 15.76 % of cases, was mainly related to lack of indications for pacing but also to phrenic nerve injuries during the surgical procedure or to local complications (infection) after the procedure. Thoracic implantation of monopolar electrodes was associated with the lowest risk of nerve injury and local complications (less electrode breakage and local infections) compared to implantation at a cervical level. In 17 patients, an incorrect indication of pacing was retrospectively identified, leading to 82.86 % pacing failure among them. When considering good indications for pacing, the rate of failure decreased to 6.06 %. Definite peripheral phrenic nerve damage is a contraindicate diaphragm pacing.

The long-term follow-up demonstrated that about 64 % of paced patients were living at home at the time they died or when this survey was done; of those who were still paced, 82 % required no or minimal supplemental support. Concerning their activity level, before death or at the termination of this study, about 42 % were working, going to school or were normally or moderately active. The removal of tracheostomies was analyzed: in the 32 cases in which closure was achieved, 75 % of tracheostomies were reopened leading the authors to recommend keeping the

Table 37.2 Series of diaphragm pacing

Authors (year)	N	Series	Type of study	Ratio children/adult/NA	Indications (%)	Approach	Types of electrodes	Mode of pacing — Implant
Thoracic or cervical approach								
Glenn et al. [3] (1988)	477	MultiC InterN	R	NA	CSCI (46)[a] Brain stem (28.3)[a] Idiopathic (13)[a] Congenital (9.5)[a] Peripheral (3.3)[a]	NA/CT	BiP MonoP	Mainly U
Weese Mayer et al. [4] (1996)	64	MultiC InterN	Q	35/24	CSCI CCHS	4 C 60 T	QuadriP	60 B 4 U
Hirschfeld et al. [10] (2008)	64	64	P	NA	CSCI	NA/CT	QuadriP	NA
Khong et al. [10] (2010)	19	MonoC	R	4/13/2	14 CSCI 1 CCHS 1 encephalithis 3 NA	10 C 6 T 3 NA	MonoP	15 B 2 U 2 NA
Le Pimpec-Barthes et al. [6] (2011)	20	MonoC	R	10/10	19 CSCI 1 CCHS	20 T	QuadriP	20 B
Ponikowski et al, [16] (2012)	16	MultiCInterN	P	0/16	Sleep Central Apnea	Transvenous	Endovascular	16 B
Laparoscopic approach								
Onders et al. [12] (2009)	88	MultiC InterN	P	All adults	50 CSCI 38 ALS	Abd	Intra diaphragmatic	88 B

Legends: *N* number of patients, *MultiC* Multicentric, *MonoC* Monocentric, *R* Retrospective, *P* prospective, *Q* questionnaire, *InterN* International, *C* cervical approach, *T* Thoracic approach, *NA* not available, *Bilat* Bilateral, *UniL* Unilateral, *CSCI* Cervical spinal cord injury, *CCHS* Congenital Central Hypoventilation Syndrome, *QuadriP* Quadripolar, *MonoP* Monopolar, *Abd* abdominal

[a]Among 477 patients, 368 had available data

tracheostomy intact (often closed with a button). In tetraplegic patients with full-time pacing, keeping the tracheostomy in place with a tracheal button is recommended. The number of years with pacing was up to 5 years in 263 patients, 5–10 years in 55 patients, 10–15 years in 17 patients and 15–20 years in four patients. In summary, bilateral diaphragm pacing gives excellent long-term results up to 20 years of active pacing.

The retrospective international study reported by Weese-Mayer included 35 children and 29 adults implanted with the quadripolar phrenic pacing system (Jukka Atrotech® Tampere, Finland) [4] (Table 37.2). DP was successful in 94 % of pediatric patients and 86 % of adult patients. Successful pacing with no complication occurred in 56 % of patients (60 % in children and 52 % adults). Morbidity included local infection in 11.4 % of pediatric patients (none in adults, total rate of 6.3 % for all patients) and 3.8 % of phrenic nerve injuries. Electrode and receiver failure was reported in 3.1 % of patients with tetraplegia and 5.9 % with CCHS (P<0.01). At a mean follow-up of 2.2 years, 95 % of patients were alive and the three deaths observed were independent from DP. This study showed that the incidence of post-operative complications was higher in pediatric patients with CCHS even though pacing complications did not increase among pediatric compared to adult patients. In summary, TDP results in full-time or part-time weaning from a ventilator in 89 % of adults and children. Compared to adult patients, a higher risk of infection is reported after DP in pediatric patients.

In 2010, the Australian experience was reported by Khong et al. [5]. This retrospective study included 19 paced patients, mainly for tetraplegia (74 %). CTP (n=11) and TDP (n=6, all bilateral) were used depending on the surgeon's preferences (Table 37.2). Avery Biomedical devices with a monopolar electrode (Commack, NY, USA) were used. Eight patients required reoperation for partial replacement; in four cases it was necessary because the original receiver had a 3–5 year lifetime, in three cases the reason was a device failure and in one case the reason was unknown. In later years of the study, the newer receivers had a longer lifetime. Eleven patients were still actively implanted with total pacing duration ranging from 1–21 years. Currently, new DP devices are available allowing long-term stimulation without the need for redo-surgical procedures.

In 2011 we reported a prospectively collected database in a retrospective monocentric study presenting our experience about 20 patients requiring full-time ventilation that underwent TDP for tetraplegia (n=19) or CCHS (n=1) [6]. We used the same quadripolar phrenic pacing system (Jukka Atrotech® Tampere, Finland) with the same surgical procedure by Video-Assisted Thoracic Surgery (VATS) for implantation performed by the same surgeon for all patients. Before implantation, the function of phrenic nerves and diaphragm muscles was ascertained by rigorous neurophysiologic tests [7]. For CSCI patients, DP was indicated if there was a persistent electromyographic response of the diaphragm to bilateral cervical magnetic stimulation and an abolished response of the diaphragm to trans-cranial magnetic stimulation. No perioperative mortality was observed and morbidity was limited to temporary lobar atelectasis. We concluded that bilateral TDP is a safe procedure with little morbidity. In 18 correctly selected patients in the preoperative period (good results by neuromuscular tests), ventilator weaning was obtained after a median reconditioning time of 6 weeks. All these patients reported a clear improvement in their quality of life. Thus, DP allows full-time ventilatory CCHS patients to improve their mobility, and allows a more normal lifestyle. Two CSCI patients did not achieve full weaning because of extreme amyotrophy: the oldest patient with no answer in preoperative stimulation tests did not get any diaphragm contraction despite reconditioning. It was a "sentimental" indication. A young woman with affected nutritional status was not able to be weaned more than 4 h. It appears that weaning from a ventilator mainly depends on the quality of the neuromuscular chain but also on the nutritional status.

A more recent personal experience since this first series, based only on more recently implanted patients, produced the same conclusions: with strict selection of patients, we can determine which patient may benefit from this technique. The improvement of quality of life was evaluated by "open interviews" of patients. An overall improvement in quality of life—comfort of breathing, better mobility, improved self-image and relationships with others by better speech—was reported by all weaned patients in our series as well as other small series not detailed here.

Of course, the criteria to evaluate the improvement of quality of life are difficult to report, especially for tetraplegic patients. This aspect and the impact on survival were recently analyzed. Romero compared two groups of high CSCI patients whether with DP (n=38) or not (n=88) [8]. By this multivariate analysis adjusted for age using a multivariate logistic correlation, even though paced patients were younger, a greater length of survival was found in this group. Compared to patients under mechanical ventilation DP improved quality of life in more social aspects for CSCI patients. An important point in "comfort" is a significant improvement of olfaction, which is very poor during mechanical ventilation, which was demonstrated in a series of ten tetraplegic patients [9]. This aspect, most often forgotten in common care for ventilator-dependent patients, is now explained to patients when DP is proposed. Patient's olfaction is improved by TDP.

The only prospective monocentric study comparing two groups of patients—paced or not—was reported by Hirschfeld et al. in 2008 [10]. It concerned 64 patients with high CSCI that were not randomized—TDP or mechanical ventilation—but selected according to the results of neurophysiologic tests. Patients with peripheral nerve injury were included in the mechanical ventilation group and patients with no nerve injury had the choice between TPD or not. A large and significant benefit on all daily aspects was observed in the paced group (n=32) compared to the mechanically ventilated group (n=32): a decrease in respiratory infections from 2 to 0 per year, running costs of respiratory treatment, improved quality of speech, and more generally an improved quality of life. Nine patients with TDP, but only two with mechanical ventilation, were employed or went back to school after rehabilitation (P=0.093). The primary investment in the respiratory device is higher with TDP, but it can be paid off within 1 year in our setting because of the reduced amount of single-use equipment, easier nursing and fewer respiratory infections compared to mechanical ventilation. Thus, compared with mechanical ventilation, TDP improves the quality of life of selected CSCI patients.

Laparoscopic Approach

Since 2002 it has been shown that the diaphragm could also be activated in humans without manipulation of the phrenic nerve, by placement of electrodes intramuscularly via laparoscopic surgery [11]. The main key to obtain a global contraction of the hemidiaphragm is the identification of the phrenic nerve motor point without viewing the nerve itself. During laparoscopy, a specialized probe (suction cup electrode giving minimal electrical stimulation) allows stimulation of multiple areas of the diaphragm to identify the motor point (causing the maximum contraction). When this area is precisely identified, two electrodes (NeuRx, Synapse Biomedical, Oberlin, Ohio) are directly implanted into each hemidiaphragm. Electrode leads are tunneled to a percutaneous exit site. A subcutaneous fifth electrode serves as an anode. All leads are connected to the external stimulator providing the pacing stimulus. After implantation, a progressive reconditioning gradually increases as tolerated, starting with 10–15 min per day. The accurate identification of the phrenic motor point is described as the crucial aspect to achieve weaning from mechanical ventilation for tetraplegic patients. The LDP, being less invasive through a laparoscopic approach, has been considered in a pilot study for ALS patients as an expansion of the indications for this approach.

In 2009, a prospective Food and Drug Administration (FDA) trial was conducted in order to evaluate all implanted patients with LDP [12]. It was a prospective non-randomized multicentric interventional trial of LDP including 88 patients (50 high CSCI and 38 ALS) implanted from March 2000 to September 2007. The motor points were clearly detectable in all patients except for 1 (implanted with pacing failure). No morbidity was reported, particularly no conversion to open surgery and no lung injury. Limited and asymptomatic pneumothorax were observed on intraoperative chest x-rays. Later, no erosion of the abdominal organs, no electrode migrations, no broken electrodes and no late change in electrode impedance were reported. ALS patients were safely extubated after surgery. ADP is thus a feasible and safe procedure in ALS patients. In the high CSCI group, pacing was successful in all patients except 1 (failure of motor point detection) leading to 98 % of success (full time or part time). ADP thus allows weaning from ventilator for selected CSCI patients. Five out of 50 patients had died from causes unrelated to the LDP or its implantation, and 44 out of 50 subjects were using their device (daily time of use not reported). For the ALS group, in all patients, fluoroscopically measured diaphragm excursion was greater with DP than with maximal voluntary effort (patients were their own control). The improvement was judged by diaphragm measurement in ultrasound, diaphragm electromyogram and vital capacity (VC).

In the article, it was not clear why only the results of a pilot subgroup were given without the results of follow-up for all ALS patients. After reconditioning of the 16 ALS patients in the initial pilot group implanted between March 2005 and March 2007, the diaphragm was significantly thicker (by ultrasound) and the average rate of monthly decline in FVC decreased (2.4–0.9 % per month). ADP clearly improves the diaphragm thickness in ALS patients giving more effective breathing. The main

goal for ALS patients was to gain time and postpone the necessity for invasive ventilation for terminal respiratory failure. The authors argued that, by maintaining
diaphragm strength, patients had delayed their need for a ventilator by up to
24 months. However no comparison with a control group was available and it is not
clear how these assertions were determined. In September 2011, the U.S. FDA
approved a DP system for patients with ALS but some clinicians and scientists were
dubious concerning the real benefit for such patients.

The impact of sleep in paced ALS patients was analyzed within an ancillary
study of the prospective non-randomized multicentric interventional trial conducted
in seven North American centers and one French center (Clinical-Trials.gov
NCT00420719). Among the 18 implanted ALS patients attending the French center
14 were selected for conditioning. The quality of sleep was compared before and
after ADP [13]. The following criteria were measured before implantation and after
4 months of conditioning: ALS functioning score, FVC, sniff nasal inspiratory pressure and polysomnographic recordings performed with the stimulator turned off. No
significant changes were observed in the sleepiness scale, sleep architecture and
percentage of nocturnal desaturation. However, sleep efficiency significantly
improved from 69 ± 15 to 75 ± 11 % ($p = 0.0394$) driven by a significant decrease in
the time spent awake after sleep onset from a mean of 182 min to 136 min
($p = 0.0032$). Therefore, ADP improves the quality of sleep in ALS patients.

Unilateral Stimulation

It is an extremely rare indication that is possible in ventilator dependent patients
with only one functional phrenic nerve. No report was found except for a short
series of 3 CSCI with unilateral phrenic nerve injury treated by a combined stimulation associating unilateral TDP and intercostal stimulation [14]. However, such an
indication may be considered in patients with high CSCI and single functional lung
(previous pneumonectomy or phrenic nerve injury).

Recently, Ponikowski reported unilateral phrenic nerve stimulation in patients
with CSA and heart failure patients [15]. The impact of CSA on cardiac function is
well known and it contributes to the increase of heart failure by stimulation of the
sympathetic system and arrhythmias. The goal of this prospective non-randomized
multicentric study was to determine the feasibility of phrenic nerve stimulation
done by a transvenous device and to evaluate its efficiency to reduce the episodes of
CSA. The transvenous placement was proposed because the transthoracic approach
was not possible in such patients. The selection of patients lied on strict apnea
hypopnea–index (AHI) ≥ 15 or central apnea index (CAI) ≥ 5 on polysomnographic
testing. The series included 16 selected patients. After introduction via axillary or
subclavian vein the therapeutic period started when the patient was asleep. The
significant benefit by unilateral phrenic stimulation was a 48 % reduction in AHI
due to a 90 % reduction in the number of CSA episodes. No significant improvement in oxygen saturation was observed comparing the mean baseline value to the

mean value during the treatment. The two adverse effects were reversible lead thrombus and an episode of ventricular tachycardia. This first study offers new ways in this particular indication requiring further study.

New indications may appear in the coming years with a preventive goal to avoid diaphragm atrophy for patients under mechanical ventilation. Indeed, since 2003, Pavlovic and Wendt [16] reviewed literature data concerning the noxious effects of prolonged mechanical ventilation and he developed the feasibility of a model of DP to train the diaphragm to synchronize to mechanical ventilation. These training methods could be applied to prevent atrophy during long-term mechanical ventilation as well as temporary ventilation of patients with a high risk of developing respiratory muscle fatigue. The common goal is to simplify the weaning procedure, shorten intubation time and finally reduce the cost of treatment. In this study the best method of DP remained undefined.

Recently an animal study reported the analysis of the biological and physiological effects of DP during mechanical ventilation [17]. Intradiaphragmatic phrenic nerve pacing electrodes were bilaterally inserted using a cervical approach in three sheep. Stimulation was performed only in one hemidiaphragm per animal. The diaphragm biopsies showed severe histological damages in the mechanically ventilated hemidiaphragm, not observed on the paced side. Lesions were lipid droplet accumulation and intense edematous infiltrates with fibers disorganization. Diaphragm fiber atrophy was noticed on both sides (paced or not) but markedly less pronounced on the paced hemidiaphragm. The pursuit of these investigations will probably help answer other questions concerning which patients may benefit from this technique, which technique can be proposed, which risk for the phrenic nerve may occur in this preventive treatment.

Conclusion

The two well-known techniques of DP (thoracic or intradiaphragmatic levels) are available and no practical comparison between them is really possible with the present limited literature. The two techniques allow weaning from ventilator and improvement in quality of life in selected patients. The ultimate goal of DP is probably to help or replace mechanical ventilation for patients with chronic respiratory disease or acute respiratory failure, in order to simplify ventilator weaning.

Summary of Recommendations

Some ventilator-dependent patients following central respiratory paralysis can be weaned from their ventilator after the institution of diaphragm pacing. Standardized neuromuscular tests are recommended to select patients for diaphragm pacing. For cervical spinal cord injury patients, diaphragm pacing is indicated if there is a persistent electromyographic response of the diaphragm to bilateral cervical magnetic stimulation and an abolished response of the diaphragm to trans-cranial magnetic stimulation. Definitive peripheral phrenic nerve damage contraindicates diaphragm pacing.

Thoracic diaphragm pacing results in full-time or part-time weaning from a ventilator in 89 % of adults and children. In full-time paced tetraplegic patients, it is recommended to keep the tracheostomy with a tracheal button. Compared to adult patients, a higher risk of infection is reported after diaphragm pacing in pediatric patients. Bilateral thoracic diaphragm pacing using bipolar or quadripolar electrodes is a safe procedure with little morbidity. Weaning from a ventilator mainly depends on the quality of the neuromuscular chain but also on the patient's nutritional status. Bilateral diaphragm pacing gives excellent long-term results up to 20 years of active pacing. Compared with mechanical ventilation, thoracic diaphragm pacing improves the quality of life of selected cervical spinal cord injury patients. Diaphragm pacing allows full-time ventilator patients with congenital central hypoventilation syndrome to improve their mobility, and allows a more normal lifestyle. Patients' olfaction is improved by thoracic diaphragm pacing.

Abdominal diaphragm pacing is a feasible and safe procedure in amyotrophic lateral sclerosis patients. It improves the diaphragm thickness in these patients, resulting in more effective breathing. Abdominal diaphragm pacing improves the quality of sleep in amyotrophic lateral sclerosis patients and allows weaning from ventilator for selected cervical spinal cord injury patients.

A Personal View of the Data

In my department, I use phrenic nerve pacing only by the VATS approach because I consider that it is the safest and most effective procedure. The main reason is that the quadripolar electrodes are precisely positioned under direct view without compression of the nerve and there is no risk of subsequent displacement. Many other reasons are listed below. VATS allows an observation of the whole phrenic nerve from its origin in the pleural cavity down to its end in the diaphragm. The thoracic surgeon can analyze the size of the nerve—a small diameter immediately evokes a concern for nerve degeneration affecting future effective pacing—and its endpoint—a bi- or trifurcated endpoint has no consequence for thoracic pacing. However, this finding represents a risk of incomplete nerve stimulation using intramuscular electrodes placed laparoscopically. The safety of stimulation is also increased by two technical aspects. First, the proximity between each electrode and the nerve allows an extremely low threshold of stimulation (about 1 mA compared to 25 for intramuscular electrodes) without risk of concomitant cardiac stimulation. Secondly, the successive stimulation done by the different electrodes around each nerve preserves the nerve fibers, avoiding fatigue. Moreover, this technique is easily reproducible for thoracic surgeons and the mini-invasive approach generally allows a short hospitalization (usually two postoperative days). Finally, the thoracic surgery environment is probably more suitable than the environment of digestive surgery for perioperative care of such patients because the problem concerns respiratory disorders and the main goal of phrenic nerve pacing is weaning from mechanical ventilation. In my 16-year experience of phrenic nerve pacing by VATS using quadripolar electrodes, I have not observed any failure related to the surgical technique in patients carefully selected by our medical team, and our group has agreed to continue this safe and effective thoracic approach.

Recommendations
- Standardized neuromuscular tests are recommended to select patients for diaphragm pacing. (Evidence quality low; weak recommendation)
- Thoracic diaphragm pacing gives a full-time or part-time weaning from a ventilator in the majority of adults and children. (Evidence quality low; weak recommendation)
- Weaning from a ventilator mainly depends on the quality of the neuromuscular chain but also on the patient's nutritional status. (Evidence quality low; weak recommendation)
- Compared with mechanical ventilation, thoracic diaphragm pacing improves quality of life in selected cervical spinal cord injury patients. (Evidence quality low; weak recommendation)
- Abdominal diaphragm pacing is a feasible and safe procedure in amyotrophic lateral sclerosis patients. (Evidence quality low; weak recommendation)
- Abdominal diaphragm pacing allows weaning from ventilator for selected cervical spinal cord injury patients. (Evidence quality low; weak recommendation)
- There is no means for determining the relative benefit of thoracic vs abdominal diaphragm pacing. (Evidence quality low; no recommendation)
- There are no current clear indications for unilateral diaphragm pacing for management of respiratory insufficiency. (Evidence quality low; weak recommendation)

References

1. Glenn WW, Holcomb WG, McLaughlin AJ, O'Hare JM, Hogan JF, Yasuda R. Total ventilatory support in a quadriplegic patient with radiofrequency. Electrophrenic respiration. N Engl J Med. 1972;286:513–6.
2. Glenn WW, Hogan JF, Loke JS, Ciesielski TE, Phelps ML, Rowedder R. Ventilatory support by pacing of the conditioned diaphragm in quadriplegia. N Engl J Med. 1984;10:1150–5.
3. Glenn WW, Brouillette RT, Dentz B, Fodstad H, Hunt CE, Keens TG, Marsh HM, Pande S, Piepgras DG, Vanderlinden RG. Fundamental considerations in pacing of the diaphragm for

chronic ventilatory insufficiency: a multi-center study. Pacing Clin Electrophysiol. 1988;11: 2121–7.

4. Weese-Mayer DE, Silvestri JM, Kenny AS, Ilbawi MN, Hauptman SA, Lipton JW, Talonen PP, Garrido Garcia H, Watt JW, Exner G, Baer GA, Elefteriades JA, Peruzzi WT, Alex CG, Harlid R, Vincken W, Davis GM, Decramer M, Kuenzle C, Terhaug AS, Schober JG. Diaphragm pacing with a quadripolar phrenic nerve electrode: an international study. Pacing Clin Electrophysiol. 1996;19:1311–9.

5. Khong P, Lazzaro A, Mobbs R. Phrenic nerve stimulation: the Australian experience. J Clin Neurosci. 2010;17:205–8.

6. Le Pimpec-Barthes F, Gonzalez-Bermejo J, Hubsch JP, Duguet A, Morelot-Panzini C, Riquet M, Similowski T. Intrathoracic phrenic pacing: a 10-year experience in France. J Thorac Cardiovasc Surg. 2011;142:378–83.

7. Similowski T, Straus C, Attali V, Duguet A, Jourdain B, Derenne JP. Assessment of the motor pathway to the diaphragm using cortical and cervical magnetic stimulation in the decision-making process of phrenic pacing. Chest. 1996;110:1551–7.

8. Romero FJ, Gambarrutta C, Garcia-Forcada A, Marín MA, Diaz de la Lastra E, Paz F, Fernandez-Dorado MT, Mazaira J. Long-term evaluation of phrenic nerve pacing for respiratory failure due to high cervical spinal cord injury. Spinal Cord. 2012;50:895–8.

9. Adler D, Gonzalez-Bermejo J, Duguet A, Demoule A, Le Pimpec-Barthes F, Hurbault A, et al. Diaphragm pacing restores olfaction in tetraplegia. Eur Respir J. 2009;34:365–70.

10. Hirschfeld S, Exner G, Luukkaala T, Baer GA. Mechanical ventilation or phrenic nerve stimulation for treatment of spinal cord injury–induced respiratory insufficiency. Spinal Cord. 2008;46:738–42.

11. DiMarco AF, Onders RP, Kowalski KE, Miller ME, Ferek, Mortimer JT. Phrenic nerve pacing in a tetraplegic patient via intramuscular diaphragm electrodes. Am J Respir Crit Care Med. 2002;166:1604–6.

12. Onders RP, Elmo MJ, Khansarinia S, Bowman B, Yee J, Road J, Bass B, Dunkin B, Ingvarsson PE, Oddsdottir M. Complete worldwide operative experience in laparoscopic diaphragm pacing: results and differences in spinal cord injured patients and amyotrophic lateral sclerosis patients. Surg Endosc. 2009;23:1433–40.

13. Gonzalez-Bermejo J, Capucine MoréLot-Panzini C, Salachas F, Redolfi S, Straus C, Becquemin M, Amulf I, Pradat P, Bruneteau G, Ignagni A, Diop M, Onders R, Nelson T, Menegaux F, Meininger V, Similowski T. Diaphragm pacing improves sleep in patients with amyotrophic lateral sclerosis. Amyotroph Lateral Scler. 2012;13:44–54.

14. DiMarco AF, Takaoka Y, Kowalski KE. Combined intercostal and diaphragm pacing to provide artificial ventilation in patients with tetraplegia. Arch Phys Med Rehabil. 2005;86:1200–7.

15. Ponikowski P, Javaheri S, Michalkiewicz D, Bart BA, Czarnecka D, Jastrzebski M, Kusiak A, Augostini R, Jagielski D, Witkowski T, Khayat RN, Oldenburg O, Gutleben KJ, Bitter T, Karim R, Iber C, Hasan A, Hibler K, Germany R, Abraham WT. Transvenous phrenic nerve stimulation for the treatment of central sleep apnea in heart failure. Eur Heart J. 2012;33:889–94.

16. Pavlovic D, Wendt M. Diaphragm pacing during prolonged mechanical ventilation of the lungs could prevent from respiratory muscle fatigue. Med Hypotheses. 2003;60(3):398–403.

17. Masmoudi H, Coirault C, Demoule A, Mayaux J, Beuvin M, Romero N, Assouad J, Similowski T. Can phrenic stimulation protect the diaphragm from mechanical ventilation-induced damage? Eur Respir J. 2013;42:280–3.

Chapter 38
Minimally Invasive Versus Open Repair of Giant Paraesophageal Hernia

Janet P. Edwards and Sean C. Grondin

Abstract This chapter reviews the literature regarding various approaches for repair of giant paraesophageal hernia (PEH) including transthoracic, open abdominal, and laparoscopic. It addresses the published mortality, complication, recurrence and reoperation rates for each operative approach. After a detailed discussion of these points of interest, evidence based recommendations are made to assist practicing surgeons in their selection of an operative approach for patients undergoing repair of giant PEH.

Keywords Giant paraesophageal hernia • Paraesophageal hernia • Hiatal hernia • Intrathoracic stomach • Repair • Operative approach • Laparoscopic • Transabdominal • Transthoracic • Minimally invasive

Introduction

Hiatal hernias are protrusions of intraabdominal content through a defect in the diaphragm at the esophageal hiatus. They can be broadly classified as either sliding or paraesophageal. Whereas only the gastroesophageal junction (GEJ) migrates through the hiatus in sliding (Type I) hiatal hernias, paraesophageal hernias (Types II, III, IV) are distinguished by the migration of part or all of the stomach above the hiatus. Types II and III paraesophageal hernia (PEH) differ according to the position of the GEJ. In Type II PEH, the normal intraabdominal position of the GEJ is maintained while the stomach migrates through the hiatus, whereas in the more common Type III PEH, the GEJ migrates through the hiatus along with some portion of the

J.P. Edwards, MD, MPH • S.C. Grondin, MD, MPH (✉)
Division of Thoracic Surgery, Foothills Medical Centre,
1403 – 29th Street NW, Room G33, Calgary, AB T2N 2T9, Canada
e-mail: janetpatriciaedwards@gmail.com; sean.grondin@albertahealthservices.ca

M.K. Ferguson (ed.), *Difficult Decisions in Thoracic Surgery*,
Difficult Decisions in Surgery: An Evidence-Based Approach 1,
DOI 10.1007/978-1-4471-6404-3_38, © Springer-Verlag London 2014

stomach. Type IV PEH involve herniation of any other abdominal organ through the hiatus along with the stomach. Published definitions of giant PEH vary, including both percentage definitions (30–50 % or more of the stomach residing in the chest) and those based on measurements (5 cm or more of stomach being intrathoracic).

Operative repair of giant PEH is a complicated endeavor for multiple reasons. The condition is often chronic, making reduction counter to the tendency of the tissues involved. This is further exacerbated in many cases by a shortened esophagus, which places traction on the repair, favoring hernia recurrence. The often large crural defects are difficult to close without undue tension, and finally the frailty or comorbid status of the typically elderly patients makes operative intervention higher risk and the tissues less robust. It is generally accepted that symptomatic giant PEH in patients fit for operation should be repaired. The steps involved in repair of PEH include reduction of the hernia content back into the abdominal cavity, excision of the hernia sac, and closure of the hiatal defect, with selective inclusion of an antireflux procedure, esophageal lengthening procedure and/or gastropexy. Significant controversy exists, however, with regard to the approach for operative repair of giant PEH as well as the use of primary repair versus tension free repair with mesh. The use of mesh for repair of PEH is discussed in Chap. 40 of this text.

The purpose of this chapter is to review the literature regarding the various approaches for repair of giant PEH including transthoracic, open abdominal, and laparoscopic. It addresses the published mortality, complication, recurrence and reoperation rates for each operative approach. After a detailed discussion of these points of interest, evidence based recommendations are made to assist practicing surgeons in their selection of an operative approach for patients requiring repair of giant PEH.

Search Strategy

The PICO method, outlined in Table 38.1, was employed to define the study question. The literature was searched using the PubMed search engine to identify studies in patients undergoing repair of giant PEH by a transthoracic, open abdominal or laparoscopic approach for the purpose of evaluating perioperative morbidity, mortality recurrence or reoperation rates. Due to the varying published criteria for defining a PEH as *giant*, an inclusive definition was used. All studies whose patient population was limited for the stated purpose of studying those with a giant Type II, III or IV hiatal hernia were included. No limitations were placed on language or year of publication. Search terms included "giant paraesophageal hernia", "paraesophageal hernia", "giant paraesophageal", "paraesophageal", "intrathoracic stomach", "laparoscopic", "transabdominal", "transthoracic", "repair", "operative repair" and "hiatal hernia". Reference lists of relevant studies and of topical review articles were also searched by hand to identify further articles for inclusion. Studies were excluded from this review for the following reasons: inclusion of Type I hiatal hernias, lack of limitation to *giant* PEH repair, definition of subgroups according to

Table 38.1 Clinical question and literature search strategy

Population	Patients with giant Type II, III or IV paraesophageal hernias
Intervention	Operative repair of PEH via a transthoracic, open abdominal or laparoscopic approach
Comparator	None necessary for inclusion. Included studies of any design including retrospective case series, prospective case series, and clinical trials of any kind. Preferred studies comparing two or more of the listed operative approaches
Outcome	Intraoperative complications, postoperative complications, mortality, recurrence rate, reoperation rate
Literature source	PubMed Central, reference lists of relevant articles and reference lists of topical reviews
Publication date	All
Language	All
Search terms	"giant paraesophageal hernia", "paraesophageal hernia", "giant paraesophageal", "paraesophageal", "laparoscopic", "transabdominal", "transthoracic", "repair", "operative repair" and "hiatal hernia"

use of prosthetic mesh (see Chap. 40), or if data were not extractable for any of the outcomes of interest. Relevant studies are detailed in Table 38.2 [1–5] and Table 38.3 [6–20]. To date, there are no randomized controlled trials comparing the various approaches for repair of giant PEH, with the overwhelming majority of the evidence consisting of retrospective case series. By definition, this study type is deemed of "low" quality according to the GRADE system. Despite that categorization, the authors of these studies provide valuable information to guide surgeons in their care of patients with giant PEH. This paucity of high quality evidence is also unlikely to change due to the many factors complicating initiation of a relevant surgical trial, including surgeon and patient preference, difficulty blinding subjects and observers, and relatively small numbers of affected patients.

Comparing the Thoracic Approach to the Open Abdominal Approach

The classic approach for repair of giant PEH is through the chest. Skinner and Belsey in their report on 632 patients undergoing transthoracic repair of PEH, provided a baseline against which future repairs were judged, publishing a 7 % rate of symptomatic recurrence [21]. Since that time, surgeons have identified several advantages to the transthoracic approach to repair of giant PEH. These include a superior ability to mobilize the esophagus from the diaphragmatic hiatus to well above the aortic arch, easy access for reduction and resection of the hernia sac, and improved visualization and preservation of both trunks of the vagus nerve. The enhanced visualization obtained through the chest also allows surgeons to optimally assess esophageal length and tension on their repair, allowing them to best determine the need for esophageal lengthening procedures such as the Collis

Table 38.2 Studies investigating thoracic and open abdominal operative approach for repair of giant paraesophageal hernia. Percentages are overall unless specified

Reference	Grade of evidence	Time frame	n	Thoracic	Abdominal	Laparoscopic (n/# converted)	Intraoperative complications	Postoperative complications	Recurrence	Reoperation	Mortality
Allen et al. [1]	Very low	1980–1990	119	111	8	0	Not stated	33 (28 %)	Not stated	Thoracic: 1 (1 %) Abdominal: 0	0
Martin et al. [2]	Very low	1977–1994	51	33	16	1 (1)	Not stated	15 (29 %)	2 (4 %)	1 (2 %)	0
Maziak et al. [3]	Very low	1960–1996	94	91	3	0	Not stated	18 (19 %)	5 (5 %)	5 (5 %)	2 (2 %)
Geha [4]	Very low	1967–1999	100	18	82	0	Not stated	Thoracic: 2 (18 %) Abdominal: 4 (5 %)	0 0	2 (18 %) 0	2 (2 %) 0
Altorki et al. [5]	Very low	1988–1997	47	46	0	1 (1)	Not stated	19 (40 %)	3 (6 %)	Not stated	1 (2 %)

Table 38.3 Studies investigating laparoscopic operative approach for repair of giant paraesophageal hernia. Percentages are overall unless specified

Reference	Grade of evidence	Time frame	n	Thoracic	Abdominal	Laparoscopic (n/# converted)	Intraoperative complications	Postoperative complications	Recurrence	Reoperation	Mortality
Hashemi et al. [6]	Very low	1985–1998	54	14	13	27 (Not stated)	Not stated	Not stated	Thoracic: 1 (7 %) / Abdominal: 2 (15 %) / Laparoscopic: 9 (33 %)	Not stated	0 / 1 (8 %) / 0
Mittal et al. [7]	Very low	2004–2009	73	7	1	65 (1)	1 (1 %)	29 (40 %)	Thoracic: 2 (29 %) / Abdominal: 0 / Laparoscopic: 2 (3 %)	0	0 / 1 (2 %) / 0
Low and Unger [8]	Low	1996–2001	72	0	72	0	0	17 (24 %)	0	0	0
Dahlberg et al. [9]	Very low	1997–2000	37	0	0	37 (2)	6 (16 %)	8 (22 %)	3 (8 %)	2 (1 %)	2 (5 %)
Terry et al. [10]	Very low	1991–1999	118	0	0	118 (not stated)	Not stated	12 (10 %)	Not stated	Not stated	3 (3 %)
Weichmann et al. [11]	Very low	1993–1997	60	0	0	60 (6)	2 (3 %)	Not stated	4 (7 %)	4 (7 %)	1 (2 %)
Pierre et al. [12]	Very low	1995–2001	203	0	0	203 (3)	9 (4 %)	53 (26 %)	Not stated	5 (2 %)	1 (.5 %)
Andujar et al. [13]	Very low	1996–2002	166	0	0	166 (2)	Not stated	14 (8 %)	6 (5 %)	10 (6 %)	Not stated
Parameswara et al. n [14]	Very low	1991–2003	49	0	0	49 (2)	2 (4 %)	11 (24 %)	1 (2 %)	Not stated	Not stated
Grotenhuis et al. [15]	Very low	1992–2006	129	0	0	129 (19)	9 (7 %)	13 (10 %)	Not stated	11 (9 %)	2 (2 %)
Morris-Stiff and Hassn [16]	Very low	2002–2005	23	0	0	23 (0)	Not stated	11 (48 %)	0	0	0
Nason et al. [17]	Very low	1997–2003	187	0	0	187 (2)	Not stated	Not stated	23 (12 %)	7 (4 %)	Not stated
Luketich et al. [18]	Very low	1997–2008	662	0	0	662 (10)	5 (1 %)	117 (17 %)	70 (16 %)	21 (3 %)	11 (2 %)

(continued)

Table 38.3 (continued)

Reference	Grade of evidence	Time frame	n	Thoracic	Abdominal	Laparoscopic (n/# converted)	Intraoperative complications	Postoperative complications	Recurrence	Reoperation	Mortality
Karmali et al. [19]	Very low	1999–2005	93	0	47	46 (7)	Abdominal: 10 (21 %) Laparoscopic: 6 (13 %)	Abdominal: 25 (53 %) Laparoscopic: 10 (22 %)	4 (9 %) 4 (9 %)	1 (2 %) 2 (4 %)	Not stated
Zehetner et al. [20]	Very low	1998–2010	146	0	73	73 (7)	Abdominal: 2 (3 %) Laparoscopic: 0	Abdominal: 26 (36 %) Laparoscopic: 8 (11 %)	18 (25 %) 9 (12 %)	Overall: 5 (3 %)	Not stated

gastroplasty. The morbidity of the transthoracic approach is a result of the thoracotomy incision as well as the need for single lung ventilation. Both of these factors increase the risk of post-operative respiratory complications and limit the application of this approach to giant PEH repair in frail patients or those with underlying cardiorespiratory disease.

Due to the morbidity of the thoracic approach, surgeons subsequently attempted to repair PEH through the abdomen. Although the laparotomy incision does not provide the same extent of visualization of the intrathoracic esophagus as the transthoracic approach, reduction of the hernia contents is often easier, and the exposure is generally considered adequate to allow safe and effective repair of giant PEH. The laparotomy incision allows easier access for performance of a gastric emptying procedure and gastropexy, as desired. This incision is also felt to be less morbid, and the lack of single lung ventilation purportedly reduced postoperative respiratory complications. This approach involves more difficult dissection of the hernia sac and esophagus. It also provides diminished visualization of the vagal trunks and arguably inferior assessment of the esophagus for tension and need for lengthening procedures. Surgeons also question whether recurrence rates are higher in patients undergoing abdominal versus transthoracic repair. The main questions when comparing these two approaches, therefore, address whether they indeed differ in terms of morbidity, mortality and recurrence rates. Unfortunately, no high grade evidence exists to answer these questions, leaving surgeons to examine retrospective case series. Studies addressing primarily the thoracic and/or open abdominal approaches to repair of giant PEH are detailed in Table 38.2 [1–5].

Maziak and colleagues [3] reported a series of 94 patients with giant PEH in which the vast majority of patients underwent elective transthoracic repair (97 %) with gastroplasty and fundoplication (80 %). In this study, the median follow-up duration was 6 years and only two patients were lost to follow up. This completeness and length of follow up is impressive when compared to other similar studies. The procedure for assessment of recurrence was not explicitly discussed and appeared to be non-uniform and symptom based. This study carried a 19 % postoperative complication rate, 2 % perioperative mortality rate, 5 % rate of reoperation for all causes and 2 % reoperation for symptomatic recurrence. Unfortunately, these rates were not reported in an approach-specific fashion, preventing any conclusions from being drawn with regard to the superiority of transthoracic or transabdominal repair of giant PEH. Two other studies report series consisting mainly of transthoracic repairs of giant PEH. Allen et al. [1] report on 147 patients with giant PEH in which the majority (93 %) underwent transthoracic repair with uncut Collis-Nissen fundoplication (66 %). There were no perioperative deaths. During follow up (median 3.5 years) with symptom driven radiologic imaging for recurrence, one patient from the thoracic repair group underwent repair of a symptomatic recurrence (1 %). In a separate series of 47 patients (98 % of whom underwent transthoracic repair without gastroplasty), Altorki and colleagues [5] experienced 2 % perioperative mortality and 42 % morbidity. With 91 % of survivors undergoing a median of 45 months of follow up, 6 % of patients were found to have recurrence. Investigation for recurrence was not standard, being performed only in symptomatic patients. A more recent series of 240 patients undergoing transthoracic repair of PEH has been published [22]. Although at first glance this study's 2 % reoperation rate for symptomatic recurrence and 2 % mortality rate appear informative, this study did not limit itself to giant PEH.

Martin et al. [2] provide a small series of 51 patients with more balanced representation of the two operative approaches (65 % thoracic, 45 % abdominal). Follow up was 94 % complete and a median of 27 months duration and again involved symptom based implementation of radiologic investigation. Rates of postoperative complications (29 %), recurrence (4 %) and reoperation (2 %) were not broken down by operative approach and no patients died in the perioperative period.

Geha and colleagues [4] reported on 100 patients with giant PEH, the majority undergoing open abdominal repair (82 %) with gastrostomy (75 %) and a loose fundoplication (65 %). Two patients in the thoracic group died postoperatively (both were emergent PEH repairs with sepsis at the time of operation), and two experienced subsequent gastric volvulus requiring reoperation. No recurrences were identified in the 86 % of patients that underwent routine follow up contrast studies. Low and Unger [8] also reported on 72 patients undergoing exclusively open abdominal repairs, finding no intraoperative complications, recurrences, or mortality.

Although these studies do not provide high level evidence comparing the thoracic and open abdominal approaches, we are left with the impression that the morbidity of the thoracic approach is higher, and the recurrence rate is not convincingly different for the less morbid open abdominal approach.

Comparing the Open Abdominal to the Laparoscopic Approach

The laparoscopic approach was introduced following the enthusiasm initially generated by laparoscopic cholecystectomy, with the hopes of further reducing the morbidity of giant PEH repair. This approach avoids the one lung ventilation of the thoracic approach, and the larger incisions of both open abdominal and thoracic approaches, while perhaps improving the visualization of the GEJ and esophagus compared to the open abdominal approach. Studies investigating the laparoscopic approach to repair of giant PEH are detailed in Table 38.3 [6–20]. Concern was raised when an early study by Hashemi et al. [6] comparing the minimally invasive approach to open abdominal and thoracic approaches found a far higher recurrence rate in the laparoscopic group (thoracic 7 %, open abdominal 15 %, laparoscopic 33 %). A more recent paper [7] performing a similar comparison of the three approaches in a retrospective case series produced very different recurrence rates according to approach (thoracic 29 %, open abdominal 0 %, laparoscopic 3 %).

Ten case series have since been published examining the laparoscopic approach to repair of giant PEH. Four of these studies involved 60 patients or less. Dahlberg and colleagues [9] present a series of 37 patients who underwent laparoscopic repair of giant PEH, with two conversions to open surgery. Complications included a death from a post-operative splenic bleed, two esophageal leaks and a pneumothorax. Median hospital stay was 4 days. Three patients (8 %) were found to have recurrence on follow up barium swallow (completed in 71 % of patients), with two patients (5 %) requiring reoperation. Weichmann et al. [11] included 60 patients with 10 % conversion to open. Radiologic assessment for recurrence was performed in 73 % of patients, with 7 % of patients having radiologic recurrence and subsequent reoperation. There was one death due to esophageal perforation. Parameswaran and colleagues [14] present their series of 46 patients, 37 % of which received mesh on-lay for crural reinforcement. Two conversions to open occurred due to esophageal perforation and difficult dissection. Only 66 % of patients underwent follow up barium swallow at a median of 19 months, with 1 % demonstrating radiologic recurrence of their PEH. Reoperation was not mentioned. The final small series of 23 patients [16] involved a formal follow up at 6 months at which time symptoms were assessed and radiologic imaging ordered accordingly. Although there was a 48 % rate of major and minor postoperative complications, there were no deaths and no documented recurrences.

Six larger case series of over 100 patients each have been conducted similarly addressing laparoscopic repair of giant PEH. Three of these do not present overall recurrence rates, making them somewhat less informative for our comparison of laparoscopic versus open abdominal giant PEH repair [10, 12, 15]. Terry et al. [10] detailed their case series of 118 patients undergoing laparoscopic repair of giant PEH. The majority of patients (85 %) received a floppy Nissen fundoplication. Three patients (3 %) died peri-operatively, two of esophageal perforation and one of gastric necrosis and perforation. Their reoperation and recurrence rates were presented along with the group undergoing surgery for GERD alone, preventing assessment of PEH specific complications. Pierre et al. [12] laparoscopically repaired 203 giant PEH, with 85 % undergoing a Collis-Nissen and 4 % conversion to open. The median length of stay was 3 days and major or minor complications occurred in 28 %. One death occurred due to esophageal perforation, and five other patients experienced nonfatal leaks. Median follow up was 18 months. Although the overall rate of recurrence and method for determining recurrence were not detailed, five patients (2 %) required reoperation for recurrence. In their series of 129 patients, Grotenhuis et al. [15] present a 9 % conversion rate primarily due to dense adhesions and/or difficulty reducing the hernia contents. The median length of stay was 5 days with 1 % mortality due to esophageal perforation. The recurrence rate was not mentioned, and the reoperation rate of 9 % was attributed to tight wraps, bleeding, slipped wrap and esophageal perforation.

Three further case studies, each examining the records of over 100 patients, provide information with regard to recurrence and reoperation rates for laparoscopic giant PEH repair [13, 17, 18]. In their series of 166 laparoscopic procedures with two conversions to open, Andujar et al. [13] performed routine evaluation for recurrence with barium swallow in 72 % of patients at a median of 15 months post operatively. They found 5 % recurrence of PEH, 20 % recurrence of a Type I PEH, and 3 % wrap failure. While a total of 10 % of patients required reoperation at a median of 7 months follow up, only two patients (1 %) received reoperation for symptomatic PEH repair. Nason et al. [17] examined the records of 187 patients undergoing laparoscopic repair of giant PEH with two conversions to open. The majority of patients (82 %) underwent clinical follow up (median 77 months) including radiographic examination for recurrence. The median duration from surgery to most recent barium swallow was 50 months. Radiographic recurrence was visualized in 23 patients, and 4.4 % of patients underwent reoperation for recurrence at a median of 44 months. A second recurrence was detected in two patients. Luketich et al. [18] provide the largest case series of laparoscopic giant PEH repair, representing 662 patients. The majority of patients (98 %) received a fundoplication (floppy Nissen or partial wrap), and esophageal lengthening (63 %), with 13 % having placement of crural mesh. Their conversion rate was 1.5 %. The majority of postoperative leaks were found to occur in those receiving a Collis gastroplasty (88 %). Major complications were more likely in patients over the age of 70 years at the time of operation, and in those with a body mass index over 35 kg/m^2. The overall mortality rate was 1.7 %. Follow up with barium swallow was available for 67 % of patients, with a median duration of 22 months. Radiographic recurrence was detected in 15.7 % of those undergoing follow up. Three percent of patients overall required reoperation, driven mainly by symptoms not radiologic recurrence. The authors identified age younger than 70 years as a significant risk factor for recurrence in multivariate analysis.

To date there are still no randomized controlled trials comparing the laparoscopic to the open abdominal approach, although two case series involving relatively balanced representation of both operative strategies provides the most direct comparison of these approaches to date. Karmali et al. [19] present 47 patients undergoing open abdominal giant PEH repair and 46 patients undergoing laparoscopic repair with seven conversions to open. The groups were similar in terms of gender, duration of symptoms, and elective vs emergent surgery. The laparoscopic cohort was significantly younger than the open group, and the operative time was significantly longer. There was no significant difference in intra-operative complication rates (laparoscopic 13 %, open 21 %). The median hospital stay was shorter in the laparoscopic group (median 5 days for laparoscopic versus 10 days for open), and the post operative complication rate was also significantly lower (laparoscopic 22 %, open 53 %). The median duration of follow up was 17 months for the laparoscopic group and 21 months for the open group. There was no difference in recurrence rates, with four patients diagnosed on upper gastrointestinal series in each group. Two patients in the laparoscopic group and a single patient in the open group underwent repair. Zehetner et al. [20] present a similar case series involving 73 open repairs of giant PEH and 73 laparoscopic with seven conversions. There were no significant demographic differences between the groups at baseline. Mesh repair was significantly more common in the laparoscopic group. Median hospital stay was shorter in the laparoscopic group (3 versus 9 days), with similar median follow up (12 months laparoscopic, 16 months open). Recurrent herniation, identified on routine videoesophagram or endoscopy, occurred in similar proportions from both groups (12 % laparoscopic, 25 % open). Reoperation for recurrence was not enumerated.

Recommendations

Operative repair of giant PEH is a challenging endeavor. High grade evidence does not exist to guide the surgeon in determining an operative approach, leaving surgeons to rely on retrospective case series. Surgeons must be familiar with the range of approaches to repair of giant PEH, as patient factors such as body habitus, medical comorbidities, and previous exposure to operative intervention may influence operative approach. From the available data, it cannot be concluded that the thoracic and open abdominal approaches differ significantly in recurrence rate, although the thoracic approach appears to entail higher perioperative morbidity. We make a weak recommendation to choose the abdominal approach over the thoracic approach due to higher morbidity of the latter, especially in patients who are frail, elderly, or likely to have difficulty tolerating one lung ventilation. In examining studies evaluating open and laparoscopic approaches to giant PEH repair, we find the balance of available evidence does not support a higher recurrence rate attributable to either approach. We make a weak recommendation to choose the laparoscopic approach over the open abdominal approach for repair of giant paraesophageal hernia. We feel this is justified due to similar recurrence rates subsequent to both approaches along with the decreased length of stay and the trend toward decreased complication rates in patients undergoing the laparoscopic approach.

A Personal View of the Data

For the majority of patients with giant PEH, the laparoscopic approach is our preferred approach due to its superior safety profile and comparable durability to the more invasive approaches. Personal experience in our center has led the senior author to change this approach when a giant PEH occurs in an obese patient. Anecdotally, the recurrence rate in this population when a laparoscopic approach is employed is considerably higher. This may be a result of the higher intraabdominal pressures exerting tension on the crural closure, or may be due to the quality of the tissues in this patient population. While some surgeons opt to use a prosthetic mesh in obese patients with giant PEH to mitigate this increased risk of recurrence, the possibility of complications arising from the mesh prosthesis, such as erosion, has led the senior author to prefer a primary tissue repair through the chest.

Recommendations

- We make a weak recommendation to choose the abdominal approach over the thoracic approach due to higher morbidity of the latter. (Evidence quality low; weak recommendation)
- We make a weak recommendation to choose the laparoscopic approach over the open abdominal approach due to similar recurrence rates along with the decreased length of stay and the decreased complication rates associated with the laparoscopic approach. (Evidence quality low; weak recommendation)

References

1. Allen MS, Trastek VF, Deschamps C, Pairolero PC. Intrathoracic stomach. Presentation and results of operation. J Thorac Cardiovasc Surg. 1993;105(2):253–9.
2. Martin TR, Ferguson MK, Naunheim KS. Management of giant paraesophageal hernia. Dis Esophagus. 1997;10:47–50.
3. Maziak DE, Todd TRJ, Pearson FG. Massive hiatus hernia: evaluation and surgical management. J Thorac Cardiovasc Surg. 1998;115:53–62.
4. Geha AS, Massad MG, Snow NJ, Baue AE. A 32-year experience in 100 patients with giant parasophageal hernia: the case for abdominal approach and selective antireflux repair. Surgery. 2000;128:623–30.
5. Altorki NK, Yankelevitz D, Skinner DB. Massive hiatal hernias: the anatomic basis of repair. J Thorac Cardiovasc Surg. 1998;115:828–35.
6. Hashemi M, Peters JH, DeMeester TR, Huprich JE, et al. Laparoscopic repair of large type III hiatal hernia: objective followup reveals high recurrence rate. J Am Coll Surg. 2000;190:553–61.
7. Mittal SK, Bikhchandani J, Gurney O, Yano F, Lee T. Outcomes after repair of the intrathoracic stomach: objective follow-up of up to 5 years. Surg Endosc. 2011;25:556–66.
8. Low DE, Unger T. Open repair of paraesophageal hernia: reassessment of subjective and objective outcomes. Ann Thorac Surg. 2005;80:287–94.
9. Dahlberg PS, Deschamps C, Miller DL, Allen MS, et al. Laparoscopic repair of large paraesophageal hiatal hernia. Ann Thorac Surg. 2001;72:1125–9.
10. Terry M, Smith CD, Branum GD, Galloway K, et al. Outcomes of laparoscopic fundoplication for gastroesophageal disease and paraesophageal hernia. Experience with 1,000 consecutive cases. Surg Endosc. 2001;15:691–9.
11. Weichmann RJ, Ferguson MK, Naunheim KS, McKesey P, et al. Laparoscopic management of giant paraesophageal herniation. Ann Thorac Surg. 2001;71:1080–7.
12. Pierre AF, Luketich JD, Fernando HC, Christie NA, et al. Results of laparoscopic repair of giant paraesophageal hernias: 200 consecutive patients. Ann Thorac Surg. 2002;74:1909–16.
13. Andujar JJ, Papasavas PK, Birdas T, Robke J, et al. Laparoscopic repair of large paraesophageal hernia is associated with a low incidence of recurrence and reoperation. Surg Endosc. 2004;18:444–7.
14. Parameswaran R, Ali A, Velmurugan S, Adjepong SE, Sigurdsson A. Laparoscopic repair of large paraesophageal hiatus hernia: quality of life and durability. Surg Endosc. 2006;20:1221–4.
15. Grotenhuis BA, Wijnhoven BPL, Bessell JR, Watson DI. Laparscopic antireflux surgery in the elderly. Surg Endosc. 2008;22:1807–12.
16. Morris-Stiff G, Hassn A. Laparoscopic paraoesophageal hernia repair: fundoplication is not usually indicated. Hernia. 2008;12:299–302.
17. Nason KS, Luketich JD, Qureshi I, Keeley S, et al. Laparoscopic repair of giant paraesophageal hernia results in long-term patient satisfaction and a durable repair. J Gastrointest Surg. 2008;12:2066–77.
18. Luketich JD, Nason KS, Christie NA, Pennathur A, et al. Outcomes after a decade of laparoscopic giant paraesophageal hernia repair. J Thorac Cardiovasc Surg. 2010;139:395–404.
19. Karmali S, McFadden S, Mitchell P, Graham A, et al. Primary laparoscopic and open repair of paraesophageal hernias: a comparison of short-term outcomes. Dis Esophagus. 2008;21:63–8.
20. Zehetner J, DeMeester SR, Ayazi S, Kilday P, et al. Laparscopic versus open repair of paraesophageal hernia: the second decade. J Am Coll Surg. 2011;212:813–20.
21. Skinner DB, Belsey RH, Russell PS. Surgical management of esophageal reflux and hiatus hernia: long-term results with 1,030 patients. J Thorac Cardiovasc Surg. 1967;53:33–54.
22. Patel HJ, Tan BB, Yee J, Orringer MB, Iannettoni MD. A 25 year experience with open primary transthoracic repair of paraesophageal hiatal hernia. J Thorac Cardiovasc Surg. 2004;127:843–9.

Chapter 39
Synthetic Reinforcement of Diaphragm Closure for Large Hiatal Hernia Repair

Katie S. Nason

Abstract Successful repair of large hiatal hernia is often based on objective recurrence rates and, as a result of several studies suggesting benefit, mesh cruroplasty is now widely used. From the patient's perspective, however, the critical outcomes are symptom relief and restoration of quality of life as well as postoperative medication use, endoscopic intervention and reoperation for recurrent symptoms and/or symptomatic hernia. Evidence supporting mesh for these outcomes and objective recurrence is low quality, recommendations for routine use of mesh for synthetic reinforcement are weak and use of mesh should remain at the surgeon's discretion until higher quality data are available.

Keywords Hernia, Paraesophageal • Surgical Mesh • Recurrence • Assessment • Outcomes • Surgical Procedures, Minimally Invasive

Introduction

Repair of large hiatal hernia is a complex operation and the best outcomes are reported from high-volume centers with expertise in benign foregut surgery. The goal of the repair is to return the stomach to the intraabdominal position with sufficient intraabdominal esophagus to minimize the axial traction of the stomach against the hiatal closure and, therefore, prevent symptomatic recurrence. The tenets of repair include complete sac reduction, extensive esophageal mobilization to reestablish at least 2–3 cm of tension-free intraabdominal esophagus, esophageal lengthening if this length cannot be achieved after extensive transhiatal esophageal

K.S. Nason, MD, MPH
Division of Thoracic and Foregut Surgery, Department of Cardiothoracic Surgery, University of Pittsburgh Medical Center, 5200 Centre Ave, Suite 715, Pittsburgh, PA 15217, USA
e-mail: nasonks@upmc.edu

M.K. Ferguson (ed.), *Difficult Decisions in Thoracic Surgery*,
Difficult Decisions in Surgery: An Evidence-Based Approach 1,
DOI 10.1007/978-1-4471-6404-3_39, © Springer-Verlag London 2014

mobilization, and tension-free hiatal closure. Similarly, because the esophagus is a dynamic structure, the hiatal opening must be wide enough that the esophagus with a food bolus can move freely through the hiatus but narrow enough that the stomach and/or adjacent organs remain below the diaphragm. Depending on the size of the hiatal opening and the integrity of the crural muscle and overlying fascia, achieving this balance can prove challenging.

Many options for management of the widely splayed crural opening, other than primary suture closure, have been described, including relaxing incisions on the diaphragm away from the crura, pledgeted sutures, and autologous tissue transplants; the most commonly used reinforcement, however, is synthetic mesh as either a bridge for a tension-free closure or, more commonly, an onlay reinforcement of a suture cruroplasty. Prior to the laparoscopic era, mesh cruroplasty was used sparingly because the diaphragm is naturally a floppy and mobile muscle and tension-free closure could be achieved in most patients. With the evolution to the laparoscopic approach, surgeons noted high rates of early- and mid-term recurrence and synthetic reinforcement of the crural closure during laparoscopic repair of large hiatal hernia repair became widespread. Data supporting this practice are mixed, however, including recent long-term follow-up of a randomized controlled trial showing no benefit [1], and reassessment of the benefit of routine mesh cruroplasty is warranted.

The aim of this chapter is to assess the literature regarding the role of mesh cruroplasty for laparoscopic repair of large hiatal hernia and to determine whether the evidence supports routine use of mesh in all patients. The clinical questions of interest are whether, in patients with large hiatal hernia, routine mesh cruroplasty, as compared to suture cruroplasty, should be used to reinforce the crural closure to: (1) reduce objective hernia recurrence; (2) improve patient symptoms and quality of life; (3) minimize the need for postoperative medication use and endoscopic intervention for symptoms (e.g. dysphagia, odynophagia, GERD); and (4) reduce the rate of reoperation for hiatal hernia recurrence.

Search Strategy

MEDLINE and EMBASE were used to perform a systematic literature review for studies comparing synthetic reinforcement to primary suture hiatal closure during repair of large hiatal hernia. Search terms included combinations of massive, large, and giant with hiatal/paraesophageal and hernia(e) (Table 39.1; n = 5,236 publications). After removing duplicates, 1,828 remained for review of titles and abstracts. Publications comparing mesh cruroplasty to suture cruroplasty for repair of large hiatal hernias and published with full-text in the English language since 1995 were considered for final inclusion. Studies reporting anti-reflux operations without a focus on or a subset analysis of large hiatal hernias, case series of less than 30 patients, studies with less than 6 months follow-up or focused on children, pelvic hernias, or posttraumatic diaphragmatic hernias, non-systematic review articles,

Table 39.1 Search terms and number of publications associated with each (as of October 12, 2013)

Search terms	Number of publications
Massive AND hiatal AND ('hernia'/exp OR hernia)	74
Massive AND hiatal AND herniae	0
Massive AND hiatal AND hernias	20
Massive AND hiatal AND (herniation/exp OR herniation)	65
Massive AND hiatus AND (hernia/exp OR hernia)	114
Massive AND hiatus AND herniae	0
Massive AND hiatus AND hernias	23
Massive AND hiatus AND 'herniation'/exp	110
Large AND hiatal AND ('hernia'/exp OR hernia)	590
Large AND hiatal AND herniae	2
Large AND hiatal AND hernias	221
Large AND hiatal AND 'herniation'/exp	590
Large AND hiatus AND hernia	1,103
Large AND hiatus AND herniae	11
Large AND hiatus AND hernias	269
Large AND hiatus AND 'herniation'/exp	1,103
Giant AND paraesophageal AND 'hernia'/exp	81
Giant AND paraesophageal AND herniae	0
Giant AND paraesophageal AND 'herniation'/exp	81
Paraesophageal AND hernia/exp	779

and letters to the editor were excluded. When the same cohort of patients was reported in more than one manuscript, the one with the longest follow-up was used. The articles meeting inclusion criteria included three randomized controlled trials, three systematic review/meta-analysis, and ten observational studies. When proportions of patients with the outcome were available in the majority of studies, relative risk of the outcome was estimated using the odds ratio and reported with a 95 % confidence interval.

Results

Use of Mesh and Objective Hernia Recurrence

To determine whether a strong recommendation can be made for routine use of mesh for crural reinforcement, it is critical to first determine whether the literature provides strong evidence that mesh improves clinically relevant outcomes. Over the past decade, hernia recurrence has become a focal point of surgical outcomes studies for large hiatal hernia, in part because it is an objective and reproducible outcome measure and, in part, because a successful operation from the surgeon's perspective is one in which the anatomic abnormality, a stomach that is partially

Table 39.2 Outcomes comparing mesh cruroplasty to primary cruroplasty for repair of large hiatal hernia

Author	Cruroplasty	Total (n)	Recurrence identified at follow-up			Reoperation for recurrence	
			Yes (n)	% recurrence	p-value	Yes (n)	p-value
Randomized controlled trials							
Carlson et al. [2]	Mesh	16	0	(0)	0.08	0	0.1012
	Suture	15	3	(19)		2	
Frantzides et al. [3]	Mesh	36	0	(0)	<0.006	0	0.0539
	Suture	36	8	(22)		5	
Oelschlager et al. [1]	Mesh	57	20	(59)	0.7	0	0.2207
	Suture	51	14	(54)		2	
Observational – prospective							
Braghetto et al. [4]	Mesh	23	0	(0)	0.055	NR	
	Suture	58	10	(18)			
Goers et al. [5]	Mesh	56	0	(0)	n/a	NR	
	Suture	33	0	(0)			
Ringley et al. [6]	Mesh	22	0	(0)	0.5045*	NR	
	Suture	22	2	(9)			
Zaninotto et al. [7]	Mesh	35	3	(8.6)	0.01	5 total (type of cruroplasty not specified)	
	Suture	19	8	(42)			
Observational – retrospective							
Dallemagne et al. [8]	Mesh n = 7	6	5	(83)	0.6399	1	0.1588
	Suture n = 78	29	18	(62)		1	
Morino et al. [9]	Mesh	37	13	(56)	0.0286*	5	0.1133
	Suture	14	10	(77)		5	
Muller-Stich et al. [10]	Mesh	16	0	(0)	0.1729*	0	1.0000
	Suture n = 40	36	7	(19)		2	
Soricelli et al. [11]	Mesh	138	3	(2)	0.0001*	3	0.0032
	Suture	37	9	(24)		6	
Observational – NOS							
Gouvas et al. [12]	Mesh	20	3	(15)	0.4112*	2	0.0834
	Suture	48	4	(8)		0	
Grubnik et al. [13]	Mesh n = 158	142	8	(4.9)	0.0488	1	0.0360
	Suture n = 103	92	12	(11.9)		5	

*p-value for difference not calculated in published manuscript

or completely herniated into the posterior mediastinum with or without volvulus, is corrected and does not recur. There are multiple publications reporting objective recurrence rates, which range from 0 to nearly 80 %, depending on the method of assessment and duration of follow-up. For the purposes of this review, only studies directly comparing suture versus mesh cruroplasty were considered; in all of the included studies, hiatal hernia recurrence was the primary outcome measure (Table 39.2). Beginning with the randomized controlled trials, Carlson and colleagues reported a trend toward a significant difference in objective recurrence, with

0/16 mesh patients having recurrence compared to 3/15 suture cruroplasty patients (p=0.008) while Frantzides and colleagues found recurrence in 8 of 36 suture cruroplasty patients compared to no recurrence in the 36 mesh repair patients (p=0.006). Similarly, Oelschlager and colleagues reported a significant difference in objective recurrence favoring the mesh patients (9 % vs. 24 %; p=0.04) at 6 months after surgery. At a mean follow-up of 5 years, however, slightly more than 50 % of patients in each group had objective recurrence, with no difference between the two groups. Taking the three randomized trials together, the likelihood for recurrence in the suture cruroplasty group is 45 % higher than in the mesh cruroplasty group, but the difference is not significant (OR 1.4448; 95 % CI 0.7449–2.8022).

In 2012, Antoniou and associates (2012) performed a meta-analysis for recurrence that included randomized trials only, and reported a stronger risk for recurrence with suture cruroplasty alone compared to mesh cruroplasty. Their study did not include the Carlson study described above, but did include a trial by Granderath and colleagues in which patients with small hiatal hernia were also included and comprised 48 % of the patients [14]. A total of 280 patients were included in the meta-analysis and follow-up (at 6–12 months) was complete for 267 patients. For the meta-analysis, the weighted mean value for recurrence after suture cruroplasty ranged from 22.2 to 26 % versus 0 to 8.9 % for mesh cruroplasty. The likelihood of recurrent hernia was four times greater after suture cruroplasty, and the difference was significant (OR 4.2; 95 % CI 1.8–9.5) When the long-term follow-up in the Oelschlager study was analyzed rather than the 6 month results (as was done with the three trials included in the current review), the likelihood of recurrent hernia decreased to two times greater after suture cruroplasty, but the difference remained significant (OR 2.3; 95 % CI 1.2–5.1; p=0.024) [15].

Two systematic reviews are also published and examined recurrence rates after repair [16, 17]. These reviews included the randomized trials discussed as well as up to 23 additional observational studies and as many as 924 patients with mesh compared to 340 patients without mesh. Both systematic reviews found significant differences in reported recurrence rates within the available studies; 14.6 % in mesh patients and 26.3 % in suture cruroplasty patients in the Furnee review and 2.6 % versus 15 %, respectively, in the subset of patients with large hiatal hernia in the Johnson review. Finally, the observational studies included in the current review also reported recurrence as the primary outcome, with rates ranging from 0 to 83 % in the mesh cruroplasty patients and 0–77 % in the suture cruroplasty patients. Overall, 7 % (35/495) of mesh cruroplasty patients in the ten observational studies were reported to have hernia recurrence compared to 21 % (80/388) of the suture cruroplasty patients. The likelihood of hernia recurrence on objective follow-up was 3.4 times greater in the suture cruroplasty group, which was statistically significant (OR 3.4137; 95 % CI 2.2371–5.2092).

Taken together, these findings suggest that objective recurrence is reduced with the use of mesh to reinforce the cruroplasty at the time of large hiatal hernia repair. Indeed, these findings have prompted many surgeons to adopt the practice as a key element to the repair. Before accepting these findings as evidence for a strong recommendation for mesh, however, it is important to determine the quality of the evidence, i.e. the quality of the studies that provide the evidence favoring mesh. Unfortunately, the quality of the evidence, overall, is low despite three randomized trials on the topic and ten observational studies. The approach to the operation, definition of large hiatal hernia, inclusion of small hiatal hernia and patients without hernia, and the approach to repair were extremely heterogeneous among the studies, with variable attention to esophageal mobilization, use of multiple types and shapes of mesh, and different locations for mesh placement. The approach to objective reassessment for recurrent hernia, time to assessment for recurrence, and definition of recurrence was also highly variable, if they were even reported (Tables 39.3 and 39.4). Only four of the ten observational studies reported time to follow-up stratified by the mesh and suture cruroplasty groups. It was common for the approach to repair to shift over time, usually from a primarily suture repair approach to a primarily mesh repair approach. As a result, the time to objective assessment was often longer in the suture repair group and lead-time bias becomes a confounding factor in the analysis given that hernia recurrences increase over time from surgery [1].

This heterogeneity within the observational studies is present even in the randomized controlled trials. In the Carlson and Frantzides trials, time to follow-up was relatively short and the randomization process was not well-described. Neither the Carlson study nor the Frantzides study provided objective follow-up at pre-specified time points, despite the prospective trial design using routine esophagrams obtained by protocol at 6 month intervals for all patients. They present, instead, a range (12–36 months) [2] and a median time (2.5 years; 6 months to 6 years) [3] for the overall study, respectively. Time to objective follow-up was not stratified for the type of repair in either study. In addition, both studies report objective recurrence assessed, but an a priori definition of objective hernia recurrence was not provided for either study. As a result, the quality of these studies for assessing the primary endpoint of recurrence is substantially reduced. In comparison, Oelschlager and associates performed objective follow-up at 6 months and 5 years in both groups of patients with an a priori definition of objective hiatal hernia recurrence to guide analysis of the postoperative imaging [1]. Even in the Oelschlager study, however, nearly half of the patients did not have objective reevaluation at 5-years, which limits the conclusions that can be made about the overall rate of objective recurrence. As such, the highest level of evidence supporting the recommendation for mesh is hampered by problems in the study design and execution, with inconsistent objective follow-up within and between studies representing the most important factor downgrading the quality of the evidence.

In summary, analysis of the available randomized controlled trials, meta-analysis and systematic review, and individual studies comparing mesh cruroplasty to suture cruroplasty reveals that the available data regarding objective recurrence are mixed. The available studies are extremely heterogeneous and lack critical information, including a priori definitions of recurrence, time to objective follow-up stratified by type of repair, and consistent approach to the operation. The definition of large hiatal hernia is also extremely variable. With these limitations in mind, the highest level data from the available randomized trials do not show a difference in the likelihood of objective hiatal hernia recurrence whereas the observational studies do

Table 39.3 Study inclusion and assessment for objective outcomes comparing mesh cruroplasty to primary cruroplasty for repair of large hiatal hernia

Author	Definition of hernia	Assessment type and schedule	Objective recurrence	Definition of recurrence	Notes
Randomized controlled trials					
Carlson et al. [2]	8 cm hiatal defect or greater	Esophagram q 6 months	12–36 months	Not defined	Randomization protocol not described
Frantzides et al. [3]	8 cm hiatal defect or greater	Esophagram at 3 months then q 6 months	Median 2.5 years (6 months to 6 years)	Not defined	Randomization protocol not described
Oelschlager et al. [1]	Greater than 5 cm	Esophagram at 6 months and 5 years	Mesh: mean 5.0 years (3.7–6.2 years; n=26) Suture: Mean 4.9 years (3.6–6.5 years; n=34)	A maximum vertical height greater than 2 cm from the level of the diaphragm adjacent to the fundoplication to the top of the wrap	Central randomization; recurrence associated with significantly more chest pain and early satiety and lower physical functioning by SF-36
Observational – prospective					
Braghetto et al. [4]	5 cm or greater received mesh and <5 cm suture only	Esophagram at 3–5 years	3–5 years	Radiologic and endoscopic evaluation demonstrate intrathoracic portion of stomach regardless of size or type	
Goers et al. [5]	30 % or more gastric herniation	Esophagram at 6 months; manometry and pH testing at 6 months and 3 years	Mesh: 6.5 months (n=40) Suture: 9.5 months (n=32)		Recurrence reported by manometry only; excluded Collis patients and patients with preoperative dysphagia
Ringley et al. [6]	Defect >5 cm	Esophagram day 1 and 6 months	Mesh: mean 6.7 months (n=15/22) Suture: mean 9.5 months (n=22/22)		Approach shifted to all mesh

(continued)

Table 39.3 (continued)

Author	Definition of hernia	Assessment type and schedule	Objective recurrence	Definition of recurrence	Notes
Zaninotto et al. [7]	1/3rd or more gastric herniation	Esophagram at 1 month; endoscopy at 12 months and q2 years	Mesh: Median 33 months Suture: Median 64 months		Symptoms in only 12 % of patients at follow-up
Dallemagne et al. [8]	50 % or more gastric herniation	Esophagram beginning 2007	99 months (17–186); (n = 35/85)	Evidence of new paraesophageal herniation or proximal migration of the cardia. Disruption or slippage of the fundoplication alone with no reherniation was noted but not classified as a recurrence	Manuscript considered pledgeted sutures as 'reinforced' repair – these patients considered 'suture' repair for this table consistent with other papers
Morino et al. [9]	6 cm or greater length; 50 % or more herniation; or 5 cm hiatal defect intraoperatively	Esophagram at 3 months and 18 months and by symptoms; EGD at 6 months; pH and manometry at 3 and 12 months	3 months in 16 patients; not reported in remaining 7 patients; not reported by group	Any evidence denoting herniation of the stomach above the level of the diaphragm	Surgical technique evolved over study period. Initially primary closure with no gastroplasty, then mesh 'tension-free' hiatoplasty with U-shaped bridging of the crural defect. Collis gastroplasty with Nissen for short esophgus added in the last 14 patients, 3 of whom also had mesh reinforcement

Muller-Stich et al. [18]	Not reported	Esophagram (scheduled assessment not specified)	Mesh: 20 months (10–60) Suture: 67 months (9–117)	Not defined	Evolution of type of hiatoplasty from primary closure to bridge hiatoplasty to primary closure with mesh onlay for all hernias larger than 3 cm; not all of the patients in this series had hernias >3 cm
Soricelli et al. [11]	Not reported	EGD 12 months then as needed	Suture: 67 months (9–117)	Not defined	Concerns with regard to functional outcome and fibrosis led to change in approach to large hiatal defects away from mesh cruroplasty
Observational – NOS					
Gouvas et al. [10]	Type II, III, or IV PEH	Esophagram: 3–12 months, 3 years, 5 years; pH and manometry: 3–12 months and as indicated	1 year	Not defined	
Grubnik et al. [19]	HSA 10–20 cm²	Esophagram, EGD and pH testing at 6, 12, and 24 months	Mean 28.6 months (10–48 months)	Migration of the stomach with or without fundoplication wrap above the diaphragm	Subset of 261 with large hiatal hernia; assessment for recurrence based on presence of symptoms or persistent dysphagia

(continued)

Table 39.4 Study description of operative procedure

Author	Sac reduction	Esophageal mobilization	Length intra-abdominal esophagus	Suture cruroplasty Location	# of sutures	Details of mesh used Type	Shape	Additional operative details
Randomized controlled trials								
Carlson et al. [2]	Yes	Yes	5 cm	Posterior	NR	Fenestrated PTFE	Keyhole	
Frantzides et al. [3]	Yes	Yes	4–5 cm	NR	NR	Fenestrated PTFE	Keyhole	
Oelschlager et al. [1]	Yes	NR	NR	Posterior	NR	SIS	U-shaped	Anterior suture and Collis at surgeon discretion
Observational – prospective								
Braghetto et al. [4]	Yes	NR	NR	NR	3–4	Vicryl Poliglecaprone-25:polypropylene composite SIS	NR	Posterior gastropexy
Goers et al. [5]	Yes	Yes	2.5–3 cm	Posterior pledgeted	NR	Biomesh NOS	Posterior onlay	Collis and partial fundoplication excluded; indication for mesh = thinning of hiatal pillars
Ringley et al. [6]	NR	Yes	NR	Posterior	2–4	Acellular dermal matrix	Posterior onlay	Begins with left crus approach to sac
Zaninotto et al. [7]	Yes	NR	NR	Posterior	2–3	Goretex: polypropylene composite	Keyhole onlay	Anterior suture added if hiatus wide
Observational – retrospective								
Dallemagne et al. [8]	Yes	Yes	NR	Posterior	NR	Polyester:collagen composite SIS	NR	'Tension-free' intraabdominal GEJ; mesh used if crura were 'poor'

Morino et al. [9]	Yes	NR	NR	Posterior pledgeted (PTFE)	5 (3–8)	PTFE	U-shaped 'tension-free' bridge	Does not specify optimal location of GEJ but assessed intraoperatively with endoscopy
Muller-Stich et al. [10]	Yes	Yes	NR	Posterior	3–4	Polypropylene PTFE:polypropylene composite; Polypropylene vicryl: polypropylene	Butterfly-shaped	Mesh in selected cases in first 33 then used routinely
Soricelli et al. [11]	Yes	Yes	4 cm	NR	2–3	Polypropylene	Posterior onlay	Mesh onlay across pillars posteriorly OR as tension-free bridge
Observational – NOS								
Gouvas et al. [12]	Yes	Yes	NR	Posterior	2–3	Polypropylene; Duo-mesh	Keyhole or U-shaped onlay	Esophageal mobilization carried to inferior pulmonary veins – length otherwise not specified
Grubnik et al. [13]	Yes	Yes	3 cm	Posterior	2–3	Poliglecaprone-25:polypropylene composite	"Sandwich" technique	Mesh for 8 cm defect in early experience then suture only; anterior suture added if hiatus wide

NR Not reported, *NOS* not otherwise specified, *PTFE* polytetrafluoroethylene, *SIS* porcine small intestinal submucosa, *GEJ* gastroesophageal junction

show a statistically significant difference. Based on this low level evidence, a weak recommendation is made for routine use of mesh to reduce objective recurrence.

Use of Mesh and Symptoms, Quality of Life

Given that the goal of paraesophageal hernia repair is to restore nearly normal foregut function while reducing the patient's risk for catastrophic complications resulting from an incarcerated stomach, focusing on outcomes that are important to the patient, including improvement in symptoms, return to normal daily life, and durable improvement in quality of life should be paramount [18]. The critical clinical question, therefore, is not whether mesh cruroplasty reduces objective hernia recurrence rates, but whether mesh cruroplasty improves patient symptoms, daily life function and quality of life compared to suture cruroplasty alone. These improvements must be weighed against the potential adverse impact of mesh, which includes mesh erosion and fibrosis with stricture. Optimally, studies comparing outcomes would provide preoperative symptom assessment using standardized symptom questionnaires and validated quality of life measures to determine patient baseline status. Serial assessments would then be performed at intervals that are similar between groups to allow paired analysis of resolved symptoms, stable symptoms (present or absent pre- and postoperatively) and new symptoms. The balance between desirable and undesirable effects would then be objectively assessed by comparing the two therapeutic interventions.

With this approach in mind, the included studies were evaluated for their approach to symptom assessment and symptom outcomes (Table 39.5). Of the three randomized trials investigating the role of mesh in hiatal closure, only one reported symptom outcomes using standardized symptom assessment prior to repair and in follow-up [1, 19]. The other two randomized trials by Carlson and colleagues (1999) and Frantzides and colleagues (2002) reported recurrence and reoperation rates only. Preoperative and postoperative symptoms were not reported except to describe whether or not recurrences were symptomatic. Neither study provided a list of the symptoms assessed and all reported recurrences were 'symptomatic,' although 'symptomatic' was not defined. Reoperation was required for 7 of 11 recurrences [2, 3]. In contrast, Oelschlager and colleagues utilized a standardized symptom questionnaire preoperatively and then reevaluated patients with the same questionnaire postoperatively (Table 39.4). Symptom severity was scored using a visual analog score. Quality of life was evaluated using the 36-item Health Survey (SF-36). Symptom severity was reported and was similar at baseline between the mesh and suture groups. Laparoscopic repair of large hiatal hernia resulted in significant reduction in symptom frequency and severity and significant improvement in quality of life at 6 months; this improvement persisted at 5 years for all symptoms, except dysphagia in the suture cruroplasty group which was improved but not significantly different from baseline in the available patients. When the severity of symptoms were compared between the suture cruroplasty and the mesh groups,

Table 39.5 Approach to symptom assessment and reporting by study

	Postoperative symptom assessment			Symptoms reported				Paired analysis	Outcomes	Long-term adverse outcomes
Author	Scheduled	Reported time to symptom assessment	Standardized assessment used	Pre-operatively	Post-operatively	Scale				
Carlson et al. [2]	1 and 2 weeks, 1 and 3 months, then q 6 months	NR	No	NR	NR	None	No	NR	NR	
Frantzides et al. [3]	1 and 2 weeks, 3 months then q year	Median 2.5 years (6 months to 6 years)	No	NR	NR	None	No	NR	No mesh-related strictures, erosions or infections
Oelschlager et al. [1]	pre-op, 2–4 weeks, 6 months and 5 years	Median 59 months (40–78 months); n=33 SIS n=39 suture	Yes – pre- and post-operatively	Heartburn, regurgitation, chest pain, dysphagia, abdominal pain, bloating, nausea, postprandial pain, and early satiety	Severity		No	Significant improvement both groups from baseline and no differences between groups at follow-up	NR	
Observational – prospective										
Braghetto et al. [4]	3–5 years	3–5 years	Yes	Heartburn, regurgitation, chest pain, dyspnea, cardiac (tachycardia, arrhythmias), anemia, vomiting, dysphagia	Heartburn, vomiting, dysphagia	Present or absent	No	Not stratified by cruroplasty type; heartburn improved with stable dysphagia rate	NR	

(continued)

Table 39.5 (continued)

Author	Postoperative symptom assessment			Symptoms reported		Scale	Paired analysis	Outcomes	Long-term adverse outcomes
	Scheduled	Reported time to symptom assessment	Standardized assessment used	Pre-operatively	Post-operatively				
Goers et al. [5]	3–4 weeks; 6 months	Mesh: 6.5 months (n=40) Suture: 9.5 months (n=32)	Yes	Assessed per methods but not reported in manuscript	Reflux, heartburn, dysphagia	Frequency and/or severity (scale 0–4)	No	Frequency and severity assessed but reported as present/absent; heartburn, chest pain, abdominal pain and inability to belch more likely in non-mesh patients	NR
Ringley et al. [6]	6 months	Mesh: 6.7 months (n=15/22) Suture: 9.5 months (n=22/22)	Yes	Regurgitation, chest pain/discomfort, dysphagia, heartburn, hoarseness		Frequency	No	Comparing pre- to postoperative mean scores – improved within both groups	NR
Zaninotto et al. [7]	1, 6, and 12 months, q2 years	Median 71 months (IQR 39–97)	No	NR	Dysphagia, retrosternal discomfort, regurgitation	Present or absent	No	Not stratified by cruroplasty type; overall rate of postoperative symptoms = 22 %	1 esophagectomy for mesh erosion

Observational – retrospective

Study	Follow-up method	Follow-up duration	Prospective	Symptoms assessed	Quality of life measure	Classification	Recurrence	Results	
Dallemagne et al. [8]	Telephone and clinic beginning 2007	151 months (21–186) in mesh group and 65 months (17–143) in suture only group	Yes – postoperative only	Heartburn, regurgitation, dysphagia, chest pain, respiratory symptoms, anemia	Gastrointestinal quality of life index and satisfaction scale	Preoperative: variable by symptom; postoperative: 5-pt Likert scale	No	Significant improvement for preop symptoms in all patients; No difference in postoperative GIQLI or satisfaction scale between groups	Not reported
Morino et al. [9]	1, 3, 12, 24, and 36-months	Median 58 months (12–124)	Yes	Assessed using Gastroesophageal Reflux Health-Related Quality of Life scale but results not reported for either pre- or postoperative symptoms		Visick classification (I–IV)	No	Not stratified by cruroplasty type; outcomes reported as single measure using Visick classification	Not reported
Muller-Stich et al. [10]	Scheduled assessment not specified	Mesh: 20 months (10–60) Suture: 67 months (9–117)	Yes – postoperative only	Reflux, epigastric pain, cough, fullness, dysphagia, vomiting, anemia, thoracic pain, dyspnea, nausea, postprandial collapses		Present or absent	No	Rates of symptom free or only mild gas bloat not significantly different between groups; good or very good in ~95 % in both groups with no difference in rate of patients reporting willingness to undergo operation again	Not reported

(continued)

Table 39.5 (continued)

Author	Postoperative symptom assessment			Symptoms reported		Scale	Paired analysis	Outcomes	Long-term adverse outcomes
	Scheduled	Reported time to symptom assessment	Standardized assessment used	Pre-operatively	Post-operatively				
Soricelli et al. [11]	1 months, 6 months, 12 months, then yearly	Mean 95.1 months (87 %)	Yes	DeMeester grading scale for reflux symptoms, GERD health-related quality of life		Severity	No	Not stratified by cruroplasty type; significant improvement in GERD-HRQL scores for all patients compared to baseline; mesh only had significantly lower GERD-HRQL than suture only (4 vs 2.6; p=0.03)	1 mesh related complication requiring removal
Observational – NOS									
Gouvas et al. [12]	3, 6, 12, and 36 months	3 years (45 pts)	Yes	Heartburn, regurgitation, dyspshagia, chest pain, epigastric or chest discomfort, abdominal bloating, respiratory and cardiovascular symptoms		Frequency and severity (absent, mild and occasional, moderate and frequent, constant, severe and incapacitating)	Yes	Significant reduction in the proportion of patients with all symptoms at follow-up; dysphagia, chest discomfort, cardiac and respiratory symptoms significantly more likely in mesh patients at 12 months	Late dysphagia (n=4) with esophageal stenosis due to mesh-induced fibrosis
Grubnik et al. [13]	6, 12, and 24 months	Mean 28.6 months (10–48 months)	No	NR	Reflux, dysphagia	Present or absent	No	No difference in rate of reflux symptom recurrence or persisting dysphagia	No mesh erosions seen

NR Not reported

there was no significant difference between the two groups at a median of 5 years of follow-up.

The three meta-analysis/systematic reviews were also assessed with regard to symptom reporting. The meta-analysis by Antoniou looked only at dysphagia reporting as an adverse quality of life outcome and did not assess other symptom outcomes. They found that only one of the three included studies reported the rate of postoperative dysphagia and none addressed long-term adverse effects of the mesh [15]. Symptom and quality of life outcomes were assessed in the systematic review by Furnee and Hazebroek [16], but summary statistics could only be generated for mesh patients as the data were insufficient for summary in the suture cruroplasty patients. Of the 27 studies, 10 reported symptom outcome for the mesh group, with successful outcome in 275/317 mesh patients (86.6 %). Only 1 study reported symptom outcomes for the suture cruroplasty group, with successful outcome in 32/33 patients (97 %). The second review by Johnson and colleagues (2006), with a total of 228 patients undergoing mesh repair compared to 153 with suture cruroplasty alone, did not report symptom or quality of life outcomes. Both reviews examined the reporting of long-term adverse outcomes of erosions, finding that more than 50 % of the studies did not report on this long-term outcome [16].

Finally, examining the individual studies included in the current review, eight out of ten studies state in the methods that standardized symptom assessment is routinely performed at varying time-intervals postoperatively (Table 39.4). When standard measures were used, the types of measures range from symptom questionnaires to validated gastrointestinal quality of life measures. Symptoms were assessed as present/absent, by frequency of symptoms, by severity of symptoms, by composite frequency and severity scales and by specific symptom scales as constructed by the authors. In eight of the ten studies, preoperative symptom assessment was performed for a variety of gastrointestinal symptoms. Only one study performed a paired analysis comparing preoperative symptoms to postoperative symptoms to determine whether symptoms in each patient were resolved, unchanged (i.e. still present or still absent), or new [12]. They reported only symptoms resolution and not new symptoms. Four of the remaining seven studies that assessed symptoms both preoperatively and postoperatively did not stratify symptom outcomes by type of cruroplasty [4, 7, 9, 11]. The other three studies reported significant improvements in gastrointestinal complaints in all patients, with conflicting results regarding differences between mesh cruroplasty and suture cruroplasty (Table 39.5). Goers and colleagues found that heartburn, chest pain, abdominal pain, and inability to belch were more likely in the suture cruroplasty at a mean follow-up time of 9.5 months in comparison to a mean follow-up time of 6.7 months for the mesh cruroplasty group [5]. In contrast, Gouvas and associates report that mesh cruroplasty patients were significantly more likely to have dysphagia, chest discomfort, cardiac and respiratory complaints at 12 months than were suture cruroplasty patients. The remaining studies by Ringley et al. [6], Dallemagne et al. [8], Muller-Stich et al. [10], and Grubnik and Malynovskyy [13] reported similar rates of symptom improvement in both groups. Only two studies used validated gastrointestinal quality of life measures to assess postoperative complaints; Soricelli reported that GERD health-related quality of life was significantly improved in all patients compared to baseline, with a statistically significant but not clinically meaningful difference comparing suture cruroplasty (mean 4 out of 50) and mesh cruroplasty (mean 2.6 of 50; p=0.03) [11]. In contrast, Dallemagne found no difference between groups in the postoperative gastrointestinal quality of life index or satisfaction scale [8].

In summary, analysis of the available randomized controlled trials, meta-analysis and systematic review, and individual studies comparing mesh cruroplasty to suture cruroplasty reveals that the available evidence assessing symptom response to surgery is of low quality and does not provide sufficient data to determine the balance between the desired result of durable symptom relief and the undesired result of new or persistent symptoms. Limitations in the study design with regard to symptom assessment were present in all of the studies and the result was inconsistency in the findings. A weak recommendation is made for routine use of hiatal mesh for crural reinforcement for the goal of improving patient symptoms, daily life function and quality of life based on this evidence.

Use of Mesh and the Incidence of Symptomatic Hiatal Hernia Recurrence

Based on the data presented above, there are good to excellent symptomatic results in most patients after both types of repair despite a significantly higher rate of objective recurrence in the observational studies comparing the two cohorts. This raises the question as to whether objective recurrence is the appropriate outcome measure for 'successful' surgery or whether the focus should be on differences in the rate of symptomatic recurrence only, comparing mesh cruroplasty to suture cruroplasty alone. Similar to the limitations associated with symptom assessment, symptomatic recurrence is not systematically addressed in the available studies. In the randomized trials, Frantzides and colleagues reported that all eight of the recurrences in their study were symptomatic and two out of three in the Carlson study were symptomatic whereas Oelschlager and colleagues reported that recurrence at 6 months was associated with significantly more chest pain and early satiety and lower physical functioning by SF-36, but they did not report symptom outcomes stratified by hernia recurrence in their 5 year follow-up publication. It is important to note, however, that Frantzides and Carlson did not report comprehensive symptom assessment preoperatively and postoperatively and it is unclear from the studies what proportion of patients had objective follow-up.

In the observational studies, three of ten did not report symptoms associated with objective recurrence [4–6]. The remaining studies reported with variable comprehensiveness; Morino and colleagues reported only on dysphagia as a symptom prompting reoperation in patients with recurrence [9], while Gouvas (4/7;57 %), Muller-Stich (4/7; 57 %), and Zaninotto (11/15; 73 %) provided rates of symptomatic hernia for the overall cohort [7, 10, 12]. Only Grubnik provided rates of symptomatic recurrence stratified by type of cruroplasty repair with 11 of 12 suture cruroplasty and 7 of 8 mesh cruroplasty patients experiencing symptoms in the setting of recurrence [13]. Only one study, by Dallemagne and colleagues, compared outcomes between patients with and without recurrence. In their study, the Gastrointestinal Quality of Life score was 116 in the patients without objective recurrence and 115 in the patients with objective recurrence (p = 0.36). They did not stratify these findings by type of cruroplasty [8]. None of the studies compared pre- and postoperative symptom complaints using paired analysis in patients with and without recurrence to determine whether the symptom complaints were new from prior to surgery, unchanged from surgery (present/not present), or resolved.

In summary, the data regarding symptom assessment in the setting of objective hernia recurrence are of low quality. In the studies that reported symptomatic complaints with recurrence, the proportion with symptoms was at least 50 % and ranged as high as 100 %. These data suggest that recurrences are symptomatic, but do not show whether the patients with recurrence are more symptomatic than those without recurrence and, based on the Dallemagne study, quality of life is preserved regardless of objective recurrence. As such, the data are inconclusive and a recommendation for routine use of hiatal mesh for crural reinforcement to reduce the incidence of symptomatic hiatal hernia recurrence cannot be made.

Use of Mesh Minimizes the Need for Reflux Medication and Endoscopic Intervention

Postoperative intervention for symptoms, including need for medication use, dilation, or endoscopic management for mesh erosions was rarely reported in any of the available studies. Most commonly, individual cases were discussed rather than a priori assessment of the outcome. Of the three randomized controlled trials, only Oelschlager and colleagues reported on proton pump inhibitor (PPI) use during follow-up. In their study, 77 % of patients were using PPI prior to surgery; 17 % at 6 months; and 44 % at 5 years with no difference between mesh and suture cruroplasty patients. Endoscopic interventions were not reported. Similarly, the rates of postoperative PPI use and endoscopic intervention were not evaluated in the meta-analysis [15] and systematic reviews [16, 17]. In the observational studies, five of the ten studies did not report on postoperative medication use or endoscopic intervention [5, 7–9, 13]. Only two of ten studies reported postoperative reflux medication use; Muller-Stich found that 31 % of mesh cruroplasty patients were using PPI postoperatively compared to 11 % of suture cruroplasty patients (p = 0.109) while Soricelli reported use in nine patients (9/175; 5 %), but did not specify cruroplasty type [10, 11]. Four studies reported the need for endoscopic intervention with dilation, but differences in dilation requirements between groups were reported in only two of the studies [4, 6, 11, 12]; Ringley and colleagues reported 1/22 (4.5 %)

patients in each group and Gouvas reported four cases, all of whom were repaired with mesh (4/20; 20 %) [6, 12].

In summary, analysis of the available randomized controlled trials and individual studies comparing mesh cruroplasty to suture cruroplasty reveals that the quality of evidence is very low. A recommendation for the routine use of hiatal mesh for crural reinforcement for the goal of minimizing the need for postoperative reflux medication use and endoscopic intervention for symptoms (e.g. dysphagia, odynophagia, GERD) based on this evidence cannot be made.

Use of Mesh Reduces the Rate of Reoperation for Hiatal Hernia Recurrence

Reoperation for anatomic and/or symptomatic recurrence after repair of large hiatal hernia is associated with worse outcomes than primary repair. In some patients, esophagectomy is required due to an inability to restore normal gastroesophageal anatomy for performance of a fundoplication or because of injury to the stomach and/or esophagus that render it unusable. As such, minimizing the need for reoperation due to recurrent hernia or symptoms is a critically important consideration when discussing operative techniques at the primary operation. Reoperation rates were reported for all 3 of the randomized controlled trials, with no reoperations in the mesh cruroplasty group and 9 of 102 patients in the suture cruroplasty cohort [1–3] (Table 39.2). Neither the meta-analysis by Antoniou nor the two systematic reviews reported reoperation rates [15–17]. Similarly, reoperations were not reported in three of ten observational studies [4–6] and were not stratified by type of cruroplasty in the study by Zaninotto [7]. The remaining 6 studies provided reoperation rates stratified by type of cruroplasty. Reoperations were required in 12 of 495 patients who had mesh cruroplasty and in 19 of 388 patients who had suture cruroplasty alone [8–13] (Table 39.2). The likelihood of reoperation is two times higher after suture cruroplasty, but the difference did not reach statistical significance (OR 2.07; 95 % CI 0.9935–4.3235).

When considering the need for reoperation comparing mesh cruroplasty to suture cruroplasty, it is important to consider reoperations due to mesh-related complications. It is known that mesh at the hiatus can lead to catastrophic complications, including erosion of the mesh into the esophagus or stomach or a severe reactive fibrosis leading to esophageal stricture. The available studies were analyzed for reporting on these known complications to determine the rate of mesh-related complications; only one of three randomized trials and four of ten observational studies addressed the issue of mesh-associated adverse events (Table 39.5). In their respective studies, Frantzides and Grubnik reported that there were no mesh-related erosions or fibrosis during follow-up [3, 13], while one patient in the Zaninotto study suffered mesh migration requiring reoperation and ultimately esophagectomy [7]. Late dysphagia at 1 year was reported in the study by Gouvas and was due to mesh-induced fibrosis; three of four patients required reoperation with mesh removal [12]. Finally, Soricelli reported 1 'mesh-related' complication requiring removal [11].

In summary, analysis of the available randomized controlled trials, meta-analysis/ systematic reviews and individual studies comparing mesh cruroplasty to suture cruroplasty suggests that reoperation rates may be reduced in mesh cruroplasty patients compared to suture only patients. Reporting is variable, however, and the total numbers of reoperations reported are small. As a result of these limitations, the evidence is low quality, with future research highly likely to provide important new information that may change the direction of the association. In addition, mesh-related complications requiring reoperation are rarely reported, but are an important factor in the debate. As such, the data appear to favor the routine use of hiatal mesh for crural reinforcement for the goal of reducing the rate of reoperation for hiatal hernia recurrence, but the recommendation based on this evidence is weak. Long-term follow-up is needed, including reoperations for mesh-related complications.

Recommendation

Determining whether or not routine use of mesh for crural reinforcement should be standard of care in the repair of large hiatal hernia depends upon the balance between a desirable outcome of sustained relief of symptoms and the undesirable outcomes of symptomatic hernia recurrence requiring reoperation and adverse effects of the mesh. Over the past decade, many surgeons have adopted routine mesh cruroplasty based on the short-term outcomes data showing higher rates of objective recurrence in the setting of suture cruroplasty alone compared to mesh cruroplasty. However, the level of evidence supporting routine mesh for crural reinforcement to minimize hernia recurrence is weak. More importantly, in the absence of symptoms, objective recurrence from the patient's perspective is not an important outcome of interest [18]. Sustained relief of symptoms, on the other hand, is a critically important outcome and the level of evidence to support the routine use of mesh for crural reinforcement in repair of large hiatal hernia is also low. Two of three randomized trials do not provide a systematic assessment of pre- and post-operative symptoms while the third compares proportions of patients with and without symptoms, but does not provide paired comparisons which would allow the patient and clinician to understand the likelihood of symptom relief versus symptom stability and, more importantly, new symptom onset. Similarly, use of postoperative medications and need for endoscopic intervention may also be important and undesirable outcomes from the patient's perspective and the level of evidence supporting routine mesh use for reducing these outcomes is very low. The majority of studies do not report on these important but not critical outcomes, limiting clinician ability to counsel patients on the likelihood of medication use or endoscopic intervention in the future. Finally, the level of evidence supporting routine use of mesh to minimize the risk of reoperation, another critical outcome from the patient perspective is low. The data suggest that reoperation for symptomatic recurrence may be lower in mesh cruroplasty patients, but the majority of studies failed to report on mesh-related complications requiring intervention.

Overall, the data supporting routine mesh cruroplasty for repair of large hiatal hernia is low because the quality of evidence in the outcomes that are critical from the patient's perspective, relief of symptoms and return to a normal quality of life, is low. Well-designed randomized trials and observational studies are needed to address these clinical questions. These studies, at a minimum, require a specific time-table for objective assessment with barium esophagram and at least 5 years of follow-up, consistent operative procedure that includes strict adherence to the tenets of repair, and adequate power based on patient-oriented outcomes will likely have an important impact on our understanding of the risk of recurrent hernia. Based on the available evidence, a weak recommendation is made for routine use of mesh reinforced cruroplasty for the repair of large hiatal hernia.

A Personal View of the Data

In our center, crural closure is considered to be only one of a number of critical steps in the operation [20]. The anatomic factors influencing hernia recurrence include axial forces from a foreshortened esophagus exerting pressure on the hiatal closure as well as tension on the closure created by tethering of the crura by the phrenosplenic and phrenogastric attachments which have developed over time. Restoration of normal anatomy is key to successful and durable closure. We begin the operation with stringent attention to reduction of the entire hernia sac. If the sac is not fully reduced, the gastroesophageal junction, by definition, cannot be reduced. The hernia sac is the attenuated phrenoesophageal ligament, which is an extension of the peritoneal and thoracic fascia onto the esophagus and stomach at the gastroesophageal junction. In Type III paraesophageal hernia, foreshortening of the esophagus exerts axial forces on the proximal stomach and increased intra-abdominal pressures push the stomach into the widening crural defect; this results in stretching of the phrenoesophageal ligament as it is pulled with the gastroesophageal junction into the posterior mediastinum. It is also important to pay close attention to maintaining the peritoneal coverage on the diaphragmatic crura, as this provides the strength layer for the sutured cruroplasty. If the muscle is denuded, the sutures will tear through when the muscles contract.

We begin our sac reduction in the anterior aspect of the sac and reduce the sac from the mediastinum with dissection under direct vision inside the sac. The lateral aspects of the sac are not divided until the apex of the sac has been reduced; once this is completed, the lateral sac is dissected from the crura with attention to leaving the crural muscle covered with peritoneum. Similarly, during esophageal mobilization, we are careful to remain aware of the impact of the dissecting instruments on the crural muscle; if the instruments are causing trauma to the muscle, we will switch ports so that the dissecting instrument is not exerting pressure on the crural muscle. Once the sac is fully reduced and extensive esophageal mobilization and/or gastroplasty has ensured 2–3 cm of intraabdominal esophagus lying tension-free below the diaphragmatic crus, the hiatus is examined. We perform complete dissection of the diaphragmatic crura free from the surrounding organs, thus releasing the attachments of the spleen and stomach so that both can return to their normal anatomic positions. This aggressive dissection untethers the diaphragmatic crura and substantially improves mobility of the left limb of the crura. Extensive esophageal mobilization and a willingness to perform Collis gastroplasty if an adequate (2–3 cm) length of tension-free abdominal esophagus cannot be achieved is also critical for restoring normal anatomic relationships between the crura, esophagus and stomach. Suture cruroplasty is performed with 0–0 polyester, non-absorbable suture using the Endostitch device. We typically use two to three sutures posteriorly. If additional suture is needed for a residual defect, anterior sutures are placed.

With these maneuvers, we successfully accomplished suture cruroplasty in 85 % of our cases between 1997 and 2010. Our objective recurrence rate at a median of 22 months (interquartile range 11–39 months) was 15.7 % [21]. Since 2010, we have modified our approach to the suture cruroplasty; because the insufflation that is necessary to perform laparoscopy causes an artificial distraction of the diaphragm toward the head, there is added tension on the crural closure. To counter this distraction, we now place a 5 mm port into the left hemithorax in approximately the ninth intercostal space in the anterior axillary line. The tonsil clamp is inserted slowly while being observed transabdominally to ensure that the diaphragm is not punctured. The 5 mm laparoscopic port is then inserted and a 5 mm camera used to ensure that the port is intrathoracic. Once confirmed, CO_2 is insufflated to create a 'floppy diaphragm'. Insufflation is stopped as soon as the diaphragm flops into the laparoscopic field, which minimizes cardiopulmonary compromise. With this maneuver, the hiatal defect collapses and the muscles can be easily reapproximated without tension. With this stringent attention to the tenets of repair in our center, focusing on all of the key steps as critical elements in a durable repair, mesh use is limited to situations where the crural integrity is compromised, either because it has been denuded or because the crural muscle has been damaged with the dissection. As others have published, this approach yields good to excellent results in 90 % of patients at medium term follow-up. Reoperation for recurrent hernia or symptoms was performed in 3.2 % and radiographic recurrence was not associated with a difference in gastroesophageal health-related quality of life score [21].

Recommendation

- Routine use of mesh reinforced cruroplasty is recommended for the repair of large hiatal hernia. (Evidence quality low; weak recommendation)

References

1. Oelschlager BK, Pellegrini CA, Hunter JG, Brunt ML, Soper NJ, Sheppard BC, et al. Biologic prosthesis to prevent recurrence after laparoscopic paraesophageal hernia repair: long-term follow-up from a multicenter, prospective, randomized trial. J Am Coll Surg. 2011;213(4):461–8.
2. Carlson MA, Richards CG, Frantzides CT. Laparoscopic prosthetic reinforcement of hiatal herniorrhaphy. Dig Surg. 1999;16(5):407–10.
3. Frantzides CT, Madan AK, Carlson MA, Stavropoulos GP. A prospective, randomized trial of laparoscopic polytetrafluoroethylene (PTFE) patch repair vs simple cruroplasty for large hiatal hernia. Arch Surg. 2002;137(6):649–52.
4. Braghetto I, Korn O, Csendes A, Burdiles P, Valladares H, Brunet L. Postoperative results after laparoscopic approach for treatment of large hiatal hernias: is mesh always needed? Is the addition of an antireflux procedure necessary? Int Surg. 2010;95(1):80–7.
5. Goers TA, Cassera MA, Dunst CM, Swanstrom LL. Paraesophageal hernia repair with bio-mesh does not increase postoperative dysphagia. J Gastrointest Surg. 2011;15(10):1743–9.
6. Ringley CD, Bochkarev V, Ahmed SI, Vitamvas ML, Oleynikov D. Laparoscopic hiatal hernia repair with human acellular dermal matrix patch: our initial experience. Am J Surg. 2006;192(6):767–72.
7. Zaninotto G, Portale G, Costantini M, Fiamingo P, Rampado S, Guirroli E, et al. Objective follow-up after laparoscopic repair of large type III hiatal hernia. Assessment of safety and durability. World J Surg. 2007;31(11):2177–83.
8. Dallemagne B, Kohnen L, Perretta S, Weerts J, Markiewicz S, Jehaes C. Laparoscopic repair of paraesophageal hernia: long-term follow-up reveals good clinical outcome despite high radiological recurrence rate. Ann Surg. 2011;253(2):291–6.
9. Morino M, Giaccone C, Pellegrino L, Rebecchi F. Laparoscopic management of giant hiatal hernia: factors influencing long-term outcome. Surg Endosc. 2006;20(7):1011–6.
10. Muller-Stich BP, Holzinger F, Kapp T, Klaiber C. Laparoscopic hiatal hernia repair: long-term outcome with the focus on the influence of mesh reinforcement. Surg Endosc. 2006;20(3):380–4.
11. Soricelli E, Basso N, Genco A, Cipriano M. Long-term results of hiatal hernia mesh repair and antireflux laparoscopic surgery. Surg Endosc. 2009;23(11):2499–504.
12. Gouvas N, Tsiaoussis J, Athanasakis E, Zervakis N, Pechlivanides G, Xynos E. Simple suture or prosthesis hiatal closure in laparoscopic repair of paraesophageal hernia: a retrospective cohort study. Dis Esophagus. 2011;24(2):69–78.
13. Grubnik VV, Malynovskyy AV. Laparoscopic repair of hiatal hernias: new classification supported by long-term results. Surg Endosc. 2013;27(11):4337–46.
14. Granderath FA, Schweiger UM, Kamolz T, Asche KU, Pointner R. Laparoscopic Nissen fundoplication with prosthetic hiatal closure reduces postoperative intrathoracic wrap herniation: preliminary results of a prospective randomized functional and clinical study. Arch Surg. 2005;140(1):40–8.
15. Antoniou SA, Antoniou GA, Koch OO, Pointner R, Granderath FA. Lower recurrence rates after mesh-reinforced versus simple hiatal hernia repair: a meta-analysis of randomized trials. Surg Laparosc Endosc Percutan Tech. 2012;22(6):498–502.

16. Furnee E, Hazebroek E. Mesh in laparoscopic large hiatal hernia repair: a systematic review of the literature. Surg Endosc. 2013;27(11):3998–40081.
17. Johnson JM, Carbonell AM, Carmody BJ, Jamal MK, Maher JW, Kellum JM, et al. Laparoscopic mesh hiatoplasty for paraesophageal hernias and fundoplications: a critical analysis of the available literature. Surg Endosc. 2006;20(3):362–6.
18. Kamolz T, Pointner R. Expectations of patients with gastroesophageal reflux disease for the outcome of laparoscopic antireflux surgery. Surg Laparosc Endosc Percutan Tech. 2002;12(6):389–92.
19. Oelschlager BK, Pellegrini CA, Hunter J, Soper N, Brunt M, Sheppard B, et al. Biologic prosthesis reduces recurrence after laparoscopic paraesophageal hernia repair: a multicenter, prospective, randomized trial. Ann Surg. 2006;244(4):481–8.
20. Nason KS, Luketich JD, Witteman BP, Levy RM. The laparoscopic approach to paraesophageal hernia repair. J Gastrointest Surg. 2012;16(2):417–26.
21. Luketich JD, Nason KS, Christie NA, Pennathur A, Jobe BA, Landreneau RJ, Schuchert MJ. Outcomes after a decade of laparoscopic giant paraesophageal hernia repair. J Thorac Cardiovasc Surg. 2010;139(2):395–404. e391.

Chapter 40
Diaphragmatic Plication for Eventration

Eitan Podgaetz and Rafael S. Andrade

Abstract Diaphragmatic eventration is a congenital defect of the muscular portion of a hemidiaphragm that eventually leads to hemidiaphragm elevation and dysfunction. The clinical diagnosis is established solely by hemidiaphragmatic elevation of unknown etiology on imaging studies. The clinical presentation of symptomatic diaphragmatic eventration and paralysis may be indistinguishable and diaphragmatic plication is the treatment of choice for both conditions.

Minimally invasive diaphragm plication techniques are effective alternatives to open transthoracic plication and result in significant improvement in dyspnea and quality of life in appropriately selected patients.

Keywords Diaphragmatic paralysis • Eventration • Laparoscopic plication • Thoracoscopic plication • Phrenic nerve injury

Introduction

Diaphragmatic eventration is a congenital muscular malformation of a hemidiaphragm that eventually leads to hemidiaphragmatic elevation and dysfunction. The clinical diagnosis is established solely by hemidiaphragmatic elevation of unknown etiology on imaging studies. The presence of an elevated hemidiaphragm on chest imaging may be an incidental finding in an asymptomatic patient, or may be identified during the work-up of a dyspneic patient. The clinical presentation of symptomatic diaphragmatic eventration and paralysis may be indistinguishable and diaphragmatic plication is the treatment of choice for both conditions. Minimally

E. Podgaetz, MD • R.S. Andrade, MD (✉)
Section of Thoracic and Foregut Surgery,
Division of Cardiothoracic Surgery, University of Minnesota,
420 Delaware St. SE, MMC 207, Minneapolis, MN 55455, USA
e-mail: eitanp@umn.edu; andr0117@umn.edu

M.K. Ferguson (ed.), *Difficult Decisions in Thoracic Surgery*,
Difficult Decisions in Surgery: An Evidence-Based Approach 1,
DOI 10.1007/978-1-4471-6404-3_40, © Springer-Verlag London 2014

invasive diaphragm plication techniques are effective alternatives to open transthoracic plication and result in significant improvement in dyspnea and quality of life in adequately selected patients.

Symptomatic diaphragmatic eventration and paralysis are uncommon conditions and experience with diaphragmatic plication is limited, the majority of reports published in the medical literature are small retrospective case series or case reports. This review focuses on the etiology, pathophysiology, diagnosis, and treatment of unilateral diaphragmatic eventration in adults.

Search Strategy

PICO terms that were used for this review include a population of adults with symptomatic diaphragmatic eventration. The intervention was diaphragmatic plication and the comparator was other surgical techniques. The target outcomes were symptomatic improvement by respiratory questionnaire and pulmonary function tests.

The literature search was performed including the terms: diaphragmatic paralysis, eventration, plication, laparoscopic, thoracoscopic. Due to a paucity of published reports on diaphragmatic plication, we considered all pertinent publications from the English language medical literature dating back to 1950 for historical reference and for comparison with current minimally invasive techniques. Based on lack of prospective trials, all evidence for this evaluation is considered to be of low quality.

Background

Etiology

True diaphragmatic eventration is a developmental defect of the muscular portion of the diaphragm with preservation of the diaphragmatic attachments to the sternum, ribs, and dorsolumbar spine [1]. Diaphragmatic eventration is rare (incidence <0.05 %), is more common in males, and more often affects the left hemidiaphragm [2–4]. In contrast to true diaphragmatic eventration, diaphragmatic paresis or paralysis is more common, acquired, and generally results from tumor- or trauma-related phrenic nerve injury [5–9].

Pathology

Diaphragmatic eventration can be bilateral, unilateral, total, and localized (anterior, posterolateral, and medial) [6]. Microscopically, the eventrated portion has diffuse fibroelastic changes and a lack of muscle fibers, while a paralyzed diaphragm has a normal amount of muscle fibers, albeit atrophic.

Pathophysiology and Clinical Presentation

Most adult patients are asymptomatic and are generally diagnosed incidentally with a chest x-ray demonstrating unilateral diaphragmatic elevation. Eventration of the hemidiaphragm results in a gradual elevation of the diaphragm over time as a result of the pressure gradient between the abdominal and thoracic cavities. Symptomatic patients with diaphragmatic eventration tend to present in adulthood due to weight gain or due to a change in lung or chest wall compliance [7, 8].

Dyspnea on exertion and orthopnea (because of further cranial displacement of the affected hemidiaphragm when supine) are the main symptoms of an elevated hemidiaphragm. Some patients, especially those with left hemidiaphragm eventration, can develop nonspecific gastrointestinal symptoms such as epigastric pain, bloating, heartburn, regurgitation, belching, nausea, constipation, and inability to gain weight [9].

Diagnosis

The evaluation of a symptomatic patient with diaphragmatic eventration (or paralysis) includes an objective assessment of dyspnea, physical examination, pulmonary function tests, and imaging studies. The diagnosis of symptomatic hemidiaphragm eventration (or paralysis) is primarily clinical, and relies on history, chest x-ray, and the physician's clinical acuity.

Symptom Evaluation

A careful history of the duration and progression of dyspnea and orthopnea is critical. Additional causes for dyspnea (e.g., morbid obesity, primary lung disease, heart failure etc.) must be investigated and treated, since dyspnea secondary to diaphragmatic eventration or paralysis is a diagnosis of exclusion. All patients with dyspnea secondary to diaphragmatic eventration (or paralysis) should fill out a standardized respiratory questionnaire to objectively document the severity of their symptoms and to assess response to treatment.

Pulmonary Function Tests

Diaphragm dysfunction and elevation reduce chest wall compliance. Pulmonary function tests (PFTs) frequently demonstrate a restrictive pattern (i.e., low forced vital capacity [FVC] and forced expiratory volume in 1 s [FEV_1]) [4]. Pulmonary function tests should be assessed in the upright and supine position. In healthy individuals a decrease in FVC of up to 20 % may be observed in the supine position

E. Podgaetz and R.S. Andrade

when compared to upright values [10]; in symptomatic patients with diaphragmatic eventration or paralysis supine FVC may decrease by 20–50 % when compared to upright values [10–13]. The main value of PFTs in the evaluation of symptomatic patients with hemidiaphragmatic elevation is to provide an objective evaluation of the response to surgery; however, changes in PFT values are variable and don't always correlate well with clinical improvement.

Imaging Studies

Chest X-Ray

On a standard full-inspiration postero-anterior and lateral (PA/LAT) chest x-ray, the right hemidiaphragm is normally 1–2 cm higher than the left [14]. Hemidiaphragm elevation can be a sign of diaphragmatic eventration or paralysis, however it is a nonspecific finding.

Fluoroscopic Sniff Test

The fluoroscopic sniff test documents diaphragmatic movement during inspiration. Patients are instructed to sniff and diaphragmatic excursion is assessed with fluoroscopy. Normally, both hemidiaphragms move caudally, but in patients with hemidiaphragmatic *paralysis*, the affected hemidiaphragm may (paradoxically) move cranially. Fluoroscopy findings should be interpreted with caution, since about 6 % of normal individuals exhibit paradoxical motion on fluoroscopy [15]. To increase the specificity of the fluoroscopic sniff test, at least 2 cm of paradoxical motion should be observed [16]. Additionally, an eventrated or paralyzed hemidiaphragm may move very little or not at all, without paradoxical motion, making the interpretation of the sniff test and the distinction between paralysis and eventration even more challenging.

Ultrasound

Ultrasound (US) can be used to assess the thickness and the change of thickness of the diaphragm during respiration; it has about 80 % concordance with fluoroscopy findings [7–18]. However, US has not been validated in clinical practice and its applicability may be hampered by obesity and operator dependency.

Computed Tomography (CT)

The principal utility of CT scans is to exclude the presence of a cervical or intrathoracic tumor as the cause of phrenic nerve paralysis and to evaluate the possibility of a subphrenic processes as the cause of hemidiaphragm elevation. CT also helps differentiate between hemidiaphragmatic elevation and diaphragmatic hernia. However, a CT scan is not routinely required if the clinical suspicion of an alternate process is low.

Magnetic Resonance Imaging (MRI)

Dynamic MRI can be used to assess diaphragmatic motion [19]. As compared with fluoroscopy, which can assess only motion of the highest points of the diaphragm, it has the advantage of enabling the study of the motion of segments of the diaphragm in multiple planes [17]. Dynamic MRI plays no role in the routine clinical evaluation of symptomatic patients with an elevated hemidiaphragm.

Treatment: Diaphragmatic Plication

Open diaphragmatic plication for hemidiaphragmatic eventration was first described in 1923 [20]. Since then, a variety of open and minimally invasive diaphragm plication techniques have been described for treatment of symptomatic hemidiaphragm elevation in patients with eventration (or paralysis). This section reviews diaphragm plication for unilateral hemidiaphragm eventration with particular emphasis on laparoscopic diaphragm plication.

Operative Indications

The **only** goal of diaphragm plication is to treat dyspnea; hence, operative intervention is indicated *exclusively* for symptomatic patients. An elevated hemidiaphragm or paradoxical motion per se does not warrant surgery in the absence of significant dyspnea. For adults with phrenic nerve injury from cardiac surgery, a 1- to 2-year period of observation is often recommended, since phrenic nerve function may improve with time [6, 21–23]; however, severe symptoms may be an indication for minimally invasive plication even after only 6 months, since dyspnea from diaphragm paralysis can significantly impact quality of life and rehabilitation.

Relative contraindications to diaphragm plication are morbid obesity and certain neuromuscular disorders. Ideally, morbidly obese patients should be evaluated for medical or surgical bariatric treatment prior to plication since dyspnea may improve after significant weight loss and a plication may no longer be warranted.

Surgical Approaches

The diaphragm can be approached from the thorax or the abdomen with open or minimally invasive techniques.

Open Transthoracic Plication

Open transthoracic plication is the traditional approach to treat symptomatic patients with hemidiaphragm eventration or paralysis is. A posterolateral thoracotomy is performed through the 6th [24, 25], 7th [26–29], or 8th [30] intercostal space. A variety of plication techniques have been described, including hand-sewn U stitches [24, 25, 30, 31], mattress sutures [26, 28], running sutures with or without pledgets, and stapling [32] techniques with or without mesh [25, 33]. Another technique includes resecting the redundant portion of diaphragm and reapproximating the tissue in overlapping layers [8, 9].

Multiple single-institution studies have demonstrated significant improvement in symptoms and respiratory function after open transthoracic plication [24, 25, 27, 29, 30, 34, 35]. In a study of 17 patients with unilateral paralysis, Graham et al. demonstrated that open transthoracic plication led to significant subjective improvement in dyspnea and orthopnea. PFTs improved as well: FVC increased by 19 % in the upright position and by 42 % in the supine position [29]. Five to 10-year follow-up data was available for six patients: durable improvement in dyspnea scores and PFTs was observed [26]. In a study of 19 patients, Higgs et al. also demonstrated durable improvements in dyspnea scores and PFTs after open transthoracic plication at 5- to 10-year follow-up. Calvinho recently reported on a series of 20 patients operated though a posterolateral thoracotomy with good results but point out that chronic surgical pain can be a challenge to manage [27].

Cumulative experience with open transthoracic plication suggests that plicating the diaphragm for symptomatic eventration or paralysis provides short- and long-term benefits. Unfortunately, open transthoracic plication is very invasive, which can preclude the option of plication in patients with multiple comorbidities. Consequently, alternative approaches to diaphragmatic plication have been developed to minimize the disadvantages of the open transthoracic approach.

Thoracoscopic Plication

Thoracoscopic plication can be performed using two ports with a mini-thoracotomy [36, 37], three ports [38–40], or four ports [41]. Plication techniques including continuous sutures [37, 41], interrupted stitches [38, 40], or stapling [42] have been described. Single-institution studies have demonstrated improvement in dyspnea and PFTs with thoracoscopic plication [36, 38, 40]. Freeman et al., initially reported a series of 25 patients with unilateral diaphragm paralysis; thoracoscopic plication was successfully performed in 22 patients, and three required conversion to thoracotomy. Follow-up at 6 months demonstrated a significant improvement in dyspnea scores and a significant increase in forced vital capacity (FVC), forced expiratory volume in 1 s (FEV1), functional residual capacity (FRC) and in total lung capacity (TLC): FVC (19 %), FEV1 (23 %), FRC (21 %), and TLC (19 %). He then reported long term follow up (57 ± 10 months) in 41 patients (31 thoracoscopic and 10 thoracotomy) with demonstrable improvement in PFTs in FVC (17 %), FEV1 (21 %), FRC (20 %), and TLC (20 %) [38, 39].

Thoracoscopic diaphragm plication is an excellent minimally invasive alternative to open transthoracic plication; mid- and long-term follow-up data suggest that it is as effective as the open approach. Workspace limitation by the ribcage and the elevated hemidiaphragm is the main disadvantage of this approach.

Open Transabdominal Plication

Open transabdominal plication has been described for unilateral or bilateral diaphragmatic eventration or paralysis in the pediatric population [43]. Little outcome data are available on the results of open transabdominal plication in adults. Advantages of an open transabdominal approach are access to both sides of the diaphragm and that it does not require selective ventilation. Additionally, a laparotomy is generally a less morbid incision than a thoracotomy. Disadvantages include an open approach and difficult access to the most posterior portion of the diaphragm.

Laparoscopic Plication

Laparoscopic diaphragm plication was initially described in a report of three patients by Hüttl et al.; all patients improved clinically and by PFT parameters [44]. Laparoscopic diaphragm plication with interrupted stitches is our preferred approach for symptomatic hemidiaphragm eventration or paralysis. We evaluate all patients with the St. George's Respiratory Questionnaire (SGRQ; total score 0–100, normal is 1–6), PA/LAT chest x-ray, and PFTs preoperatively and postoperatively. Our early experience in 25 patients with 1 year follow-up showed an average decrease in SGRQ score of 20 points (≥ 4 points is considered clinically significant), and pulmonary function tests improved on average by about 10 % (Table 40.1) [45–47]. Technical advantages of laparoscopic diaphragm plication include non-selective ventilation and ample working space. Central obesity (BMI >35) is the main relative contraindication to laparoscopic diaphragm plication.

Complications of Plication

Reported complications include pneumonia [24, 36], pleural effusions, abdominal compartment syndrome [48], conversion to open (for minimally invasive approaches) [16], abdominal organ injury, deep venous thrombosis [26] pulmonary emboli,, and acute myocardial infarction [30].

Table 40.1 Comparison of SGRQ score, FVC, and FEV₁ before and 1 year after laparoscopic diaphragm plication in 25 patients

	Preop	1 year postop
SGRQ total	59.3 ± 26.8	30.8 ± 18.8[a]
FVC (% pred)	59.2 ± 11.7	61.0 ± 10.6[a]
FEV₁ (% pred)	55.4 ± 12.9	60.9 ± 10.7[a]

The SGRQ score changes dramatically, while FVC and FEV1 change only modestly; this is an indication that PFTs do not correlate well with symptoms in patients with hemidiaphragmatic eventration or paralysis [45–47]

SGRQ St. George Respiratory Questionnaire, *% pred* percent of predicted value, *FVC* forced vital capacity, *FEV1* forced expiratory volume in 1 s, *PFTs* pulmonary function tests

[a]$p < 0.05$ vs. preop

Comparison of Surgical Approaches for Diaphragm Plication

No studies exist on the comparative safety and efficacy of different surgical techniques of diaphragm plication. Regardless of technique, the principles of diaphragm plication for symptomatic hemidiaphragm eventration or paralysis are proper patient selection, and a safely performed tight plication. The surgical approach is secondary and a matter of surgeon preference.

Conclusions Based on the Data

Symptomatic hemidiaphragmatic eventration is an uncommon condition and is sometimes impossible to distinguish clinically from paralysis. Asymptomatic patients require no treatment; symptomatic patients benefit significantly from diaphragm plication. The choice of plication approach is dependent upon the expertise of the surgeon.

A Personal View of the Data

I approach patients with dyspnea and an elevated hemidiaphragm with basic principles. Preoperatively, I first ensure that any other potential causes of dyspnea are excluded or medically optimized; second, I routinely evaluate the patient with a CXR and pulmonary function tests only; third, I obtain a chest CT only if diaphragmatic hernia is in the differential diagnosis; fourth, I offer a laparoscopic plication if the BMI is <35.

Intraoperatively I emphasize a tight posterior plication for maximum symptom improvement, and the immediate postoperative CXR must show that the plicated hemidiaphragm is lower than the contralateral hemidiaphragm to guarantee a satisfactory result. A chest tube must remain in place until the drainage is <200 ml/24 h to prevent a delayed effusion. At 1 month both hemidiaphragms should be at about the same level on the CXR. Following these basic principles ensures the best symptomatic relief.

Recommendations

- Surgical treatment for diaphragmatic paralysis is reserved exclusively for symptomatic patients (evidence quality low; weak recommendation)
- Patients with phrenic nerve injury after cardiac surgery should wait 1-2 years before operative intervention unless severely symptomatic (evidence quality low; weak recommendation)
- Morbidly obese patients ought to attempt to lose weight before plication of the diaphragm (evidence quality low; weak recommendation)
- Respiratory questionnaires should be used pre- and postoperatively to follow patients with diaphragmatic paralysis, as they are often the most objective assessment of response to treatment (evidence quality low; weak recommendation)

References

1. Deslauriers J. Eventration of the diaphragm. Chest Surg Clin N Am. 1998;8(2):315–30.
2. Chin EF, Lynn RB. Surgery of eventration of the diaphragm. J Thorac Surg. 1956;32(1):6–14.
3. Christensen P. Eventration of the diaphragm. Thorax. 1959;14:311–9.
4. McNamara JJ, Paulson DL, Urschel Jr HC, Razzuk MA. Eventration of the diaphragm. Surgery. 1968;64(6):1013–21.
5. Riley EA. Idiopathic diaphragmatic paralysis; a report of eight cases. Am J Med. 1962;32:404–16.
6. Efthimiou J, Butler J, Woodham C, Benson MK, Westaby S. Diaphragm paralysis following cardiac surgery: role of phrenic nerve cold injury. Ann Thorac Surg. 1991;52(4):1005–8.
7. Thomas TV. Nonparalytic eventration of the diaphragm. J Thorac Cardiovasc Surg. 1968;55(4):586–93.
8. Thomas TV. Congenital eventration of the diaphragm. Ann Thorac Surg. 1970;10(2):180–92.
9. Shah-Mirany J, Schmitz GL, Watson RR. Eventration of the diaphragm. Physiologic and surgical significance. Arch Surg. 1968;96(5):844–50.
10. Allen SM, Hunt B, Green M. Fall in vital capacity with posture. Br J Dis Chest. 1985;79(3):267–71.
11. McCredie M, Lovejoy FW, Kaltreider NL. Pulmonary function in diaphragmatic paralysis. Thorax. 1962;17:213–7.
12. Clague HW, Hall DR. Effect of posture on lung volume: airway closure and gas exchange in hemidiaphragmatic paralysis. Thorax. 1979;34(4):523–6.
13. Gould L, Kaplan S, McElhinney AJ, Stone DJ. A method for the production of hemidiaphragmatic paralysis. Its application to the study of lung function in normal man. Am Rev Respir Dis. 1967;96(4):812–4.
14. Wynn-Willaims N. Hemidiaphragmatic paralysis and paresis of unknown aetiology without any marked rise in level. Thorax. 1954;9:299–303.
15. Alexander C. Diaphragm movements and the diagnosis of diaphragmatic paralysis. Clin Radiol. 1966;17(1):79–83.
16. Gibson GJ. Diaphragmatic paresis: pathophysiology, clinical features, and investigation. Thorax. 1989;44(11):960–70.
17. Gierada DS, Slone RM, Fleishman MJ. Imaging evaluation of the diaphragm. Chest Surg Clin N Am. 1998;8(2):237–80.

18. Houston JG, Fleet M, Cowan MD, McMillan NC. Comparison of ultrasound with fluoroscopy in the assessment of suspected hemidiaphragmatic movement abnormality. Clin Radiol. 1995;50(2):95–8.
19. Slone RM, Gierada DS. Radiology of pulmonary emphysema and lung volume reduction surgery. Semin Thorac Cardiovasc Surg. 1996;8(1):61–82.
20. Morrison JMW. Eventration of the diaphragm due to unilateral phrenic nerve paralysis. Arch Radiol Electrother. 1923;28:72–5.
21. Curtis JJ, Nawarawong W, Walls JT, Schmaltz RA, Boley T, Madsen R, et al. Elevated hemidiaphragm after cardiac operations: incidence, prognosis, and relationship to the use of topical ice slush. Ann Thorac Surg. 1989;48(6):764–8.
22. Summerhill EM, El-Sameed YA, Glidden TJ, McCool FD. Monitoring recovery from diaphragm paralysis with ultrasound. Chest. 2008;133(3):737–43.
23. Gayan-Ramirez G, Gosselin N, Troosters T, Bruyninckx F, Gosselink R, Decramer M. Functional recovery of diaphragm paralysis: a long-term follow-up study. Respir Med. 2008;102(5):690–8.
24. Kuniyoshi Y, Yamashiro S, Miyagi K, Uezu T, Arakaki K, Koja K. Diaphragmatic plication in adult patients with diaphragm paralysis after cardiac surgery. Ann Thorac Cardiovasc Surg. 2004;10(3):160–6.
25. Simansky DA, Paley M, Refaely Y, Yellin A. Diaphragm plication following phrenic nerve injury: a comparison of paediatric and adult patients. Thorax. 2002;57(7):613–6.
26. Graham DR, Kaplan D, Evans CC, Hind CR, Donnelly RJ. Diaphragmatic plication for unilateral diaphragmatic paralysis: a 10-year experience. Ann Thorac Surg. 1990;49(2):248–51; discussion 252.
27. Calvinho P, Bastos C, Bernardo JE, Eugenio L, Antunes MJ. Diaphragmatic eventration: long term follow up and results of open chest plicature. Eur J Cardiothorac Surg. 2009;36(5):883–7.
28. Wright CD, Williams JG, Ogilvie CM, Donnelly RJ. Results of diaphragmatic plication for unilateral diaphragmatic paralysis. J Thorac Cardiovasc Surg. 1985;90(2):195–8.
29. Higgs SM, Hussain A, Jackson M, Donnelly RJ, Berrisford RG. Long term results of diaphragmatic plication for unilateral diaphragm paralysis. Eur J Cardiothorac Surg. 2002;21(2):294–7.
30. Versteegh MI, Braun J, Voigt PG, Bosman DB, Stolk J, Rabe KF, et al. Diaphragm plication in adult patients with diaphragm paralysis leads to long-term improvement of pulmonary function and level of dyspnea. Eur J Cardiothorac Surg. 2007;32(3):449–56.
31. Schwartz MZ, Filler RM. Plication of the diaphragm for symptomatic phrenic nerve paralysis. J Pediatr Surg. 1978;13(3):259–63.
32. Maxson T, Robertson R, Wagner CW. An improved method of diaphragmatic plication. Surg Gynecol Obstet. 1993;177(6):620–1.
33. Di Giorgio A, Cardini CL, Sammartino P, Sibio S, Naticchioni E. Dual-layer sandwich mesh repair in the treatment of major diaphragmatic eventration in an adult. J Thorac Cardiovasc Surg. 2006;132(1):187–9.
34. Ciccolella DE, Daly BD, Celli BR. Improved diaphragmatic function after surgical plication for unilateral diaphragmatic paralysis. Am Rev Respir Dis. 1992;146(3):797–9.
35. Ribet M, Linder JL. Plication of the diaphragm for unilateral eventration or paralysis. Eur J Cardiothorac Surg. 1992;6(7):357–60.
36. Mouroux J, Venissac N, Leo F, Ailfano M, Guillot F. Surgical treatment of diaphragmatic eventration using video-assisted thoracic surgery: a prospective study. Ann Thorac Surg. 2005;79(1):308–12.
37. Mouroux J, Padovani B, Poirier NC, Benchimol D, Bourgeon A, Deslauriers J, et al. Technique for the repair of diaphragmatic eventration. Ann Thorac Surg. 1996;62(3):905–7.
38. Freeman RK, Wozniak TC, Fitzgerald EB. Functional and physiologic results of video-assisted thoracoscopic diaphragm plication in adult patients with unilateral diaphragm paralysis. Ann Thorac Surg. 2006;81(5):1853–7; discussion 1857.
39. Freeman RK, Woerkom JV, Vyverberg A, Ascioti AJ. Long-term follow up of the functional and physiologic results of diaphragm plication in adults with unilateral diaphragm paralysis. Ann Thorac Surg. 2009;88:1112–7.

40. Suzumura Y, Terada Y, Sonobe M, Nagasawa M, Shindo T, Kitano M. A case of unilateral diaphragmatic eventration treated by plication with thoracoscopic surgery. Chest. 1997;112(2):530–2.
41. Hwang Z, Shin JS, Cho YH, Sun K, Lee IS. A simple technique for the thoracoscopic plication of the diaphragm. Chest. 2003;124(1):376–8.
42. Moon SW, Wang YP, Kim YW, Shim SB, Jin W. Thoracoscopic plication of diaphragmatic eventration using endostaplers. Ann Thorac Surg. 2000;70(1):299–300.
43. Kizilcan F, Tanyel FC, Hiçsönmez A, Büyükpamukçu N. The long-term results of diaphragmatic plication. J Pediatr Surg. 1993;28(1):42–4.
44. Huttl TP, Wichmann MW, Reichart B, Geiger TK, Schildberg FW, Meyer G. Laparoscopic diaphragmatic plication: long-term results of a novel surgical technique for postoperative phrenic nerve palsy. Surg Endosc. 2004;18(3):547–51.
45. Groth SS, Andrade RS. Diaphragmatic eventration. Thorac Surg Clin. 2009;19(4):511–9.
46. Groth SS, Andrade RS. Diaphragm plication for eventration or paralysis: a review of the literature. Ann Thorac Surg. 2010;89(6):S2146–50.
47. Groth SS, Rueth NM, Kast T, D'Cunha J, Kelly RF, Maddaus MA, Andrade RS. Laparoscopic diaphragmatic plication for diaphragmatic paralysis and eventration: an objective evaluation of short term and midterm results. J Thorac Cardiovasc Surg. 2010;139(6):1452–6.
48. Phadnis J, Pilling JE, Evans TW, Goldstraw P. Abdominal compartment syndrome: a rare complication of plication of the diaphragm. Ann Thorac Surg. 2006;82(1):334–6.

Chapter 41
Management of Minimally Symptomatic Recurrent Hiatal Hernia

Brant K. Oelschlager and Robert B. Yates

Abstract Recurrent hiatal hernias are a common and challenging clinical problem. The goal of this chapter is to provide guidance on the management of patients with minimally symptomatic recurrent hiatal hernias. To this end, we review the epidemiology and mechanisms of these recurrences and discuss the clinical features that are necessary to consider when deciding the appropriate management for patients with recurrent hiatal hernias.

Keywords Hiatal hernia • Paraesophageal hernia • Recurrent hiatal hernia

Introduction

Definitions: Hiatal Hernia, Paraesophageal Hernia, and Recurrent Hernias

There are four types of hernias that occur at the esophageal hiatus. Type I is the most common and occurs when the gastroesophageal junction (GEJ) is displaced above the esophageal hiatus and resides in the posterior mediastinum. Type II, the least common hiatal hernia, exists when the gastric fundus is located above the hiatus and

B.K. Oelschlager, MD (✉)
Department of Surgery, Center for Videoendoscopic Surgery,
University of Washington, Center for Esophageal and Gastric Surgery,
1959 NE Pacific St., 356410, Seattle, WA 98195, USA
e-mail: brant@u.washington.edu

R.B. Yates, MD
Department of Surgery, Center for Videoendoscopic Surgery,
University of Washington, 1959 NE Pacific St., 356410, Seattle, WA 98195, USA

M.K. Ferguson (ed.), *Difficult Decisions in Thoracic Surgery*,
Difficult Decisions in Surgery: An Evidence-Based Approach 1,
DOI 10.1007/978-1-4471-6404-3_41, © Springer-Verlag London 2014

the GEJ resides in its normal anatomic location in the abdomen. Type III combines characteristics of Types I and II: Both the GEJ and the fundus of the stomach are located above the hiatus. Finally, in Type IV, an organ other than the stomach – frequently the colon, small bowel, spleen, and pancreas – is located above the hiatus in the mediastinum. Type I hernia is often referred to as a "sliding hiatal hernia"; Types II–IV are referred to as "paraesophageal hernias" (PEH).

Beyond their anatomic differences, the four types of hernias at the esophageal hiatus have differences in the clinical presentation and natural history. For example, Type I hernias are frequently asymptomatic or associated with symptoms of gastro-esophageal reflux disease (GERD). For that reason, repair of Type I hernias is most commonly performed as part of an antireflux operation that is completed for the management of GERD. Paraesophageal hernias, however, are frequently associated with foregut symptoms that may significantly impact patient quality of life. These symptoms, which include epigastric and chest pain, dysphagia, early satiety, and regurgitation, result from two features of the hernia: One, the amount of stomach that lies within the mediastinum; and/or two, the extent to which the stomach adopts an abnormal anatomic orientation in the mediastinum. In addition to chronic foregut symptoms, PEH can lead to acute gastric volvulus, gastric outlet obstruction, and even life-threatening gastric strangulation. Because of these differences in the ana-tomic configuration and clinical manifestations of primary hernias at the esophageal hiatus, the nomenclature that differentiates hiatal hernias from paraesophageal her-nias is useful and practical.

Unlike the well-defined terms used to describe primary hernias at the esopha-geal hiatus, there are no well-accepted definitions and no formal classification systems to describe recurrent hernias. Consequently, the terms used to describe primary hernias at the esophageal hiatus have been applied to recurrent hernias. This is incorrect and should be avoided. First, the terms "recurrent hiatal hernia" and "recurrent PEH" should not be used interchangeably. Because primary hiatal hernia and primary PEH have different anatomic definitions and different symp-tom profiles, in the setting of recurrent hernias, the use of these terms as syn-onyms causes confusion.

Second, small recurrent hernias are frequently referred to as "sliding" type her-nias. In reality, unlike primary Type I hiatal hernias, these recurrent hernias do not move between the abdominal and thoracic cavities. This relative fixation of recur-rent hernias occurs due to the deliberate division of the phrenoesophageal mem-brane at the time of the initial operation and the postoperative adhesions that develop around the esophageal hiatus. Regardless of the resulting symptoms – they may be asymptomatic or associated with GERD symptoms – anatomically these are not Type I sliding hiatal hernias.

Finally, confusion has resulted from attempts to classify recurrent hernias at the esophageal hiatus as PEHs. Following the repair of a primary PEH, surgeons, radi-ologists, and gastroenterologists will often label any stomach herniating above the esophageal hiatus as a recurrent PEH. At the time of the initial operation, if a fun-doplication has been performed correctly, gastric fundus should be located above the GEJ. If there is a recurrent opening of the hiatus, gastric fundus will always move above the hiatus, thereby fulfilling the anatomic definition of PEH. However, because postoperative adhesions secure these hernias in a relatively fixed position, these recurrent hernias do not carry the same risk of acute gastric volvulus. In a recurrent hiatal hernia, the stomach may adopt an anatomic configuration that constitutes a PEH. However, the clinical implications of this anatomic configuration are not the same as a primary PEH and, consequently (in our opinion), should not be labeled as recurrent PEH.

To avoid the confusion that results from the use of the terms noted above, and to maintain consistency when discussing hernia recurrence at the esophageal hiatus, in this chapter we will refer to any hernia at the esophageal hiatus that develops after a prior repair as a recurrent hiatal hernia. We will use this term regardless of the hernia that was initially repaired (i.e. Type I sliding hiatal hernia or Types II–IV PEH). In this chapter, we will briefly review the repair of PEH and mechanisms of failure after their repair as well as the epidemiology of recurrent hiatal hernia. Our focus will be on the clinical factors to consider during the evaluation and management of patients with recurrent hiatal hernias.

Repairing Paraesophageal Hernia and Mechanisms of Failure

There are five steps to the standard operative repair of hernias at the esophageal hiatus: (1) Reduction of the hernia contents into the abdomen; (2) Excision of the hernia sac from the mediastinum; (3) Mobilization of the esophagus to obtain a minimum of 3 cm of intraabdominal esophageal length; (4) Closure of the hiatus; and (5) Completion of an antireflux operation. Although these operative steps are the same whether they are performed open or laparoscopically, multiple authors have reported that laparoscopic repair of hiatal hernias provides exceptional visualization, improves quality of life, provides excellent relief from preoperative symptoms [1–3], and is associated with less pain, fewer complications, and shorter recovery times [4–6]. Despite these advancements in PEH repair, studies have called into question the durability of these repairs, and more authors are reporting their experience with recurrent hiatal hernias.

There are several mechanisms that are thought to underlie the development of recurrent hiatal hernia. Inadequate mobilization of the esophagus at the time of primary hiatal and PEH repairs – frequently referred to as a "short esophagus" – generates a force that pulls the GEJ above the hiatus. While gastroplasty can increase the effective length of the esophagus, laparoscopy offers excellent visualization of the posterior mediastinum, which allows the experienced minimally invasive surgeon to sufficiently mobilize the esophagus to achieve the accepted 3 cm of intraabdominal esophageal length. Incomplete excision of the hernia sac also places unwanted force on the hernia repair that tends to pull the stomach into the mediastinum and increase the risk of recurrence. Therefore, mobilization of the hernia sac and complete hernia sac excision are necessary to reestablish a tension-free intraabdominal GEJ.

Even without these unwanted forces, patients may be at increased risk of developing a recurrent hiatal hernia when the repair at the hiatus is subjected to a sudden increase in intraabdominal pressure. This can result from straining associated with lifting heavy objects, constipation, and vomiting, as well as acute gastric distention due to overeating and rapid ingestion of carbonated beverages. Patients who experience very early postoperative recurrences frequently report antecedent vomiting and retching [7–9], though it is unclear whether this is the direct cause of the recurrent hernia. Laparoscopy is associated with less pain, so patients require less time before they feel ready to return to activities, such as lifting, that promote increased intraabdominal pressure. The small size and rapid healing of laparoscopic incisions lower the risk for the development of an abdominal wall hernia. However, the hiatal hernia repair remains susceptible to becoming disrupted due to acute increases in intraabdominal pressure, particularly during the early postoperative period while scar tissue is developing between the stomach, distal esophagus, and hiatus. Laparoscopy is associated with the development of less intraabdominal scar tissue, and some surgeons have suggested that laparoscopic repairs are more susceptible to recurrence [10], however this notion has since been contradicted by the same proponents [11]. Regardless, most surgeons restrict patients from lifting in the early postoperative period (4–6 weeks).

Epidemiology: How Often Do Hiatal and Paraesophageal Hernia Repairs Fail?

Recurrence After Type I Hiatal Hernia Repair

Type I hiatal hernias are frequently associated with GERD symptoms, and these hernias are commonly repaired during antireflux surgery. Over the past 20 years, the adoption of laparoscopic antireflux surgery has expanded considerably [12], and long-term outcomes of these operations are becoming available. There are two common mechanisms for failure of antireflux surgery: Failure of the fundoplication, and failure of the hiatus. The fundoplication can either become disrupted or it can migrate distally around the body of the stomach (i.e. "slipped Nissen"). Both of these anatomic complications occur due to incorrect construction of the fundoplication; most commonly, incorrect construction occurs when surgeons inappropriately incorporate the gastric body into the fundoplication. Fundoplication disruption and slipped Nissen are the cause of 25–35 % of failed antireflux operations [9, 13, 14].

The second mechanism for failed antireflux operation, and the most common, is the development of a recurrent hiatal hernia. We reviewed three studies that evaluated their experience with reoperation after failed antireflux surgery. Coelho and colleagues reviewed 1,698 patients that underwent laparoscopic treatment for GERD [14]. Of this cohort, 53 patients (3.1 %) underwent late reoperation for failed primary antireflux surgery. Twenty-four of 53 (45 %) patients that underwent reoperation were found to have recurrent hiatal hernia, and in 83 % of patients with a recurrent hernia, GERD was the indication for reoperation. Seelig and colleagues reviewed their experience with laparoscopic antireflux surgery in 720 patients and identified seven (0.9 %) patients that required reoperation for recurrent hiatal hernia [15]. In these seven patients, four underwent evaluation for dysphagia, and none reported GERD symptoms. Finally, Smith and colleagues reviewed their experience with 1,892 primary laparoscopic antireflux operations [9]. In the 54 patients required reoperation for recurrent symptoms, the most commonly reported symptoms were dysphagia (56 %) and GERD (48 %). A recurrent hiatal hernia was found in 33/54 (61 %) patients that underwent reoperation.

These results suggest that, following primary antireflux surgery, a very small number of patients require reoperation for recurrent hiatal hernia. While these studies evaluate a large number of patients, the true incidence of recurrent hiatal hernia following antireflux surgery may be underrepresented in these investigations. These authors only reported patients that required a reoperation, and none of these studies employed systematic radiographic follow-up to evaluate for anatomic abnormalities in the absence of symptoms. Therefore, a limitation to these studies is selection bias for patients with recurrent symptoms. Additionally, the initial operations were carried out at large volume centers with experienced foregut surgeons, so the incidence of recurrent hiatal hernia may be lower than if the index operation is performed outside of these centers. To determine the true incidence of recurrent hiatal hernia would require routine use of barium esophagram in all patients that have undergone antireflux surgery.

Recurrence After Paraesophageal Hernia Repair

Numerous studies have reported recurrent hiatal hernia following primary PEH repair [10, 16–20]. The reported rates of recurrence vary according to several factors, including the duration of follow-up, whether radiographic evaluation is performed routinely on all patients or selectively in patients with recurrent foregut symptoms, and the physician reading the radiographic study (blinded, specialized GI radiologist or surgeon). In short-term follow-up studies that radiographically evaluate only patients with foregut symptoms, recurrent hiatal hernia have been found in as few as 2 % of patients [21]. In long-term follow-up studies that evaluate patients with routine barium esophagram, overall recurrence rates are reported as high as 57 % [22].

Although recurrent hiatal hernia is common, several studies have called into question the clinical significance of these radiographic findings [23]. At a mean follow-up of 11.3 years, White and colleagues reported a 32 % hiatal hernia recurrence rate in 31 patients [23]. Despite this high rate of hernia recurrence, all patients with recurrent hiatal hernia reported improvement in heartburn, chest pain, dysphagia, and regurgitation. In another study [21], nine hiatal hernia recurrences were found in 99 patients who underwent laparoscopic PEH repair, however only two of nine recurrences were symptomatic, and only one symptomatic recurrence required reoperation. For patients with radiographic evidence of recurrent hiatal hernia and uncontrollable, life-limiting symptoms (e.g. dysphagia, regurgitation, heartburn, epigastric pain), reoperative hiatal hernia repair is an appropriate, albeit challenging, endeavor. The more common, and arguably more challenging, scenario is the patient with a minimally symptomatic recurrent hiatal hernia.

In the remainder of this chapter, we will provide recommendations for the management of patients with minimally symptomatic recurrent hiatal hernias. Specifically, we will discuss each of the clinical factors that we believe important to consider when determining the optimal treatment of such a patient: (1) Patient symptoms; (2) Presence of a well-constructed fundoplication; (3) Size of recurrent hernia; (4) Number hiatal hernia operations; and (5) Patient obesity.

Search Strategy

To develop recommendations for the management of patients with minimally symptomatic recurrent hiatal hernia, a PubMed search was completed using combinations of the following terms: "recurrent", "paraesophageal hernia", "reoperation", and "hiatal hernia". These searches produced 430 results. Only full-text articles of primary studies published in English and after 1990 were reviewed. Studies of patients undergoing primary antireflux operations were included if they discussed incidence and/or management of recurrent hiatal hernias. No randomized studies were identified. The studies analyzed were retrospective reviews (n=28), one prospective trial, and one metaanalysis. Table 41.1 displays the incidence of radiographic recurrence after open and laparoscopic PEH repair.

Evaluation of Patients with Recurrent Hiatal Hernia

Patient Symptoms

The evaluation of patients with recurrent hiatal hernias requires the surgeon assess the severity of patient symptoms. Several studies report that patients have minimal symptoms and good quality of life despite high rates of radiographic recurrent hiatal hernia [1, 24–26]. Other studies show relatively low rates of recurrence, however higher rates of symptoms among those patients identified with a recurrent hernia [27, 28]. In both groups, the most common indication for operative management of recurrent hiatal hernia is symptoms insufficiently managed with non-operative therapies (e.g. acid suppression medication and esophageal dilation).

Andujar and colleagues retrospectively reviewed their experience with laparoscopic PEH repair in 166 patients [25]. A barium esophagram was completed in 120 patients (72 %) at a mean of 15 months postoperatively and revealed 30 patients (25 %) with recurrent hiatal hernia. In 18/30 patients, pre- and postoperative symptom scores were available. Despite the presence of a recurrent hiatal hernia, these

Table 41.1 Summary of studies reporting recurrent hiatal hernia following primary paraesophageal hernia repair

Study	Total patient number	Operation type	UGI indication	Patients with UGI	Follow up duration	Recurrence rate (%)	Symptomatic recurrences (%)	Reoperations	GRADE of evidence
Dallemagne et al. [1]	64	Laparoscopic PEH	Routine	35	Median 99 months	65.7	13	0	Moderate
Dahlberg et al. [18]	37	Laparoscopic PEH	Routine	22	Median 15 months	13.8	66	2	Moderate
Low and Unger [46]	72	Open PEH	Routine	60	≥12 months	18.3	na	0	Moderate
Targarona et al. [24]	44	Laparoscopic PEH	Routine	30	≥6 months	20	50	1	Moderate
Khaitan et al. [47]	31	Laparoscopic PEH	Routine	15	Mean 25.2 months	6.7	100	1	Moderate
Lubezky et al. [35]	59	Laparoscopic PEH	Routine	45	Mean 28.4 months	46.7	71	0	Moderate
Oelschlager et al. [22]	72	Laparoscopic PEH	Routine	60	Median 58 months	56.7	na	2	Moderate
Wiechmann et al. [2]	6-	Laparoscopic PEH	Routine	44	6 months	6.8	100	3	Moderate
Aly et al. [3]	100	Laparoscopic PEH	Routine	60	Mean 3.9 years	30	70	4	Moderate
Luketich et al. [17]	662	Laparoscopic PEH	Routine	445	≥3 months	15.7	na	21	Moderate
Wu et al. [19]	38	Laparoscopic PEH	Routine	35	≥3 months	22.8	12	1	Moderate
Zaninotto et al. [16]	54	Laparoscopic PEH	Routine	53	Median 71 months	28.3	Na	5	Moderate
Andujar et al. [25]	166	Laparoscopic PEH	Routine	120	Mean 15 months	25	50	12	Moderate

(continued)

Table 41.1 (continued)

Study	Total patient number	Operation type	UGI indication	Patients with UGI	Follow up duration	Recurrence rate (%)	Symptomatic recurrences (%)	Reoperations	GRADE of evidence
Lidor et al. [20]	101	Laparoscopic PEH	Routine	58	≥12 months	20.7	na	1	Moderate
Gibson et al. [21]	100	Laparoscopic PEH	Routine	99	Mean 18 months	9	22	1	Moderate
Diaz et al. [26]	96	Laparoscopic PEH	Routine	66	≥6 months	31.8	62	3	Moderate
Jobe et al. [28]	52	Laparoscopic PEH	Routine	34	Mean 37 months	32.3	64	2	Moderate
Gangopadhyay et al. [48]	171	Laparoscopic PEH	Routine	84	Mean 35 months	25	50	1	Moderate
Trus et al. [27]	76	Laparoscopic PEH	Symptoms	na	Median 6 months	na	100	4	Low
Pierre et al. [49]	200	Laparoscopic PEH	Symptoms	na	Median 18 months	na	100	5	Low
Edye et al. [8]	55	Laparoscopic PEH	Symptoms	9	Mean 20 months	100	100	4	Low
White et al. [23]	52	Laparoscopic PEH	Symptoms	9	Mean 11.3 years	100	100	2	Moderate

na Not available, *PEH* Paraesophageal hernia, *UGI* Upper gastrointestinal series

patients had significant improvement in heartburn, regurgitation, dysphagia, and chest pain at 6 and 24 months postoperatively. Furthermore, when these 18 patients with recurrent hiatal hernias were compared to patients without postoperative hiatal hernia (n = 76), there were no differences in symptom severity at 24 months postoperatively. Only three patients with recurrent hiatal hernia required reoperation. In these three patients, the indication for operation was GERD symptoms that were insufficiently improved with medical management.

Lidor and colleagues reported their results of 101 patients who underwent laparoscopic PEH repair [20]. At 12 months postoperatively, 58 patients underwent barium esophagram and an assessment of symptoms and quality of life. Despite a recurrent hiatal hernia rate of 27.6 %, all patients had improvement in reported foregut symptoms. However, when patients with recurrent hiatal hernia were compared to those without hiatal hernia, patients with recurrence had worse symptom scores for early satiety, dysphagia, odynophagia, and bloating/gas. Despite these findings, overall patient satisfaction was reported to be excellent. One patient required reoperation for obstructive symptoms recalcitrant to dilation therapy.

After a patient is identified with a recurrent hiatal hernia, the surgeon must carefully evaluate the patient's symptoms. In patients with symptomatic recurrent hiatal hernia, a concerted attempt should be made at non-operative management of symptoms. In most cases, proton-pump inhibitor therapy will ameliorate symptoms of GERD. On the other hand, obstructive symptoms are more likely to require operative intervention. In the end, when non-operative therapy fails to provide adequate control of symptoms, reoperative hiatal hernia repair should be considered.

Presence of a Well-Constructed Fundoplication

We routinely perform a 360-degree Nissen fundoplication at the time of primary PEH repair, a practice advocated for in the literature by us and others [29, 30]. There are several reasons that we believe a fundoplication is a key step to PEH repair. Theoretically, it provides reinforcement of the hernia repair by securing the stomach below the diaphragm, particularly if the fundoplication is sutured to the diaphragmatic crura, which effectively creates a gastropexy. The fundoplication also provides an additional surface to which adhesions can develop, which may assist to secure the stomach to the hiatus and prevent the gastric body from migrating into the chest.

If a recurrent hiatal hernia develops, an appropriately created fundoplication can be protective against both obstructive and GERD related symptoms. By incorporating the gastric fundus into a fundoplication, the fundus is unable to migrate into the posterior mediastinum where, if it distends, it can create angulation to the esophagus resulting in dysphagia or other obstructive symptoms. If the fundoplication remains intact, even in the setting of a recurrent hiatal hernia, then it often will retain its competency as an anti-reflux valve and counteract GERD symptoms.

For a fundoplication to provide these protective effects, it must be constructed with the correct part of the stomach, and it must be positioned around the distal esophagus. Frequently, recurrent hiatal hernias consist of a mild (2–4 cm) widening of the esophageal hiatus and cephalad displacement of the fundoplication into the posterior mediastinum. If the fundoplication is inappropriately constructed (i.e. fundus sutured to gastric body, or the fundoplication is created too loose or "floppy") the result is a redundant fundus that lies behind the esophagus. When this occurs, a disproportionately large amount of stomach can herniate through a relatively small recurrent hiatal hernia. The result is a symptomatic recurrent hiatal hernia that is due to a poorly constructed fundoplication rather than a widening of the hiatus, per se.

We believe that our investigation of the long-term outcomes of laparoscopic PEH repair indirectly supports the protective effect of a well-constructed fundoplication [22]. All patients in this study underwent 360-degree Nissen fundoplication. The geometry of our Nissen fundoplication is created by expert foregut surgeons in a very standardized manner, ensuring that only fundus is used. This approach prevents the creation of Nissen that is too loose or "floppy", decreasing the likelihood of postoperative heartburn and/or obstructive symptoms. In that study, we reported a high rate of recurrent hiatal hernia following primary laparoscopic PEH repair (>50 %). However, the patients with hernia recurrence maintained an overall quality of life similar to patients without recurrence. While heartburn was more common in patients with recurrent hiatal hernia, the severity was usually mild, most patients were adequately controlled on medication, and need for reoperation was rare. We believe that an appropriately constructed Nissen fundoplication minimized the symptoms associated with these recurrent hiatal hernias.

Size of Recurrent Hiatal Hernia

Traditionally, patients found to have large asymptomatic primary PEH were recommended to undergo repair to prevent acute gastric volvulus and the need for emergent repair [31, 32]. Unlike primary PEH, large recurrent hiatal hernias are more likely to be symptomatic and, for that reason, require repair. These severe recurrences almost always are associated with intraoperative evidence of an inadequate primary PEH repair – for example, incomplete sac excision, insufficient mobilization of the esophagus, and/or poor construction of the fundoplication. Therefore, reoperation for these very large recurrent hiatal hernias has a greater likelihood of correcting a persistent anatomic problem and creating a long-term durable repair. While some authors have advocated for routine repair of larger asymptomatic recurrent hiatal hernias [24], compared to primary PEH repair, reoperative hiatal hernia repair is more technically challenging and associated with greater risk. So, the question remains whether size alone should be considered in determining need for recurrent hiatal hernia repair.

As part of our prospective multi-institutional study of laparoscopic PEH repair, we assessed the relationship between recurrent hiatal hernia size and patient symptoms [22]. Recurrent hernia size was measured vertically above the diaphragm using barium esophagram; patient symptoms were assessed using standardized patient questionnaires. Long-term clinical and radiographic data were available for 60 of

108 (56 %) patients. Twenty-six (43 %) patients had a recurrent hernia measuring <20 mm, 14 (24 %) patients measuring 20–39 mm, and 20 (33 %) patients measuring ≥40 mm (though rarely larger). Patients with large (≥40 mm) recurrent hernias had greater heartburn severity compared to patients without hiatal hernia (<20 mm) (p=0.046). Importantly, operative repair was required in only two of these patients, and symptoms, not size, was the criterion used to determine need for repair.

While there is a belief that hiatal hernias grow over time, this was not consistently seen in our study. Thirteen patients were identified to have a recurrent hiatal hernia on routine barium esophagram at 6 months postoperatively. At long-term follow-up (median 58 months, range 40–78 months), there was no significant change in hernia size for these patients (31 mm vs. 30 mm; p=0.84). This suggests that continued hernia growth is not inevitable, supporting our practice to re-operate for the management of patient symptoms and not to prevent development of future symptoms or complications of larger hernias (e.g. gastric volvulus).

Due to the long-term follow-up and systematic use of barium esophagram as well as quality of life and symptom evaluations, we believe that our study is particularly illustrative of the natural history of primary PEH repair. Consequently, except for extremely large recurrent hernias, in which it is likely primary hernia repair was inadequate, size should not be an independent criterion for reoperation.

Number of Prior Hiatal Hernia Operations

The first attempt at PEH repair is the best opportunity for the surgeon to perform a durable repair. Reoperation at the esophageal hiatus is challenging due to obscured tissue planes and adhesive disease. One study reported a 31 % incidence of visceral injury during reoperative hiatal hernia repair [33]. At reoperation, the crura are less pliable, and creation of a tension-free hiatal herniorrhaphy is more difficult; consequently, additional procedures are frequently required to close the hiatus, such as lateral diaphragmatic relaxing incisions [34] or mesh reinforcement of the hiatus [35]. Despite these difficulties, when comparing the outcomes of primary and recurrent hiatal hernia repair, two studies found similar improvement in symptoms and freedom from hernia recurrence [33, 35]. However, some patients that undergo recurrent hiatal hernia repair will develop subsequent hernia recurrences. For these patients with multiply recurrent hiatal hernias, the question must be asked: How many times should a recurrent hiatal hernia be repaired?

Smith and colleagues reviewed their experience with reoperation for failed primary PEH repair and antireflux surgery [9]. Their results demonstrate diminished symptomatic and anatomic improvement with subsequent reoperations. In this study, 241 patients underwent reoperation, 59 underwent a second redo, 6 underwent a third redo, and 1 underwent a fourth redo. The failure rate increased with each subsequent repair, with the rate of second (7.1 %) and third (6.8 %) redo operations more than twice the rate of initial reoperation (2.8 %). For patients undergoing reoperation, the most common mechanism of failure was recurrent hiatal hernia. Furthermore, the incidence of recurrent hernia increased with each subsequent reoperation (50 % at first redo vs. 72 % at second redo, P<0.05), and the presence of a recurrent hiatal hernia at the first operation was an independent predictor for the need for a subsequent operation (OR 4.0, CI 1.2–12.4). Two-thirds of patients that underwent a second reoperation did so for the same symptoms that lead to their initial reoperation, suggesting that the initial reoperation did not provide long-term improvement in these symptoms. Therefore, with each subsequent operation, the chance of long-term anatomic repair and symptom improvement decreases while the technical aspects of reoperation become more challenging due to more extensive fibrotic tissues. Of the six patients who required three reoperations, one ultimately underwent a fourth operation. Based on these results, the authors concluded that alternative management strategies should be considered (e.g. esophagectomy) if recurrence occurs after three reoperations.

In general, we agree with these authors' conclusions. However, it is likely the extent of dissection at prior reoperation, rather than the absolute number of reoperations, that precludes repair of a subsequent hiatal hernia. In some patients that have undergone multiple repairs, one or even two of the reoperations may have included a very limited dissection and therefore may not preclude the performance of a successful subsequent repair. On the other hand, there are many patients with two prior operations who will have a hiatus and/or stomach too damaged to permit a durable repair. Therefore, a surgeon considering reoperation should know if an expert laparoscopic foregut surgeon completed the prior repair(s) and meticulously review all operative notes to determine what impact those repairs might have on subsequent reoperation. If the surgeon determines that prior attempts at repair prohibit the benefit of a subsequent repair, an alternative management strategy (e.g. esophagectomy or gastrectomy) should be considered. This should be the surgeon's approach, regardless of the absolute number of prior repairs the patient has undergone.

Patient Obesity

Obesity is a risk factor for both the development of primary PEH [36] and for recurrent hiatal hernia [37], presumably as a result of increased intraabdominal pressure. Repair of primary and recurrent hiatal hernias are technically more challenging in obese patients, because visualization is impaired secondary to increased visceral fat (which may also contribute to failure). In obese patients that present with recurrent hiatal hernia, a standard reoperative hiatal hernia repair may not be a durable approach for long-term symptomatic management and prevention of recurrence. Moreover, reoperative hiatal hernia repair does not address the patients underlying obesity. In these cases, bariatric surgery should be considered. Options for a bariatric operation include laparoscopic Roux-en-Y gastric bypass and laparoscopic sleeve gastrectomy.

Bariatric surgery for management of recurrent hiatal hernia offers several advantages over standard recurrent hiatal hernia repair. First, it is the most effective treatment for obesity and obesity-related comorbidities. By treating the patient's obesity, this operation directly addresses one of the common underlying causes of hiatal hernia recurrence in obese patients. Second, bariatric surgery alters gastroesophageal anatomy so that, in the event of a recurrent widening of the esophageal hiatus, it is unlikely that the fundus and body of the stomach will re-herniate into the mediastinum. This anatomic change decreases the chance of developing a symptomatic recurrent hiatal hernia and essentially eliminates the opportunity of developing gastric volvulus and strangulation.

Several authors have demonstrated the safety and utility of laparoscopic Roux-en-Y gastric bypass in obese patients with hiatal and paraesophageal hernia [38–40]. In these reports, patients demonstrated significant loss of excess weight and demonstrated no evidence of recurrent hiatal hernia on barium esophagram at 6 and 18 month follow-up. Further, all patients had improvement in GERD symptoms and remained off acid suppression therapy. While these studies support the use of gastric bypass to manage patients with obesity and primary PEH, at the time this chapter was published, there were no published reports of laparoscopic gastric bypass for the management of *recurrent* hiatal hernia.

Unlike gastric bypass, sleeve gastrectomy has been used for the management of both primary PEH and recurrent hiatal hernias [41–43]. We published the first report of simultaneous recurrent hiatal hernia repair and laparoscopic sleeve gastrectomy [44]. At 18 months postoperatively, our patient remained free of all foregut symptoms, had no clinical evidence of a recurrent hernia, and lost 57 lb. Rodriguez and colleagues reported their experience with laparoscopic sleeve gastrectomy in addition to PEH repair in 14 obese and morbidly obese patients with symptomatic PEH and five patients with recurrent hiatal hernia [45]. At a mean follow-up of 13 months, 89.5 % of patients were available for evaluation. Compared to preoperatively, these patients reported significant improvement in their symptoms and reduction in acid-suppression medication use. Additionally, 14 patients experienced excess weight loss of mean 29 ± 23 % (range 17–89 %). Despite no evidence of recurrent hiatal hernia, one patient, who had two prior attempts at hiatal hernia repair, failed to have any improvement in symptoms with sleeve gastrectomy. This patient underwent revision to Roux-en-Y gastric bypass.

Compared to Roux-en-Y gastric bypass, sleeve gastrectomy is easier and safer to construct, and postoperative alterations in diet may be less dramatic than with a bypass. These advantages may be particularly beneficial in patients with recurrent hiatal hernia, as many of these patients are older. The weakness of sleeve gastrectomy is the propensity for it to potentiate GERD symptoms, particularly heartburn and regurgitation.

In summary, obese patients present an additional challenge to the operative repair of recurrent hiatal hernia. In these patients, performance of a bariatric operation—either laparoscopic Roux-en-Y gastric bypass or laparoscopic sleeve gastrectomy—in combination with recurrent hiatal hernia repair can provide durable anatomic repair and improvement in symptoms. In the event of breakdown of the hiatal repair, the anatomy of the foregut following these operations makes it less likely that patients experience recurrent symptoms, and greatly reduces the risk of life-threatening complications of gastric volvulus. Finally, these operations can provide durable weight loss and management of obesity-related comorbidities.

Conclusions

The goal of this chapter is to provide recommendations for the management of patients with minimally symptomatic recurrent hiatal hernia. Patients with symptomatic recurrent hiatal hernia warrant careful clinical evaluation by an experienced foregut surgeon. Particular attention should be paid to several key features: Severity of symptoms, presence of an appropriately constructed fundoplication, size of the hernia, number of prior operations, and patient body habitus. Despite high rates of recurrent hiatal hernia, most of these patients do not require operative repair. When a reoperation is indicated, and performed by an experienced surgeon, repair of recurrent hiatal hernia can be safely performed with acceptable improvement in patient symptoms.

Recommendations

Reoperative hiatal hernia repair should be considered for patients with symptoms that can be attributed to the recurrent hernia and are uncontrollable with maximal non-operative therapy. At the time of primary hiatal and paraesophageal hernia repair, a correctly constructed fundoplication should be created to mitigate the symptoms associated with recurrent hiatal hernia. An incorrectly constructed fundoplication can potentiate patient symptoms in the setting of a recurrent hiatal hernia. Except for extremely large recurrences, which are associated with inadequate primary repair, size of recurrent hiatal hernia should not be used as an independent criterion for reoperation. For patients who present with multiply recurrent hiatal hernias, the surgeon must determine if the prior hernia repairs prohibit the likelihood of a successful subsequent reoperation. After three recurrent hiatal hernia operations, esophagectomy or gastrectomy should be strongly considered over a fourth repair. In obese patients with recurrent hiatal hernias that warrant operative repair, bariatric surgery (i.e. Roux-en-Y gastric bypass or sleeve gastrectomy) should be considered.

A Personal View of the Data

As we demonstrate in this chapter, surgeons must consider multiple factors when deciding the appropriate management of minimally symptomatic recurrent hiatal hernia. When faced with a patient with a recurrent hiatal hernia, several key questions that need answered:

- Does the patient have symptoms unmanageable despite maximal non-operative therapy, and are those symptoms attributable to a defined anatomic abnormality that can be corrected with an operation?
- At the time of the patient's initial operation, was a fundoplication correctly constructed?

- Is the patient presenting with a very large recurrent hiatal hernia that suggests the initial repair was inadequate?
- How many prior repairs of the hiatus has the patient undergone, who performed the repairs, and what specifically was done during those operations?
- Is the patient a candidate for a bariatric operation to manage the recurrent hiatal hernia?

For each patient with a primary or recurrent hiatal hernia, we routinely perform several diagnostic studies, including a barium esophagram, upper gastrointestinal endoscopy, esophageal manometry, and if symptoms of GERD then a 24-h pH study. We believe that these studies provide the operative surgeon with a comprehensive understanding of the patient's gastroesophageal anatomy and physiology. The results of these studies also provide some objectivity to the patient's symptoms that may assist the surgeon in identifying patients that will benefit from reoperation.

Finally, reasonable expectations must be discussed with the patient regarding the outcome of reoperative hiatal hernia repair, especially symptom improvement. Both the surgeon and the patient must understand that reoperations follow the law of diminishing returns: With each repair, the opportunity to improve symptoms and create a durable anatomic repair decreases. For patients that have undergone two or three prior hiatal hernia repairs and continue to have gastroesophageal symptoms, it is important to consider alternative operations. In obese patients, this includes Roux-en-Y gastric bypass and sleeve gastrectomy; in non-obese patients, alternative operations are esophagectomy and total gastrectomy.

Recommendations

- Reoperative hiatal hernia repair should be considered for patients with symptoms that can be attributed to the recurrent hernia and are uncontrollable with maximal non-operative therapy. (Evidence quality low; weak recommendation)
- At the time of primary hernia repair, a correctly constructed fundoplication should be created to mitigate the symptoms associated with recurrent hiatal hernia. (Evidence quality very low; weak recommendation)
- Except for extremely large recurrences, recurrent hiatal hernia size should not be used as an independent criterion for reoperation. (Evidence quality low; weak recommendation)
- After multiple hiatal hernia operations, esophagectomy or gastrectomy should be strongly considered over a fourth repair. (Evidence quality low; weak recommendation)
- In obese patients with recurrent hiatal hernias that warrant operative repair, bariatric surgery should be considered. (Evidence quality low; weak recommendation)

References

1. Dallemagne B, Kohnen L, Perretta S, Weerts J, Markiewicz S, Jehaes C. Laparoscopic repair of paraesophageal hernia. Long-term follow-up reveals good clinical outcome despite high radiological recurrence rate. Ann Surg. 2011;253(2):291–6.
2. Wiechmann RJ, Ferguson MK, Naunheim KS, McKesey P, Hazelrigg SJ, Santucci TS, et al. Laparoscopic management of giant paraesophageal herniation. Ann Thorac Surg. 2001;71(4):1080–6; discussion 1086–7.
3. Aly A, Munt J, Jamieson GG, Ludemann R, Devitt PG, Watson DI. Laparoscopic repair of large hiatal hernias. Br J Surg. 2005;92(5):648–53.
4. Fullum TM, Oyetunji TA, Ortega G, Tran DD, Woods IM, Obayomi-Davies O, et al. Open versus laparoscopic hiatal hernia repair. JSLS. 2013;17(1):23–9.
5. Nguyen NT, Christie C, Masoomi H, Matin T, Laugenour K, Hohmann S. Utilization and outcomes of laparoscopic versus open paraesophageal hernia repair. Am Surg. 2011;77(10):1353–7.
6. Fisichella PM, Patti MG. Laparoscopic repair of paraesophageal hiatal hernias. J Laparoendosc Adv Surg Tech A. 2008;18(4):629–32.
7. Mattar SG, Bowers SP, Galloway KD, Hunter JG, Smith CD. Long-term outcome of laparoscopic repair of paraesophageal hernia. Surg Endosc. 2002;16(5):745–9.
8. Edye MB, Canin-Endres J, Gattorno F, Salky BA. Durability of laparoscopic repair of paraesophageal hernia. Ann Surg. 1998;228(4):528–35.
9. Smith CD, McClusky DA, Rajad MA, Lederman AB, Hunter JG. When fundoplication fails: redo? Ann Surg. 2005;241(6):861–9; discussion 869–71.
10. Hashemi M, Peters JH, DeMeester TR, Huprich JE, Quek M, Hagen JA, et al. Laparoscopic repair of large type III hiatal hernia: objective followup reveals high recurrence rate. J Am Coll Surg. 2000;190(5):553–60; discussion 560–1.
11. Zehetner J, Demeester SR, Ayazi S, Kilday P, Augustin F, Hagen JA, et al. Laparoscopic versus open repair of paraesophageal hernia: the second decade. J Am Coll Surg. 2011;212(5):813–20.
12. Finlayson SR, Laycock WS, Birkmeyer JD. National trends in utilization and outcomes of antireflux surgery. Surg Endosc. 2003;17(6):864–7.
13. Musunuru S, Gould JC. Perioperative outcomes of surgical procedures for symptomatic fundoplication failure: a retrospective case-control study. Surg Endosc. 2012;26(3):838–42.
14. Coelho JC, Goncalves CG, Claus CM, Andrigueto PC, Ribeiro MN. Late laparoscopic reoperation of failed antireflux procedures. Surg Laparosc Endosc Percutan Tech. 2004;14(3):113–7.
15. Seelig MH, Hinder RA, Klingler PJ, Floch NR, Branton SA, Smith SL. Paraesophageal herniation as a complication following laparoscopic antireflux surgery. J Gastrointest Surg. 1999;3(1):95–9.
16. Zaninotto G, Portale G, Costantini M, Fiamingo P, Rampado S, Guirroli E, et al. Objective follow-up after laparoscopic repair of large type III hiatal hernia. Assessment of safety and durability. World J Surg. 2007;31(11):2177–83.
17. Luketich JD, Nason KS, Christie NA, Pennathur A, Jobe BA, Landreneau RJ, et al. Outcomes after a decade of laparoscopic giant paraesophageal hernia repair. J Thorac Cardiovasc Surg. 2010;139(2):395–404. e1.
18. Dahlberg PS, Deschamps C, Miller DL, Allen MS, Nichols FC, Pairolero PC. Laparoscopic repair of large paraesophageal hiatal hernia. Ann Thorac Surg. 2001;72(4):1125–9.
19. Wu JS, Dunnegan DL, Soper NJ. Clinical and radiologic assessment of laparoscopic paraesophageal hernia repair. Surg Endosc. 1999;13(5):497–502.
20. Lidor AO, Kawaji Q, Stem M, Fleming RM, Schweitzer MA, Steele KE, et al. Defining recurrence after paraesophageal hernia repair: correlating symptoms and radiographic findings. Surgery. 2013;154(2):171–8.
21. Gibson SC, Wong SC, Dixon AC, Falk GL. Laparoscopic repair of giant hiatus hernia: prosthesis is not required for successful outcome. Surg Endosc. 2013;27(2):618–23.

22. Oelschlager BK, Petersen RP, Brunt LM, Soper NJ, Sheppard BC, Mitsumori L, et al. Laparoscopic paraesophageal hernia repair: defining long-term clinical and anatomic outcomes. J Gastrointest Surg. 2012;16(3):453–9.

23. White BC, Jeansonne LO, Morgenthal CB, Zagorski S, Davis SS, Smith CD, et al. Do recurrences after paraesophageal hernia repair matter?: Ten-year follow-up after laparoscopic repair. Surg Endosc. 2008;22(4):1107–11.

24. Targarona EM, Novell J, Vela S, Cerdan G, Bendahan G, Torrubia S, et al. Mid term analysis of safety and quality of life after the laparoscopic repair of paraesophageal hiatal hernia. Surg Endosc. 2004;18(7):1045–50.

25. Andujar JJ, Papasavas PK, Birdas T, Robke J, Raftopoulos Y, Gagne DJ, et al. Laparoscopic repair of large paraesophageal hernia is associated with a low incidence of recurrence and reoperation. Surg Endosc. 2004;18(3):444–7.

26. Diaz S, Brunt LM, Klingensmith ME, Frisella PM, Soper NJ. Laparoscopic paraesophageal hernia repair, a challenging operation: medium-term outcome of 116 patients. J Gastrointest Surg. 2003;7(1):59–66. discussion -7.

27. Trus TL, Bax T, Richardson WS, Branum GD, Mauren SJ, Swanstrom LL, et al. Complications of laparoscopic paraesophageal hernia repair. J Gastrointest Surg. 1997;1(3):221–7. discussion 8.

28. Jobe BA, Aye RW, Deveney CW, Domreis JS, Hill LD. Laparoscopic management of giant type III hiatal hernia and short esophagus. Objective follow-up at three years. J Gastrointest Surg. 2002;6(2):181–8. discussion 8.

29. Horgan S, Eubanks TR, Jacobsen G, Omelanczuk P, Pellegrini CA. Repair of paraesophageal hernias. Am J Surg. 1999;177(5):354–8.

30. Furnee EJ, Draaisma WA, Gooszen HG, Hazebroek EJ, Smout AJ, Broeders IA. Tailored or routine addition of an antireflux fundoplication in laparoscopic large hiatal hernia repair: a comparative cohort study. World J Surg. 2011;35(1):78–84.

31. Hill LD. Incarcerated paraesophageal hernia. A surgical emergency. Am J Surg. 1973;126(2):286–91.

32. Willwerth BM. Gastric complications associated with paraesophageal herniation. Am Surg. 1974;40(6):366–9.

33. Juhasz A, Sundaram A, Hoshino M, Lee TH, Mittal SK. Outcomes of surgical management of symptomatic large recurrent hiatus hernia. Surg Endosc. 2012;26(6):1501–8.

34. Greene CL, Demeester SR, Zehetner J, Worrell SG, Oh DS, Hagen JA. Diaphragmatic relaxing incisions during laparoscopic paraesophageal hernia repair. Surg Endosc. 2013;27:4532–8.

35. Lubezky N, Sagie B, Keidar A, Szold A. Prosthetic mesh repair of large and recurrent diaphragmatic hernias. Surg Endosc. 2007;21(5):737–41.

36. Wilson LJ, Ma W, Hirschowitz BI. Association of obesity with hiatal hernia and esophagitis. Am J Gastroenterol. 1999;94(10):2840–4.

37. Perez AR, Moncure AC, Rattner DW. Obesity adversely affects the outcome of antireflux operations. Surg Endosc. 2001;15(9):986–9.

38. Kasotakis G, Mittal SK, Sudan R. Combined treatment of symptomatic massive paraesophageal hernia in the morbidly obese. JSLS. 2011;15(2):188–92.

39. Amini A, Vaziri K, Nagle AP. Simultaneous laparoscopic type III paraesophageal hernia repair with porcine small intestine submucosa and Roux-en-Y gastric bypass. Surg Obes Relat Dis. 2008;4(6):764–7.

40. Salvador-Sanchis JL, Martinez-Ramos D, Herfarth A, Rivadulla-Serrano I, Ibanez-Belenguer M, Hoashi JS. Treatment of morbid obesity and hiatal paraesophageal hernia by laparoscopic Roux-en-Y gastric bypass. Obes Surg. 2010;20(6):801–3.

41. Varela JE. Laparoscopic biomesh hiatoplasty and sleeve gastrectomy in a morbidly obese patient with hiatal hernia. Surg Obes Relat Dis. 2009;5(6):707–9.

42. Korwar V, Peters M, Adjepong S, Sigurdsson A. Laparoscopic hiatus hernia repair and simultaneous sleeve gastrectomy: a novel approach in the treatment of gastroesophageal reflux disease associated with morbid obesity. J Laparoendosc Adv Surg Tech A. 2009;19(6):761–3.

43. Merchant AM, Cook MW, Srinivasan J, Davis SS, Sweeney JF, Lin E. Comparison between laparoscopic paraesophageal hernia repair with sleeve gastrectomy and paraesophageal hernia repair alone in morbidly obese patients. Am Surg. 2009;75(7):620–5.

44. Cuenca-Abente F, Parra JD, Oelschlager BK. Laparoscopic sleeve gastrectomy: an alternative for recurrent paraesophageal hernias in obese patients. JSLS. 2006;10(1):86–9.
45. Rodriguez JH, Kroh M, El-Hayek K, Timratana P, Chand B. Combined paraesophageal hernia repair and partial longitudinal gastrectomy in obese patients with symptomatic paraesophageal hernias. Surg Endosc. 2012;26(12):3382–90.
46. Low DE, Unger T. Open repair of paraesophageal hernia: reassessment of subjective and objective outcomes. Ann Thorac Surg. 2005;80(1):287–94.
47. Khaitan L, Houston H, Sharp K, Holzman M, Richards W. Laparoscopic paraesophageal hernia repair has an acceptable recurrence rate. Am Surg. 2002;68(6):546–51; discussion 551–2.
48. Gangopadhyay N, Perrone JM, Soper NJ, Matthews BD, Eagon JC, Klingensmith ME, et al. Outcomes of laparoscopic paraesophageal hernia repair in elderly and high-risk patients. Surgery. 2006;140(4):491–8; discussion 498–9.
49. Pierre AF, Luketich JD, Fernando HC, Christie NA, Buenaventura PO, Litle VR, et al. Results of laparoscopic repair of giant paraesophageal hernias: 200 consecutive patients. Ann Thorac Surg. 2002;74(6):1909–15; discussion 1915–6.

Part V
Airway

Chapter 42
Stenting for Benign Airway Obstruction

Septimiu Murgu

Abstract In patients suffering from benign central airway obstruction (CAO), airway stents improve dyspnea, lung function, quality of life and potentially survival. These prostheses, however, are foreign objects within the airways, have expected adverse events and therefore should only be used when curative open surgical interventions are not feasible or are contraindicated. This chapter is a systematic review of the published literature on histologically benign CAO including post intubation, post tracheostomy, tuberculosis and transplant-related strictures, tracheobronchomalacia and extrinsic compression due to benign thyroid disease. Evidence-based recommendations are provided for each of these clinical entities.

Keywords Airway stents • Stenting • Laryngotracheal stenosis • Tracheal stenosis • Bronchial stenosis • Airway obstruction • Tracheobronchomalacia • Bronchomalacia • Tracheomalacia

Introduction

Airway stents have been shown to improve symptoms, lung function, quality of life and potentially survival in patients suffering from histologically benign central airway obstruction (CAO). The frequency and severity of adverse events depend on patient-related factors, stent biomechanics and specific stent-tissue interactions. The bronchoscopist must determine the expected benefits of airway stenting, alternatives, and immediate and long-term expected adverse events. A first step during this process is to objectively classify CAO based on confirmed histology,

S. Murgu, MD
Department of Medicine, Section of Pulmonary and Critical Care Medicine,
The University of Chicago, 5841 S Maryland Ave, MC 6076,
Chicago, IL 60637, USA
e-mail: smurgu@medicine.bsd.uchicago.edu

M.K. Ferguson (ed.), *Difficult Decisions in Thoracic Surgery*,
Difficult Decisions in Surgery: An Evidence-Based Approach 1,
DOI 10.1007/978-1-4471-6404-3_42, © Springer-Verlag London 2014

Table 42.1 Central airway
obstruction classification
based on quantitative and
qualitative criteria

Qualitative criteria	Quantitative criteria
Histology	**Extent (vertical length)**
Benign	Normal
Malignant	Focal
	Multifocal
	Diffuse
Mechanism	**Severity of airway narrowing**
Extrinsic	Normal
Intraluminal	Mild (<50 %)
Exophytic	Moderate (50–75 %)
Infiltrative	Severe (75–100 %)
Strictures	
Mixed	
Dynamic features	**Functional impairment**
Fixed	Normal
Dynamic	Mild
	Moderate
	Severe

mechanism of obstruction and dynamic features. An accurate assessment of the extent, severity of airway narrowing and impact on patient's functional status are necessary prior to interventions (Table 42.1). This chapter will address the common causes of benign CAO with emphasis on adult post intubation/tracheostomy tracheal stenosis and tracheobronchomalacia (TBM) for the following reasons: (1) post intubation (PITS) and post tracheostomy tracheal stenosis (PTTS) are the most common causes of histologically benign CAO; (2) surgical management of these entities may be contraindicated, not feasible or not available, in which case airway stents can be used to palliate symptoms and improve quality of life; (3) airway stents in PITS and PTTS could results in significant complications which may preclude subsequent curative open surgical intervention; (4) TBM is a disease of the central airways characterized by weakened airway cartilaginous structures but is often confused with excessive dynamic airway collapse (EDAC), characterized by excessive bulging of the posterior membranous wall inside the airway lumen in the lack of cartilaginous abnormalities; and (5) patients with significant symptoms from TBM may benefit form airway stent insertion; EDAC, however, is generally caused by peripheral airway disease (asthma, COPD, bronchiolitis) or morbid obesity and does not represent a true central airway abnormality. The literature search for this systematic review was performed to identify studies specifically focused on the benefits and potential adverse effects of stent insertion strategies designed to palliate symptoms from histologically benign CAO. Four Population Intervention Comparator Outcome (PICO) questions were developed to guide the review (Table 42.2).

Table 42.2 Investigation/Intervention Comparator Outcome (PICO) questions for the role of airway stent insertion in benign central airway obstruction

PICO question 1	Among patients with CAO from benign tracheal or bronchial stenosis, does airway stent insertion improve health outcomes (defined as performance status, quality of life, frequency and duration of hospitalizations, incidence of respiratory failure, need for repeat bronchoscopic procedures, and survival)?
PICO question 2	Among patients with CAO from benign tracheal or bronchial stenosis, does airway stent insertion adversely affect health outcomes (defined as performance status, quality of life, frequency and duration of hospitalizations, incidence of respiratory failure, need for repeat bronchoscopic procedures, and survival)?
PICO question 3	Among patients with CAO from tracheobronchomalacia, does airway stent insertion improve health outcomes (defined as performance status, quality of life, frequency and duration of hospitalizations, incidence of respiratory failure, need for repeat bronchoscopic procedures, and survival)?
PICO question 4	Among patients with CAO from tracheobronchomalacia, does airway stent insertion adversely affect health outcomes (defined as performance status, quality of life, frequency and duration of hospitalizations, incidence of respiratory failure, need for repeat bronchoscopic procedures, and survival)?

Search Strategy

Study Identification

Systematic methods were used to find relevant studies, assess their eligibility for inclusion, and evaluate study quality. An attempt was made to retrieve all published studies that reported on post-stent insertion outcomes for patients with benign CAO since the introduction of dedicated airway stents. The online database MEDLINE was searched for papers published in English between January 1st, 1990 and September 10th, 2013. The start date was selected in order to assure inclusion of relevant studies on the subject matter at the time of the introduction of the dedicated silicone airway stent in the early 1990s in Europe. The following terms were used in Pubmed advanced search engine: Search details: (((((((((("stents"[MeSH Terms] OR stenting[Text Word]) AND "airway obstruction"[MeSH Terms]) OR "tracheal stenosis"[MeSH Terms]) OR bronchial stenosis[Text Word]) OR laryngotracheal stenosis[Text Word]) OR subglottic stenosis[Text Word]) OR "tracheomalacia"[MeSH Terms]) OR "tracheobronchomalacia"[MeSH Terms]) OR "bronchomalacia"[MeSH Terms]) AND English[Language]) AND ("1990/01/01"[EDAT] : "3000"[EDAT])) AND "adult"[MeSH Terms]. Additional articles were captured by reviewing the reference lists from identified studies and pertinent review articles.

Stenting for benign airway obstruction Systematic Review

Study Eligibility Form

Aim: to determine the outcomes of patients with benign airway obstruction after airway stent insertion

Reviewer Name:

Publication identification (paste or write in reference)

Type of study (check all that apply)	Yes	Unclear	No

Q1

	Yes	Unclear	No
Randomized Controlled Clinical Trial	☐	☐	☐
Cohort Study (unselected, consecutive patients)	☐	☐	☐
Case Control Study	☐	☐	☐
Before and after Trial	☐	☐	☐
Interrupted Time series Analysis	☐	☐	☐
Cross Sectional Study	☐	☐	☐
Case Series (selected or non-consecutive patients)	☒	☐	☐
other: _____	☐	☐	☐

GO   TO   Q2 (if yes to one of these)

	Yes	Unclear	No
Systematic or Narrative Review	☐	☐	☐
other: _____	☐	☐	☐

EXCLUDE (if yes to one of these, or if unclear

Study Participants	Yes	Unclear	No
Q2 Adult patient population	☒	☐	☐
Q3 Patients with airway stents **AND**	☒	☐	☐
Central airway obstruction fistulas*			

*at least 80% of sample had benign disease **OR** separate data was reported for patients with benign disease

GO   TO   NEXT   EXCLUDE if
Question (only if yes)   no/unclear

Interventions/outcomes	Yes	Unclear	No
Q4 Surveillance/Intervention described	☒	☐	☐
e.g. CT, CXR, bronehouopy, clinic viaits, etc.			
Q5 Outcome described	☒	☐	☐
e.g. mortality, morbidity, PS, QOL, etc.			

GO   TO   FINAL   EXCLUDE if
DECISION (if yes to both)

Comments: _____
_____

Final Decision	INCLUDE	Unclear	EXCLUDE
	☒	☐	☐

Fig. 42.1 Study inclusion form illustrating inclusion and exclusion criteria

Study Eligibility and Data Abstraction

Articles deemed potentially eligible for inclusion were reviewed and assessed according to predefined criteria (Fig. 42.1). Data were summarized in a table of evidence (Table 42.3) based on the type of study, patient demographics, type of benign CAO, stent type, length of follow up, and reported outcomes including benefits and harms [1–56]. Specific outcomes including performance status, lung function, quality of life, incidence of respiratory failure, need for repeat bronchoscopic

Table 42.3 PICO table of evidence summarizing original research articles on stent insertion for benign central airway obstruction for years 2004–2013

Reference	Study design	Patients (indications)/follow up time	Type of intervention/comparison	Primary outcome	Adverse events/risk factors	Evidence quality
Redmond et al. [1]	Retro; case series	N = 22 lung **transplant** BM; BS Mean 285 days	Metallic stents (N = 43) via rigid bronch Comparison: none	42 % (18/43) complications 9 % (4/43) required stent removal	Stent collapse, fracture, migration, granulation tissue, and coughing up pieces of stent	Very low
Terra et al. [2]	Retro; cohort study	N = 92 with benign, **inoperable TS** Mean 34.3 +/– 33.9 months	T tubes Dumon stents Y stents Comparison: none	Successful decannulation (no need for intervention for >6 months) achieved in 19/92	Tracheostomy before stent : threefold increase in the likelihood of the patient remaining with a tracheal stent	Low
Chen et al. [3]	Case series	N = 21 with **PITS**; 20 pts had stent removal Median for stent placement = 5 months	Covered SEMS (N = 27) inserted fluoroscopically CT and bronch follow up Comparison: none	Improved airway patency, FEV1 and Hugh-Jones classification of greater than one grade post stent removal	Complications in 19 (91 %): granulation tissue formation (n = 18), stent migration and stent expectoration (n = 2), mucus plugging (n = 1), and halitosis (n = 6)	Very low
Verma et al. [4]	Retro; case series	N = 17 inoperable, **post TB stenosis** Median 72 months (12–114)	Silicone stents (N stent) Comparison: none	Increase in the FEV1% and FVC% (Δ26.5 % and Δ16.5 %, respectively) in the long term; The median duration for which N-stents tolerated 7.9 (3–11) years	Granulation tissue formation (76 %), migration (70 %), and mucostasis (17 %)	Very low

(continued)

Table 42.3 (continued)

Reference	Study design	Patients (indications)/follow up time	Type of intervention/comparison	Primary outcome	Adverse events/risk factors	Evidence quality
Gallo et al. [5]	Retro; case series	N = 70 with **LTS**	T tube (either a single dilation or with endoscopic/open neck surgery)	77.1 % (54/70) were decannulated	13 % were decannulated after more than 5 surgical procedures; patients over 60 years of age and with a higher grade of stenosis had a significantly lower success rate	Very low
		Iatrogenic 55	Total of 257 surgeries	72.2 % underwent 3 or fewer surgical procedures; no significant correlation between the rate of decannulation and gender, etiology, site of stenosis or surgery		
		Post traumatic 11	Comparison: none			
		Others 4				
Jeong et al. [6]	Retro; case series	N = 30 patients with inoperable **post op stenosis** 19/30 (63 %) had stent placement	106 procedures (balloon, bouginage, Nd:YAG, and stent insertion)	37 % had stents removed at a median of 7 months after insertion	Stent-related late complications (70 %): restenosis (43 %), granulation tissue (33 %), migration (32 %), mucostasis (30 %), and malacia after stent removal (16 %)	Very low
		Median 34 months	Follow up bronch			
			Comparison: N/A			
Lim et al. [7]	Retro, case series	N = 55 patients with **inoperable PITS**	Silicone stent placement after laser and mechanical dilation	Stent removal in 40 % of the patients after median 12 months	The stent could be removed in those pts without cardiac disease ((OR) = 12.195] and the intervention was performed within 6 months after intubation (OR = 13.029)	Very low
		Median 12 months	Comparison: none	In 60 %, surgery was needed after initial stabilization		

Chen and Ruan [8]	Retro; case series N = 13 pts with **LTS**; 9 with 1 stent; 4 with two stents Follow up: N/R	Nickel-titanium alloy stent (SEMS) Comparison: none	Glottic and/or subglottic extension of cervical tracheal stenosis (n=6), new tracheal stricture (n=4), severe left bronchial stricture with massive left pulmonary collapse (n=1), and cervical tracheoesophageal fistula (n=2)	6 patients with glottic and/or subglottic to cervical tracheal stenosis underwent successful laryngotracheal reconstruction; 1 patient with tracheoesophageal fistula died from massive hemorrhage and asphyxiation induced by the stent	Very low
Lari et al. [9]	Retro; case series N = 12 pts with **post transplant airway complications** (BI stenosis or malacia) Follow up: N/R	T-Tube in BI Comparison: N/A	FEV_1 improved post stent placement	Migration (33 %)	Very low
Perotin et al. [10]	Retro; case series N = 23 pts with weblike (61 %) or complex (39 %) **TS**, located in the upper part of the trachea Follow up: 41±34 months post treatment	Stent placement (18 %): 2 for weblike and 2 for complex strictures when the stricture was at 3 +/−1 cm below the cords Comparison: N/A	Recurrences were frequent (30 % at 6 months, 59 % at 2 years, and 87 % at 5 years) with a delay of 14+/−16 months N = 2 recurred in the stent group (50 %)	No correlation between the risk or the number of recurrence and the type (weblike versus complex), the severity of obstruction, the height of stenosis (<1 cm versus >1 cm), the distance from the vocal cords or the endoscopic treatment performed	Very low
Lim et al. [11]	Retro; case series N = 71 pts with **Post TB** stenosis Median 12.5 months	Silicone stents Comparison: none	Stent removal in 40/71 pts at a median of 12.5 months; in 27, stent was re-inserted; 4 had surgery	Predictors of successful stent removal: atelectasis <1 month before bronchoscopic intervention, and absence of complete lobar atelectasis	Very low

(continued)

Table 42.3 (continued)

Reference	Study design	Patients (indications)/follow up time	Type of intervention/comparison	Primary outcome	Adverse events/risk factors	Evidence quality
Chung et al. [12]	Retro; cohort study	N = 72 with **benign** and 77 with malignant **CAO**: 429 days for the benign group	SEMS (N = 116) placed for benign disorders Comparison: none	Symptoms improved more after SEMS insertion for benign than in malignant disease (76.7 % vs. 51.6 %; p < 0.0001)	Complication rate after SEMS in patients with benign conditions was higher than that in patients with malignancy (42.2 % vs. 21.1 %; p = 0.001)	Low
Fernandez-Bussy et al. [13]	Retro; cohort study	N = 223 pts with 345 anastomoses N = 70 (20.23 %) anastomoses complications **post transplant** Follow up: N/R	Stent insertion after failed balloon dilation N = 631 bronchoscopic interventions in 52 pts N = 33 had BS and BM N = 18 with BS N = 47 had stent placement Comparison: none	FEV1 improved post stent insertion	Granulation 57.3 % of patients	Low
Charokopos et al. [14]	Retro; case series	N = 12 with **PTTS** 3 with subglottic stenosis Follow up: 6–96 months	SEMS in 11pts; follow up bronchoscopy and CT Comparison: none	Immediate improvement in all 11/12 pts	2 migration post procedure 4 granulation tissue 12–43 months requiring electrocautery or tracheostomy	Very low
Tan et al. [15]	Retro; case series	N = 3 pts with **post transplant BI** strictures Follow up: N/R	SEMS (covered) n = 6 Comparison: none	5/6 migrated immediately post placement Secretions in 6/6	Stent retrieval successful in 3/5	Very low
Fruchter et al. [16]	Retro; case series	N = 24/305 (7.8 %) pts with **post transplant** BM and BS Follow up: 30 months	SEMS retrieval via flexible bronch using moderate sedation Comparison: none	25 % required stent removal due to granulation and obstruction by mucus	Stent was removed in 5/6 patients	Very low

Yu et al. [17]	Retro; case series N=32 pts with **TS** Median 865 days	SEMS follow up with CT (3D recon) Comparison: none	17/32 had stent fracture detected by 3D recon CT	Fracture of SEMS can be predicted by CT measurements	Very low
Alazemi et al. [18]	Retro; case series N=46 pts with SEMS; 80 % were for **benign CAO** Mean in situ SEMS 292 days	SEMS removal (N=55) Comparison: none	Median no of removal procedures/encounter = 1 Median no of total procedures/encounter = 2 Hospitalization and ICU admission in 78 % and 39 % of the encounters with a median length of stay of 3.5 and 0 days, respectively	The estimated median total cost per encounter to remove the stents was $10,700 The measured outcomes were statistically significantly better when in situ stent duration was < or = 30 days ($P<0.05$)	Very low
Kim et al. [19]	Retro; case series N=41 pts with **TS** Follow up: N/R	T tube placement Comparison: none	Successful decannulation Age, sex, and multiplicity and severity of stenoses were not significantly related to successful decannulation	Predictors of decannulation failure: The longitudinal extent of stenosis and greater circumferential involvement	Very low
Chung et al. [20]	Retro; case series N=67 pts with **benign TS and TM** Median = 106 days	SEMS placement (N=75) Comparison: none	47.8 % had granulation Time to granulation tissue detection was shorter in patients with structural airway obstruction before SEMS implantation (structural airway obstruction vs. dynamic collapse airway: median (IQR) 95 (38–224, n=26] vs. 396 days (73–994, n=9]; $P=0.02$)	Structural airway obstruction prior to SEMS implantation predicts obstructive granulation tissue formation after SEMS implantation (odds ratio: 3.84; 95 % CI: 1.01–8.7; $P=0.04$)	Very low

(continued)

Table 42.3 (continued)

Reference	Study design	Patients (indications)/follow up time	Type of intervention/comparison	Primary outcome	Adverse events/risk factors	Evidence quality
Melkane et al. [21]	Retro; cohort study	N = 33 consecutive patients with **Post intubation LTS**; The endoscopic candidates were chronically ill patients presenting with simple, strictly TS not exceeding 4 cm in length Follow up: 6 months	N = 19 endoscopic treatments Stents were placed if the stenosis was associated with TM or exceeded 2 cm in total length Comparison: N = 14 surgical treatment: healthy patients presenting with complex TS, subglottic involvement or associated TM	50 % of the patients were decannulated in the surgically treated group versus 84.2 % in the endoscopically treated group (p = 0.03)	In the surgically treated group, 2/14 patients needed more than one procedure versus 8/19 patients in the endoscopically treated group	Low
Rahman et al. [22]	Retro; case series	N = 115 pts with **benign TS** due to **PTTS** (N = 76) **PTTS** (N = 30), Wegener's granulomatosis (N = 2), sarcoidosis (N = 2), amyloidosis (N = 2) and **ITS** (N = 3) Stent was placed in 33 pts of whom 28 also underwent brachytherapy Median 51 months	Flexible bronchoscopy balloon dilatation and laser treatment (N = 98) Comparison: none	The overall success rate was 87 %	26 % died, mostly due to exacerbation of their underlying conditions	Very low
Ko et al. [23]	Retro; case series	N = 55 procedures for **TS** Follow up: N/R	T tubes N = 46 Dumon silicone stent N = 9 Comparison: none	Granulation (23 procedures, 41.82 %)	The granulation complication rate was higher in those with a stent-to-vocal fold distance of <10 mm	Very low

Study	Design	Population	Intervention	Results	Complications	Quality
Nam et al. [24]	Retro; case series	N=11 pts with carinal stenosis included **post TB stricture** in 7 pts (64 %), **PITS** in 2 (18 %), postoperative **TM** in 2 (18 %). Median duration of stent placement=439 days	Balloon dilation; Nd:YAG laser resection, or bougienation (by rigid bronchoscopy) to dilate the airway, followed by placement of the Natural Y stent. Comparison: none	100 % subjective symptomatic relief immediately after stent placement	No procedurally related deaths or immediate major complications occurred. Stent-related late complications included granulation (64 %) and mucostasis (18 %)	Very low
Fernandez-Bussy et al. [25]	Retro; cohort study	N=24 consecutive pts with **post transplant bronchial anastomoses complications** **BS** in 12, bronchomalacia in 12, BS plus **BM** in 20, and partial bronchial dehiscence in 5	SEMS N=49 (hybrid) via flexible bronchoscopy. Adjunctive procedures included EC in 1, balloon dilatation in 7, and EC plus balloon dilatation in 4. Comparison: none	The average degree of stenosis decreased from 80 % to 20 %. The average increase was 0.28 L in FVC and 0.44 l in FEV_1	Complications included granulation in 10 stents, migration in 9, mucus in 2, and fracture in 3	Low
Abi-Jaoudeh et al. [26]	Retro; case series	N=41 pts with **post transplant BS**. 10–40 months	Stent placed when balloon dilation failed; 56 % received a stent because of balloon dilation failure or stenosis recurrence. Comparison: balloon dilation	After the first treatment, airway patency was higher in patients treated with stents (71 %) than in those who underwent bronchoplasty (19 %) ($P=0.037$). Airway patency: 40 months for stented strictures versus 10 months for strictures treated with bronchoplasty ($P<0.02$). Dyspnea and cough were improved after intervention ($P<0.001$), and FEV_1 was improved by 17 % ($P<0.00003$) at last follow-up	Mean survival in patients with stents was longer than that in those who underwent bronchoplasty (82 vs 22 months, respectively) stent insertion: associated with a 66 % reduction in the risk of death ($P<0.02$)	Low

(continued)

Table 42.3 (continued)

Reference	Study design	Patients (indications)/follow up time	Type of intervention/ comparison	Primary outcome	Adverse events/risk factors	Evidence quality
Gottlieb et al. [27]	Retro; cohort study	N=65 (9.2 %) out of 706 lung transplant	111 (91 % uncovered) SEMS were inserted a median (range) 133 (55–903) days after lung transplantation	Clinical improvement in 80 % of pts	Re-stenosis occurred in 34 (52 %) out of 65 pts at 85 (7–629) days after insertion	Very low
		Recipients with **post transplant BS**	Comparison: none	The FEV_1 increased by 21+/–33 % (mean +/– SD)	Stent insertion before post-operative day 90 was independently associated with an increased risk of re-stenosis (HR 3.29, 95 % CI 1.50–7.18; p=0.003); 40 % of pts had new bacterial airway colonization after SEMS insertion	
		777 (7–3.655) days			In SEMS patients, 5-year survival was significantly lower than in the total cohort (60 % versus 76 %; p=0.02)	
Park et al. [28]	Retro; case series	N=32 pts with **PITS**	Silicone stent (N stent)	100 % symptomatic and spirometric improvement without immediate complications	Late complications were migration (34 %), mucostasis (31 %), granulation (38 %) and re-stenosis (40 %)	Very low
		Median 22 months	Nd:YAG laser, ballooning or bougienage was followed by N stent insertion	Removal of the stent without re-stenosis was successful in 38 % of pts at a median time of 7 months after insertion		
			Comparison: none	The stent could not be removed or needed reinsertion in 31 % of patients; 16 % of pts had surgery after initial stenting		

Carretta et al. [29]	Retro; cohort study	N = 75 pts with **benign TS** complex lesions or comorbidities N = 7 had undergone unsuccessful treatment with Dumon stents Follow up: 5 years	T-tube in 51 pts with contraindication to surgery (group I), a temporary measure in 15 pts prior to surgery (group II), and in 9 pts (group III) for complications of airway reconstruction Comparison: none	In group I, the T-tube was removed in 24 % of pts after 35.3 +/− 8.2 months following resolution of the stenosis In group II, the T-tubes were maintained in place before surgery for 17.1 +/− 4.8 months In group III, 3 stents were removed following tracheal healing after 115.3 +/− 3.7 months After 5 years the stents were in place in 82 %, 7 % and 100 % of the pts, respectively in groups I, II and III	Migration in 3 (4 %) pts, granulation in 14 (19 %), subglottic edema in 3 (4 %), and mucus retention in 7 (9 %); Treatment of complications (tracheostomy cannula, steroid infiltration, Argon/laser coagulation bronchoscopy) was required in 27 % of pts	Low
Dooms et al. [30]	Retro; case series	N = 17 pts with 10 stents were deployed in a structural **PITS** Other indications were multinodular goiter, anastomotic stricture, **Post TB stenosis**, damaged cartilage and relapsing polychondritis Follow up: 12 weeks	7 Silmet, 8 Alveolus stents Comparison: none	Short-term (<12 weeks after stent deployment) complication rate was 75 %, requiring stent removal in 60 %	Migration 65 % Stent fracture 15 % Shriveling of the stent in 10 % Granulation 10 %	Very low

(continued)

Table 42.3 (continued)

Reference	Study design	Patients (indications)/follow up time	Type of intervention/ comparison	Primary outcome	Adverse events/risk factors	Evidence quality
Thistlethwaite et al. [31]	Retro, cohort study	N = 20/240 (8.3 %) pts with **post transplant BS** (>50 % narrowing) Follow up: 4.9 +/− 3.5 years after stent removal	Dilation and silicone stent placement Comparison: none	The mean time to diagnosis of BS was 81.5 +/− 26.9 days Airway patency and symptom improvement in 18/20 pts N = 16 pts were able to have their stents removed at a mean of 362.3 +/− 126.4 days with permanent resolution of airway stenosis; Overall survival was similar for patients with and without BS	Pulmonary aspergillosis and pseudomonal infection, age less than 45 years, and early rejection correlated with BS; ischemic time, side of transplant, and preoperative disease did not	Low
Galluccio et al. [32]	Retro; cohort study	N = 209 consecutive pts with **PITS** (N = 167) and **PTTS** (N = 34) 8 other benign TS Follow up: 2 years	Mechanical dilatation, laser resection and placement of a silicone stent Comparison: none	Simple stenoses (N = 167) treated by 346 endoscopic procedures (mean of 2.07/patient), 16 stents and 1 end-to-end anastomosis N = 38 granulomas treated by 59 procedures (1.56/patient) N = 97 concentrical stenoses by 228 procedures (2.35/patient) and 32 web-like lesions with 59 operative endoscopies (1.84/ patient) Overall success rate was 96 %	Among the 42 complex stenoses, 9 were immediately treated by surgical resection and the remaining 33 lesions underwent 123 endoscopic procedures (3.27/patient), with 34 stents and 1 end-to-end anastomosis subsequent to recurrence after stent removal In this group the success rate was 69 %	Low

Shlomi et al. [33]	Cohort study	N = 19 pts with benign obstructions and 11 with **post transplant stenosis** on immunosuppressive therapy Follow up: 2 years	SEMS in transplant Comparison: SEMS in other benign strictures	Granulation was significantly lower in the transplant recipients than in the non-transplant pts at 3, 15 and 18 months	Transplant recipients underwent significantly fewer laser resections and brachytherapy treatments for stent granulation	Low
Chan et al. [34]	Retro; case series	N = 35 pts with **inoperable benign CAO** Follow up: N/R	82 SEMS (67 % Ultraflex, 33 % Wallstent) Comparison: none	83 % of patients showed immediate symptomatic improvement Reversible complications developed in 9 % of pts within 24 h of stent placement	Late complications (>24 h) occurred in 77 % of pts, of which 37 % were significant or required a procedure; migration (12.2 %), fracture (19.5 %), or granulomas (24.4 %) The overall granuloma rate of 57 % was higher at tracheal sites (59 %) than bronchial ones (34 %), but not significantly different between Ultraflex and Wallstents Wallstents were associated with higher rates of bleeding (5 % vs. 30 %, $p=0.005$) and migration (7 % vs. 26 %, $p=0.026$)	Very low
Murgu et al. [35]	Retro; case series	N = 15 with **TBM and EDAC** Mean 188 days	Silicone stents Comparison: none	Mean functional class and severity and extent of airway collapse significantly improved within 48 h after treatment ($p<0.05$) Stent-related complications within 48 h after stent insertion occurred in 3 patients (1 granulation, 1 migration, and 1 mucus plugging)	N = 26 stent-related complications (12 mucus plugs, 8 migrations, and 6 granulation tissues) were seen in 10 of the 12 patients No perioperative deaths	Very low

(continued)

Table 42.3 (continued)

Reference	Study design	Patients (indications)/follow up time	Type of intervention/comparison	Primary outcome	Adverse events/risk factors	Evidence quality
Terra et al. [36]	Prospective case series	N=16 pts with **inoperable** **TS** secondary to **PTTS** (n=12), neoplasia (n=3), or Wegener's granulomatosis (n=1) Mean 7.45 months	Polyflex (Self-expanding stent made of polyester mesh with silicon coating) via suspension laryngoscopy Comparison; none	Symptoms resolved in 100 % of pts Immediate postoperative complications were dysphonia (n=2, 12.5 %) and odynophagia (n=2 12.5 %)	Late complications were cough (n=10, 62.5 %), migration (n=7, 43.75 %), granuloma (in n=2, 12.5 %), and pneumonia (n=1 6.25 %)	Very low
Ernst et al. [37]	Prospective, observational	N=58 pts with **TBM** Follow up: 10–14 days	Rigid bronchoscopy with silicone stent placement Comparison: none	45 of 58 pts, symptomatic improvement; quality of life scores improved in 19 of 27 patients (p=0.002) Dyspnea scores improved in 22 of 24 patients (p=0.001); functional status scores improved in 18 of 26 patients (p=0.002)	N=49 complications: 21 partial stent obstructions, 14 infections, and 10 stent migrations	Low
Cavaliere et al. [38]	Retro; cohort study	N=73 pts with **PITS** Granulomas, pseudoglottic stenosis excluded 13 (18 %) web-like and 60 (82 %) complex stenoses Follow up: 28–78 months	LAMD and stent insertion Comparison: none	Web-like stenoses were successfully treated with LAMD alone; for complex stenoses LAMD was sufficient to treat 13 pts (22 %); 47 pts (78 %) required stent placement: N=22 had their stent removed after 1 year and did not require any further therapy, 13 inoperable pts required permanent stent and 12 were referred to surgery after failure of multiple endoscopic treatments	No permanent complications due to endoscopic treatment; 48 patients (66 %) received a stable, good result with the endoscopic procedure, 13 (18 %) required a permanent stent while 12 patients (16 %) were referred to surgery	Very low

Study	Study type	Population / Follow-up	Stent type / Comparison	Results	Complications	Quality
Kapoor et al. [39]	Retrospective case series	N = 25 transplant pts requiring stent insertion for 27 **post transplant** airway complications (9 **BM** and 12 **BS**, 3 **BS with BM** and 3 dehiscence); Follow up: 1–69 months	SEMS; Comparison: none	Technical success was 100 %; 84 % of pts had immediate relief in dyspnea; The mean percentage change in FEV_1 and FVC at 12 months was not significant	The overall complication rate following stent placement was 0.049 per patient per month (23 complications/471 patient months); Migration and granulation: the most frequent complications	Very low
Kim et al. [40]	Retro; case series	N = 24 pts with **benign CAO** requiring 30 stents; Mean 24 months	Covered SEMS under fluoro; Comparison: none	A high symptomatic recurrence rate of 62.5 % was found after stent removal; Granulation, migration, and bronchial obstruction of the left upper lobe occurred in 36.7 %, 13.3 %, and 3.3 % of pts, respectively	Duration of stent placement (p = 0.002) and the occurrence of granulation (p = 0.026) were associated with maintained patency after temporary stenting	Very low
Gildea et al. [41]	Retrospective case series	N = 12 pts with 16 stents; **post transplantation BS** (4); **TS** (3); **TBM** (2); chondroplastica (1); relapsing polychondritis (1); bronchopleural fistula (1); Follow up: N/R	Polyflex stent self-expanding, thin-walled, silicone stent; Comparison: none	Immediate palliation was established in most cases (90 %); Incidence of complications was 75 %; The complication rate was 100 % in pts with BS	Migration was the most common complication, with time to the event ranging from <24 h to 7 months. N = 1 stent was expectorated within <24 h; N = 1 patient coughed up a portion of the stent; Emergent bronchoscopy was required in 4 patients for mucous impaction	Very low

(continued)

Table 42.3 (continued)

Reference	Study design	Patients (indications)/follow up time	Type of intervention/comparison	Primary outcome	Adverse events/risk factors	Evidence quality
Cheng and Kao [42]	Prospective case series	N=9 pts with **PITS** Mean 18.6 months	Bougienage, followed by SEMS insertion 2 bare metal 7 covered stents Comparison: none	100 % successful discharge back to the chronic care unit	N=2 episodes of granulation in one bare-stent patient and in one coated-stent patient, respectively In another covered SEMS patient, complications arose from a broken stent	Low
Ryu et al. [43]	Retro; case series	N=94 pts required stents for **post-TB stenosis** (74 %), **PITS** (21 %) Follow up: 42 months	N=100 stents (43 Dumon and 57 Natural) Comparison: Dumon vs. Natural stent	Dyspnea improved in pts who underwent Dumon (90 %) and Natural (86 %) stenting Stents could be successfully removed in pts who underwent Dumon (54 %) or Natural (49 %)	Similar complications rates for the two stents	Low
Ryu et al. [44]	Retro; case series	N=75/80 pts with **post TB stenosis** after failed dilation required stent Median 41 months	Ballooning, Nd:YAG laser resection and/or bougienation as first-line methods of dilatation Silicone stents Comparison: none	88 % of the pts had symptoms and lung function improvement Stents could be removed successfully in 65 % pts at a median of 14 months	Acute complications included: excessive bleeding (1); pneumothorax (5); and pneumomediastinum without mortality (2) Migration (51 %), granuloma (49 %), mucostasis (19 %) and re-stenosis (40 %)	

Madden et al. [45]	Retro; case series	N=31 TBM (n=7), PTTS (n=8), posttracheostomy rupture (n=2), post pneumonectomy bronchopleural fistula (n=2), stricture post transplant (n=3), lobectomy (n=3), post TB, traumatic injury to right main bronchus (n=1 patient each), extrinsic compression Follow up: 1 week to 96 months	Rigid bronchoscopy with SEMS (Ultraflex) Comparison: none	Complications included granulation (11) treated with Nd: YAG laser, migration (1); stent removed, another deployed, metal fatigue (1), stent removal (1), mucus plugging (2), halitosis (6)	N=13 patients died of unrelated causes between 1 week and 15 months after stent deployment	Very low
Thornton et al. [46]	Retro; case series	N=40 pts with benign stenosis included post transplant BS (n=13), PTTS (n=10), inflammation (n=6), TBM (n=4), infection (n=3), and extrinsic compression (n=4) Follow up: 6–2,473 days	SEMS Comparison: none	Symptoms improved in 39/40 cases Survival at 1, 2, 3, 4, 5, and 6 years was 79, 76, 51, 47, 38, and 23 %, respectively Loss of patency was most rapid during the 1st year With repeat intervention, patency was 90 % at 6.8 years	N=18 had died of comorbid causes, 1 had died of uncertain causes, 3 had undergone subsequent airway surgery, 2 had undergone airway stent retrieval, and 2 was lost to follow-up	Very low
Noppen et al. [47]	Retro; cohort study	N=15 pts with benign CAO and respiratory failure TM, PTTS, extrinsic compression intrathoracic (substernal) goiter and post-pneumonectomy syndrome with BM and obstruction of left main bronchus Follow up: 1–54 months	Rigid bronchoscopy, dilatation and Dumon and SEMS (covered Ultraflex) Offered for surgery refusal, medical or surgical inoperability, or absence of alternative treatment options Comparison: none	93.3 % were successfully and permanently extubated/decanulated immediately after the bronchoscopy	Minor complications occurred in 6 patients (40 %) leading to a second intervention, managed bronchoscopically, long-term follow up was uneventful	Very low

(continued)

Table 42.3 (continued)

Reference	Study design	Patients (indications)/follow up time	Type of intervention/comparison	Primary outcome	Adverse events/risk factors	Evidence quality
Eller et al. [48]	Retro; case series	N=16 pts with benign **TS** (81 % **PITS**) Mean follow up 20 months	N=26 SEMS Comparison: none	Each stent remained functional for an average of 12.4 months	87 % had a complication that required surgical intervention to maintain patent airway; granulation causing restenosis (81 %), and 5 pts (31 %) required tracheotomy as a result of restenosis around the stent; N=14 of the stents (56 %) were removed or expelled from the patients	Very low
Marel et al. [49]	Prospective case series	N=80 pts with benign TS (62 **PITS** and **PITS**) 18 others N=38 surgery; 42 interventional bronchoscopy with stent Follow up: N/R	Nd-YAG laser, EC, stent Comparison: surgery	8/42 surgical patients had recurrence; 2 reoperation; 6 interventional bronchoscopy; For 35/42, interventional bronchoscopy was successful The median survival=9 months	N=65 patients were alive at the time of evaluation, 15 patients died; N=5 died from a disease other than airway stenosis; N=10 non-resected pts died, with 1 exception, due to a disease other than airway stenosis	Low
Lunn et al. [50]	Retro; case series	N=25 pts with SEMS requiring removal 80 % **benign CAO** Follow up: N/R	Rigid bronchoscopy and SEMS removal Comparison: none	N=30 SEMS successfully removed	Complications were as follows: retained stent pieces (n=7), mucosal tear with bleeding (n=4), re-obstruction requiring temporary silicone stent placement (n=14), need for postoperative mechanical ventilation (n=6), and tension pneumothorax (n=1)	Very low

Noppen et al. [51]	Retro; case series	N = 39 pts with **benign CAO**; stent removal for excessive or recurrent granulation (n = 5), recurrence of stenosis after stent failure (n = 1), stent fracture (n = 2), and end of treatment (n = 2) Follow up: 16.2 +/− 17.5 months duration of stent placement prior to removal	N = 10 of 39 pts (25.6 %), bearing 12 covered stents, presented with an indication for stent removal Comparison: none	Removal was successful without major complications	No complications	Very low
Ciccone et al. [52]	Retro; case series	N = 18 pts with **subglottic stenosis (SGS)** Follow up: 2–9 years	N = 4 pts (Group I) had laser and stenting by a Dumon stent as the only treatment N = 6 had laser and stenting followed after 1–6 months by laryngotracheal resection (Group II) N = 8 surgery (Group III) Comparison: Laser and stent vs surgery	In Group I, 1 patient required repositioning of the stent and in 2 the stent was removed; 2 pts died of their underlying disease; at a follow-up of 2–9 years pts required aerosolized therapy and periodical bronchoscopy In Group II, there were 2 wound infections	In Group III, 2 pts developed anastomotic postoperative stenosis, treated by laser (2) and stenting (1), and 1 patient with previous tracheostomy had a wound infection Overall, in the 14 surgical patients (Groups II and III) stenosis occurred in 14.2 % and infection in 21.3 %. After a follow up of 15 months to 12 years, all surgical patients breathe and speak well	Very low

(continued)

Table 42.3 (continued)

Reference	Study design	Patients (indications)/follow up time	Type of intervention/comparison	Primary outcome	Adverse events/risk factors	Evidence quality
Low et al. [53]	Retro cohort study	N=21 consecutive patients with **post TB stenosis** trachea and mainstem bronchus (not suitable for surgery) Median 25 months	Rigid bronchoscopy with Dumon stent after dilation and NdYAG laser Comparison: none	All pts had immediate symptomatic improvement	Repeat procedures in 19 % of patients for stent related complications	Low
Sesterhenn et al. [54]	Retro; case series	N=11 pts with **PITS** (6), **PTTS** (4) and chondropathia (1) Mean follow up 67.5 weeks	SEMS under flouroscopy Comparison: none	52 % (11 out of 21) remained asymptomatic No immediate complications	N=1 recurrent dyspnea 3 months after implantation and N=1 granulation	Very low
Pereszlenyi et al. [55]	Retro; cohort study	N=163 pts with **PTTS** and **PITS** in 111 cases Follow up: 2–18 months	Segmental tracheal resection in 87 cases, stenting in 68 cases (modified T-tube in 65 cases and by other traditiional stents in 3) Comparison: surgery and stents	N=27 pts (41.6 %) were successfully treated by T tube modality	Segmental tracheal resection (n=87) was successful in almost all the cases (96 %)	Low
Noppen et al. [56]	Retro; cohort study	N=30 consecutive pts with **inoperable benign** 17 and malignant 13 **thyroid disease** due to **TM, extrinsic compression**, and/or tracheal ingrowth Follow up: 46.4+/−34.4 months	Dilatation, stenting and/or Nd-YAG laser N=21 stents in 17 pts with benign disease; Stent types included silicone stents (Dumon, Tygon-Noppen) and SEMS (Ultraflex) Comparison: none	In the benign group, immediate (100 % relief of dyspnea) and long-term (88 % relief of dyspnea) after airway stenting (21 stents used in 17 patients) No procedure related complications	There was one unrelated death 1 week after stenting There were 6 % and 30 % short-term and long-term complications, respectively; these could be managed bronchoscopically	Low

BI bronchus intermedius, *BM* bronchomalacia, *BS* bronchial stenosis, *TS* tracheal stenosis, *PITS* post intubation tracheal stenosis, *TB* tuberculosis, *LTS* laryngotracheal stenosis, *CAO* central airway obstruction, *Nd:YAG* neodymium-yttrium aluminum garnet, *LAMD* laser-assisted mechanical dilation, *PTTS* post intubation tracheal stenosis, *PTTS* post tracheostomy tracheal stenosis, *ITS* idiopathic tracheal stenosis, *Retro* retrospective, *N/R* not reported, *N/A* not available, *SEMS* Self-expendable metallic stent, *OR* odds ratio, *hrs* hours, *pts* patients, *EC* electrocautery

procedures, and survival were included when available. The population of interest for this systematic review was adult patients. Stent insertion options included silicone, metal and hybrid stents inserted using rigid, flexible bronchoscopic and fluoroscopic techniques.

Study Quality and Statistical Analysis

The GRADE system was applied to assess the quality of the evidence. Odds ratios, median values and ranges for summary statistics are reported, when available, based on information provided in each of the original studies. Because of the heterogeneity in outcome measures and populations studied, and because a few studies provided raw data that would be necessary for quantitative synthesis, no attempt was made to pool data across studies.

Results

A total of 1,523 abstracts were generated from the search for possible inclusion in the final review. An analysis of these abstracts detected 150 potentially relevant original research articles; these articles were reviewed and included in the table of evidence if found relevant. Studies limited to a few patients with benign CAO, those studying devices no longer available on the market, those with poorly defined or unclear outcomes were not included in the table of evidence. Although the published literature from 1990 to 2013 was reviewed and taken into account for providing the recommendations, Table 42.3 summarizes the original articles addressing the role of stent insertion for patients with benign CAO published between 2004 and 2013. The vast majority of the studies were retrospective case series or cohort studies without a comparison and thus of very low and low quality. The literature search identified a few reports on stent insertion for strictures due to granulomatosis with polyangiitis (former Wegener's granulomatosis), amyloidosis, sarcoidosis, ulcerative colitis, or Klebsiella rhinoscleromatis infection; there are rare reports on the role of stent insertion for extrinsic compression from benign mediastinal adenopathy, cysts, vascular abnormalities and for recurrent respiratory papillomatosis. The evidence is anecdotal, however, and no recommendation can be provided for these entities. The vast majority of studies described the role of stent insertion for symptomatic PITS/PTTS and transplant-related strictures not amenable to open surgical interventions. Few studies reported on the role of stent insertion for post TB strictures, idiopathic tracheal stenosis (ITS) or laryngotracheal stenosis (LTS) and pure extrinsic compression due to benign thyroid disease. The evidence for stent insertion is summarized the based on specific etiology.

Tracheal Stenosis (Post Intubation and Post Tracheostomy)

Straight Silicone Stents

Because of their easy removability, silicone stents are preferable in benign tracheal stenosis (TS). Evidence suggests that for PITS and PTTS, stent placement should be considered only in inoperable symptomatic patients. Stricture extent and morphology impact management. Both surgery and bronchoscopy improve functional outcomes if the treatment strategy is based on predefined objective criteria [21]. For example, a simple web-like stricture (vertical extent <1 cm), without chondritis which is dilated and without recurrence will not require a stent; a complex stricture (defined as extensive scar >1 cm in vertical length) however, often has associated chondritis, and because the cartilaginous frame is affected, dilation alone is not successful in restoring airway patency long term and thus a stent would be required in nonsurgical candidates [32]. Some authors suggest that the bronchoscopic treatment of PITS can be considered a safe first-line therapy, leaving selected cases and the recurrent strictures for surgical resection. Stent-related complications, however, are not uncommon (>30 %) and include migration, obstruction from secretions, infection and significant granulation tissue formation at the proximal or distal extremities of the stent. Thus curative open surgery is preferable but not always feasible. In a study of 42 patients with complex strictures, only 9 were surgical candidates; 33 patients were treated with silicone stent insertion, with a success rate of 69 % [32]. Maintained airway patency after stent removal in complex stenosis (usually after at least 6 months) is reportedly low (17.6 %) suggesting the need for long-term indwelling airway stent in this patient population. A higher rate of airway stability after stent removal (46.8 %), however, has been reported when stents remained in place for a longer period of time (mean of 11.6 months), with more than 50 % of patients having their stents in place for more than 12 months. While several silicone stent designs have been described, the most commonly used straight silicone stent for PITS and PTTS is the studded silicone stent (Dumon type) (Table 42.3).

Silicone T-Tubes (Montgomery T Tubes)

T-tubes are warranted in the few patients with critical airway narrowing who are neither candidates for surgery or indwelling airway stent insertion or who develop recurrence or complications after such interventions. In a case series of 53 patients with complex tracheal stenosis (N=24 PTTS), T-tube insertion was considered effective in 70 % of patients [57]. Risks factors for T-tube induced granulation tissue include the sharp edge of the proximal aspect of the T tube, suboptimal tracheostomy tract (i.e. non-midline stoma), and placement within 0.5–1 cm from the vocal cords [57]. The longitudinal (vertical) extent and the circumferential involvement of stenosis were found to negatively correlate with successful T-tube decannulation. Treatment of complications including tracheostomy, steroid infiltration, argon/laser coagulation may be required in approximately one fourth of patients with T-tubes. Some physicians perform 3–4 biweekly follow up bronchoscopies in patients with T-tubes, followed by once every 4 weeks once good stent patency has been documented [29, 57].

Self-Expandable Metallic Stents (SEMS)

The SEMS brands studied to date are to be avoided, if possible, in benign TS. Immediate symptomatic improvement is expected, but the long-term complications are common and may be life threatening [58]. A stent fracture rate of ~50 % (detected by CT scanning) was observed after a median of 2.5 years of follow up in one case series. SEMS placement for benign disease continues to be reported even after the US Food and Drug Administration warned against their use in 2005 [58]. While bronchoscopic removal of SEMS is feasible, it could be associated with significant complications and health care-related costs [18]. In one series using fully covered SEMS, the short-term (<12 weeks after stent insertion) complication rate was 75 %, requiring stent removal in 60 %. Overall, stent migration was observed in 65 %, stent fracture in 15 % and granulation formation in 10 % of patients. The reproducible evidence of high complications in benign disorders led many physicians abandon the use of SEMS (including the fully covered types) for benign airway strictures. In addition to potentially very rare fatal complications such as airway perforation and massive hemoptysis, a feared adverse event is the extension of benign inflammatory strictures induced by SEMS placement, which may preclude further surgical interventions. In one series, the Ultraflex and Wallstents were used in ten patients with PITS and five with other indications. Stricture and granulations within previously normal airway had developed in all patients after stent insertion, with new subglottic strictures resulting from the stent in four patients and esophago-respiratory fistula in another two patients. Primary surgical reconstruction, judged to have been possible before stent insertion in ten patients, was performed after stenting in only seven and failed in two. The authors of this study suggest that the studied generation of SEMS should be avoided in benign strictures [59]. In another case series, 87 % of patients had a complication that required surgical intervention to maintain a patent airway. Complications included granulation tissue formation at the ends of the stent causing restenosis (81 %), with 31 % of patients requiring tracheotomy as a result of restenosis around the stent [48].

Self-Expandable Silicone Stents

This type of stent (i.e. Polyflex) is easily inserted and removed and has been studied in benign CAO including TS and TBM [41]. While immediate symptom palliation was established in most cases, the incidence of complications was high (75 %) with stent migration occurring in 69 % of cases, especially in patients with PITS [41].

Tracheobronchomalacia (TBM)

The decision to insert an airway stent in TBM is complicated by the lack of standardized definitions and cut off values to define abnormal airway narrowing and by the lack of clear understanding if this entity is truly responsible for airflow limitation. EDAC, due to bulging of the posterior membrane within the airway lumen during exhalation in the presence of intact cartilage is not a true central airway disease. It is, however, often confused and treated as TBM with stenting or tracheoplasty.

Silicone Stents

The limited published evidence suggests that in the very short term (~2 weeks) quality of life (QOL) and functional status are improved in 70 % and dyspnea in 90 % of patients post stent insertion, but the lung function as measured by FEV_1 has not been consistently reported to improve after stent insertion or other forms of central airway stabilization (i.e. membranous tracheoplasty) [35, 37]. Stent-related complications in TBM include obstruction from mucus plugging and migration, and in one series, almost 10 % of patients had complications related to the bronchoscopic procedure itself [37]. Although not life threatening, these stent-related adverse events require multiple repeat bronchoscopies [35]. In one series, adverse effects from silicone stent insertion were very common with a total of 26 stent-related adverse events noted in 10 of 12 patients (83 %), a median of 29 days after intervention [35]. TBM due to relapsing polychondritis (RP) is one disease for which one or more stents are necessary due to a diffuse lack of airway cartilaginous support.

Self-Expandable Metallic Stents

There are several case series reporting on the use of SEMS for TBM. Airway patency and symptoms improve and in the short-term there are no major complications. There are reports, however, of patients who underwent insertion of one or more SEMS (Gianturco) stents for TBM and required removal within the first 6 months for stent-related complications including stent fracture [60].

Idiopathic Tracheal Stenosis (ITS)

In ITS the use of stent is mainly limited by the proximity of lesions to the vocal cords. Bronchoscopic management is a therapeutic option but long-term results are not well established. Laser assisted resection with or without stenting has been used as an alternative to surgery or optimize the timing of operation in patients with subglottic stenosis [61]. Although most studies support the use of surgery as the treatment of choice for ITS, some reports suggest bronchoscopy as the initial management, with open surgery by laryngoplasty or laryngotracheal resection and anastomosis being recommended for complex lesions longer than 1 cm and after repeated endoscopic failures [61].

Post Tuberculosis Tracheal and Bronchial Stenosis (Post TB Stenosis)

Silicone Stents

In a retrospective case series, the Natural airway stent (a type of silicone stent) was found to be as effective and safe as the Dumon stent for the management of 94 patients (of whom 74 % had post TB stenosis). Both stent types could be successfully removed in half of the patients during a 42-months follow-up period. Complication rates were similar in patients who underwent Dumon or Natural stenting [43]. These results seem to be reproducible. In another series of post TB stenosis, silicone stents were required in 75 out of 80 (94 %) patients to maintain airway patency and improve lung function. After a median of 14 months post insertion, 49 out of 75 (65 %) of patients had their stents successfully removed without difficulty. Stent-related late complications, such as migration (51 %), granuloma formation (49 %), mucostasis (19 %) and re-stenosis (40 %), were controllable with bronchoscopy during a median follow-up of 41 months.

Post Transplant Bronchial Stenosis (BS) and Bronchomalacia (BM)

Patients with airway complications after lung transplantation may have a higher mortality than patients without airway complications. A small number of patients with post transplant BS respond to dilatation alone and thus airway stenting may be warranted.

Self-Expandable Metallic Stents

Most studies for post transplant BS and BM used SEMS. Some centers and operators, however, are reluctant to use SEMS since their removal is sometimes needed, and may be difficult requiring the use of rigid bronchoscopy. In one study, re-stenosis occurred in 34 (52 %) out of 65 recipients at 85 days after insertion. Stent insertion before post-operative day 90 was independently associated with an increased risk of re-stenosis [27]. The complication rate after the use of hybrid SEMS (fully covered SEMS) in this population is comparable with other airway stents but this stent has the advantage of removability with flexible bronchoscopy. Clinical outcome and FEV$_1$ improve after SEMS placement and, in one series, longer survival and bronchial patency were observed after stent insertion. For bronchus intermedius strictures in lung transplant recipients, however, one series suggested that the use of covered SEMS may not offer a therapeutic advantage over balloon dilation alone.

Biodegradable Stents

Pilot studies suggest that biodegradable (polydioxanone) stents are a safe, effective and reliable alternative to metallic stents in patients with BS after lung transplantation, and may avoid the need for permanent stenting [62]. As of this writing, the experience with this type of stent is very limited.

Silicone Stents

For post-transplant BM and BS, silicone stent insertion after dilation may be a less traumatic alternative to SEMS insertion. Removal of these stents with long-term airway patency (mean follow-up of ~5 years after stent removal) was shown to be achievable in most lung transplant recipients with airway stenosis [31].

Extrinsic Compression from Benign Disorders

The most frequent cause of thyroid-induced airway obstruction is the presence of a substernal (benign or malignant) goiter compressing the trachea, with or without associated tracheomalacia. In patients with benign thyroid disease causing tracheal compression, stent placement can serve as an effective bridge to surgery. Immediate and long-term relief of dyspnea was achieved in 100 and 88 %, respectively. This series reports 6 and 30 % short-term and long-term complications, respectively, which could be managed by bronchoscopy. Bronchoscopic procedures including stenting may be valuable alternatives to surgery in inoperable thyroid-induced tracheal obstruction [51].

Summary of Recommendations

As evident in Table 42.3, most published studies are of very low-low quality mainly due to being retrospective, uncontrolled case series or cohort studies. For most disease entities addressed in this review, however, the benefits of stent insertion were considered to outweigh the risk of no intervention. For inoperable patients with symptomatic complex post intubation, post tracheostomy, and post tuberculosis tracheobronchial stenosis, silicone stent insertion is recommended to improve dyspnea. Stent removal should be considered after 6–12 months post insertion. T-tubes could be used for inoperable patients who are not candidates or develop complications after silicone stent insertion. For patients with symptomatic benign tracheobronchial strictures, metallic stent insertion is not recommended to improve dyspnea or quality of life. For patients with high tracheal stenosis or subglottic stenosis, metallic stents are contraindicated. For patients with severe, diffuse and symptomatic tracheobronchomalacia, silicone stent insertion is suggested to improve dyspnea and quality of life. Such stents may be used as a bridge to membranous tracheoplasty or as a definitive therapy in non-surgical candidates. For patients with tracheobronchomalacia, metallic stents are not recommended to improve dyspnea or quality of life. For patients with symptomatic post transplant anastomotic bronchial stenosis or malacia, stent insertion is recommended to improve lung function and dyspnea. Silicone stents may be preferred in these patients due to easy removability, and stent insertion is reserved for symptomatic patients who fail bronchoscopic dilation. For patients with symptomatic extrinsic tracheal obstruction due to compression by benign thyroid disease, stent insertion is recommended to improve dyspnea in inoperable patients. Silicone stents may be preferred to covered SEMS, and stent insertion may be considered prior to surgical resection.

A Personal View of the Data

Physiologic Basis

Stent insertion may be lifesaving and allows successful withdrawal from mechanical ventilation, hospitalization in a lower level of care environment, relief of symptoms, and extended survival in critically ill patients with benign CAO. For symptomatic but stable patients with fixed CAO, a stent is inserted to improve the lumen to less than 50 % obstruction. For symptomatic patients with TBM, stents are inserted to stabilize the airway at the collapsible segment responsible for flow limitation (also known as the "choke point"). A trial and error approach is still used for these patients. A stent is placed temporarily and clinical improvement is assessed; if symptoms improve, a surgeon could perform an external splinting procedure; if there is no improvement, the stent should be removed. Evidence suggests that choke point location may need to be identified using physiologic studies, including intraluminal pressure measurements, because a collapsible airway may not be flow limiting, as is the case with EDAC due to COPD or obesity. By measuring airway pressure in each aspect of the airway narrowing (proximal and distal) during quiet breathing intra-operatively, the site of physiologically relevant CAO can be determined objectively. This allows intra-operative estimation of the outcomes of a particular interventional bronchoscopic procedure, including stent insertion.

Stent Biomechanics and Airway Morphology

Stent-tissue interactions depend on the airway morphology (tortuous versus straight). Stents also differ in terms biomechanics and hydrophilic properties. These details are still considered proprietary information. Regulatory bodies do not mandate their reporting. Manufactures should probably describe some biomechanical properties including the resistance to angulation, radial expansive force, compression force and mechanical failure to help physicians predict successful airway patency restoration and stent-related complications. The future of stenting in benign disease, however, may see the incorporation of bio-absorbable stents. In theory, these stents are ideal as they can support the airway wall and dissolve after the remodeling process is completed. Only pilot human studies have been published to date.

Airway Wall Integrity

In complex PITS and PTTS, cartilage integrity or lack thereof is not always easily assessed on white light bronchoscopy, mainly because of the overlying stenotic hypertrophic tissues. To assess the integrity of the cartilage, high frequency endobronchial ultrasound (20 MHz balloon based radial probe) can be used during the bronchoscopic intervention. The high-resolution image allows visualization of the hypertrophic stenotic tissues and the cartilaginous structures. In complex stenoses, there is partial or total destruction of cartilage histologically which can be identified by EBUS but not always by white light bronchoscopy. In these cases, the contractile force of the scar is stronger than the expansile force of the impaired cartilage and thus it is unlikely that a dilation technique will reliably restore airway patency (as supported by published literature). With radial EBUS, a decision can be taken immediately during a rigid bronchoscopy. If the cartilage is destroyed on EBUS and patient is not a surgical candidate, a stent can be inserted immediately and avoid repeated dilations. This hypothesis needs validation.

Patient Education and Follow up Post Stent Insertion

Immediately after stent insertion, a chest radiograph is performed to confirm its location. Because stents are associated with significant problems, a stent alert card should be given to the patient. This provides information for patients and for the doctors that may encounter patients with airway stents. The card includes the patient's name, indication for stent insertion, type, location and size of stent inserted, contact information, and instructions for both patients and physicians in case of stent-related complications. Also, while not a universal practice, saline nebulization is offered by many bronchoscopists to keep the stent humidified in order to avoid excessive mucus plugging. One study showed that routine surveillance bronchoscopy every 2–3 months after stent insertion did not detect a high incidence of stent-related complications among patients without new respiratory symptoms [63]. Only silicone stents were studied in this paper, however, and most patients had a fixed stenosis. Based on the severity of complications that can occur long term, difficulty in removing some fractured stents or stents obstructed by granulation, and based on the median time to complications of ~6 weeks post insertion, a bronchoscopic follow-up at 4–6 weeks is warranted followed by repeated exams every 2–3 months while the patient has the indwelling airway stent.

Recommendations

- For inoperable patients with symptomatic complex post intubation, post tracheostomy, and post tuberculosis tracheobronchial stenosis, silicone stent insertion is recommended. (Evidence quality low; weak recommendation)
- For patients with symptomatic benign tracheobronchial strictures, metallic stent insertion is not recommended. (Evidence quality low; weak recommendation)
- For patients with severe, diffuse and symptomatic tracheobronchomalacia, silicone stent insertion is suggested. (Evidence quality low; weak recommendation)
- For patients with tracheobronchomalacia, metallic stents are not recommended. (Evidence quality low; weak recommendation)
- For patients with symptomatic post transplant anastomotic bronchial stenosis or malacia, stent insertion is recommended in symptomatic patients who fail bronchoscopic dilation. (Evidence quality low; weak recommendation)
- For patients with symptomatic extrinsic tracheal obstruction due to compression by benign thyroid disease, stent insertion is recommended in inoperable patients. (Evidence quality low; weak recommendation)

References

1. Redmond J, Diamond J, Dunn J, Cohen GS, Soliman AM. Rigid bronchoscopic management of complications related to endobronchial stents after lung transplantation. Ann Otol Rhinol Laryngol. 2013;122(3):183–9.
2. Terra RM, Bibas BJ, Minamoto H, Waisberg DR, Tamagno MF, Tedde ML, Pêgo-Fernandes PM, Jatene FB. Decannulation in tracheal stenosis deemed inoperable is possible after long-term airway stenting. Ann Thorac Surg. 2013;95(2):440–4.
3. Chen G, Wang Z, Liang X, Wang Y, Wang Y, Wang Z, Xian J. Treatment of cuff-related tracheal stenosis with a fully covered retrievable expandable metallic stent. Clin Radiol. 2013;68(4):358–64.

4. Verma A, Um SW, Koh WJ, Suh GY, Chung MP, Kwon OJ, Kim H. Long-term tolerance of airway silicone stent in patients with post-tuberculosis tracheobronchial stenosis. ASAIO J. 2012;58(5):530–4.
5. Gallo A, Pagliuca G, Greco A, Martellucci S, Mascelli A, Fusconi M, De Vincentiis M. Laryngotracheal stenosis treated with multiple surgeries: experience, results and prognostic factors in 70 patients. Acta Otorhinolaryngol Ital. 2012;32(3):182–8.
6. Jeong BH, Um SW, Suh GY, Chung MP, Kwon OJ, Kim H, Kim J. Results of interventional bronchoscopy in the management of postoperative tracheobronchial stenosis. J Thorac Cardiovasc Surg. 2012;144(1):217–22.
7. Lim SY, Kim H, Jeon K, Um SW, Koh WJ, Suh GY, Chung MP, Kwon OJ. Prognostic factors for endotracheal silicone stenting in the management of inoperable post-intubation tracheal stenosis. Yonsei Med J. 2012;53(3):565–70.
8. Chen W, Ruan Y. Late complications of nickel-titanium alloy stent in tracheal stenosis. Laryngoscope. 2012;122(4):817–20.
9. Lari SM, Gonin F, Colchen A. The management of bronchus intermedius complications after lung transplantation: a retrospective study. J Cardiothorac Surg. 2012;7:8.
10. Perotin JM, Jeanfaivre T, Thibout Y, Jouneau S, Lena H, Dutau H, Ramon P, Lorut C, Noppen M, Vergnon JM, Vallerand H, Merol JC, Marquette CH, Lebargy F, Deslee G. Endoscopic management of idiopathic tracheal stenosis. Ann Thorac Surg. 2011;92(1):297–301.
11. Lim SY, Park HK, Jeon K, Um SW, Koh WJ, Suh GY, Chung MP, Kwon OJ, Kim H. Factors predicting outcome following airway stenting for post-tuberculosis tracheobronchial stenosis. Respirology. 2011;16(6):959–64.
12. Chung FT, Chen HC, Chou CL, Yu CT, Kuo CH, Kuo HP, Lin SM. An outcome analysis of self-expandable metallic stents in central airway obstruction: a cohort study. J Cardiothorac Surg. 2011;6:46.
13. Fernández-Bussy S, Majid A, Caviedes I, Akindipe O, Baz M, Jantz M. Treatment of airway complications following lung transplantation. Arch Bronconeumol. 2011;47(3):128–33.
14. Charokopos N, Foroulis CN, Rouska E, Sileli MN, Papadopoulos N, Papakonstantinou C. The management of post-intubation tracheal stenoses with self-expandable stents: early and long-term results in 11 cases. Eur J Cardiothorac Surg. 2011;40(4):919–24.
15. Tan JH, Fidelman N, Durack JC, Hays SR, Leard LL, Laberge JM, Kerlan RK, Golden JA, Gordon RL. Management of recurrent airway strictures in lung transplant recipients using AERO covered stents. J Vasc Interv Radiol. 2010;21(12):1900–4.
16. Fruchter O, Raviv Y, Fox BD, Kramer MR. Removal of metallic tracheobronchial stents in lung transplantation with flexible bronchoscopy. J Cardiothorac Surg. 2010;5:72.
17. Yu CT, Chou CL, Chung FT, Wu JT, Liu YC, Liu YH, Lin TY, Lin SM, Lin HC, Wang CH, Kuo HP, Chen HC, Liu CY. Tracheal torsion assessed by a computer-generated 3-dimensional image analysis predicts tracheal self-expandable metallic stent fracture. J Thorac Cardiovasc Surg. 2010;140(4):769–76.
18. Alazemi S, Lunn W, Majid A, Berkowitz D, Michaud G, Feller-Kopman D, Herth F, Ernst A. Outcomes, health-care resources use, and costs of endoscopic removal of metallic airway stents. Chest. 2010;138(2):350–6.
19. Kim SC, Kim SH, Kim BY. Successful decannulation of T-tubes according to type of tracheal stenosis. Ann Otol Rhinol Laryngol. 2010;119(4):252–7.
20. Chung FT, Lin SM, Chou CL, Chen HC, Liu CY, Yu CT, Kuo HP. Factors leading to obstructive granulation tissue formation after ultraflex stenting in benign tracheal narrowing. Thorac Cardiovasc Surg. 2010;58(2):102–7.
21. Melkane AE, Matar NE, Haddad AC, Nassar MN, Almoutran HG, Rohayem Z, Daher M, Chalouhy G, Dabar G. Management of postintubation tracheal stenosis: appropriate indications make outcome differences. Respiration. 2010;79(5):395–401.
22. Rahman NA, Fruchter O, Shitrit D, Fox BD, Kramer MR. Flexible bronchoscopic management of benign tracheal stenosis: long term follow-up of 115 patients. J Cardiothorac Surg. 2010;5:2.
23. Ko PJ, Liu CY, Wu YC, Chao YK, Hsieh MJ, Wu CY, Wang CJ, Liu YH, Liu HP. Granulation formation following tracheal stenosis stenting: influence of stent position. Laryngoscope. 2009;119(12):2331–6.

24. Nam HS, Um SW, Koh WJ, Suh GY, Chung MP, Kwon OJ, Kim J, Kim H. Clinical application of the natural Y stent in the management of benign carinal stenosis. Ann Thorac Surg. 2009; 88(2):432–9.
25. Fernandez-Bussy S, Akindipe O, Kulkarni V, Swafford W, Baz M, Jantz MA. Clinical experience with a new removable tracheobronchial stent in the management of airway complications after lung transplantation. J Heart Lung Transplant. 2009;28(7):683–8.
26. Abi-Jaoudeh N, Francois RJ, Oliva VL, Giroux MF, Therasse E, Cliche A, Chaput M, Ferraro P, Poirier C, Soulez G. Endobronchial dilation for the management of bronchial stenosis in patients after lung transplantation: effect of stent placement on survival. J Vasc Interv Radiol. 2009;20(7):912–20.
27. Gottlieb J, Fuehner T, Dierich M, Wiesner O, Simon AR, Welte T. Are metallic stents really safe? A long-term analysis in lung transplant recipients. Eur Respir J. 2009;34(6):1417–22.
28. Park HY, Kim H, Koh WJ, Suh GY, Chung MP, Kwon OJ. Natural stent in the management of post-intubation tracheal stenosis. Respirology. 2009;14(4):583–8.
29. Carretta A, Casiraghi M, Melloni G, Bandiera A, Ciriaco P, Ferla L, Puglisi A, Zannini P. Montgomery T-tube placement in the treatment of benign tracheal lesions. Eur J Cardiothorac Surg. 2009;36(2):352–6.
30. Dooms C, De Keukeleire T, Janssens A, Carron K. Performance of fully covered self-expanding metallic stents in benign airway strictures. Respiration. 2009;77(4):420–6.
31. Thistlethwaite PA, Yung G, Kemp A, Osbourne S, Jamieson SW, Channick C, Harrell J. Airway stenoses after lung transplantation: incidence, management, and outcome. J Thorac Cardiovasc Surg. 2008;136(6):1569–75.
32. Galluccio G, Lucantoni G, Battistoni P, Paone G, Batzella S, Lucifora V, Dello Iacono R. Interventional endoscopy in the management of benign tracheal stenoses: definitive treatment at long-term follow-up. Eur J Cardiothorac Surg. 2009;35(3):429–33.
33. Shlomi D, Peled N, Shitrit D, Bendayan D, Amital A, Kramer MR. Protective effect of immunosuppression on granulation tissue formation in metallic airway stents. Laryngoscope. 2008;118(8):1383–8.
34. Chan AL, Juarez MM, Allen RP, Albertson TE. Do airway metallic stents for benign lesions confer too costly a benefit? BMC Pulm Med. 2008;8:7.
35. Murgu SD, Colt HG. Complications of silicone stent insertion in patients with expiratory central airway collapse. Ann Thorac Surg. 2007;84(6):1870–7.
36. Terra RM, Minamoto H, Tedde ML, Almeida JL, Jatene FB. Self-expanding stent made of polyester mesh with silicon coating (Polyflex) in the treatment of inoperable tracheal stenoses. J Bras Pneumol. 2007;33(3):241–7.
37. Ernst A, Majid A, Feller-Kopman D, Guerrero J, Boiselle P, Loring SH, O'Donnell C, Decamp M, Herth FJ, Gangadharan S, Ashiku S. Airway stabilization with silicone stents for treating adult tracheobronchomalacia: a prospective observational study. Chest. 2007; 132(2):609–16.
38. Cavaliere S, Bezzi M, Toninelli C, Foccoli P. Management of post-intubation tracheal stenoses using the endoscopic approach. Monaldi Arch Chest Dis. 2007;67(2):73–80.
39. Kapoor BS, May B, Panu N, Kowalik K, Hunter DW. Endobronchial stent placement for the management of airway complications after lung transplantation. J Vasc Interv Radiol. 2007;18(5):629–32.
40. Kim JH, Shin JH, Song HY, Shim TS, Yoon CJ, Ko GY. Benign tracheobronchial strictures: long-term results and factors affecting airway patency after temporary stent placement. AJR Am J Roentgenol. 2007;188(4):1033–8.
41. Gildea TR, Murthy SC, Sahoo D, Mason DP, Mehta AC. Performance of a self-expanding silicone stent in palliation of benign airway conditions. Chest. 2006;130(5):1419–23.
42. Cheng YJ, Kao EL. Expandable metal stents as an alternative treatment of cuff-related tracheal stenosis in tracheostomy-dependent ventilated patients: a prospective study of nine cases and description of the complications. Langenbecks Arch Surg. 2007;392(4):479–83.
43. Ryu YJ, Kim H, Yu CM, Choi JC, Kwon YS, Kim J, Suh SW. Comparison of natural and Dumon airway stents for the management of benign tracheobronchial stenoses. Respirology. 2006;11(6):748–54.

44. Ryu YJ, Kim H, Yu CM, Choi JC, Kwon YS, Kwon OJ. Use of silicone stents for the management of post-tuberculosis tracheobronchial stenosis. Eur Respir J. 2006;28(5):1029–35.
45. Madden BP, Loke TK, Sheth AC. Do expandable metallic airway stents have a role in the management of patients with benign tracheobronchial disease? Ann Thorac Surg. 2006;82(1): 274–8.
46. Thornton RH, Gordon RL, Kerlan RK, LaBerge JM, Wilson MW, Wolanske KA, Gotway MB, Hastings GS, Golden JA. Outcomes of tracheobronchial stent placement for benign disease. Radiology. 2006;240(1):273–82.
47. Noppen M, Stratakos G, Amjadi K, De Weerdt S, D'Haese J, Meysman M, Vincken W. Stenting allows weaning and extubation in ventilator- or tracheostomy dependency secondary to benign airway disease. Respir Med. 2007;101(1):139–45.
48. Eller RL, Livingston 3rd WJ, Morgan CE, Peters GE, Sillers MJ, Magnuson JS, Rosenthal EL. Expandable tracheal stenting for benign disease: worth the complications? Ann Otol Rhinol Laryngol. 2006;115(4):247–52.
49. Marel M, Pekarek Z, Spasova I, Pafko P, Schutzner J, Betka J, Pospisil R. Management of benign stenoses of the large airways in the university hospital in Prague, Czech Republic, in 1998–2003. Respiration. 2005;72(6):622–8.
50. Lunn W, Feller-Kopman D, Wahidi M, Ashiku S, Thurer R, Ernst A. Endoscopic removal of metallic airway stents. Chest. 2005;127(6):2106–12.
51. Noppen M, Poppe K, D'Haese J, Meysman M, Velkeniers B, Vincken W. Interventional bronchoscopy for treatment of tracheal obstruction secondary to benign or malignant thyroid disease. Chest. 2004;125(2):723–30.
52. Ciccone AM, De Giacomo T, Venuta F, Ibrahim M, Diso D, Coloni GF, Rendina EA. Operative and non-operative treatment of benign subglottic laryngotracheal stenosis. Eur J Cardiothorac Surg. 2004;26(4):818–22.
53. Low SY, Hsu A, Eng P. Interventional bronchoscopy for tuberculous tracheobronchial stenosis. Eur Respir J. 2004;24(3):345–7.
54. Sesterhenn AM, Wagner HJ, Alfke H, Werner JA, Lippert BM. Treatment of benign tracheal stenosis utilizing self-expanding nitinol stents. Cardiovasc Intervent Radiol. 2004;27(4):355–60.
55. Pereszlenyi A, Igaz M, Majer I, Harustiak S. Role of endotracheal stenting in tracheal reconstruction surgery-retrospective analysis. Eur J Cardiothorac Surg. 2004;25(6):1059–64.
56. Noppen M, Stratakos G, D'Haese J, Meysman M, Vinken W. Removal of covered self-expandable metallic airway stents in benign disorders: indications, technique, and outcomes. Chest. 2005;127(2):482–7.
57. Liu HC, Lee KS, Huang CJ, Cheng CR, Hsu WH, Huang MH. Silicone T-tube for complex laryngotracheal problems. Eur J Cardiothorac Surg. 2002;21:326–30.
58. U.S. Food and Drug Administration. Metallic tracheal stents in patients with benign airway disorders. 02 Aug 2005. Available at: http://www.fda.gov/safety/medwatch/safetyinformation/safetyalertsforhumanmedicalproducts/ucm153009.htm. Accessed 20 Oct 2013.
59. Gaissert HA, Grillo HC, Wright CD, Donahue DM, Wain JC, Mathisen DJ. Complication of benign tracheobronchial strictures by self-expanding metal stents. J Thorac Cardiovasc Surg. 2003;126:744–7.
60. Hramiec JE, Haasler GB. Tracheal wire stent complications in malacia: implications of position and design. Ann Thorac Surg. 1997;63:209–12.
61. Giudice M, Piazza C, Foccoli P, Toninelli C, Cavaliere S, Peretti G. Idiopathic subglottic stenosis: management by endoscopic and open-neck surgery in a series of 30 patients. Eur Arch Otorhinolaryngol. 2003;260:235–8.
62. Lischke R, Pozniak J, Vondrys D, Elliott MJ. Novel biodegradable stents in the treatment of bronchial stenosis after lung transplantation. Eur J Cardiothorac Surg. 2011;40:619–24.
63. Matsuo T, Colt HG. Evidence against routine scheduling of surveillance bronchoscopy after stent insertion. Chest. 2000;118:1455–9.

Chapter 43
Bioengineered Tissues for Tracheal Reconstruction

Philipp Jungebluth and Paolo Macchiarini

Abstract Extended (>6 cm) reconstruction of the trachea is an unmet clinical need, and all conventional surgical approaches thus far have failed to provide any definitive solutions to this common problem. Tissue engineering, including cell-seeded scaffolds using a bioreactor, has recently became a promising therapeutic option. Despite its successful use in initial clinical compassionate cases, an understanding of the underlying mechanisms of in situ regeneration remain unclear and routine clinical applications are still far away. Early outcomes suggest that specific clinical scenarios require different approaches and additional strategies aside from tissue engineering might be necessary. There is no evidence-based medicine available for this emerging field, hence we provide an overview of hitherto investigated concepts and applied procedures.

Keywords Trachea tissue engineering • Clinical transplantation • Tracheal reconstruction • Scaffold

Introduction

Malignant and benign diseases of the trachea are treated conventionally by surgical resection and subsequent reconstruction using an end-to-end anastomosis [1] with curative intent. This is, unfortunately, only possible with diseased tracheal segments of less than 6 cm in length in adults and one third of the entire tracheal length in

The authors declare no competing financial interests.

P. Jungebluth, MD • P. Macchiarini, MD, PhD (✉)
Division of Ear, Nose, and Throat (CLINTEC), Advanced Center for Translational
Regenerative Medicine (ACTREM), Karolinska Institutet,
Alfred Nobels Allé 8, Huddinge, Stockholm SE-141 86, Sweden
e-mail: jungebluthp@aol.com; paolo.macchiarini@ki.se

Table 43.1 Symptoms of tracheal disorders

Symptoms
Wheezing
Stridor
Dyspnea
Cough
Hoarseness and other voice changes
Hemoptysis
Dysphagia
Pneumonia

children. Diseases extending longer cannot be surgically treated and palliation is the standard of care. Due to unspecific symptoms (Table 43.1), the majority of primary malignant diseases are diagnosed in a locally advanced stage and therefore only palliative strategies are possible, such as tumor debulking, stenting and radiotherapy [1, 2]. The treatments of choice for long segment benign diseases are also limited to endoluminal strategies but seldom solve or cure these problems [1, 3].

The next logical therapeutic step – tracheal replacement – was performed by Rose and colleagues for the first time in man in 1979 using an allogeneic trachea [4]. However, both experimental and clinical data revealed irreconcilable challenges in the following years, such as the need for lifelong immunosuppressive medication and/or technical difficulties [5–8]. Among them, the immunogenicity of the trachea is more clinically important than initially assumed [8, 9]. To reduce this immunogenicity, various techniques have been investigated and partly clinically applied, such as cryopreservation, irradiation or chemical fixation [10–13]. Beside the additional need of local reconstructive tissue and/or partial stenting for some of the these techniques [11, 14], the impact on immunogenicity is controversial, at least for cryopreserved tissues [10, 12, 15, 16].

Aside from using tracheal tissue for reconstruction, other tissues have been attempted. Fonkalsrud and colleagues performed [17, 18] a few cases of autologous esophagus transposition for tracheal replacement in 1963 and 1971. However, the intermediate and long-term outcomes were unsatisfying. Wurtz and colleagues introduced the aorta as a new approach to reconstruction of the trachea with initial promising clinical outcomes that were stent dependent [19, 20]. Modifications of this technique might extend the applications of this method [21]. Similarly, another surgical approach using an autologous fascio-cutaneous flap reinforced by rib cartilages has entered the clinical realm with a reasonable outcome [22]. Even though various techniques have been investigated, so far none has been emerged as the gold-standard treatment, hence, further alternatives are desired.

Tissue engineering may offer novel possibilities for the field of tracheal reconstruction (Table 43.2.). This chapter addresses the different strategies of tissue engineering, the potential clinical benefit and early clinical data.

Table 43.2 Indications, contraindications and eligibility for surgical interventions

Indication for tracheal intervention	
Benign disorders:	
Idiopatic, iatrogenic and trauma related stenosis	
Polychondritis	
Tuberculosis	
Amyloidosis	
Osteochondroplastica	
Agenesis	
Tumors	
Malignant disorders:	
Tumors	
Postlaryngectomy recurrences or diseases	
Contraindication for conventional tracheal reconstruction	**Eligibility criteria for tracheal replacement**
More than 6 cm of the entire length of the trachea affected in adults	Benign and malignant diseases with extended length
More than 1/3 of the entire length of the trachea affected in children	Previous maximal conventional treatment
Mediastinal invasion of unresectable organs	Age 2–75 year
Many positive lymph nodes	No metastasis
Distant metastases in squamous cell carcinoma	No micro-metastasis (bone marrow sampling proven)
Radiation <60 Gy on mediastinum	No definite surgical contraindications
	No psychological/psychiatric abnormalities
	Written patient consent
	Ethical permit (local, national ethic and transplantation board)

Search Strategy

A systematic literature search of English, German, Spanish and Italian languages on PubMed, Scopus, Science Citation Index/Social Sciences Citation Index, Ovid, was used to identify all publications, including clinical trials, meta-analyses, and reviews, with the terms such as "trachea reconstruction", "tracheal graft", "tracheal tissue engineering", "trachea replacement", "trachea and stem cells". Since tissue engineering for tracheal reconstruction is a very young field, there are no randomized controlled trials or comparative or cohort studies – only extensive experimental studies and initial single clinical cases. Therefore the chapter does not aim to give clear evidence-based recommendations but *only* provides the various possibilities in order to help in clinical decision-making.

Tissue Engineering—The Concept

Tissue engineering (TE) is the current most promising alternative for patients suffering from long-segmental tracheal lesions [1, 23]. For other organs and tissues, such as the urine bladder, lungs, heart and heart valves and other tubular structures, TE seems to be an interesting strategy for tissue regeneration and replacement [24–28]. Basically three components are combined in TE: cells seeded on a scaffold and cultured in a bioreactor. Moreover, novel technologies have been introduced into TE using bioactive molecules to alter in situ tissue regeneration.

Cells

The need of cell seeding prior tracheal replacement has been shown to avoid graft contamination and mechanical impairments [29, 30]. Due to their significant ethical and/or immunological concerns, pluripotent cells such as human embryonic (hECs) and induced pluripotent stem cells (iPSCs) are, for the time being, not of interest for clinical use in tracheal reconstruction. However, their capacity to differentiation into airway specific cells has been proven elsewhere [31, 32].

In contrast to the applications of allogeneic adult stem cells in other scenarios, such as for burn injuries (NCT01443689), acute myeloid leukemia (NCT00606723), end-stage heart failure (NCT01759212) and many others, only autologous cells have been clinically used in the field of tracheal tissue engineering. To date, bone marrow derived mesenchymal stem cells (MSCs) and mononuclear cells (MNCs) with a heterogeneous cell population including MSCs and hematopoietic stem cells (HSCs), have been used in the clinical scenario [14, 30, 33, 34]. The actual mechanism of how these cells contribute to the regeneration of the airways is currently controversial. Potentially they can differentiate into tracheal specific cell types, such as epithelial cells or chondrocytes [35, 36]. Aside from adult stem cells, terminally differentiated cells have been utilized in the clinic. In 2004 smooth muscle and fibroblast were utilized to engineer a tracheal vascularized patch for clinical application in a patient [37, 38]. Autologous epithelial cells were obtained from both the bronchial mucosa [33, 39], tracheal [40] mucosa, and/or the right inferior turbinate mucosa and used for tracheal engineering in a patient.

In a more time consuming procedure, autologous buccal mucosa was transferred to a tracheal graft, heterotopically placed into the forearm and subsequently implanted into the orthotopic position [41]. However, the first clinical cases showed various efficiency for the processing outcome [42]. Chondrocytes have been terminally differentiated from MSCs and seeded on the scaffold [33] or differentiation has been initiated after seeding [34, 39]. As described before, preoperative cell seeding seems to be crucial, however, evidence has been provided that bone marrow derived MSCs contribute to tracheal in situ regeneration [43].

The existence of tracheal niche stem/progenitor cells and their contribution for in situ airway regeneration has been demonstrated in animals [44–46]. One may

Table 43.3 Optimal tracheal graft

Characteristics
Non-toxic and/or immunogenic
Liquid- and air-tight seals
Biocompatibility to allow cell attachment, viability and differentiation
Mechanical properties similar to the human trachea to react to longitudinal and lateral forces allow for swallowing, coughing and respiratory function

suppose that these cells can be most likely detected in human trachea as well, but so far only lung tissue stem/progenitor cells have been described, and remain controversial [47].

Scaffolds—Biological and Synthetic

The scaffold, regardless of what materials it is made of, presents the basic structure to give structural integrity to the tracheal graft. The ideal tracheal graft requires several specific properties (Table 43.3). In general two different approaches have been introduced to the clinic: *biological-* and *synthetic-based scaffolds*.

Biological Scaffold

To date, two different *biological scaffolds* have been applied in the clinical setting. Donated organs, the tracheae [33, 39, 48] and porcine jejunum [37, 38] have been decellularized in order to remove all immunological relevant cellular components, in particular the major histocompatibility complexes I and II. Different techniques can be applied to obtain a non-immunogenic scaffold, such as enzymatic and detergent solutions (alkaline, acidic, zwitterionic, ionic, nonionic, resolvent or chelating agents), thermic (cryopreservation) strategies and physical effects (agitation, perfusion or static). Despite the removal of the donor DNA and immunogenic components, the basic nano-fiber structure of the extracellular matrix (EXM) can be preserved by these decellularization techniques. The ECM-associated proteins, such as elastin, collagen, lamin, etc., demonstrated their impact on cell proliferation and differentiation [49] but also the beneficial influences on healing processes by host immune response modulation and reestablishing homeostasis [50].

The hitherto clinically utilized donated tracheal scaffolds have all been prepared with a detergent-enzymatic method of DNase and deoxycholate. The scaffolds were evaluated in detail prior to cell seeding and subsequently implanted in a patient without the need of immunosuppressive medication [33, 39, 48]. When porcine jejunum was used clinically in 2004, the tissue was decellularized via a similar protocol except with the additional of initial mechanical removal of the small bowel mucosa. The xenogenic tissue did also not provoke any adverse immune response.

Synthetic Scaffold

In order to avoid human donations or xenogenic-derived scaffolds, synthetic-based scaffolds have been introduced into the clinical setting. In addition to the non-donation dependent method of developing the graft from scratch, the synthetic scaffold can be custom-made in a fast and reproducible way. Moreover, the final product is sterilisable on a clinical grade. The decellularization of biological tissues lasts several weeks and is therefore inapplicable in patients with malignancies.

However, the trachea is not *only* a tubular structure between the larynx and the lungs that transports air in between but holds also immunological properties that protect the lungs from simple infections. Further challenges for synthetic based graft engineering are the mechanical characteristics of the trachea and its vascularization [1].

Different synthetic materials (both degradable and non-degradable), such as Marlex mesh, polyhydroxyacids, poly-ε-caprolactone, polypropylene mesh, polyester urethane, gelatin sponge, polyethylene oxide/polypropylene oxide copolymer, poly-actic/glycolic acid, alginate gel have been studied for their potential use clinically [1]. However, only *polyethylene terephthalate* (PET), polyurethane (PU) and polyhedral oligomeric silsesquioxane poly(carbonate-urea) urethane (POSS-PCU) have been processed in the context of tissue engineering by combing material with cell seeding [30, 34, 51].

Innovative solutions using composite scaffolds made of biological and synthetic components may provide promising results in smaller defects of the trachea (<50 mm), such as the approach Omori and colleagues proposed by combining Marlex mesh tube covered by collagen sponge [52]. Scaffold-free solutions using cell sheets have no clinical relevance at this stage for longer and/or circumferential defects due to the absence of mechanical strength.

Tissue engineering strategies may help to overcome the drawbacks of synthetic materials. Stem cells, in particular MSCs, have significant bioactive capacities and act beneficially via immunomodulation and cell homing in various respiratory conditions [53]. For clinical applications, synthetic materials are therefore seeded with MSCs prior transplantation in order to reduce inflammatory responses and increase cell homing to the surgical site.

The most important future aim of tissue engineering must be the further improvement of graft vascularization in order to guarantee cell viability and tissue in situ regeneration. Currently vascularization of the neo-trachea can be obtained through various purely surgical techniques, e.g. *latissimus dorsi* and musculofascial flaps and/or omentum major transposition. The latter option was used in the first clinical cases of synthetic-based trachea replacement [34, 51].

Bioreactor

Bioreactors have an essential role in most of the processing steps in tissue engineering, such as decellularization, 3-D cell-scaffold seeding and culture. Various bioreactors are available for different tissues and organs to mimic the appropriate physiological and biological conditions. In the field of tracheal tissue engineering nearly all clinically applied grafts have been processed with a bioreactor similar to the one developed by Asnaghi and colleagues [54]. The environment provided by the bioreactor allows for safe and controlled cell attachment, proliferation and differentiation. Further improvements are currently under investigation to provide more detailed information regarding cell surface coverage, cell viability, proliferation and differentiation status.

Aside from this, in vivo tracheal tissue engineering, avoiding any in vitro culture, has been clinically applied using either a *single-* [40, 55] or dual-*staged approach* [41].

Bioactive Molecules

Engineered organs/tissues further regenerate within the body after transplantation via neovascularization, cell-cell interaction, and cell differentiation. However, the regeneration capacity has its limitations and must be supported by either adding bioactive substances into the culture conditions, incorporating molecules into the scaffold or by the external administration of pharmaceutical interventions. Some strategies already have been applied in the clinical setting [34, 40], while others are still at a preclinical level [56, 57]. The application of erythropoietin (EPO) appears to have a positive effect on the reduction of cell apoptosis, as described by Brines and Cerami [58]. Clinical findings showed up-regulation of anti-apoptotic genes, such as Janus tyrosine kinase-2 (JAK-2), STAT5 (signal transducer and activator of transcription 5), Bcl-2, phosphatidylinositol 3, protein kinase B, mitogen-activated protein kinase, and nuclear factor-κB, after systemic EPO administration (for 14 days postoperative). No negative side-effects have been clinically observed [34]. Circulating stem and progenitor cells have been found to be involved in tissue regeneration and would healing [59, 60]. To this end, mobilization strategies of stem cells from their bone marrow niche may further improve in situ regeneration and wound healing.

The use of granulocyte colony stimulating factor (G-CSF) resulted not only in the increase of circulating endothelial progenitor cells (EPCs) but also CXCR-4 positive MSCs and HSCs [34]. The mobilized MSCs can potentially contribute to wound healing through their strong immunomodulatory properties. Besides, cell homing to the surgical site is supported by different MSC-related chemokines and activating products, as well as through the SDF-1/CXCR4 axis. The mobilized EPCs are essential for neovascularization of the implanted tracheal construct and can therefore further alter the graft's integrity. Currently efforts are made to further understand and improve homing pathways and regenerative mechanisms.

Clinical Overview

To our knowledge, 11 patients have been treated worldwide with engineered airway tissue but only 10 patients have received a circumferential engineered graft. The recent 5-year follow-up report provides definitive evidence about the tissue engineering technology [48], although there is much room for improvement. The overall

Table 43.4 World-wide outcome of transplanted engineered tracheal tissue (segmental and patches)

Characteristics	Biological scaffolds	Bioartificial scaffolds	Total
Indications			
Benign	7	6	13
Malignant	4	2	6
N. of patients	11	8	19
Age (years)	11–72	2–42	2–72
Gender (male vs. female)	5 *vs* 6	3 vs 5	8 *vs* 11
Status (alive vs. death)	5 *vs* 6	6 vs 2	11 *vs* 8
Cause of death (all confirmed by autopsy)	Systemic metastasis (n=4)	Gastrointestinal bleeding (n=1)	
	Pulmonary embolism (n=1)	Myocardial infarction and cerebral hemorrhage, respiratory failure with pulmonary infarction, but airway with normal epithelium (n=1)	
	Cardiac arrest (n=1)		

outcomes thus far suggest that long-segment replacement of the trachea using biological decellularized trachea results in unpredictable mechanical impairments (Table 43.4). However, biological scaffolds are excellent alternatives for short segmental replacement.

To date eight patients have been managed with synthetic-based scaffolds with somewhat promising early and intermediate outcomes (Table 43.4). Vascularization and re-epithelialization strategies must be further investigated.

Conclusions

After decades of investigating a variety of surgical techniques, using various graft materials and obtaining contradictory results, tissue engineering has become a clinical reality. Early and intermediate data from patients provide evidence for its potential clinical relevance in the future. Both biological and synthetic solutions seem to be appropriate graft materials for tracheal replacement. However, more efforts will be necessary to further understand underlying pathways of trachea regeneration before this technology can become clinical routine.

Recommendations

• Circumferential long-length tracheal reconstruction is not currently appropriate for routine clinical use. (Evidence quality low; weak recommendation).

References

1. Grillo HC. Tracheal replacement: a critical review. Ann Thorac Surg. 2002;73:1995–2004.
2. Macchiarini P. Primary tracheal tumours. Lancet Oncol. 2006;7:83–91.
3. Nakahira M, Nakatani H, Takeuchi S, Higashiyama K, Fukushima K. Safe reconstruction of a large cervico-mediastinal tracheal defect with a pectoralis major myocutaneous flap and free costal cartilage grafts. Auris Nasus Larynx. 2006;33:203–6.
4. Rose K, Sesterhenn K, Wustrow F. Tracheal allotransplantation in man. Lancet. 1979;1:433.
5. Lenot B, Macchiarini P, Dulmet E, Weiss M, Dartevelle P. Tracheal allograft replacement. An unsuccessful method. Eur J Cardiothorac Surg. 1993;7:648–52.
6. Macchiarini P, Lenot B, De Montpreville V, Dulmet E, Mazmanian GM, Fattal M, et al. Heterotopic pig model for direct revascularization and venous drainage of tracheal allografts. Paris-Sud University Lung Transplantation Group. J Thorac Cardiovasc Surg. 1994;108:1066–75.
7. Levashov YN, Yablonsky PK, Cherny SM, Orlov SV, Shafirovsky BB, Kuznetzov IM. One-stage allotransplantation of thoracic segment of the trachea in a patient with idiopathic fibrosing mediastinitis and marked tracheal stenosis. Eur J Cardiothorac Surg. 1993;7:383–6.
8. Delaere PR, Liu Z, Sciot R, Welvaart W. The role of immunosuppression in the long-term survival of tracheal allografts. Arch Otolaryngol Neck Surg. 1996;122:1201–8.
9. Shaari CM, Farber D, Brandwein MS, Gannon P, Urken ML. Characterizing the antigenic profile of the human trachea: implications for tracheal transplantation. Head Neck. 1998;20:522–7.
10. Kunachak S, Kulapaditharom B, Vajaradul Y, Rochanawutanon M. Cryopreserved, irradiated tracheal homograft transplantation for laryngotracheal reconstruction in human beings. Otolaryngol Head Neck Surg. 2000;122:911–6.
11. Jacobs JP, Quintessenza JA, Andrews T, Burke RP, Spektor Z, Delius RE, et al. Tracheal allograft reconstruction: the total North American and worldwide pediatric experiences. Ann Thorac Surg. 1999;68:1043–51.
12. Hisamatsu C, Maeda K, Tanaka H, Okita Y. Transplantation of the cryopreserved tracheal allograft in growing rabbits: effect of immunosuppressant. Pediatr Surg Int. 2006;22:881–5.
13. Seguin A, Radu D, Holder-Espinasse M, Bruneval P, Fialaire-Legendre A, Duterque-Coquillaud M, et al. Tracheal replacement with cryopreserved, decellularized, or glutaraldehyde-treated aortic allografts. Ann Thorac Surg. 2009;87:861–7.
14. Elliott MJ, Haw MP, Jacobs JP, Bailey CM, Evans JN, Herberhold C. Tracheal reconstruction in children using cadaveric homograft trachea. Eur J Cardiothorac Surg. 1996;10:707–12.
15. Liu Y, Nakamura T, Sekine T, Matsumoto K, Ueda H, Yoshitani M, et al. New type of tracheal bioartificial organ treated with detergent: maintaining cartilage viability is necessary for successful immunosuppressant free allotransplantation. ASAIO J. 2002;48:21–5.
16. Yokomise H, Inui K, Wada H, Goh T, Yagi K, Hitomi S, et al. High-dose irradiation prevents rejection of canine tracheal allografts. J Thorac Cardiovasc Surg. 1994;107:1391–7.
17. Fonkalsrud EW, Martelle RR, Maloney JV. Surgical treatment of tracheal agenesis. J Thorac Cardiovasc Surg. 1963;45:520–5.
18. Fonkalsrud EW, Sumida S. Tracheal replacement with autologous esophagus for tracheal stricture. Arch Surg. 1971;102:139–42.
19. Wurtz A, Porte H, Conti M, Dusson C, Desbordes J, Copin MC, et al. Surgical technique and results of tracheal and carinal replacement with aortic allografts for salivary gland-type carcinoma. J Thorac Cardiovasc Surg. 2010;140:387–93.e2.
20. Wurtz A, Porte H, Conti M, Desbordes J, Copin MC, Azorin J, et al. Tracheal replacement with aortic allografts. N Engl J Med. 2006;355:1938–40.
21. Wurtz A, Hysi I, Kipnis E, Zawadzki C, Hubert T, Jashari R, et al. Tracheal reconstruction with a composite graft: fascial flap-wrapped allogenic aorta with external cartilage-ring support. Interact Cardiovasc Thorac Surg. 2013;16:37–43.
22. Fabre D, Kolb F, Fadel E, Mercier O, Mussot S, Le Chevalier T, et al. Successful tracheal replacement in humans using autologous tissues: an 8-year experience. Ann Thorac Surg. 2013;96:1146–55.

23. Haag JC, Jungebluth P, Macchiarini P. Tracheal replacement for primary tracheal cancer. Curr Opin Otolaryngol Head Neck Surg. 2013;21:171–7.
24. Atala A, Bauer SB, Soker S, Yoo JJ, Retik AB. Tissue-engineered autologous bladders for patients needing cystoplasty. Lancet. 2006;367:1241–6.
25. Petersen TH, Calle EA, Zhao L, Lee EJ, Gui L, Raredon MB, et al. Tissue-engineered lungs for in vivo implantation. Science. 2010;329:538–41.
26. Ott HC, Matthiesen TS, Goh S-K, Black LD, Kren SM, Netoff TI, et al. Perfusion-decellularized matrix: using nature's platform to engineer a bioartificial heart. Nat Med. 2008;14:213–21.
27. Cebotari S, Lichtenberg A, Tudorache I, Hilfiker A, Mertsching H, Leyh R, et al. Clinical application of tissue engineered human heart valves using autologous progenitor cells. Circulation. 2006;114:I132–7.
28. Olausson M, Patil PB, Kuna VK, Chougule P, Hernandez N, Methe K, et al. Transplantation of an allogeneic vein bioengineered with autologous stem cells: a proof-of-concept study. Lancet. 2012;6736:1–8.
29. Go T, Jungebluth P, Baiguero S, Asnaghi A, Martorell J, Ostertag H, et al. Both epithelial cells and mesenchymal stem cell-derived chondrocytes contribute to the survival of tissue-engineered airway transplants in pigs. J Thorac Cardiovasc Surg. 2010;139:437–43.
30. Jungebluth P, Haag JC, Lim ML, Lemon G, Sjöqvist S, Gustafsson Y, et al. Verification of cell viability in bioengineered tissues and organs before clinical transplantation. Biomaterials. 2013;34(16):4057–67.
31. Ghaedi M, Calle EA, Mendez JJ, Gard AL, Balestrini J, Booth A, et al. Human iPS cell-derived alveolar epithelium repopulates lung extracellular matrix. J Clin Invest. 2013;123(11):4950–62.
32. Coraux C, Nawrocki-Raby B, Hinnrasky J, Kileztky C, Gaillard D, Dani C, et al. Embryonic stem cells generate airway epithelial tissue. Am J Respir Cell Mol Biol. 2005;32:87–92.
33. Macchiarini P, Jungebluth P, Go T, Asnaghi MA, Rees LE, Cogan TA, et al. Clinical transplantation of a tissue-engineered airway. Lancet. 2008;372:2023–30.
34. Jungebluth P, Alici E, Baiguera S, Le Blanc K, Blomberg P, Bozóky B, et al. Tracheobronchial transplantation with a stem-cell-seeded bioartificial nanocomposite: a proof-of-concept study. Lancet. 2011;378:1997–2004.
35. Kokubun K, Pankajakshan D, Kim MJ, Agrawal DK. Differentiation of porcine mesenchymal stem cells into epithelial cells as a potential therapeutic application to facilitate epithelial regeneration. J Tissue Eng Regen Med. 2013. doi: 10.1002/term.1758 (in press); Epub ahead of print.
36. Alves da Silva ML, Costa-Pinto AR, Martins A, Correlo VM, Sol P, Bhattacharya M, et al. Conditioned medium as a strategy for human stem cells chondrogenic differentiation. J Tissue Eng Regen Med. 2013. doi: 10.1002/term.1812 (in press); Epub ahead of print.
37. Macchiarini P, Walles T, Biancosino C, Mertsching H. First human transplantation of a bioengineered airway tissue. J Thorac Cardiovasc Surg. 2004;128:638–41.
38. Walles T, Giere B, Hofmann M, Schanz J, Hofmann F, Mertsching H, et al. Experimental generation of a tissue-engineered functional and vascularized trachea. J Thorac Cardiovasc Surg. 2004;128:900–6.
39. Berg M, Ejnell H, Kovács A, Nayakawde N, Patil PB, Joshi M, et al. Replacement of a tracheal stenosis with a tissue-engineered human trachea using autologous stem cells: a case report. Tissue Eng Part A. 2014;20(1-2):389–97.
40. Elliott MJ, De Coppi P, Speggiorin S, Roebuck D, Butler CR, Samuel E, et al. Stem-cell-based, tissue engineered tracheal replacement in a child: a 2-year follow-up study. Lancet. 2012;380:994–1000.
41. Delaere P, Vranckx J, Verleden G, De Leyn P, Van Raemdonck D. Tracheal allotransplantation after withdrawal of immunosuppressive therapy. N Engl J Med. 2010;362:138–45.
42. Delaere PR, Vranckx JJ, Meulemans J, Vander Poorten V, Segers K, Van Raemdonck D, et al. Learning curve in tracheal allotransplantation. Am J Transplant. 2012;12:2538–45.
43. Seguin A, Baccari S, Holder-Espinasse M, Bruneval P, Carpentier A, Taylor DA, et al. Tracheal regeneration: evidence of bone marrow mesenchymal stem cell involvement. J Thorac Cardiovasc Surg. 2013;145(5):1297–1304.e2.

44. Kim CF, Jackson EL, Woolfenden AE, Lawrence S, Babar I, Vogel S, et al. Identification of bronchioalveolar stem cells in normal lung and lung cancer. Cell. 2005;121:823–35.
45. Mailleux AA, Kelly R, Veltmaat JM, De Langhe SP, Zaffran S, Thiery JP, et al. Fgf10 expression identifies parabronchial smooth muscle cell progenitors and is required for their entry into the smooth muscle cell lineage. Development. 2005;132:2157–66.
46. Reya T, Morrison SJ, Clarke MF, Weissman IL. Stem cells, cancer, and cancer stem cells. Nature. 2001;414:105–11.
47. Kajstura J, Rota M, Hall SR, Hosoda T, D'Amario D, Sanada F, et al. Evidence for human lung stem cells. N Engl J Med. 2011;364:1795–806.
48. Gonfiotti A, Jaus MO, Barale D, Baiguera S, Comin C, Lavorini F, 9913, et al. The first tissue-engineered airway transplantation: 5-year follow-up results. Lancet. 2014;383:238–44.
49. Mittag F, Falkenberg EM, Janczyk A, Götze M, Felka T, Aicher WK, et al. Laminin-5 and type I collagen promote adhesion and osteogenic differentiation of animal serum-free expanded human mesenchymal stromal cells. Orthop Rev (Pavia). 2012;4:e36.
50. Piterina AV, Cloonan AJ, Meaney CL, Davis LM, Callanan A, Walsh MT, et al. ECM-based materials in cardiovascular applications: inherent healing potential and augmentation of native regenerative processes. Int J Mol Sci. 2009;10:4375–417.
51. Jungebluth P, Macchiarini P. Airway transplantation. Thorac Surg Clin. 2014;2(12):975–82.
52. Omori K, Tada Y, Suzuki T, Nomoto Y, Matsuzuka T, Kobayashi K, et al. Clinical application of in situ tissue engineering using a scaffolding technique for reconstruction of the larynx and trachea. Ann Otol Rhinol Laryngol. 2008;117:673–8.
53. Weiss DJ. Current status of stem cells and regenerative medicine in lung biology and diseases. Stem Cells. 2014;32(1):16–25.
54. Asnaghi MA, Jungebluth P, Raimondi MT, Dickinson SC, Rees LEN, Go T, et al. A double-chamber rotating bioreactor for the development of tissue-engineered hollow organs: from concept to clinical trial. Biomaterials. 2009;30:5260–9.
55. Bader A, Macchiarini P. Moving towards in situ tracheal regeneration: the bionic tissue engineered transplantation approach. J Cell Mol Med. 2010;14:1877–89.
56. Del Gaudio C, Baiguera S, Boieri M, Mazzanti B, Ribatti D, Bianco A, et al. Induction of angiogenesis using VEGF releasing genipin-crosslinked electrospun gelatin mats. Biomaterials. 2013;34:7754–65.
57. Lemon G, Gustafsson Y, Haag JC, Lim ML, Sjöqvist S, Ajalloueian F, et al. Modelling biological cell attachment and growth on adherent surfaces. J Math Biol. 2014;68(4):785–813.
58. Brines M, Cerami A. Erythropoietin-mediated tissue protection: reducing collateral damage from the primary injury response. J Intern Med. 2008;264:405–32.
59. Ohno S, Hirano S, Kanemaru S, Mizuta M, Ishikawa S, Tateya I, et al. Role of circulating MSCs in vocal fold wound healing. Laryngoscope. 2012;122:2503–10.
60. Mansilla E, Marín GH, Drago H, Sturla F, Salas E, Gardiner C, et al. Bloodstream cells phenotypically identical to human mesenchymal bone marrow stem cells circulate in large amounts under the influence of acute large skin damage: new evidence for their use in regenerative medicine. Transplant Proc. 2006;38:967–9.

Chapter 44
Percutaneous Versus Standard Tracheostomy in the Critically Ill Adult

Mara B. Antonoff and Varun Puri

Abstract The development of percutaneous dilational tracheostomy (PDT) has provided a feasible alternative to conventional surgical tracheostomy (ST). In this review we examine the current body of literature comparing PDT versus ST in terms of short-term, mid-term, and long-term outcomes. PDT is associated with slightly fewer early complications than ST and comparable intermediate outcomes. There is a minor trend toward more frequent tracheal stenosis following PDT. With regard to resource utilization, PDT tends to provide moderate cost savings compared to ST. We recommend use of PDT as a preferred modality if the institution has adequate resources and appropriately trained personnel.

Keywords Tracheostomy • Percutaneous tracheostomy • Surgical tracheostomy • Bedside tracheostomy • Complications • Outcomes • Resource utilization

Introduction

Creating a tracheostomy for airway access is often assumed to be a relatively minor procedure, but it involves careful planning, coordination of ventilation strategy, and attention to detail in the technical conduct of the operation to ensure an optimal outcome. Over the last two decades, development of percutaneous dilational tracheostomy (PDT) has provided a viable and attractive alternative to conventional surgical tracheostomy (ST). The two procedures differ not only technically in the incision and degree of dissection involved, but often also in the

M.B. Antonoff, MD • V. Puri, MD (✉)
Division of Cardiothoracic Surgery, Washington University School of Medicine,
660 South Euclid Avenue, Campus Box 8234, St. Louis, MO 63110, USA
e-mail: antonoffm@wudosis.wustl.edu; puriv@wudosis.wustl.edu

M.K. Ferguson (ed.), *Difficult Decisions in Thoracic Surgery*,
Difficult Decisions in Surgery: An Evidence-Based Approach 1,
DOI 10.1007/978-1-4471-6404-3_44, © Springer-Verlag London 2014

venue of the operation. The majority of STs are performed in the operating room under general anesthetic, while most PDT procedures are performed at the bedside in the intensive care unit using deep sedation without inhalational agents. The advent of PDT has also allowed intensivists and pulmonologists to perform the procedure in some settings without the involvement of thoracic surgeons or otorhinolaryngologists. As one may expect, the relative novelty of the procedure and variety of practitioners performing it has generated a wide range of literature where the definition of PDT is not standardized. For the purpose of this review, we examine the comparative evidence for PDT and ST as standard of care at the current time.

Search Strategy

In order to review currently published data on the topic of interest, electronic literature searches were performed on 8/3/2013 using PubMed (www.ncbi.nlm.nih.gov/pubmed). Search terms included "percutaneous tracheostomy" and "surgical tracheostomy," with each of these terms paired with "outcomes" and "complications." An additional search was performed using "percutaneous versus surgical tracheostomy." Filters were used to limit the findings to English-language publications. Studies were included from as far back as 1996, with all but one paper in the set published between 2000 and 2013. Additional filters were used in order to limit the resultant papers only to those pertaining to adult patients and to those individuals undergoing tracheostomy in the setting of respiratory failure/critical illness. Studies pertaining to tracheostomies for alternative indications (such as laryngeal malignancy) were not included. Case reports and case series were not included due to their very low quality of evidence.

Early techniques for percutaneous dilational tracheostomy were variable with regard to the use of bronchoscopic guidance; however, in the current era, real-time bronchoscopic visualization during percutaneous tracheostomy is considered standard of care [1]. It is well established that use of bronchoscopy as a procedural adjunct decreases the risks of inadvertent extubation, injury to the posterior membranous tracheal wall, and tracheal ring/cricoid fracture [2]. As such, we did not include any studies reporting outcomes of percutaneous tracheostomy if it was performed in the absence of bronchoscopic guidance.

The literature includes studies comparing various commercially available kits for percutaneous tracheostomy. For the purposes of this review, we did not differentiate among the manufacturers' products in our analyses. However, we limited our review to studies that reported on percutaneous tracheostomies placed via needle stick, wire guidance, and dilation using Seldinger-technique. Applicable procedures utilized the Ciaglia sequential dilational kit or Ciaglia Blue Rhino single-step dilation kit with tapered dilator (Cook Medical, Bloomington, IN), the Portex Uni-Perc (Smiths Medical, Dubin, OH), as well as any other kits with similar over-the-wire dilational strategies. Those studies which specifically compared various percutaneous dilational kits to one another were not included, as these papers provided data stratified by brand of kit rather than in a combined fashion. For the majority of the publications, the kits types were not specified. We did not include papers in which percutaneous tracheostomy was performed by means other than using dilation over a wire. Consequently, we excluded those infrequent reports on the Fantoni translaryngeal retrograde technique, the Portex Griggs' guidewire dilating forceps (Smiths Medical, Dubin, OH), the PercuTwist kit (Rusch Teleflex-Medical, Research Triangle Park, NC), or the Ciaglia Blue Dolphin balloon dilation kit (Cook Medical, Bloomington, IN).

Evidence

Early Outcomes

In assessing overall early complications, it is not overtly clear that either surgical tracheostomy or PDT has an obvious advantage. Single cohort studies evaluating early complication rates following PDT have been reported in the range of 8–9 % [3–5]. In a prospective randomized controlled trial of 53 adults requiring tracheostomy, Friedman et al. found that postoperative complications were less frequent for patients undergoing PDT, with an incidence of 12 %, compared to 41 % among patients undergoing ST (P=0.008) [6]. (Table 44.1) The authors of this study acknowledge a relatively high complication rate, especially for ST, which they attribute to strict definitions and an intense search for complications. While the authors recognize that some of the included complications may be of minimal clinical significance (such as transient hypoxia or minimal bleeding requiring no intervention), it is clear that identical definitions were applied to both study groups, with a significant difference seen between them.

In contrast, another prospective randomized trial, performed by Massick and colleagues in 2001, evaluated 164 patients in the medical intensive care unit selected for tracheostomy and found a higher rate of overall short-term complications among patients receiving PDT [7]. The incidence of postoperative complications for PDT was 16 %, compared to 2 % for ST (P<0.05). However, it should be noted that this study compared bedside PDT to bedside ST, with a separate population of patients who underwent ST in the operating room, whose complications were not included with those considered as part of the comparative bedside groups. Thus, any complications secondary to transfer to the operating room or the general anesthetic are not included, and, in order to replicate the circumstances of this study, one would need to have adequate resources to perform a full surgical tracheostomy at the bedside. Providing no further clarity on the issue, Beltrame's 2008 case-cohort study found that, among 528 patients undergoing tracheostomy, there was no significant difference between short-term complication rates in the two groups, with an incidence of 14.7 % for PDT and 19.2 % for ST (NS) [8].

Table 44.1 Published data

Author	Year	Study type	N	Early outcomes	Intermediate outcomes	Long-term outcomes	Resource utilization	Quality of evidence
Friedman et al. [6]	1996	Prospective randomized controlled trial	53	Bleeding 8 % PDT vs 15 % ST; stomal infx 0 PDT vs 15 % ST; accidental decannulation 4 % PDT vs 15 % ST; 1 death (3.7 %) directly related to ST vs 0 PD–otal complications 12 % PDT vs 41 % ST (p=0.008)	Decannulation rate 19.2 % PDT vs 18.5 % ST (NS); trend toward earlier stomal closure in PDT (4.0 vs 12.2 days)		Wait time until procedure 28.5 h PDT vs 100.4 h ST (P<0.001); PDT procedure 8.2 min vs ST 33.9 min (P<0.0001)	High
Freeman et al. [10]	2000	Comparative meta-analysis	136	PDT with less bleeding (OR 0.39, CI 0.17–0.88; PDT with less stomal infection (OR 0.02, CI 0.01–0.07)			Operative time shorter for PDT (9.84 min shorter than ST, 95 % CI 7.83–10.85)	High
Massick et al. [7]	2001	Prospective randomized controlled trial	164	Bleeding 4 % PDT vs 2 % ST (NS); site infection 2 % PDT vs 0 ST (NS); death secondary to complication of trach 2 % of PDT vs 0 ST (NS); overall postoperative complications 16 % PDT vs 2 % ST (P<0.05)			Bedside procedure $1,760 less than OR procedure	High

Polderman et al. [9]	2003	Comparative retrospective review	211	Bleeding 3.3 % for PDT vs 12.5 % ST; respiratory deterioration lasting >12 h 3 % PDT vs 12.5 % ST; stomal infection 0.7 % PDT vs 7.5 % ST	Mid-term complications included intermittent tracheal kinking in 3.3 % PDT vs 2.5 % ST	Tracheal stenosis 0 % PDT vs 12.5 % ST	Similar wait time for procedure	Moderate
Bacchetta et al. [16]	2005	Comparative retrospective review	86	No complications due to PDT or ST; median ICU LOS for PDT 35 days vs 36 days ST			PDT \$325 vs ST \$1,200; ICU LOS for ST 1 day greater (\$2,250)	Moderate
Koitschev et al. [14]	2006	Comparative observational study	146			Suprastomal stenosis seen in 58.1 % PDT vs 24.4 % ST, p=0.0004; Severe suprastomal stenosis 23.8 % PDT vs 7.3 % ST, p=0.033		Moderate
Higgins et al. [12]	2007	Meta-analysis	973	Less wound infection for PDT (OR 0.37, CI 0.22–0.62, P<0.0002); No difference in minor hemorrhage (OR for PDT 1.09, CI 0.61–1.97, P=0.77), No difference in major hemorrhage (OR for PDT 0.60, CI 0.28–1.26, P=0.17)	Decannulation/obstruction more common in PDT (OR 2.79, CI 1.29–6.03, P=0.009); PDT with less unfavorable scarring (OR 0.44, CI 0.23–0.83, P <0.01)	Subglottic stenois equal (PTD OR 0.59, CI 0.27–1.29, P=0.19)	Cost for PDT \$456.61 USD less than ST; PDT with less time utilization (4.59 min less than ST)	High

(continued)

Table 44.1 (continued)

Author	Year	Study type	N	Early outcomes	Intermediate outcomes	Long-term outcomes	Resource utilization	Quality of evidence
Beltrame et al. [8]	2008	Case-cohort	528	Short term complications PDT 14.7 % vs ST 19.2 % (NS); minor bleeding PDT 0 vs ST 5.0 % (P<0.01); major bleeding PDT 0 vs ST 1.9 % (P<0.05); stomal infection PDT 0 vs ST 5.0 % (P<0.01)	Canula dislodgement PDT 0 vs ST 1.9 % (P<0.05)	Granulomas PDT 0.5 % vs ST 0 (NS); tracheal stenosis PDT 5.4 % vs ST 1.9 % (NS); dysphagia PDT 1.1 % vs ST 3.1 % (NS)	PDT shorter procedure time 5.4±5.2 min vs ST 19±10 min STs (P<0.05)	Moderate
Kost et al. [4]	2009	Prospective single-cohort observation	500	9.2 % complication rate; bleeding 2.4 %; stomal infection 0.8 %; posterior tracheal wall abrasion 0.6 %	Inadvertent decannulation 1 %	36.5 % decannulated		Low
Zagli et al. [5]	2010	Retrospective single-cohort review	509	Intraoperative bleeding 9.1 %, stomal infection 1.2 %; tracheal ring fracture 7.5 %;				Low
Pappas et al. [11]	2010	Multi-institutional historical cohort comparison	1,175	Bleeding 6.6 % PDT vs 1.9 % ST (P<0.002);	Accidental decannulation 0.5 % PDT vs 0.9 % ST; tracheitis 1.0 % PDT vs 0.9 % ST			Moderate
Deppe et al. [3]	2013	Retrospective single cohort study	213	8 % complications; 6.1 % bleeding complications				Low
Park et al. [13]	2013	Prospective comparative observational study	640	Stomal infection less frequent in PDT 3.4 % vs ST 7.0 % (P=0.04)				High

CI confidence interval, *OR* odds ratio, *PDT* percutaneous dilational tracheostomy, *ST* surgical tracheostomy

Complications

One of the reasons for the outcomes disparities in randomized trials may be the variable classification of minor events as identifiable complications. In order to tease out any true differences, it is helpful to consider specific named complications.

Bleeding

Bleeding is a commonly reported short-term complication following tracheostomy. While, theoretically, hemostasis may be easier to achieve in a surgical setting with maximal exposure, PDT requires less dissection and the tracheostomy appliance fits snugly via the small incision, thus minimizing the propensity to bleed. In Friedman's 1996 trial, clinically noted bleeding occurred among 8 % of PDT patients and 15 % of ST patients, although this did not reach statistical significance [6]. A 2003 retrospective review of 211 patients found the incidence of bleeding to be 3.3 % for PDT and 12.5 % for ST, although this study was inadequately powered to show a difference [9]. While Massick found bleeding to be more likely among PDT (4 % versus 2 %), this also failed to reach significance [7]. A comparative meta-analysis performed by Freeman et al. included 136 patients and found that PDT was likely to have less bleeding events than ST, with an odds ratio (OR) of 0.39 (95 % confidence interval [CI] 0.17–0.88) [10].

In contrast, Pappas and colleagues conducted a 2010 multi-institutional review of nearly 1,200 patients, finding that bleeding occurred after 6.6 % of PDT and 1.9 % of ST procedures ($P < 0.002$) [11]. The wide range of incidences would suggest inconsistent parameters for labeling bleeding as clinically relevant. Further obscuring the issue, some investigators have chosen to categorize bleeding events into major and minor hemorrhage. In Higgins' 2007 meta-analysis reviewing outcomes in 973 patients, no differences were seen in minor (OR for PDT 1.09, 95 % CI 0.61–1.97) or major hemorrhage (OR for PDT 0.60, 95 % CI 0.28–1.26) [12]. A 2008 case-cohort study, however, reviewed 528 patients' charts and found that hemorrhagic complications were significantly less frequent among patients who received PDT, with no bleeding events for the PDT group and incidence of minor and major bleeding for ST 5.0 % and 1.9 %, respectively ($P < 0.01$) [8]. Further supporting PDT, a retrospective review of 213 patients demonstrated that PDT could be safely performed among patients with coagulation disorders [3].

Stomal Infection

Stomal infection is another notable short-term complication following tracheostomy, and several studies have shown a tendency toward fewer wound infections among patients undergoing PDT [6, 8–10, 12]. Freeman reported a significant reduction in risk of wound infection for PDT compared to ST, with an OR of 0.02, CI 0.01–0.07.10 Likewise, similar findings emerged from Higgins' meta-analysis, with OR of

0.37, CI 0.22–0.62 (P < 0.0002) for PDT compared to ST [12]. More recently, a prospective study of 640 patients performed by Park et al. in 2013 demonstrated less frequent stomal infections in PDT, at 3.4 %, compared to 7.0 % for ST (P=0.04) [13]. Among papers included in this systematic review, only one study found a higher rate of wound infection among PDT, and this was not statistically significant [7].

Decannulation

Several authors comment on rates of inadvertent decannulation in the early postoperative period, but this is of unclear clinical relevance. Mechanistically, in ST some surgeons place stay sutures through the tracheal rings and anchor them to the skin, thus theoretically making inadvertent decannulation somewhat less likely. However, inadvertent loss of airway is in all likelihood more a function of patient body habitus, positioning, and bedside handling and care of the airway. In the prospective study out of Ohio State, Massick and colleagues describe a case in which otolaryngology was consulted to perform an emergent ST in a patient who had undergone PDT, experienced inadvertent tube removal, and then failed translaryngeal intubation [7]. This patient subsequently suffered cardiopulmonary arrest and death 4 h after the event. Based on this isolated incident, the authors report a 2 % incidence of deaths secondary to complications of PDT, which is not statistically significant; however, interpretation of this single severe complication and its generalizable applicability are not immediately apparent. Inadvertent extubation and resulting consequences seem to be inadequately reported in literature.

Intermediate Outcomes

Among mid-term complications, our review did not demonstrate any consistent strengths of one technical approach over the other. The most commonly reported intermediate outcomes included tube dislodgement, tracheitis, unfavorable scarring, and time to tracheal closure [4, 6, 8, 9, 11, 12]. Many investigators reported similar outcomes for PDT and ST and statistically significant findings were rare. Intermediate outcomes were reported for 6 of the 13 studies, with only 2 authors showing significant findings.

In their mid-term analysis, Higgins and colleagues found that patients who underwent PDT had less unfavorable scarring than those who underwent ST (OR 0.44, CI 0.23–0.83, P < 0.01), favoring PDT [12]. However, in their study, problems with decannulation and tracheostomy tube obstruction were more common following PDT (OR 2.79, CI 1.29–6.03, P=0.009). In contrast, another large study of over 500 patients found opposing results. Beltrame reported no cases of cannula dislodgement for PDT, whereas the rate for ST was 1.9 % (P < 0.05) [8]. Again, it is not obvious that such differences would depend on the operative strategy employed, and results of mid-term outcomes are unlikely to guide overall recommendations.

Late Outcomes

While essentially all authors provided early complication rates following tracheostomy, fewer investigators followed the patients for longer periods of time to provide insight into differences in long-term outcomes. Results from those studies with prolonged follow-up are particularly useful in discerning whether there is a difference in tracheal stenosis, the most important long-term complication of endotracheal intubation.

Two papers in this review demonstrated significant differences in rates of tracheal stensosis. In a German study, 146 patients with previous tracheostomies underwent endoscopic assessment of the presence and severity of tracheal stenosis, with mean interval of 52.5 days between tracheostomy and surveillance [14]. Authors found that all cases of stenosis were suprastomal. The incidence of severe suprastomal stenosis (more than 50 % of the lumen) was 23.8 % after PDT and 7.3 % following ST (P=0.033). The authors concluded that PDT may be associated with an increased risk of severe suprastomal tracheal stenosis compared to ST. However, this methodology of this study ought to be considered: these patients all underwent surveillance regardless of symptomology, and the clinical relevance of the findings is unclear. After a mean follow-up duration of 14 months (range 6–29 months), Polderman and colleagues found no cases of *clinically evident* tracheal stenosis after PDT, compared to a rate of 12.5 % for ST, although this did not reach significance [9]. In meta-analysis evaluation, Higgins also found that rates of subglottic stenosis tended toward less frequency with PTD without statistical significance (OR 0.59, CI 0.27–1.29, P=0.19) [12].

Due to the limited long-term follow-up presently published following PDT versus ST, this remains an important consideration for further investigation. Variations in the nature of long-term complications following surgical versus percutaneous tracheostomy have been uncovered and recently described, further fueling the importance of ongoing follow-up in this realm [15].

Resource Utilization

There are several key differences in resource utilization between PDT and ST, with the majority favoring PDT. While PDT typically involves a disposable, commercially produced, single-use kit, ST is performed using a standard operative set with reusable instruments (which can be reused, but do incur the costs and man-power of reprocessing). ST is usually performed in the operating room, with a full team of personnel, including anesthesia providers, nurses, and surgical technologists; PDT may be performed in the operating room, but is more often conducted in the intensive care unit. Bedside PDT can often be performed by the surgeon with sedation provided by an intensivist, without the need for involvement of any additional health-care providers or the use of expensive and scarce operating room time. While resource utilization is not always taken into consideration when determining the best possible approach for optimizing patient outcomes, in the setting of similar outcomes and acceptable complication rates with both strategies, resource utilization should perhaps be addressed. Further, issues with resource allocation do directly impact individual patients; for example, limited operating room availability may prolong a patient's wait for ST, whereas a PDT may potentially be performed earlier, allowing more rapid rehabilitation [6].

After the point of determining that a given patient needed tracheostomy, Friedman and colleagues found that wait time for PDT averaged 28.5 h, just over 1 day, compared to 100.4 h (more than 4 days) for ST (P < 0.001) [6]. Further, they reported that the actual procedure duration for PDT was shorter, at a mean of 8.2 min versus 33.9 min for ST (P < 0.0001). Subsequently, Freeman, Higgins, and Beltrame also found similar results, with significantly shorter operative times for PDT [8, 10, 12].

With regard to cost, authors have used varying schema to evaluate differences between PDT and ST; regardless of disparities in study methodology, definitions in elements of cost, and institutional/geographical factors, PDT has consistently been found to be less expensive. In a prospective randomized controlled trial, Massick et al. found that the cost of bedside PDT was $1,760 less than ST in the operating room [7]. Likewise, in 2005, Bachetta reported PDT to be nearly $900 cheaper than ST [16]. Higgins' meta-analysis also found that ST cost an average of $457 more than bedside PDT [12]. Despite the disposable single-use kit required for PDT, the relatively more intense resource utilization required for ST in the operating room resulted in greater costs in all studies reviewed.

Recommendations

PDT is associated with slightly fewer immediate and early complications including bleeding and surgical site infection, when compared to ST. There appears to be no significant difference in intermediate outcomes between the two approaches and a minor trend is seen toward a higher incidence of tracheal stenosis with PDT. We recommend that PDT can be utilized as a preferred modality if the institution is adequately equipped and well-trained personnel perform the procedure. Additionally, contraindications including difficult body habitus should be specifically sought out before planning PDT. Finally, PDT tends to provide moderate cost savings compared to ST.

A Personal View of the Data

We have, over the last 5–7 years, adopted PDT as our technique of choice for creating a tracheostomy. At our center, we perform the procedure in the intensive care unit (ICU) with attending cardiothoracic anesthesiologists (who also staff the cardiothoracic ICU) providing sedation. For patients who have a short neck and poor neck extension, or morbidly obese individuals where anatomic landmarks are difficult to palpate, we still perform a conventional ST. When, based upon clinical examination, it is felt that an extra-long appliance would be required, we prefer ST. All PDT procedures are carried out with real-time, continuous, bronchoscopic guidance. For PDT, we believe that meticulous attention to detail is required in choosing the initial needle puncture site on the anterior wall of the airway. We stay strictly in the midline, between the second and third tracheal rings and avoid coming through a cartilaginous ring. This tends to deform the anterior wall of the airway the least and, in our opinion, leads to a lower incidence of delayed stenosis.

Recommendation

- We recommend percutaneous dilational tracheostomy as opposed to conventional open surgical tracheostomy if an appropriate team is available and no specific contraindications exist. (Evidence quality moderate; weak recommendation)

References

1. Hsia DW, Ghori UK, Musani AI. Percutaneous dilational tracheostomy. Clin Chest Med. 2013;34(3):515–26.
2. Cools-Lartigue J, Aboalsaud A, Gill H, Ferri L. Evolution of percutaneous dilatational tracheostomy–a review of current techniques and their pitfalls. World J Surg. 2013;37(7):1633–46.
3. Deppe AC, Kuhn E, Scherner M, Slottosch I, Liakopoulos O, Langebartels G, et al. Coagulation disorders do not increase the risk for bleeding during percutaneous dilatational tracheotomy. Thorac Cardiovasc Surg. 2013;61(03):234–9.
4. Kost KM. Endoscopic percutaneous dilatational tracheotomy: a prospective evaluation of 500 consecutive cases. Laryngoscope. 2009;115(S107):1–30.
5. Zagli G, Linden M, Spina R, Bonizzoli M, Cianchi G, Anichini V, et al. Early tracheostomy in intensive care unit: a retrospective study of 506 cases of video-guided Ciaglia Blue Rhino tracheostomies. J Trauma. 2010;68(2):367–72.
6. Friedman Y, Fildes J, Mizock B, Samuel J, Patel S, Appavu S, et al. Comparison of percutaneous and surgical tracheostomies. Chest. 1996;110(2):480–5.
7. Massick DD, Yao S, Powell DM, Griesen D, Hobgood T, Allen JN, et al. Bedside tracheostomy in the intensive care unit: a prospective randomized trial comparing open surgical tracheostomy with endoscopically guided percutaneous dilational tracheotomy. Laryngoscope. 2001;111(3):494–500.
8. Beltrame F, Zussino M, Martinez B, Dibartolomeo S, Saltarini M, Vetrugno L, et al. Percutaneous versus surgical bedside tracheostomy in the intensive care unit: a cohort study. Minerva Anestesiol. 2008;74(10):529–35.
9. Polderman KH, Spijkstra JJ, de Bree R, Christiaans HM, Gelissen HP, Wester JP, et al. Percutaneous dilatational tracheostomy in the ICU: optimal organization, low complication rates, and description of a new complication. Chest. 2003;123(5):1595–602.

10. Freeman BD, Isabella K, Lin N, Buchman TG. A meta-analysis of prospective trials comparing percutaneous and surgical tracheostomy in critically ill patients. Chest. 2000; 118(5):1412–8.
11. Pappas S, Maragoudakis P, Vlastarakos P, Assimakopoulos D, Mandrali T, Kandiloros D, et al. Surgical versus percutaneous tracheostomy: an evidence-based approach. Eur Arch Otorhinolaryngol. 2010;268(3):323–30.
12. Higgins KM, Punthakee X. Meta-analysis comparison of open versus percutaneous tracheostomy. Laryngoscope. 2007;117(3):447–54.
13. Park H, Kent J, Joshi M, Zhu S, Bochicchio GV, Henry S, et al. Percutaneous versus open tracheostomy: comparison of procedures and surgical site infections. Surg Infect (Larchmt). 2013;14(1):21–3.
14. Koitschev A, Simon C, Blumenstock G, Mach H, Graumüller S. Suprastomal tracheal stenosis after dilational and surgical tracheostomy in critically ill patients. Anaesthesia. 2006;61(9):832–7.
15. Jacobs JV, Hill DA, Petersen SR, Bremner RM, Sue RD, Smith MA. "Corkscrew stenosis": defining and preventing a complication of percutaneous dilatational tracheostomy. J Thorac Cardiovasc Surg. 2013;145(3):716–20.
16. Bacchetta MD, Girardi LN, Southard EJ, Mack CA, Ko W, Tortolani AJ, et al. Comparison of open versus bedside percutaneous dilatational tracheostomy in the cardiothoracic surgical patient: outcomes and financial analysis. Ann Thorac Surg. 2005;79(6):1879–85.

Chapter 45
Carinal Resection for Non Small Cell Lung Cancer

Timothy M. Millington and Henning A. Gaissert

Abstract Modern surgical and anesthetic technique permits the resection of non-small cell lung cancers involving the tracheal carina. Retrospective reviews suggest a surgical mortality below 10 % and 5-year survival approaching 40 % in selected patients. Despite the use of induction therapy, fewer than 15 % of patients with mediastinal lymph node metastases survive 5 years and patients not responsive to induction should not be considered for surgery. The most serious complications are anastomotic dehiscence and acute respiratory distress syndrome (ARDS), which may be minimized with careful patient selection, surgical technique and airway management intra- and post-operatively.

Keywords Carinal resectional • Carinal pneumonectomy • Bronchogenic carcinoma • Non-small cell lung cancer

Introduction

Despite more than 50 years of experience with carinal resection worldwide, lung cancers invading the tracheal carina were regarded as marginally resectable, reflected until recently in their stage IIIB designation. Although carinal invasion is still staged T4 in the 7th edition of the International Association for the Study of Lung Cancer TNM staging system, T4N0M0 tumors are now categorized as IIIA. This revision reflects the fact that patients with non-small cell lung cancer (NSCLC) involving the carina should be considered as candidates for surgical resection.

T.M. Millington, MD • H.A. Gaissert, MD (✉)
Department of Thoracic Surgery, Massachusetts General Hospital,
55 Fruit Street, Boston, MA 02114, USA
e-mail: hgaissert@partners.org

M.K. Ferguson (ed.), *Difficult Decisions in Thoracic Surgery*,
Difficult Decisions in Surgery: An Evidence-Based Approach 1,
DOI 10.1007/978-1-4471-6404-3_45, © Springer-Verlag London 2014

At experienced centers employing modern surgical and anesthetic technique, carefully selected patients with NSCLC involving the carina may undergo surgical resection with operative mortality of less than 10 % and 5-year survival reaching 40 %.

Carinal resection alone should be considered separately from resections including lobectomy or pneumonectomy, as the operative technique increases in complexity with the number of anastomoses while operative risk is related to the extent of parenchymal resection.

Search Strategy

To determine the evidence basis for carinal resection, we developed a search query using the PICO methodology. Our PICO terms were as follows:

- Patient/problem = Non-small cell lung cancer, bronchogenic carcinoma
- Intervention = Carinal resection, carinal pneumonectomy
- Comparison = N/A
- Outcome = Surgical mortality, morbidity, long-term survival

We are not aware of a randomized controlled trial of carinal resection versus nonoperative management and so no comparison term was selected. The PICO methodology led to the following query: ("non-small cell lung cancer" OR "bronchogenic carcinoma" OR "non-small cell lung cancer") AND ("carinal resection" OR "carinal pneumonectomy") AND (mortality OR morbidity OR "long-term survival"). We excluded three papers in languages other than English, three review articles, one case report and nine case series addressing other problems and including fewer than ten carinal resections. A total of 15 publications ranging from 1982 to 2009 were identified.

Review of the Evidence

The publications reviewed described carinal resections carried out between 1957 and 2006 (Table 45.1). Each article was a single-center, retrospective study. Although the studies drew conclusions from a range of eras, there was a clear tendency toward reduced operative mortality in those series drawing on patients primarily after 1990. For this reason we focused our review and recommendations on series published after 2000.

Technical Considerations

The technical aspects of carinal resection have been well described elsewhere [3, 7, 12] and are beyond the scope of this article. There is some variability in anesthetic and surgical technique between centers that deserves mention.

Table 45.1 Published cases series of carinal resection for bronchogenic carcinoma

Author	Year of publication	Patients[a]	Years	Morbidity (%)	30 day mortality (%)	5-year survival (%)
Jensik et al. [1]	1982	34	1964–1981		29	15
Watanabe et al. [2]	1990	12			17	NR
Mathisen and Grillo et al. [3]	1991	37	1973–1991		19	19
Roviaro et al. [4]	1994	28	1983–1992		4	20
Ayabe et al. [5]	1995	15	1957–1993	93	13.3	NR
Dartevelle et al. [6]	1996	60			7	43
Mitchell et al. [7]	1999	58	1962–1996		15.5	
Mitchell et al. [8]	2001	60	1973–1998		15	42
Porhanov [9]	2002	151	1979–2001	35.6[b]	16[b]	24.7
Regnard et al. [10]	2005	65	1983–2002	51	7.7	26.5
de Perrot et al. [11]	2006	103	1981–2004	47	7.8	44
Macchiarini et al. [12]	2006	50	1999–2004	37	4	51
Yamamoto et al. [13]	2007	35	1987–2004	22.8	8.5	28.3
Rea et al. [14]	2008	49	1982–2005	28.6	6.1	27.5
Jiang et al. [15]	2009	41	1982–2006		2.4	26.8

[a]Excludes patients undergoing carinal resections for indications other than NSCLC
[b]Overall rate, including additional patients undergoing carinal resection for indications other than NSCLC

Anesthetic Technique

Various ventilation techniques during carinal resection have been described including sterile cross-field ventilation [8, 11], high-frequency jet ventilation (HFJV) [9, 10, 14], and apneic hyperoxygenation [12]. Because most reports of carinal resection come from single institutions, comparative studies have not been conducted. There may be an increased rate of acute respiratory distress syndrome (ARDS) with HFJV [9] although this observation has not been supported by other groups [10]. Planned cardiopulmonary bypass (CPB) is not routinely required and emergency use of CPB is uncommon [11]. There may be a decreased incidence of barotrauma-related ARDS with apneic hyperoxygenation [12].

Choice of Approach

For anatomic reasons, right-sided carinal resections are more common than left-sided procedures [7, 11]. Whereas right-sided carinal resection is approached preferably via right posterolateral thoracotomy, the much less common left-sided carinal resection may be approached via left thoracotomy or bilateral anterior thoracotomy [7]. Median sternotomy [11, 12] affords access to carinal resection alone and to resections combined with right or left parenchymal resections.

Anastomotic Considerations

In order to achieve a tension-free anastomosis, the majority of authors limit tracheo-bronchial resection to 4 cm [7, 11, 15]. This distance refers to the maximal resectable airway length that still allows acceptable tension between trachea and left main bronchus. Hilar release of the left main stem bronchus by pericardial circumcision of the pulmonary veins is useful to reduce anastomotic tension but laryngeal release does not transfer additional tracheal length to the carina [11]. The use of a guardian stitch (a stitch between the chin and anterior chest wall to prevent neck extension postoperatively) varies among institutions. Anastomotic complications increase with each additional anastomosis; end-to-side reimplantation of a main or intermedius bronchus has a greater incidence of leak and separation. Variation in postoperative morbidity and mortality by length of trachea resected is not described in these series. At least 13 configurations for reconstructing the carina have been described [7] and the choice of anastomosis is dictated by the anatomy of the individual resection.

Resection of Additional Mediastinal Structures

Resection and reconstruction of various other mediastinal structures including the pulmonary artery, left atrium and superior vena cava were included in several series [11, 14, 15]. Evidence for increased mortality with more extensive resections is not presented but may be assumed if vascular anastomoses are added. Involvement of these structures by the primary tumor is not a contraindication to carinal resection.

Postoperative Considerations

The most frequent causes of early postoperative death in these series were anastomotic complication and respiratory failure due to ARDS. The mortality of anastomotic dehiscence or ARDS approach or exceed 50 % [11, 13]. A higher incidence of anastomotic complications appears to correlate with operative mortality (Table 45.2). Greater anastomotic complexity must therefore be balanced with the aim to preserve lung parenchyma. In the majority of published cases a viable tissue wrap (usually pericardium or intercostal muscle) is used to protect the anastomosis [7, 14, 15]. Comparative rates of anastomotic dehiscence or stenosis with or without a wrap are not described.

It is speculated that postoperative pulmonary edema, which frequently precedes ARDS, is caused by ventilator-induce barotrauma [11]. The use of apneic hyper-oxygenation as an alternative to traditional cross-field ventilation has been advocated as a means of avoiding barotrauma [12]. Hypercapnia develops during the apneic period used to construct the anastomosis, but according to its proponents is rapidly reversed when ventilation is reestablished [16]. The lower rate of operative mortality and ARDS in more recent reports suggests that the coinciding use of

Table 45.2 Incidence of anastomotic complications and operative mortality

Author	Year of publication	Operative mortality (%)	Anastomotic complication (%)
Mitchell et al. [8]	2001	12.7	17.2
Porhanov et al. [9]	2002	16	35.4
Regnard et al. [10]	2005	7.7	15.3
de Perrot et al. [11]	2006	7.6	10.1
Macchiarini et al. [12]	2006	4	16
Yamamoto et al. [13]	2007	8.5	11.4
Rea et al. [14]	2008	6.1	2
Jiang et al. [15]	2009	2.4	2.4

modern ventilating algorithms during operation may protect the contralateral lung. Other common postoperative complications included pneumonia and atrial tachyarrhythmias.

Oncologic Considerations

Nodal Status and Survival

The presence of mediastinal lymph node metastases has a marked impact on the survival of patients undergoing carinal resection (Table 45.3). The effect of hilar lymph node metastases is unclear. Positive N1 nodes may also portend poorer 5-year survival [7, 14] but other series fail to reflect a significant difference [11]. N1 status should not be used to exclude potential surgical candidates. Radical mediastinal lymph node dissection devascularizes the adjacent airway and is therefore relatively contraindicated in carinal resections; understandably, no systematic study of this topic exists.

Mediastinal Staging

Modalities for staging the mediastinum include PET-CT, endobronchial ultrasound with transbronchial needle aspiration and mediastinoscopy. In addition to precise nodal staging, mediastinoscopy at the time of proposed resection has been advocated to determine the extent of extraluminal disease and mobilize the pretracheal plane while sparing the lateral blood supply and recurrent laryngeal nerves [7]. An alternative approach is to use preoperative CT-PET imaging to identify possible N2 disease [12, 14] with confirmatory preoperative mediastinoscopy for patients with PET-avid mediastinal nodes. The role of endobronchial ultrasound (EBUS) in staging the mediastinum prior to carinal resection is unclear; its potential advantage would consist of preserving pretracheal tissue planes when mediastinal evaluation precedes carinal resection.

Table 45.3 Nodal status and 5-year survival

Author	Year of publication	Overall 5-year survival (%)	5-year survival, N0-N1 patients (%)	5-year survival, N2+ patients (%)
Mitchell et al. [8]	2001	42	51 (N0)/32 (N1)	12
Porhanov et al. [9]	2002	24.7	32	7.5
Regnard et al. [10]	2005	26.5	38	5.3
de Perrot et al. [11]	2006	44	55 (N0)/50 (N1)	15
Yamamoto et al. [13]	2007	28.3	44.4	0
Rea et al. [14]	2008	27.5	56 (N0)/17 (N1)	0
Jiang et al. [15]	2009	26.8	37.0	7.1

Adjuvant Therapy

If metastatic disease is detected in the mediastinal nodes before operation, induction chemotherapy should be considered. The addition of induction radiotherapy is controversial as radiation increases the risk of tracheal dehiscence [11, 12]. Re-staging after induction therapy is by repeat CT-PET and re-do mediastinoscopy is not performed [12]. It is not clear that induction chemotherapy increase perioperative mortality and some groups advocating routinely administering it to nearly all NSCLC patients undergoing planned carinal resection [11]. Others proceed directly to surgery in the absence of N2 disease [12] while some consider induction chemotherapy a relative contraindication to carinal resection [13]. Postoperative adjuvant chemoradiotherapy may be given to patients with N2 disease detected at the time of resection [12].

Recommendations

Patients with non-small cell lung cancer involving the carina should undergo a complete staging evaluation including whole-body PET CT and brain MRI. Patients with non-small cell lung cancer involving the carina should undergo a careful cardiopulmonary assessment to determine their fitness for potential pneumonectomy. Physiologically fit patients with clinical T4N0M0 lesions involving the carina should undergo invasive mediastinal staging followed by carinal resection in the absence of nodal metastases. Physiologically fit patients with PET-avid hilar or mediastinal lymph nodes should undergo invasive mediastinal staging, and selected patients with T4N1-N2 should be treated with induction chemotherapy. Responders should undergo carinal resection. Patients with T4N2 NSCLC involving the carina who do not respond to induction chemotherapy should not be considered for surgical resection. Carinal resection should be performed at high-volume centers with surgeons and thoracic anesthesiologists experienced in complex ventilation strategies for airway surgery.

Summary

Advances in surgical technique, anesthesiology and critical care have helped to improve the mortality of complex airway procedures and extended the boundaries of resectability for lung cancer. Studies from North America, Europe and Asia demonstrate that centrally located NSCLC with mediastinal invasion may frequently be resected with a 30-day mortality not markedly exceeding that of conventional pneumonectomy. In selected patients without metastatic disease, long-term survival is possible. In the presence of mediastinal lymph node metastases, long-term outcomes after mediastinal resection remain poor despite the addition of induction chemotherapy.

Many of the technical aspects of carinal resection, including the need for a well-vascularized, tension-free anastomosis protected by a viable tissue buttress, are well established. The optimum intraoperative and postoperative ventilation strategy for preventing post-pneumonectomy pulmonary edema and ARDS is a promising target for future study.

A Personal View of the Data

Under general anesthesia, a bronchoscopy is performed to determine the extent of tumor. Usually, biopsies from a prior endoscopy have secured the outline of tumor and tumor-free margins. The patient is then reintubated with a long single-lumen tube that reaches into the left main bronchus and is more pliable than a double-lumen tube; an armored 6.6 or 7.0 mm tube (Rusch Inc., Duluth, GA) is adequate.

We prefer the anterior transsternal approach to carinal resection. This incision allows a bilateral pericardial release and access to trachea, right main and the upper half of the left main bronchus. The pretracheal and prebronchial planes are completely mobilized. Once cross-table ventilating tubing is set up, the airway is divided below tumor across the main bronchus selected for ventilation; the endotracheal tube is withdrawn into the trachea. The tumor-bearing carina is resected with narrow margins. No formal lymph node dissection is conducted. A sliver of airway is sent from the patient side of each airway for frozen section to confirm freedom from tumor.

Lateral traction sutures of 2-0 Vicryl are placed in each end of the airway. The best reconstructive configuration of the neo-carina is now determined. Y-reconstruction is selected with resection of short carinal segments. An end-to-end anastomosis between the trachea and left main bronchus is otherwise created for right carinal pneumonectomy. If the right lung is preserved, the anastomosis of the right bronchus is performed to the anterolateral trachea at least 2 cm above the tracheal end. The airway ends are joined with interrupted 4-0 Vicryl, first placed in a circumferential manner and then tied. Each anastomosis is tested for leaks and circumferentially wrapped with pedicled, vascularized tissue, usually pericardial fat pad or thymus.

The sternum is closed. While neck flexion does not translate to additional tracheal length at the carina, a chin stitch in selected patients prevents upward traction on the trachea. The anastomosis is assessed with bronchoscopy 7 days after the operation.

Recommendations

- Physiologically fit patients with clinical T4N0M0 lesions involving the carina should undergo invasive mediastinal staging followed by carinal resection in the absence of nodal metastases. (Evidence quality low; weak recommendation)
- Physiologically fit patients with PET-avid hilar or mediastinal lymph nodes should undergo invasive mediastinal staging. Selected patients with T4N1-N2 should be treated with induction chemotherapy, and responders should undergo carinal resection. (Evidence quality low; weak recommendation)
- Patients with T4N2 NSCLC involving the carina who do not respond to induction chemotherapy should not be considered for surgical resection. (Evidence quality low; weak recommendation)
- Carinal resection should be performed at high-volume centers with surgeons and thoracic anesthesiologists experienced in complex ventilation strategies for airway surgery. (Evidence quality low; weak recommendation)

References

1. Jensik RJ, Faber LP, Kittle CF, Miley RW, Thatcher WC, El-Baz N. Survival in patients undergoing tracheal sleeve pneumonectomy for bronchogenic carcinoma. J Thorac Cardiovasc Surg. 1982;84(4):489–96.
2. Watanabe Y, Shimizu J, Oda M, Hayashi Y, Watanabe S, Yazaki U, Iwa T. Results in 104 patients undergoing bronchoplastic procedures for bronchial lesions. Ann Thorac Surg. 1990;50(4):607–14.
3. Mathisen DJ, Grillo HC. Carinal resection for bronchogenic carcinoma. J Thorac Cardiovasc Surg. 1991;102(1):16–22.
4. Roviaro GC, Varoli F, Rebuffat C, Scalambra SM, Vergani C, Sibilla E, Palmarini L, Pezzuoli G. Tracheal sleeve pneumonectomy for bronchogenic carcinoma. J Thorac Cardiovasc Surg. 1994;107(1):13–8.
5. Ayabe H, Tagawa Y, Tsuji H, Kawahara K, Akamine S, Takahashi T, Hara S, Tomita M. Results of carinal resection for bronchogenic carcinoma. Tohoku J Exp Med. 1995;175(2):91–9.
6. Dartevelle P, Macchiarini P. Carinal resection for bronchogenic cancer. Semin Thorac Cardiovasc Surg. 1996;8(4):414–25.
7. Mitchell JD, Mathisen DJ, Wright CD, Wain JC, Donahue DM, Moncure AC, Grillo HC. Clinical experience with carinal resection. J Thorac Cardiovasc Surg. 1999;117(1):39–52.

8. Mitchell JD, Mathisen DJ, Wright CD, Wain JC, Donahue DM, Allan JS, Moncure AC, Grillo HC. Resection for bronchogenic carcinoma involving the carina: long-term results and effect of nodal status on outcome. J Thorac Cardiovasc Surg. 2001;121(3):465–71.

9. Porhanov VA, Poliakov IS, Selvaschuk AP, Grechishkin AI, Sitnik SD, Nikolaev IF, Efimtsev JP, Marchenko LG. Indications and results of sleeve carinal resection. Eur J Cardiothorac Surg. 2002;22(5):685–94.

10. Regnard J, Perrotin C, Giovannetti R, Schussler O, Petino A, Spaggiari L, Alifano M, Magdeleinat P. Resection for tumors with carinal involvement: technical aspects, results, and prognostic factors. Ann Thorac Surg. 2005;80:1841–6.

11. de Perrot M, Fadel E, Mercier O, Mussot S, Chapelier A, Dartevelle P. Long-term results after carinal resection for carcinoma: does the benefit warrant the risk? J Thorac Cardiovasc Surg. 2006;131(1):81–9.

12. Macchiarini P, Altmayer M, Go T, Walles T, Schulze K, Wildfang I, Haverich A, Hardin M, Hannover Interdisciplinary Intrathoracic Tumor Task Force Group. Technical innovations of carinal resection for nonsmall-cell lung cancer. Ann Thorac Surg. 2006;82(6):1989–97.

13. Yamamoto K, Miyamoto Y, Ohsumi A, Imanishi N, Kojima F. Results of surgical resection for tracheobronchial cancer involving the tracheal carina. Gen Thorac Cardiovasc Surg. 2007;55(6):231–9; discussion 238–9.

14. Rea F, Marulli G, Schiavon M, Zuin A, Hamad AM, Feltracco P, Sartori F. Tracheal sleeve pneumonectomy for non small cell lung cancer (NSCLC): short and long-term results in a single institution. Lung Cancer. 2008;61(2):202–8.

15. Jiang F, Xu L, Yuan F, Huang J, Lu X, Zhang Z. Carinal resection and reconstruction in surgical treatment of bronchogenic carcinoma with carinal involvement. J Thorac Oncol. 2009;4(11):1375–9.

16. Go T, Altmayer M, Richter M, Macchiarini P. Decompressing manubriectomy under apneic oxygenation to release the median thoracic outlet compartment in Bechterew disease. J Thorac Cardiovasc Surg. 2003;126(3):867–9.

Part VI
Pleura and Pleural Spaces

Chapter 46
Management of Persistent Postoperative Air Leaks

Robert E. Merritt

Abstract The management of postoperative alveolar air leaks (AALs) continues to be a challenge for thoracic surgeons who routinely perform pulmonary resections. In order to ameliorate the impact of postoperative AALs, surgeons have incorporated the use of buttressed staple lines and topical sealants to manage intraoperative air leaks. In order to manage prolonged postoperative air leaks, surgeons have implemented Heimlich valves, pleurodesis, and blood patches. The direct clinical implications and evidence based use of these therapies are reviewed in this chapter. AALs can increase length of stay (LOS) and direct healthcare costs; however, these therapies used to mitigate AALs may be ineffective and may increase healthcare costs even more. This chapter provides a review of the current evidence-based literature that attempts to analyze the efficacy of the current therapeutic options that are available to prevent and reduce intraoperative and postoperative alveolar air leaks.

Keywords Air leak • Alveolar air leak • Thoracostomy • Pneumothorax • Emphysema • Stapling devices • Pulmonary lobectomy • Lung sealants

Introduction

Alveolar air leaks (AALs) that occur after pulmonary resections are a significant clinical problem in the practice of thoracic surgery. AALs that persist beyond the immediate postoperative period are associated with a variety of complications, and they can result in increased hospital length of stay (LOS) and increased costs. For

R.E. Merritt, MD
Department of Surgery,
Ohio State University – Wexner Medical Center,
Columbus, OH, USA
e-mail: rmerritt@stanford.edu

M.K. Ferguson (ed.), *Difficult Decisions in Thoracic Surgery*,
Difficult Decisions in Surgery: An Evidence-Based Approach 1,
DOI 10.1007/978-1-4471-6404-3_46, © Springer-Verlag London 2014

these reasons, multiple studies have been published in recent years to evaluate the products and techniques designed to prevent or ameliorate ALLs. Many of the methods proposed to minimize postoperative AALs can add substantial cost to lung resections. The author carried out an evidenced-based review of all of the available literature to determine which management techniques for intraoperative and postoperative air leaks have the greatest scientific support.

Search Strategy

A systematic review of the management of postoperative air leaks and intraoperative air leaks after lung resection was conducted. The specific key word "alveolar air leak" was entered into a PubMed search with the dates January 1, 1990 to August 1, 2013. The search was limited to articles written in the English language and involved human subjects. A total of 57 articles were identified in Pubmed. An additional 20 articles were identified from the reference sections of the 57 articles identified from Pubmed. A total of 50 articles were considered relevant for review for the chapter.

Results

Intraoperative Management of Air Leaks

Postoperative air leaks may occur directly at staple lines, from tissues adjacent to staple lines, from sites where pleural adhesions have been taken down, and from areas of dissection such as within fissures and around lymph nodes. The optimal time to manage these AALs is intraoperatively. Beyond simple suture repair of the areas of visible air leaks, several other intraoperative techniques have been introduced to in an attempt to minimize the risk postoperative prolonged air leaks. The two most recent techniques introduced are buttressing the staple line and using lung sealant agents to close leaks from visceral pleural breaches.

Cooper et al. first reported the utilization of bovine pericardium in buttressing staple lines in patients undergoing major lung resection to control air leaks following lung volume reduction surgery (LVRS) [1]. Subsequently, a number of researchers have further supported the use of bovine pericardium to control air leaks not only in patients with emphysema but also in non-emphysematous patients undergoing pulmonary resection [2]. Many other materials are also utilized as buttresses including excised parietal pleura, polydioxane ribbon, Teflon felt, expanded polytetrafluoroethylene, and collagen patches [3]. There are four randomized studies which compared buttressed to non-buttressed stapling of lung parenchyma during a lung resection, two in LVRS patients [4, 5] and two in lobectomy patients [6, 7].

Buttressed Staple Lines in Patients with Severe Emphysema

Two randomized studies in patients undergoing pulmonary resection predominately for lung cancer evaluated bovine pericardium for staple line reinforcement. Venuta et al. (n = 30) demonstrated decreased AALs and shorter hospital stay while Miller et al. (n = 80) demonstrated reduced duration of AAL but no significant difference in hospital length of stay [6, 7]. In the Venuta study, the lung fissures were completed with either a GIA™ stapler buttressed with bovine pericardial sleeves (n = 10), TA-55 staplers alone (n = 10), or clamps and silk ties (n = 10). Postoperative alveolar air leaks persisted for 2 days in the group with buttressed staple lines compared to 5 days in the other two groups. The mean length of stay was significantly shorter at 4 days compared to 7 days in the non-buttressed resections (p = 0.0001). The lack of the ideal control group using un-buttressed GIA™ staplers and the small numbers in this study limits the conclusions one can draw from it.

Miller et al. performed a multicenter trial consisting of 80 patients undergoing pulmonary resection, randomly assigned to the un-buttressed control group or staple line reinforcement with bovine pericardium [6]. Increased alveolar air leak duration was associated with assignment to the control group (r = 0.27, p = 0.02), but there were no statistical differences noted in the mean intensive care unit length of stay (p = 0.9), number of days with a chest drain (p = 0.6), or total length of stay (p = 0.24).

Although both of these studies of buttressing staple lines in patients without severe chronic obstructive pulmonary disease (COPD) suggest that buttressing reduces duration of alveolar air leaks slightly, the larger and better-controlled trial did not identify a significant benefit of staple line reinforcement in terms of length of stay or chest tube duration. Given unclear benefits, buttressing staple lines during pulmonary resection is not currently recommended for the routine use for patients with less than moderate emphysema.

Buttressing Staple Lines in Patients with Severe Emphysema

Management of AALs is particularly challenging in LVRS patients, who have severe emphysema. Two randomized clinical trials in patients with severe emphysema demonstrate a benefit from buttressing staple lines [4, 5]. A randomized two-center study by Hazelrigg et al. involving 123 patients undergoing unilateral thoracoscopic LVRS shows a significant decrease in the duration of postoperative air leaks, earlier chest drain removal, and a shorter hospital stay in patients receiving bovine pericardial strips compared to patients without such buttressing [4]. The costs were unchanged, as the costs of the pericardial sleeves offset the savings in hospital days. Stammberger et al. presented a randomized three-center study evaluating buttressing in LVRS [5]. Sixty-five patients underwent bilateral LVRS by video-assisted thoracoscopy using endoscopic staplers either with or without bovine pericardium for buttressing. There was a significant decrease in the incidence of initial AAL: 77 % vs. 39 %. Seven patients (three in the treatment group) needed a re-operation because of persistent alveolar air leak. The median duration of AALs was shorter in the treatment group (0 vs. 4 days; p < 0.001), and there was a shorter median drainage time in this group (5 vs. 7.5 days; p = 0.045). Hospital stay was comparable between the two groups (9.5 vs. 12.0 days; p = 0.14).

In summary, the evidence from randomized studies suggests that using buttresses on staple lines in emphysematous patients reduces the incidence of AALs when performing non-anatomic pulmonary resections such as LVRS. This permits the earlier removal of chest drains and shortens hospital length of stay.

Use of Topical Sealants

A variety of surgical sealants have been developed in an effort to prevent alveolar air leaks. They are applied directly to the lung surfaces where violation of the visceral pleura has occurred during a lung resection. The sealants used include: fibrin glues, synthetic polyethylene glycol-based hydrogel sealants, and fleece-bound sealants. Surgical sealants can be effective in reducing the percentage of patients who have a visible AAL at the conclusion of an operation. However, their overall benefit has not been established. Studies do not consistently show that sealants reduce the time to removal of chest drains, decrease the hospital length of stay, or reduce the duration of postoperative air leaks. Serra-Mitjans et al. [8] and Tambiah et al. [9] performed comprehensive reviews of the literature evaluating sealants to prevent AAL after pulmonary resections in patients with lung cancer. These reports identified several published and unpublished trials in which standard closure techniques plus a sealant were compared with the same intervention without a sealant. The outcomes measured included morbidity, mortality, postoperative chest drain time, and postoperative hospital time. The 2005 report from Serra-Mitjans and colleagues identified 12 randomized controlled trials with a total of 1,097 patients [8].

These studies describe a host of sealants following pulmonary resections. Fibrin glue, a sealant that consists of fibrinogen, factor XIII, fibronectin, aprotinin, plasminogen and a thrombin solution was evaluated in six trials [10–14]. A synthetic sealant consisting of polyethylenglycol, trimethylene carbonate and acrylate was used in two trials [15, 16]. A water soluble polyethylene glycol-based gel photopolymerizable was used in one trial [17]. A polymeric biodegradable sealant (polyethylenglycol-based cross-linker, functionalized with succinate groups, PEG-(SS), with human serum albumin-USP) was used in one trial and a different polymeric sealant with used in another similar report [18, 19]. TachoComb, an absorbable patch consisting of an equine-collagen fleece coated with human fibrinogen and human thrombin, was used in one study [20]. A slightly different human fibrinogen and thrombin mix (TachoSil) was used in three other reports [21–23]. Vivostat is an autologous fibrin sealant that was evaluated in two trials [24, 25]. Finally, Tansley et al. [26] used a mixture of bovine serum albumin and glutaraldehyde (BioGlue) in a prospective, randomized trial of efficacy in treating AAL.

Serra-Mitjans et al. determined that the quality and methodology in these trials were variable [8]. In the majority of the trials, there was no standard definition of AAL. In addition, the investigators made no attempt to quantify the degree of AAL in the perioperative period. In three trials, patients were randomized after checking for the presence of intraoperative alveolar air leak. In nine of trials, the staple lines and cut surfaces of the lung parenchyma in the experimental group were routinely covered with topical sealant regardless of the presence of AAL.

In 11 trials, a significantly lower percentage of patients had AAL at the conclusion of the operation when sealants were utilized. Serra-Mitjans and Tambiah each point out; however, that many of these trials do not demonstrate a reduction in number of chest tube days with the use of sealants. The limiting factor in removing chest drains in these patients was often the volume of fluid drainage rather than the presence or absence of AAL. There are only three studies with sealants that demonstrate a reduction in the number of chest tube days. Fabian et al. found mean time to chest drain removal in the treatment group was 3.5 days and in the control group was 5 days [10]. Tansley et al. [26] reported that patients who were treated with BioGlue had significantly shorter median duration of chest drainage; 4 versus 5 days (p=0.012). In a more recent report by Anegg et al. [23], the authors attempted to seal grade 1–2 alveolar air leaks visualized in the operating room with a fleece-bound collagen product after routine fissure management. The results also demonstrated significantly reduced number of chest tube days with the product (p<0.02).

Hospital length of stay has also not been generally reduced by topical lung sealants; however, there are randomized clinical trials demonstrating some benefit. Allen et al. demonstrated that the hospital length of stay was significantly reduced in patients treated with an albumin based lung sealant (Progel), but there was no reduction in time of chest drain duration [18]. This seemingly contradictory result may be related to the use of Heimlich valves. This study also failed to demonstrate a reduction in the incidence of AAL requiring a Heimlich valve in the sealant group. The Tansley et al. study of BioGlue showed a shorter median hospital length of stay: 6 versus 7 days (p=0.004), compared with controls [26].

In patients who did have an AAL postoperatively regardless of whether or not a surgical sealant was utilized, there was a reduction in mean AAL duration time in four of the trials. Air leaks in Porte et al. trial lasted a mean 33.7 h in the treatment group and 63.2 h in control group, and 30.9 h and 52.3 h respectively in the Wain et al. trial [15, 17]. Air leaks lasted a mean of 1.1 and 3.1 days, respectively in the treatment versus control group in Fabian's trial [10]. Interestingly, in that trial there was a significantly higher rate of prolonged AALs in those patients who were not treated by sealants (2 % versus 16 %, p=0.015). D'Andrilli et al. [21] described a randomized study to evaluate a polymeric sealant (CoSeal) in 203 patients with moderate/severe intraoperative air leaks after anatomical pulmonary resections (n=110) or minor resections (n=93). Patients were randomly assigned to suture/stapling or suture/stapling plus Coseal sealant. Air leak rates at 24 h and 48 h were significantly lower in the Coseal group (19.6 % versus 40.6 %, p=0.001 at 24 h; 23.5 % versus 41.6 %, p=0.006 at 48 h) and the duration of air leaks was significantly shorter in the Coseal group (p=0.01).

Moser et al. reported a prospective, randomized, blinded study evaluating lung sealants in 25 patients undergoing bilateral thoracoscopic LVRS [25]. In each patient, an autologous fibrin sealant was applied along the staple line on one side of the chest only. The incidence of prolonged AALs and mean duration of drainage were significantly reduced on the sealant side (4.5 % and 2.8 days versus 31.8 % and 5.9 days).

Sealants Combined with Electrocautery

Beyond the use of sealants after traditional parenchymal stapling, there have been recent reports that a particular type of sealant combined with electrocautery dissection of fissures may be superior to the use of stapler devices to divide fissures. Rena et al. [22] conducted a randomized trial of 60 patients with COPD and fused fissures. They reported that collagen patches coated with human fibrinogen and thrombin (TachoSil) following electrocautery dissection is more effective than stapling fissures in terms of length of chest tube drainage (mean 3.5 versus 5.9 days, P=0.0021) and length of stay (5.9 versus 7.5 days; p=0.01). Another study randomized 40 patients to stapler dissection versus electrocautery dissection plus collagen patches coated with fibrinogen and thrombin [21]. In this study, there was a reduction in the duration of AALs in the electrocautery plus collagen group (1.7 versus 4.5 days, p=0.003). This approach may in fact prove to be more advantageous economically to adding sealants to standard staplers since it has the advantage of eliminating the costs of the staplers.

Summary

In summary, most of the sealants studied appear to reduce the percentage of patients with a visible intraoperative air leaks present at the end of an operative procedure. The vast majority of these sealants, however, do not appear to alter the mean duration of AAL or mean duration of chest tube drainage to a clinically significant degree. A total of 4 of 16 randomized studies show significantly reduced hospital length of stay in the sealant group, and four randomized studies clearly show a reduced air leak duration and chest tube duration with the use of lung sealants (Table 46.1). Only one randomized study of a lung sealants included patients with substantial emphysema. This study showed a benefit to its sealant (autologous fibrin), giving us a hint that perhaps that lung sealants might be appropriately applied to a select group of patients with substantial emphysema. Given the inconsistent results of the clinical trials of lung sealants, it would seem appropriate to use lung sealants in selective cases when an intraoperative air leak is detected. There is no current evidence to support the routine use of lung sealants for reducing the incidence of prolonged postoperative air leaks.

Postoperative Management of Prolonged Air Leaks

It is rare that aggressive re-interventions are required to treat prolonged postoperative air leaks. The most common treatment of prolonged postoperative air leaks is watchful waiting with continued chest tube drainage. More than 90 % of prolonged postoperative air leaks stop within several weeks following operation with this form of management alone.

With continuing pressure to minimize the length of hospitalization, clinical management strategies have evolved that allow treatment of prolonged postoperative air leaks in

Table 46.1 Randomized clinical trials for use of lung sealants

Author	N	Study design	Product	Outcome	Quality of evidence
Fabian et al. [10]	113	Randomized	Fibrin glue	Decreased overall incidence of AAL, chest tube duration, and duration of AAL No significant difference in LOS	Moderate
Porte et al. [15]	124	Randomized	Synthetic lung sealant	Decrease in mean duration of AAL. No significant difference in LOS	Moderate
Wain et al. [17]	172	Randomized	Synthetic lung sealant	Decrease in mean duration of AAL. No significant difference in LOS	Moderate
Allen et al. [18]	161	Randomized	Progel	Significant decrease in LOS	Moderate
D'Adrilli et al. [21]	203	Randomized	Coseal	Decrease in mean duration of AAL. No significant decrease in LOS	Moderate
Anegg et al. [23]	173	Randomized	Tachosil	Decrease in mean duration of AAL. Significant decrease in LOS	Moderate
Tansely et al. [26]	52	Randomized	Bioglue	Decrease in mean duration of AAL, chest tube days, and LOS	Moderate

AAL alveolar air leak, *LOS* length of stay

the outpatient setting. These strategies involve using a one-way valve attached to the chest drain and regular outpatient visits to monitor cessation of the prolonged postoperative air leak [27–30]. A valved, out-patient system such as a Heimlich valve can only be considered in patients who have no more than a small, stable, asymptomatic pneumothorax on water seal. Portable, closed one-way egress devices [31] are likely to be equally effective but have not been as well studied in this setting. There are a combined 148 patients described within the six publications that report results of out-patient, one-way valves for prolonged postoperative air leaks. Of these patients, all but 5 (3.4 %) had their leak successfully managed in this manner. Three patients (2.0 %) were readmitted with increasing pneumothorax or subcutaneous air leading to a change in therapy, and three patients developed infectious problems – none requiring reoperation.

It is not unusual to have a patient with a Heimlich valve or other portable, one-way device in place who demonstrates persistent evacuation of a few bubbles from the drain when coughing but who remains without leak on tidal breathing. Kato et al. reported six patients with this sort of prolonged postoperative air leak and all had at least some degree of residual post-resectional pleural space [32]. In four of these patients the tube thoracostomy was clamped, and three of these four had the drain successfully removed 3–5 days after clamping. In the remaining two patients, the tube was successfully removed without a trial of test clamping at 11 and 21 days postoperatively. Kirschner described a similar approach in an undisclosed number of patients with PAL beyond the first postoperative week [33]. He coined the term "provocative clamping" in this report.

If a period of watchful waiting is unsuccessful in treating prolonged postoperative air leaks, one must consider active interventions to mechanically seal the site of alveolar air leak. Multiple methods to accomplish pleurodesis have some support in the literature. The instillation of sclerosing materials into the pleural space through the thoracostomy tube may promote symphysis of visceral and parietal pleura and leak closure. Tetracycline/Doxycycline and talc are effective for pleurodesis in some cases [34, 35]. The potential for microscopic contamination of the pleural space after a prolonged period with a Heimlich valve mitigates against the routine use of a foreign body such as talc. An antibiotic such as doxycycline may thus be preferable for pleurodesis in this scenario.

Autologous blood patch is another non-surgical option to treat prolonged postoperative air leak following operation or spontaneous pneumothorax [36–41]. Blood-patch pleurodesis involves the instillation of autologous blood into the pleural space through a chest catheter. It is simple, relatively painless, and often effective, but some information suggests that blood-patch pleurodesis may also carry an increased risk of intra-thoracic infection [40, 41]. It may be that the infection rate will be higher if the blood patch is used after a Heimlich valve that has been in place for several weeks.

Invasive procedures are indicated to treat of prolonged postoperative air leaks if more conservative measures like watchful waiting, chemical pleurodesis or blood patch pleurodesis are not effective. Additionally some patients may not be candidates for instillation of materials through the thoracostomy tube. Pneumoperitoneum instilled via a transabdominal catheter has been reported to be effective in some cases [42, 43]. Surgical options to accomplish pleural symphysis and/or control the source of an alveolar air leak include Video-Assisted Thoracoscopy (VATS) with parenchymal stapling, VATS with chemical pleurodesis, VATS with pleural abrasion [44, 45], VATS with application of topical sealants [46, 47], and VATS with laser sealing of the site of leak [48]. These procedures should ideally be carried out promptly after it is clear that bedside pleurodesis has failed so that an evolving partial pleurodesis does not complicate the operation.

Some support for recently introduced bronchoscopic techniques also exists in the literature but with limited levels of evidence. Ferguson and co-authors, for example, suggest that an endobronchial artificial valve may limit prolonged postoperative air leaks after lung volume reduction procedures [49]. Other rarely used interventions have been reported to successfully treat prolonged postoperative air leaks in special circumstances. For example, patients with prolonged postoperative air leaks from incompletely resected pulmonary malignancy may benefit from radiation therapy to both treat the malignancy and limit the air leak [50].

In summary, prolonged postoperative alveolar air leaks will usually stop with conservative therapy alone that most appropriately consists of out-patient management with a Heimlich valve. Gradual escalation of therapy is indicated after a period of a few weeks, and choices for therapy run a spectrum from sclerosing agents instilled via tube thoracostomy to recently propose bronchoscopic interventions, to VATS or thoracotomy for direct repair of the leak site and/or pleurodesis or to tissue flap transposition. Of the more aggressive interventions described for treatment of prolonged postoperative air leaks, one technique cannot be recommended over another based on the available evidence. Clinical judgment taking into consideration individual patient factors and knowledge of all available options offers the best solution to complex management of prolonged postoperative air leaks.

Recommendations

Evidence from randomized studies suggests that using buttresses on staple lines in emphysematous patients reduces the incidence of AALs when performing non-anatomic pulmonary resections such as LVRS. This permits the earlier removal of chest drains and shortens hospital length of stay. Most of the sealants appear to reduce the percentage of patients with a visible intraoperative air leaks present at the end of an operative procedure. The vast majority of these sealants, however, do not appear to alter the mean duration of AAL or mean duration of chest tube drainage to a clinically significant degree. Given the inconsistent results of the clinical trials of lung sealants, use of lung sealants should be restricted to cases in which an intraoperative air leak is detected. There is no current evidence to support the routine use of lung sealants for reducing the incidence of prolonged postoperative air leaks. Prolonged postoperative alveolar air leaks will usually stop with conservative therapy alone. Of the more aggressive interventions for prolonged postoperative air leaks, one technique cannot be recommended over another based on the available evidence.

A Personal View of the Data

Postoperative air leak is a difficult management issue that greatly impacts the length of stay after a pulmonary resection. I personally attempt to identify patients that are the highest risk for developing postoperative air leaks. Patients with chronic obstructive lung disease (COPD) are the most likely to develop prolonged air leaks due the poor tissue integrity of the lung parenchyma. In addition, these patients are often treated with corticosteroid therapy which inhibits normal wound healing. When faced with performing a lung resection in this patient population, I routinely use endoscopic staplers that are buttressed with bovine pericardium to minimize the risk of prolonged air leak from the staple line. In addition, I will often apply a layer of an albumin based topical lung sealant on the visceral pleura surface of the lung that was disrupted by dissection. I consider a prolonged postoperative air leak to be present if there are detectable air bubbles in the Pleur-evac chamber on postoperative number 5. I will often wait at least 14 days after the lung resection to allow the air leak to resolve. At that time, I will connect Heimlich valve to the chest tube and discharge the patient home with the chest tube. Fortunately, I have never had to re-operate on a patient with a prolonged air leak. All of the patients have resolved their prolonged air leak without operative intervention within 21 days of the lung resection.

Recommendations

- Staple lines in emphysematous patients should be buttressed to reduce the incidence of air leak when performing non-anatomic pulmonary resections such as LVRS. (Evidence quality moderate; weak recommendation)
- Use of lung sealants should be restricted to cases in which an intraoperative air leak is detected. There is no current evidence to support the routine use of lung sealants for reducing the incidence of prolonged postoperative air leaks. (Evidence quality moderate; weak recommendation)
- Of the more aggressive interventions for prolonged postoperative air leaks, one technique cannot be recommended over another based on the available evidence. (Evidence quality low; no recommendation)

References

1. Cooper JD. Technique to reduce air leaks after resection of emphysematous lung. Ann Thorac Surg. 1994;57:1038–9.
2. Vaughn CC, Wolner E, Dahan M, Grunenwald D, Vaughn CC, Klepetko W, et al. Prevention of air leaks after pulmonary wedge resection. Ann Thorac Surg. 1997;63:864–6.
3. Thomas P, Massard G, Porte H, Doddoli C, Ducrocq X, Conti M. A new bioabsorbable sleeve for lung staple-line reinforcement (FOREseal): report of a three-center phase II clinical trial. Eur J Cardiothorac Surg. 2006;29:880–5.
4. Hazelrigg SR, Boley TM, Naunheim KS, Magee MJ, Lawyer C, Henkle JQ, et al. Effect of bovine pericardial strips on air leak after stapled pulmonary resection. Ann Thorac Surg. 1997;63:1573–5.
5. Stammberger U, Klepetko W, Stamatis G, Hamaher J, Schmid RA, Wisser W, et al. Buttressing the staple line in lung volume reduction surgery: a randomized three-center study. Ann Thorac Surg. 2000;70:1820–5.
6. Miller Jr JI, Landreneau RJ, Wright CE, Santucci TS, Sammons BH. A comparative study of buttressed versus nonbuttressed staple line in pulmonary resections. Ann Thorac Surg. 2001;71:319–22; discussion 323.
7. Venuta F, Rendina EA, De Giacomo T, Flaishman I, Guarino E, Ciccone AM, et al. Technique to reduce air leaks after pulmonary lobectomy. Eur J Cardiothorac Surg. 1998;13:361–4.
8. Serra-Mitjans M, Belda-Sanchis J, Rami-Porta R. Surgical sealant for preventing air leaks after pulmonary resections in patients with lung cancer. Cochrane Database Syst Rev. 2005;3: CD003051.
9. Tambiah J, Rawlins R, Robb D, Treasure T. Can tissue adhesives and glues significantly reduce the incidence and length of postoperative air leaks in patients having lung resections? Interact Cardiovasc Thorac Surg. 2007;6:529–33.
10. Fabian T, Federico JA, Ponn RB. Fibrin glue in pulmonary resection: a prospective, randomized, blinded study. Ann Thorac Surg. 2003;75:1587–92.
11. Fleisher AG, Evans KG, Nelems B, Finley RJ. Effect of routine fibrin glue use on the duration of air leaks after lobectomy. Ann Thorac Surg. 1990;49:133–4.
12. Wong K, Goldstraw P. Effect of fibrin glue in the reduction of postthoracotomy alveolar air leak. Ann Thorac Surg. 1997;64:979–81.
13. Mouritzen C, Dromer M, Keinecke HO. The effect of fibrin gluing to seal bronchial and alveolar leakages after pulmonary resections and decortications. Eur J Cardiothorac Surg. 1993;7: 75–80.

14. Wurtz A, Chambon JP, Sobecki L, Bartrouni R, Huart JJ, Burnouf T. Use of a biological glue in partial pulmonary excision surgery. Results of a controlled trial in 50 patients. Ann Chir. 1991;45:719–23.
15. Porte HL, Jany T, Akkad R, Conti M, Gillet PA, Guidat A, et al. Randomized controlled trial of a synthetic sealant for preventing alveolar air leaks after lobectomy. Ann Thorac Surg. 2001;71:1618–22.
16. Macchiarini P, Wain J, Almy S, Dartevelle P. Experimental and clinical evaluation of a new synthetic, absorbable sealant to reduce air leaks in thoracic operations. J Thorac Cardiovasc Surg. 1999;117:751–8.
17. Wain JC, Kaiser LR, Johnstone DW, Yang SC, Wright CD, Friedberg JS, et al. Trial of a novel synthetic sealant in preventing air leaks after lung resection. Ann Thorac Surg. 2001;71:1623–8; discussion 1628–9.
18. Allen MS, Wood DE, Hawkinson RW, Harpole DH, McKenna RJ, Walsh GL, et al. Prospective randomized study evaluating a biodegradable polymeric sealant for sealing intraoperative air leaks that occur during pulmonary resection. Ann Thorac Surg. 2004;77:1792–801.
19. Wurtz A, Gambiez L, Chambon J. Evaluation de l'efficacité d'une colle de fibrine en chirurgie d'exérèse pulmonaire partielle. Résultats d'un nouvel essai contrôlé chez 50 malades. Lyon Chir. 1992;88:368–71.
20. Lang G, Csekeo A, Stamatis G, Lampl L, Hagman L, Marta GM, et al. Efficacy and safety of topical application of human fibrinogen/thrombin-coated collagen patch (TachoComb) for treatment of air leakage after standard lobectomy. Eur J Cardiothorac Surg. 2004;25:160–6.
21. D'Andrilli A, Andreetti C, Ibrahim M, Ciccone AM, Venuta F, Mansmann U, et al. A prospective randomized study to assess the efficacy of a surgical sealant to treat air leaks in lung surgery. Eur J Cardiothorac Surg. 2009;35(5):817–20; discussion 820–1.
22. Rena O, Papalia E, Mineo TC, Massera F, Pirondini E, Turello D, et al. Air-leak management after upper lobectomy in patients with fused fissure and chronic obstructive pulmonary disease: a pilot trial comparing sealant and standard treatment. Interact Cardiovasc Thorac Surg. 2009;9(6):973–7.
23. Anegg U, Lindenmann J, Matzi V, Smolle J, Maier A, Smolle-Juttner. Efficiency of fleece-bound sealing (TachoSil) of air leaks in lung surgery: a prospective randomized trial. Eur J Cardiothorac Surg. 2007;31(2):198–202.
24. Belboul A, Dernevik L, Aljassim O, Skrbic B, Radberg G, Roberts D. The effect of autologous fibrin sealant (Vivostat) on morbidity after pulmonary lobectomy: a prospective randomised, blinded study. Eur J Cardiothorac Surg. 2004;26:1187–91.
25. Moser C, Opitz I, Zhai W, Rousson V, Russi EW, Weder W, et al. Autologous fibrin sealant reduces the incidence of prolonged air leak and duration of chest tube drainage after lung volume reduction surgery: a prospective randomized blinded study. J Thorac Cardiovasc Surg. 2008;136(4):843–9.
26. Tansley P, Al-Mulhim F, Lim E, Ludas G, Goldstraw P. A prospective, randomized, controlled trial of the effectiveness of BioGlue in treating alveolar air leaks. J Thorac Cardiovasc Surg. 2006;132:105–12.
27. McKenna Jr RJ, Fischel RJ, Brenner M, Gelb AF. Use of the Heimlich valve to shorten hospital stay after lung reduction surgery for emphysema. Ann Thorac Surg. 1996;61:1115–7.
28. Ponn RB, Silverman HJ, Federico JA. Outpatient chest tube management. Ann Thorac Surg. 1997;64:1437–40.
29. McKenna RJ, Mahtabifard A, Pickens A, Kusuanco D, Fuller CB. Fast-tracking after video-assisted thoracoscopic surgery lobectomy, segmentectomy, and pneumonectomy. Ann Thorac Surg. 2007;84:1663–7.
30. McManus KG, Spence GM, McGuigan JA. Outpatient chest tubes. Ann Thorac Surg. 1998;66:299–300.
31. Rieger KM, Wroblewski HA, Brooks JA, Hammoud ZT, Kesler KA. Postoperative outpatient chest tube management: initial experience with a new portable system. Ann Thorac Surg. 2007;84:630–2.
32. Kato R, Kobayashi T, Watanabe M, Kawamura M, Kikuchi K, Kobayashi K, et al. Can the chest tube draining the pleural cavity with persistent air leakage be removed? Thorac Cardiovasc Surg. 1992;40:292–6.

33. Kirschner PA. "Provocative clamping" and removal of chest tubes despite persistent air leak. Ann Thorac Surg. 1992;53:740–1.
34. Read CA, Reddy VD, O'Mara TE, Richardson MS. Doxycycline pleurodesis for pneumothorax in patients with AIDS. Chest. 1994;105:823–5.
35. Kilic D, Findikcioglu A, Hatipoglu A. A different application method of talc pleurodesis for the treatment of persistent air leak. ANZ J Surg. 2006;76:754–6.
36. Droghetti A, Schiavini A, Muriana P, Comel A, DeDonna G, Beccaria M, et al. Autologous blood patch in persistent air leaks after pulmonary resection. J Thorac Cardiovasc Surg. 2006;132:556–9.
37. Shackcloth MJ, Poullis M, Jackson M, Soorae A, Page RD. Intrapleural instillation of autologous blood in the treatment of prolonged air leak after lobectomy: a prospective randomized controlled trial. Ann Thorac Surg. 2006;82:1052–6.
38. Yokomise H, Satoh K, Ohno N, Tamura K. Autoblood plus OK432 pleurodesis with open drainage for persistent air leak after lobectomy. Ann Thorac Surg. 1998;65:563–5.
39. Dumire R, Crabbe MM, Mappin FG, Fontenelle LJ. Autologous "blood patch" pleurodesis for persistent pulmonary air leak. Chest. 1992;101:64–6.
40. Cagirici U, Sahin B, Cakan A, Kayabas H, Buduneli T. Autologous blood patch pleurodesis in spontaneous pneumothorax with persistent air leak. Scand Cardiovasc J. 1998;32:75–8.
41. Lang-Lazdunski L, Coonar AS. A prospective study of autologous 'blood patch' pleurodesis for persistent air leak after pulmonary resection. Eur J Cardiothorac Surg. 2004;26:897–900.
42. De Giacomo T, Rendina EA, Venuta F, Francioni F, Moretti M, Pugliese F, et al. Pneumoperitoneum for the management of pleural air space problems associated with major pulmonary resections. Ann Thorac Surg. 2001;72:1716–9.
43. Handy Jr JR, Judson MA, Zellner JL. Pneumoperitoneum to treat air leaks and spaces after a lung volume reduction operation. Ann Thorac Surg. 1997;64:1803–5.
44. Suter M, Bettschart V, Vandoni RE, Cuttat JF. Thoracoscopic pleurodesis for prolonged (or intractable) air leak after lung resection. Eur J Cardiothorac Surg. 1997;12:160–1.
45. Torre M, Grassi M, Nerli FP, Maioli M, Belloni PA. Nd-YAG laser pleurodesis via thoracoscopy. Endoscopic therapy in spontaneous pneumothorax Nd-YAG laser pleurodesis. Chest. 1994;106:338–41.
46. Carrillo EH, Kozloff M, Saridakis A, Bragg S, Levy J. Thoracoscopic application of a topical sealant for the management of persistent posttraumatic pneumothorax. J Trauma. 2006;60:111–4.
47. Thistlethwaite PA, Luketich JD, Ferson PF, Keenan RJ, Jamieson SW. Ablation of persistent air leaks after thoracic procedures with fibrin sealant. Ann Thorac Surg. 1999;67:575–7.
48. Sharpe DA, Dixon C, Moghissi K. Thoracoscopic use of laser in intractable pneumothorax. Eur J Cardiothorac Surg. 1994;8:34–6.
49. Ferguson JS, Sprenger K, Van Natta T. Closure of a bronchopleural fistula using bronchoscopic placement of an endobronchial valve designed for the treatment of emphysema. Chest. 2006;129:479–81.
50. Ong YE, Sheth A, Simmonds NJ, Heenan S, Allan R, Glees JP. Radiotherapy: a novel treatment for pneumothorax. Eur Respir J. 2006;27:427–9.

Chapter 47
Fibrinolytics for Managing Pleural Empyema

Nirmal K. Veeramachaneni and Casey P. Hertzenberg

Abstract Parapneumonic effusions and empyema present a difficult challenge to thoracic surgeons. While early surgical intervention is successful, it can come at a significant cost in terms of morbidity, utilization of resources and hospital length of stay. The use of fibrinolytics has been extensively studied to minimize the need for surgical intervention, with varied results. There has been growing evidence for the efficacy of intrapleural fibrinolytics for treating pleural effusions and empyema, especially if the stage of the parapneumonic effusion (exudative, fibrinopurulent, organizing) is considered. Fibrinolytics are not helpful in patients with an organized pleural effusion characterized by a thick peel on the lung, with associated ingrowth of fibroblasts, but may avoid the need for surgery in earlier phases.

Keywords Fibrinolytic • Parapneumonic effusion • Empyema • Streptokinase • tPA

Introduction

Pleural empyemas have posed a difficult problem in medicine for centuries, however it was not until recently that a further understanding of the natural history of effusions and empyema was elucidated [1]. Light and colleagues defined exudative effusions as having a pleural fluid-to-serum protein ratio >0.5, pleural fluid-to-serum ratio >0.6, or pleural fluid lactate dehydrogenase >2/3 the upper limit of normal. An empyema is defined as an exudative effusion with a pH <7.2 and a positive gram stain or culture. Light further divided parapneumonic effusions into three progressive categories: *exudative phase* defined by a sterile fluid collection that has

N.K. Veeramachaneni, MD (✉) • C.P. Hertzenberg, MD
Department of Cardiothoracic Surgery, University of Kansas Hospital,
3901 Rainbow Boulevard, Kansas City, KS 66103, USA
e-mail: nveeramachaneni@kumc.edu; chertzenberg@kumc.edu

M.K. Ferguson (ed.), *Difficult Decisions in Thoracic Surgery*,
Difficult Decisions in Surgery: An Evidence-Based Approach 1,
DOI 10.1007/978-1-4471-6404-3_47, © Springer-Verlag London 2014

formed mainly by an increase in visceral pleural permeability; *fibrinopurulent phase* which is characterized by infection of the sterile exudate, often leading to fibrin deposition and formation of loculations; and *organizing phase* characterized by fibroblast ingrowth leading to a thick pleural peel and entrapped lung.

Although the general recommendation of the treatment for effusions and empyema has been complete drainage within the early stages, the means of achieving this have varied widely in terms of the invasiveness of the procedures utilized. Pleural instillation of fibrinolytics, namely streptokinase, has been in practice for over 60 years [2] mainly based upon the belief of its ability to breakdown loculations within the effusion, thus rendering thoracostomy drainage more effective. Extensive research into the use of intrapleural fibrinolytics for the treatment of parapneumonic effusions and empyema have been greeted mostly with equivocal findings in terms of overall efficacy [3]. Recently, larger trials with modifications in the type of fibrinolytic used, as well as the concomitant addition of other chemical adjuncts have shed new light on their overall benefit [4]. The forthcoming text will review the literature in regards to using intrapleural fibrinolytics for the management of empyema, highlight the shortcomings of the available studies and provide a recommendation based upon these results and our own experience.

Search Strategy

A literature review was undertaken using the following key words: intrapleural fibrinolytic; parapneumonic effusion; empyema; streptokinase; tPA. Studies older than 20 years were excluded as were studies that focused on specific bacteriologic causes of empyema such as tuberculosis. A primary focus was placed on papers that were either a randomized, prospective trial or a meta-analyses of available literature.

Published Data

Multiple studies have been performed over the last several decades reviewing the efficacy of intrapleural fibrinolytics. Many of the early reports, however, were retrospective case series [5–8] evaluating the use of streptokinase. One of the first notable randomized controlled trials was performed by Davies and colleagues [9] in 1997. Twenty-four patients with community acquired parapneumonic infections were studied. Patients were randomly assigned to receive either daily streptokinase or normal saline flushes for 3 days administered via a 14 French thoracostomy tube, in addition to IV antibiotics. The streptokinase group had more than double the amount of drainage (2.6 vs. 1.1 L) and had demonstrated improvement in chest radiographic appearance at time of discharge. A study by Chin et al. [10] demonstrated similar findings, but there was no difference in need for surgery, hospital length of stay, morbidity or mortality. Both studies mainly utilized chest x-ray as the means of evaluating the stage of empyema.

Two additional randomized trials [11, 12] evaluated the efficacy of streptokinase. Diacon and colleagues [11] evaluated 44 patients with either frankly purulent pleural drainage or pleural fluid with a pH <7.2 along with loculations noted on chest x-ray, and randomized these patients to either placebo or daily instillation of intrapleural streptokinase. They noted a higher clinical success rate in the streptokinase group (82 % vs. 48 %) defined as subjective and objective clinical improvement based upon control of systemic infection, adequate pleural drainage, and radiologic clearance. In addition, there was a reduction in referral for surgery within the streptokinase group (45 % vs. 9 %). Misthos et al. [12] performed a prospective, randomized trial including 127 patients with thoracic empyema secondary to bacterial pneumonia treated either by chest tube drainage alone or streptokinase. The stage of empyema was not taken into account. The treatment group had a higher clinical success rate (88 % vs. 67 %) defined as evacuation of the pleural space as evidenced by CT or chest x-ray, re-expansion of the lung and resolution of symptoms. They also noted a significant decrease in length of treatment (15.5 vs. 7 days) and mortality (4.2 % vs. 1.7 %) in the streptokinase group.

In a more modern series comparing streptokinase to minimally invasive video assisted thoracic surgery (VATS), Wait and colleagues [13] randomized 20 patients to either arm of the study. Eligibility was determined by patients having either pleural fluid pH <7.2 or loculated effusions as determined by chest x-ray. The VATS group had a decrease in total number of hospital days (8.7 vs. 12.8) along with a higher treatment success (91 % vs. 44 %) in regards to improvement on chest radiograph as well as resolution of fever and leukocytosis.

Despite the aforementioned promising results of streptokinase, its use could not be fully confirmed in larger studies [3, 14]. Maskell and colleagues [14] performed a randomized double-blind placebo trial in the United Kingdom titled "Multicentre Intrapleural Sepsis Trial" or "MIST-1". Four hundred and fifty-four patients with pleural infections were randomized to receive either streptokinase twice daily for 3 days versus placebo with primary endpoints being death and need for surgery. Patients were included if the pleural fluid had a positive gram stain or culture, was grossly purulent, or had a fluid pH <7.2 in patients with clinical signs of infection. Efficacy was determined by reduction in pleural opacity per chest x-ray. Ultimately, they found no difference in radiographic improvement, need for surgery, length of hospital stay or mortality. One caveat is that most of these patients were treated in hospitals without thoracic surgeon support. This study has also been criticized for multiple other reasons including their lack of more specific diagnostic modalities such as CT or ultrasound, absence of measurement of total fluid drained, and acceptance of patients in all stages of parapneumonic effusion.

Given the potential side effects of streptokinase (7 % of patients) noted by Maskell et al. [14], more recent studies began focusing on alternatives to streptokinase, namely tissue plasminogen activator (tPA) or its derivatives (i.e. alteplase, tenecteplase, etc.). In the MIST-2 trial [15], tPA was substituted for streptokinase, with or without the use of DNase. This was a randomized double-blind study of 210 patients. The primary endpoint was the change in pleural opacity on chest radiograph, as calculated by percentage of the hemithorax occupied by effusion. Upon review, they found a significant reduction in the volume of pleural opacity within the tPA + DNase group compared to placebo (29.5 % vs. 17.2 %). The other groups (either tPA or DNase given alone) had no significant decrease in the amount of pleural fluid reduction. In addition, notable findings were discovered in the secondary endpoints within the tPA + DNase group including reduction in surgical referral at 3 months (4 % vs. 16 %) and overall hospital stay. They also noted the frequency of adverse events were similar between all groups regardless of the agent used. Of note, the dose of tPA used by the investigators was less than reported by other investigators [16] which may explain the lack of efficacy of tPA.

Additional studies evaluating the effects of intrapleural alteplase are also noteworthy. Thommi and colleagues [16] performed a randomized, controlled, double-blind, crossover trial evaluating the rate of surgical decortication required in patients receiving intrapleural alteplase. Their review included 68 patients who received alteplase daily for 3 days versus placebo. Patients were evaluated by either CXR or CT to determine resolution of their effusions. If resolution did not occur, they were allowed to crossover into the other treatment arm. Overall, 95 % of patients within the intrapleural alteplase group had clinical resolution of their effusions, without the need for surgery as opposed to 12 % in the placebo group. Surgery was avoided in all patients. Ben-Or [17] and colleagues performed a retrospective review of 118 patients analyzing the efficacy and risks associated with alteplase use in multiple patient subsets including those with parapneumonic effusions, empyema thoracis, loculated effusions, hemothoraces, and malignant effusions. A thoracic surgeon was consulted, and made the decision to offer tPA treatment, after evaluating CT scans, and excluding patients with radiographic evidence of a fibrothorax. Their results showed successful resolution of effusions determined via chest radiography in 86.4 % of patients. Thus, they concluded that intrapleural alteplase can be effective in a variety of patients with pathologic pleural processes.

Lastly, two recent meta-analyses have been performed, one by Cameron and colleagues as a Cochrane Review in 2008 [3], and the other by Janda and colleagues in 2012 [4]. Cameron reviewed seven studies [11, 12, 14, 18–21] with a combined total of 761 patients. The main adjuncts of choice were streptokinase and urokinase. Ultimately, they demonstrated an overall advantage to the use of fibrinolytics. Janda and colleagues, using the Cochrane methodology, evaluated a total of seven randomized controlled studies including 801 patients [9, 11, 12, 14, 15, 19, 21]. A variety of fibrinolytics were used within these studies including streptokinase, urokinase, tPA and DNase. Overall, they had mixed results, but did find fibrinolytic therapy was beneficial for the outcomes of treatment failure and death (RR 0.5) as well as need for surgical intervention (RR 0.66). They concluded that "...fibrinolytic therapy is potentially beneficial in the management of parapneumonic effusions and empyemas in the adult population..." [4]. The summary of the studies can be found in Table 47.1.

Table 47.1 Summary of literature

Author/year	N	Design	Agents	Imaging	Effusion stage	Quality of evidence	Conclusion
Wait et al. [13]/1997	20	RCT	SK 250,000 u/day vs. VATS	CXR	Fibrino-purulent	Moderate	VATS had ↑ efficacy and ↓ hospital days in complex, loculated effusions
Chin and Lim [10]/1997	52	RCT	SK 250,000 u/day vs. thoracostomy tube alone	CT	All stages	Moderate	SK ↑ drainage volume, but no improvement in morbidity or mortality
Davies et al. [9]/1997	24	RCT	SK 250,000 u/day × 3 days vs. NS	US CXR CT	All stages	Moderate	SK ↑ drainage volume and improved CXR in SK group
Bouros et al. [19]/1999	31	RCT	UK 100,000 u/day × 3 days vs. NS	US CXR CT	Fibrino-purulent, empyema	High	UK ↓ hospital days, ↑ successful drainage (86.5 % vs. 25 %) and ↓ surgery (13.5 % vs. 37.5 %)
Diacon et al. [11]/2004	44	RCT	SK 250,000 u/day vs. NS	US CXR	Fibrino-purulent, empyema	High	SK ↑ "clinical success" (82 % vs. 48 %) and ↓ need for surgery (14 % vs. 32 %)
Misthos et al. [12]/2005	127	RCT	SK 250,000 u/day vs. thoracostomy tube alone	US CXR CT	All stages	High	SK ↑ success (87 % vs. 67 %), ↓ hospital stay and mortality
Maskell et al. [14]/2005 MIST 1 trial	454	RCT, double-blind	SK 250,000 u/day vs. Placebo	CXR	All stages	High	SK does not ↓ need for surgery, hospital stay or mortality; pop. had high % of mature empyemas
Cameron et al. [3]/2009 cochrane review	761	Meta-analysis	SK, UK	Multiple	N/A	High	Fibrinolytics ↓ the requirement for surgical intervention; however results vary

(continued)

Table 47.1 (continued)

Author/year	N	Design	Agents	Imaging	Effusion stage	Quality of evidence	Conclusion
Tuncozger et al. [21]/2011	49	RCT	UK 100,000 u/day × 3 days	US CXR CT	All stages	High	UK ↓ hospital stay (14 vs. 21 days) and need for surgery (29 % vs. 60 %)
Rahman et al. [15]/2011 MIST 2 Trial	210	RCT, double-blind	tPA 10 mg BID, DNase 5 mg BID, tPA/DNase, placebo	CXR	All stages	High	t-PA + DNase ↑ drainage volume (29 % vs. 17 %), ↓ need for surgery and hospital stay
Ben-Or et al. [17]/2011	118	Retro-spective review	AT 25 mg/day × 1–8 days vs. thoracostomy tube	CXR CT	All stages	High	AT effectively drained effusions (86.4 %) without ↑ morbidity; no benefit to using >2 doses
Thommi et al. [16]/2012	68	RCT, double-blind	AT 25 mg/day × 3 days vs. placebo	CXR CT	All stages	High	AT ↓ need for operation without ↑ morbidity; high percentage of patients crossed over
Janda et al. [4]/2012	801	Meta-analysis	SK, UK, tPA, DNase	Multiple	N/A	High	Fibrinolytics may ↓ the need for surgery in loculated pleural effusions/empyemas

RCT randomized controlled trial, *VATS* video assisted thoracoscopic surgery, *SK* streptokinase, *US* ultrasound, *CXR* chest x-ray, *CT* computed tomography, *UK* urokinase, *NS* normal saline, *DNase* deoxyribonuclease, *tPA* tissue plasminogen activator, *AT* alteplase

Summary

The use of fibrinolytics for the treatment of complicated parapneumonic effusions has evolved over the past few decades. There is an overall advantage to the use of fibrinolytics in the treatment of parapneumonic effusions to avoid the need for surgical intervention and decrease hospital length of stay. The choice of imaging has varied, although CT is emerging as the most reliable and informative modality mainly due to its ability to ascertain the presence of loculations and to characterize the underlying lung parenchyma. In terms of the treatment of choice, the use of streptokinase has all but ceased due to adverse events. As a result, t-PA or its derivatives, with or without DNase currently appear to be the most popular agent(s) to be utilized, although other fibrinolytics have appeared to be effective as well. The duration of therapy has varied in previous studies but it appears that 1–3 doses have yielded satisfactory results. Whether to proceed directly to surgery versus first attempting a trial of intrapleural therapy depends largely upon when the effusion first began. Therefore, in regards to timing, early intervention within the exudative or early fibrinoproliferative stage seems effective, especially in cases of loculated effusions. Overall, the literature supports the use of intrapleural fibrinolytic therapy in the early stages of parapneumonic effusions and empyemas within the adult population. A guideline for patient assessment and use of fibrinolytics is provided in Fig. 47.1.

A Personal View of the Data

Given the overall efficacy of tPA, we believe that intrapleural instillation of a fibrinolytic is a useful treatment modality. In patients presenting with an exudative pleural effusion, we drain the fluid and assess the pleural space radiographically. Should there be evidence of a complex pleural effusion, we obtain a CT scan to assess not only the pleural space, but the underlying lung parenchyma. Lung characterized by dense pneumonia and air bronchograms is more problematic to treat by decortication than atelectatic lung caused by pleural disease alone. Patients with a thick fibrinous peel on the lung, or evidence of chronic entrapment are offered surgical intervention, as this represents a late stage of empyema, whereas most other patients are treated with 2–3 doses of intrapleural tPA administered over subsequent days, assuming there is no contraindication to the use of lytics (low platelets, coagulopathy). We reassess patients in a manner similar to Thommi et al. [16], with a repeat CT scan of the chest after treatment to evaluate the efficacy of the intervention. Using this strategy, we have altered our own practice, and have been able to achieve satisfactory results.

Intrapleural fibrinolytics should be considered for early stage empyema.

Fig. 47.1 Recommended
guidelines for management of
pleural effusions

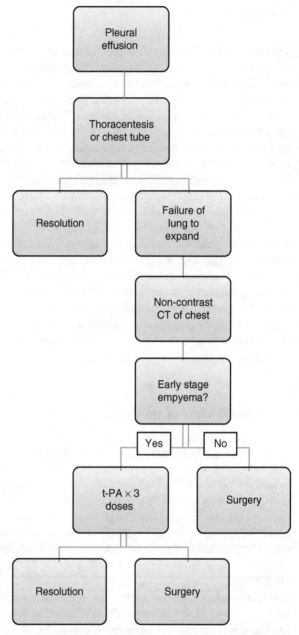

Recommendation

- We recommend the use of intrapleural fibrinolytic therapy in the early stages of parapneumonic effusions and empyemas in adults (Evidence quality high; strong recommendation).

References

1. Light RW. Parapneumonic effusion and empyema. Clin Chest Med. 1985;6:55–62.
2. Tillet WS, Sherry S. The effect in patients of streptococcal fibrinolysin (streptokinase) and streptococcal desoxyribonuclease on fibrinous, purulent and sanguinous pleural exudations. J Clin Invest. 1949;28(1):173–90.
3. Cameron R, Davies HR. Intra-pleural fibrinolytic therapy versus conservative management in the treatment of parapneumonic effusions and empyema. Cochrane Database Syst Rev. 2008;(2):CD002312.
4. Janda S, Swiston J. Intrapleural fibrinolytic therapy for treatment of adult parapneumonic effusions and empyemas: a systematic review and meta-analysis. Chest. 2012;142(2):401–11.
5. Henke CA, Leatherman JW. Intrapleurally administered streptokinase in the treatment of acute loculated nonpurulent parapneumonic effusions. Am Rev Respir Dis. 1992;145:680–4.
6. Taylor RF, Rubens MB, Pearson MC, Barnes NC. Intrapleural streptokinase in the management of empyema. Thorax. 1994;49:856–9.
7. Laisaar T, Puttsepp E, Laisaar V. Early administration of intrapleural streptokinase in the treatment of multiloculated pleural effusions and pleural empyemas. Thorac Cardiovasc Surg. 1996;44:252–6.
8. Roupie E, Bouabdallah K, Delclaux C, Brun-Buisson C, Lemaire F, Vasile N, Brochard L. Intrapleural administration of streptokinase in complicated purulent pleural effusion: a CT-guided strategy. Intensive Care Med. 1996;22:1351–3.
9. Davies RJ, Traill ZC, Gleeson FV. Randomised controlled trial of intrapleural streptokinase in community acquired pleural infection. Thorax. 1997;52(5):416–21.
10. Chin NK, Lim TK. Controlled trial of intrapleural streptokinase in the treatment of pleural empyema and complicated parapneumonic effusions. Chest. 1997;111(2):275–9.
11. Diacon AH, Theron J, Schuurmans MM, Schuurmans MM, Van de Wal BW, Bollinger CT. Intrapleural streptokinase for empyema and complicated parapneumonic effusions. Am J Respir Crit Care Med. 2004;170(1):49–53.
12. Misthos P, Sepsas E, Konstantinou M, Athanassiadi K, Skottis I, Lioulias A. Early use of intrapleural fibrinolytics in the management of postpneumonic empyema. A prospective study. Eur J Cardiothorac Surg. 2005;28(4):599–603.
13. Wait MA, Sharma S, Hohn J, Dal Nogare A. A randomized trial of empyema therapy. Chest. 1997;111(6):1548–51.
14. Maskell NA, Davies CW, Nunn AJ, Hedley EL, Gleeson FV, Miller R, et al. U.K. controlled trial of intrapleural streptokinase for pleural infection. N Engl J Med. 2005;352(9):865–74.
15. Rahman NM, Maskell NA, West A, Teoh R, Arnold A, Mackinlay C, et al. Intrapleural use of tissue plasminogen activator and DNase in pleural infection. N Engl J Med. 2011;365(6):518–26.
16. Thommi G, Shehan JC, Robison KL, Christensen M, Backemeyer LA, McLeay MT. A double blind randomized cross over trial comparing rate of decortication and efficacy of intrapleural instillation of alteplase vs. placebo in patients with empyemas and complicated parapneumonic effusions. Respir Med. 2012;106(5):716–23.
17. Ben-Or S, Feins RH, Veeramachaneni NK, Haithcock BE. Effectiveness and risks associated with intrapleural alteplase by means of tube thoracostomy. Ann Thorac Surg. 2011;91(3):860–3.
18. Bouros D, Schiza S, Patsourakis G, Chalkiadakis G, Panagou P, Siafakas NM. Intrapleural streptokinase versus urokinase in the treatment of complicated parapneumonic effusions. Am J Respir Crit Care Med. 1997;155(1):291–5.
19. Bouros D, Schiza S, Tzanakis N, Chalkiadakis G, Drositis J, Siafakas N. Intrapleural urokinase versus normal saline in the treatment of complicated parapneumonic effusions and empyema. Am J Respir Crit Care Med. 1999;159(1):37–42.
20. Davies RO, Traill ZC, Gleeson FV. Randomised controlled trial of intrapleural streptokinase in community acquired pleural infection. Thorax. 1997;52:416–21.
21. Tuncozgur B, Ustunsoy H, Sivrikoz MC, Dikensoy O, Topal M, Sanli M, et al. Intrapleural urokinase in the management of parapneumonic empyema: a randomised controlled trial. Int J Clin Pract. 2001;55(10):658–60.

Chapter 48
VATS Versus Open Management of Pleural Empyema

Udo Abah, Felice Granato, and Marco Scarci

Abstract Pleural empyema is a common and serious clinical problem. Controversy exists regarding the optimum surgical approach for debridement and decortication. The current evidence base consists of mainly retrospective observational studies and demonstrates the role for video assisted thoracoscopic surgery, with comparable success rates to conventional open surgery in many series and the associated benefits of minimally invasive surgery. There is a high conversion rate associated with chronic empyema; risk factors for conversion to open are a prolonged time from symptom onset to surgery, persistent fever, gram negative organisms and evidence of pleural thickening on imaging.

Keywords Pleural empyema • Video assisted thoracoscopic surgery • Thoracotomy • Debridement • Decortication

U. Abah, MBChB, MRCS
Department of Cardiothoracic Surgery, Papworth Hospital,
Papworth Everard, Cambridge, CB23 3RE, UK
e-mail: udoabah@nhs.net

F. Granato, MD, PhD
Department of Thoracic Surgery, Papworth Hospital,
Papworth Everard, Cambridge, CB23 3RE, UK
e-mail: felicegranato@yahoo.it

M. Scarci, MD, PGCTS, FRCS (✉)
Department of Thoracic Surgery, Papworth Hospital NHS Foundation Trust, Papworth Everard, Cambridge, CB23 3RE, UK
e-mail: marco.scarci@nhs.net

M.K. Ferguson (ed.), *Difficult Decisions in Thoracic Surgery*,
Difficult Decisions in Surgery: An Evidence-Based Approach 1,
DOI 10.1007/978-1-4471-6404-3_48, © Springer-Verlag London 2014

Introduction

Pleural empyema is a common and serious clinical problem, with increasing incidence in Western countries [1–4]. The current incidence is approximately 80,000 cases annually in the United Kingdom and USA combined [5, 6] and mortality rates vary from 10 to 20 % [1, 7]. Treatment options range from isolated antibiotic therapy, through minimally invasive drainage procedures, to radical surgery, and are largely dependent upon the stage and presentation of the condition. The disease progresses through an initial exudative stage (uncomplicated parapneumonic effusion, stage 1), through a fibropurulent stage where the pleural space becomes infected and loculation occurs (complicated parapneumonic effusion, stage 2) and finally an organized phase were a pleural peel develops (pleural empyema, stage 3). Conventionally, early stage empyema was managed with tube thoracostomy, with more advanced stages requiring open thoracotomy and decortication. Since 1991, the introduction of video assisted thoracoscopic surgery (VATS) has revolutionized the treatment of thoracic empyema. VATS has shown superior results in the treatment of the fibropurulent stage when compared to tube thoracostomy alone [8, 9] and thoracostomy in conjunction with intrapleural fibrinolytics [10]. Disagreement still remains regarding the use of minimally invasive techniques versus open thoracotomy for the management of more complex disease (stage 3).

Search Strategy

The search strategy for this review was designed based on PICO elements including patient with pleural empyema recommended to have surgical intervention who underwent either open or VATS surgery. Outcomes assessed included success rates, morbidity, mortality, hospital length of stay, and duration of chest tube drainage. PubMed was searched for the keys words "pleural empyema", "thoracic empyema", "parapneumonic effusion", "video assisted thoracoscopic surgery", "VATS", "debridement", "decortication". The search was limited to English language, and Human studies, the titles were reviewed and relevant articles read with review of their significant references.

VATS vs. Thoracotomy—The Evidence

There is no general consensus regarding the optimal surgical approach in the management of pleural empyema. The British Thoracic Society (BTS) guideline for the management of pleural infection [11] recommends surgical referral 5–8 days following failure of initial management but does not address the method of surgical intervention, whilst the American College of Chest Physicians guideline for the treatment of parapneumonic effusions states that VATS and open operations are both acceptable approaches for managing patients with advanced-stage empyema [12]. Clinicians therefore base their practice upon local preference and expertise. The evidence base consists of mainly retrospective observational series with their associated limitations; only two studies identified were conducted prospectively [13, 14] (Table 48.1). To date no randomized control trials have been conducted comparing VATS vs. open surgery for the management of empyema. The significant differences in the distinctive stages of empyema, varying etiologies, and heterogeneous mixture of patients makes interpretation of retrospective series challenging due to the implicit degree of selection bias between interventions. It is likely that preoperative factors will have influenced procedure choice, with more advanced and complex stages of empyema undergoing open debridement and decortication. Some series compare VATS cohorts with historical open cohorts [15, 16], further limiting interpretation of results. Other factors might also play a role in the comparison of VATS decortication versus open decortication; there is some debate as to the true extent of what is reported as a VATS decortication, which may in some instances migrate to an extensive debridement. A learning curve is also associated with VATS; increasing rates of success may be associated with increasing operative experience [16]. Despite the limitations of the current evidence base, conclusions can be drawn from outcomes that are common among studies.

Treatment Success

In the treatment of stage 2 pleural empyema VATS techniques have been demonstrated to have equivalent rates of treatment success to debridement via thoracotomy [17]. The management of stage 3 empyema creates a further surgical challenge, due to the requirement to decorticate the lung. A number of studies have compared outcomes in VATS and open cohorts. Chan et al. [14] prospectively compared VATS vs. open decortication, and approximately 75 % of each study arm had stage 3 empyema. A 100 % treatment success was reported in both arms with no conversion to open procedure in the VATS arm, and a reduction in operative time was demonstrated in VATS cohort [14, 15]. Muhammed and colleagues [13] also conducted a prospective study comparing VATS vs. open surgery in stage 2 and 3 empyema. VATS was associated a 92 % procedural success compare to 100 % in the thoracotomy cohort. Multiple retrospective series have demonstrated comparable success rates VATS and open cohorts in patients managed for stage 2/3 empyema [15, 18–20] and high success rates in VATS series (21. In a retrospective series of stage 3 empyema, Waller and colleagues [16] reported no re-intervention in patients managed with VATS decortication alone; in a similar series Drain et al. reported a 6 % re-intervention rate. The rate of re-intervention varies between studies with some reporting no re-intervention in either group [14]. Re-operation (4.8 % vs 1 %) was lower in the VATS cohort in another similar study [15]. The management of chronic empyema with trapped lung necessitates a different approach; however, the use of

Table 48.1 Studies comparing VATS techniques to open thoracotomy for the management of pleural empyema

Study	Stage of empyema	Procedure (no. of patients)	Op time	Chest tube drainage	Postoperative length of stay (days)	Postop morbidity	Procedure Success/ Re-intervention	Mortality	Conversion rate	Quality of evidence
Muhammed [13] (2012) (Prospective)	Stage II/III	VATS (25)	84.68±23.98	5.72±3.27	7.76±4.63	–	PS: 92%	0%	8%	Moderate
		Open (24)	137.37±26.98	7.25±2.31	8.87±2.59	–	PS: 100%	0%		
Marks et al. [18] (2012) (Retrospective)	Stage II/III	VATS (116)	–	–	5 (8–8.5) med	25.1%ᵃ	PS: 95.1%	5.7%ᵃ	14.7%	Moderate
		Open (277)	–	–	7 (5–14) med					
Tong et al. [20] (2010)ᵇ (Retrospective)	Stage II/III	VATS (326)	97	7.0±13.7	7 (median)	Look up	RI: 7.7%	7.6%	11.4%	Low
		Open (94)	155	9.7±10.1	10 (median)	Look up	RI: 10.6%	16.1%		
Shahin et al. [24] (2010) (Retrospective)	Stage II	VDB (28)	–	–	6 (med)	3.5%	–	0%	0%	Moderate
	Stage III	VDC (32)	–	–	5 (med)	9.3%	–	0%	19%	
	Stage II/III	Open (21)	–	–	8 (med)	26.1%	–	0%	–	
Casali et al. [23] (2009) (Retrospective)	Stage II	VATS (27)	100.4	4.0	6.4	24%ᵃ	–	0%	8%	Moderate
		Open (24)	115.4	7.3	9.0		–	0%		
	Stage III	Open (68)	131.5	5.7	14.6		–	2.94%		
Cardillo et al. [15] (2009) (Retrospective)	Stage II/III	VATS (185)	79.7±6.8	–	8.6±1.8	18.3%	1.62%	0%	5.9%	Moderate
		Open (123)	70.0±7.4	–	10±7.8	25.2%	0%	3.25%		
Chan et al. [14] (2007) (Prospective)	Stage II/III	VATS (41)	2.5±0.96	7.9±5.7	16±6.5	22%ᵃ	RI: 0%	0%	0%	Moderate
		Open (36)	3.8±1.4	8.5±4.4	21±14.2		RI: 0%	0%		
Lardinois et al. [19] (2005) (Retrospective)	Stage II/III	VATS (178)	–	–	–	9%ᵃ	RI: 2%	3%	44%	Moderate
		Open (150)	–	–	–		RI: 2.6%	4%		

Study	Stage	Group (n)								
Waller and Rengarajan [16] (2001) (Retrospective)	Stage III	VS (21)	78.8±6.5	–	5.5±0.6	–	RI:0 %	4.76 %	41.67 %	Moderate
		VU (15)	119.6±13.5	–	8.5±1.3	–	RI:0 %	6.67 %		
		Open (12)	109±5.5	–	8.4±0.7	–	RI:0 %	0 %		
Podbielski et al. [22] (2000) (Retrospective)	Stage II/III	VATS (16)	76.2±30.7	4.7±2.8	17.6±16.8	6.25 %	–	–	6.7 %	Low
		Open (14)	125.0±71.7	8.3±4.6	10.0±7.2	7.14 %	–	–		
Angelillo et al. [17] (1996) (Retrospective)	Stage II	VATS (31)	119+32.5	4.3+1.5	6.7+3.0	16.1 %	PS: 100 %	3.2 %	10 %	Low
		Open (33)	123+25.8	6.1+2.3	11.6+9.1	15.1 %	PS: 88 %	3 %		

VATS video assisted thoracoscopic surgery, *VS* VATS successful, *VU* VATS unsuccessful, i.e. required conversion to thoracotomy, *VDB* VATS debridement, *VDC* VATS decortication

[a]Study did not differentiate outcomes between VATS and open group

[b]Study included patients with hemothorax and recurrent/complex effusions

VATS is still plausible. Waller et al. [16] evaluated VATS vs. open decortication to re-expand entrapped lung in a series of patients with chronic postpneumonic pleural empyema. VATS decortication was successful in 21/36 patients with 15(42 %) requiring conversion to open to achieve lung expansion. Operating time was significantly longer in the thoracotomy group as was post-operative hospital stay (mean difference 2.9 days). Interestingly, the success of VATS decortication was not related to either the delay between onset of symptoms or hospital admission and surgery; in fact, the operating time decreased with increasing pre-operative delay. Drain et al. [21] report the successful management of stage 3 empyema by two-window VATS decortication in 52 patients. The mean drainage time was 3.9 days and the median time to hospital discharge was 10 days. There were no reported complications and resolution occurred in 94 % of patients.

Morbidity and Mortality

The potential advantages of the VATS approach include improved visualization, reduced surgical trauma, including postoperative pain, and an improved postoperative quality of life. These outcomes are addressed in a number of studies and favor a minimally invasive approach [20]. Lower rates of postoperative air leak [15], renal failure, blood loss [20, 22] and ventilator requirements have been demonstrated when comparing VATS to open thoracotomy. Post-operative pain has also shown to be reduced [14, 15], which may lead to reduced dyspnea [23] and increased deep breathing and lung expansion and therefore equate to reduce rates of postoperative pneumonia and respiratory complications. The reduced morbidity associated with VATS approach is reflected in shorter duration of chest tube drainage, reduced length of postoperative hospital stay [13, 15, 16, 18, 20, 24] and a quicker return to work [15]. The VATS approach is associated with greater satisfaction with the wounds and the operation overall [25]. Mortality has also been demonstrated to be lower in VATS cohorts [15, 20].

Conversion Rates in VATS

Whilst the feasibility of VATS management of stage 3 empyema has been demonstrated, various studies have shown a high conversation rate to thoracotomy. In studies of stage 2/3 empyema managed with VATS debridement and decortication, conversion rates to open thoracotomy ranged from 0 to 59 % (Tables 48.1 and 48.2). A longer delay from onset of symptoms to the operation, the presence of fever and detection of pleural thickening were independent predictors of conversion to thoracotomy [15, 26–28]. Stefani et al. [27] reported that all cases in their series with evident pleural thickening, the presence of fever and a delay above 20 days from diagnosis to surgery, required conversion to open approach. Lardinois et al. [19]

Table 48.2 Case series of VATS for pleural empyema

Study	Stage of empyema	Number of patients	Operation time (min)	Chest tube drainage	Postoperative length of stay (days)	Postop morbidity	Procedure Success/ Re-intervention	Mortality	Conversion rate	Quality of evidence
Stefani et al. [27] (2013) (Retrospective)	Stage II/III	97	146 / 162[a]	4.4 / 5.0[a]	8.3 / 8.4	5 % / 18 %	PS:100 %	0 %	59 %	Low
Solaini et al. [25] (2007) (Retrospective)	Stage II	110	–	6 days	7.1 days	11 %	PS: 99.1 %	–	8.2 %	Moderate
Drain et al. [21] (2007) (Retrospective)	Stage III	52	–	3.9 (mean) 4 (median)	10 (median)	0 %	PS: 94 % RI: 6 %	0 %	0 %	Low
Luh et al. [29] (2005) (Retrospective)	Stage II/III	234	64.3 + 22.5	7 (med)	12 (med)	7.69 %	PS: 86.3 % RI: 6.8 %	3.4 %	10.3 %	Moderate
Kim et al. [30] (2004) (Retrospective)	Stage II/III	70	–	5 + 3	5 ± 0.7	0 %	PS: 92.86 %	0 %	7.14 %	Moderate
Roberts [33] (2003) (Retrospective)	Stage II/III	172	–	10.5	15.3 (mean)	9 % / 21 %[a]	3.03 % / 3.77 %	0 % / 10 %[a]	38.37	Low
Striffeler et al. [32] (1998) (Retrospective)	Stage II	67	82.1 (mean)	4.1 (mean)	12.3 (mean)	–	RI: 4 %	4 %	28 %	Moderate
Lawrence et al. [31] (1997) (Retrospective)	Stage II/III	42	–	4.0 ± 0.3	5.3 ± 0.4	–	RI: 23.81 %	0	4.76 %	Low
Landreneau et al.[28] (1996) (Retrospective)	Stage II/III	76	–	3.3 + 2.9 (in 67 pts)	7.4 ± 7.2	–	PS: 83 % RI: 7.89 %	6.6 %	9.21 %	Moderate

[a]Data from patients who underwent conversion to thoracotomy

found that delayed referral and gram-negative microorganisms were significant independent predictors for conversion to thoracotomy; the probability was found to rise from 22 to 86 % between at an interval of 12 and 16 days from onset of symptoms to surgery. Similarly, Casali et al. [23] found a significant difference in time from onset of symptoms to surgery when studying VATS vs open cohorts, of 12 ± 6 vs 32 ± 22 days, respectively, suggesting that delayed cases were more likely to require a thoracotomy. Luh [29] and colleagues reported their series of VATS decortication and found a mean preoperative length of stay of 11.4 days in patients who achieved successful VATS debridement, in comparison to a stay of 18.4 days in those who required conversion or re-intervention. The significantly higher conversion rate demonstrated with delayed intervention likely reflects progression of the disease. This was confirmed by their report of a 21.3 % conversion rate for stage 3 disease, compared with 3.5 % for stage 2 empyema. Similarly, Shahin et al. [24] reported a higher conversion rate in patients with stage 3 empyema: 19 % vs. 3.5 % for stage 2.

Conclusion

The question of whether VATS or open surgery is superior in the management of pleural empyema should rather be: what are the key preoperative predictors to guide an appropriate surgical approach? The different physical properties between the progressive phases mandate that different approaches are required for the appropriate management of each stage. Whilst the mainstay of treatment in stage 1 is antibiotic therapy and chest tube drainage, the best approach to the management of stage 2 is VATS debridement. In stage 3 empyema multiple studies have shown that VATS is as effective as open decortication in a significant proportion of patients, with the associated benefit of a reduction in postoperative morbidity and length of hospital stay, as well as greater satisfaction with postoperative wound appearance and an earlier return to work. There is however the caveat of a high conversion rate to open decortication. The true clinical challenge is to predict which cohort of patients is more likely to require an open approach and which can be successfully treated via VATS. Whilst the benefit demonstrated in successful VATS decortication promotes an attempt at VATS decortication in all patients [30–33], the prediction of those in whom conversion is highly likely allows for appropriate preoperative planning. Reported predictors of conversion to open thoracotomy are a delay from onset of symptoms to surgical intervention, the presence of gram-positive bacteria and a persistent fever. We suggest that when these factors are present, the patients and the operative team should be made aware of the high likelihood of conversion to open thoracotomy.

The early recognition and intervention of pleural empyema will increase the success of a minimally invasive approach and will therefore reduce associated morbidity, mortality and healthcare costs [4].

Recommendations

Early referral (5–8 days following failure of thoracotomy and antibiotic therapy) and treatment (<12 days from onset of symptoms) are paramount to reduce morbidity. In patients with stage 2 or 3 empyema who are fit enough to undergo an operative procedure, surgical intervention is superior to tube thoracostomy. In patients with stage 2 empyema, VATS is recommended over open thoracotomy. In patients with stage 3 organizing empyema decortication should be attempted by VATS with a low threshold for conversation to open thoracotomy in cases of operative indication, prolonged time form onset of symptoms (>12 days), gram negative bacteria, detect of pleural thickening, persistent fever.

A Personal View of the Data

My personal approach is to study carefully the CT and determine the chances of re-expanding the lung and clearing the pleural space by VATS. If there is a long-standing effusion, evidence of a parietal and/or visceral pleura peel, and loss of volume of the hemithorax, then I would go straight for an open approach, otherwise I would go for VATS first. In case of thoracotomy, I electively remove a segment of rib (usually the 6th) to gain access to the chest. I prefer this approach, rather than force ribs open breaking them with potential for malunion and chronic pain.

There is a debate on whether to remove the parietal pleura. My preference is to remove it leaving just a small area around the spine to insert a paravertebral catheter for analgesia. Most anesthetists are reluctant to insert an epidural in an infected patient. The purpose of removing the parietal cortex is to re-expand the hemithorax and allow the physiological "bucket-handle" movement of the ribs. There is controversy regarding re-expansion of the hemithorax in the presence of a trapped lung, leaving a space-problem. I believe that this is never the case if the lung is mobilized completely and each lobe decorticated. I believe it is important to get into the fissure to allow better movement and re-expansion of the lung in each direction, otherwise the lobes will be tethered on one side and will not re-expand.

Air-leak is an unavoidable problem, but I have found this is greatly minimized by the routine use of a radiofrequency diathermy with irrigated tips. We also found that with this device the need for transfusions is minimal. During closure of thoractomy I re-approximate the intercostal muscles with an air tight running suture of 2/0 vicryl, otherwise there is a risk of significant surgical emphysema if the air leak is right under the thoracotomy wound.

Recommendations

- Early referral for and treatment of empyema are paramount to reduce morbidity.
- VATS is recommended over open decortication for stage 2 empyema.
- In patients with stage 3 organizing empyema decortication should be attempted by VATS with a low threshold for conversation to open thoracotomy.

References

1. Roxburgh CS, Youngson GG. Childhood empyema in North-East Scotland over the past 15 years. Scott Med J. 2007;52:25–7.
2. Grijalva CG, Zhu Y, Pekka Nuorti J, Griffin MR. Emergence of parapneumonic empyema in the USA. Thorax. 2011;66(8):663–8.
3. Farjah F, Symons RG, Krishnadasan B, Wood DE, Flum DR. Management of pleural space infections: a population- based analysis. J Thorac Cardiovasc Surg. 2007;133:346–51.
4. Finley C, Clifton J, Fitzgerald JM, Yee J. Empyema: an increasing concern in Canada. Can Respir J. 2008;15:85–9.
5. Light RW. Parapneumonic effusions and empyema. Clin Chest Med. 1985;6:55–62.
6. Ferguson AD, Prescott RJ, Selkon JB, Watson D, Swinburn CR. The clinical course and management of thoracic empyema. QJM. 1996;89:285–9.
7. Davies CW, Kearney SE, Gleeson FV, Davies RJ. Predictors of outcome and long-term survival in patients with pleural infection. Am J Respir Crit Care Med. 1999;160:1682–7.
8. Mandal AK, Thadepalli H, Chettipally U. Outcome of primary empyema thoracis: therapeutic and microbiologic aspects. Ann Thorac Surg. 1998;66:1782–6.
9. Bilgin M, Akcali Y, Oguzkaya F. Benefits of early aggressive management of empyema thoracis. ANZ J Surg. 2006;76:120–2.
10. Wait MA, Beckles DL, Paul M, Hotze M, Dimaio MJ. Thoracoscopic management of empyema thoracis. J Minim Access Surg. 2007;3(4):141–8.
11. Davies CW, Gleeson FV, Davies RJ, BTS Pleural Disease Group, a subgroup of the BTS Standards of Care Committee. BTS guidelines for the management of pleural infection. Thorax. 2003;58(Suppl II):ii18–28.
12. Colice GL, Curtis A, Deslauriers J. Medical and surgical treatment of parapneumonic effusions: an evidence-based guideline. Chest. 2000;118:1158–71.
13. Muhammad MI. Management of complicated parapneumonic effusion and empyema using different treatment modalities. Asian Cardiovasc Thorac Ann. 2012;20(2):177–81.
14. Chan DT, Sihoe AD, Chan S, Tsang DS, Fang B, Lee TW, et al. Surgical treatment for empyema thoracis: is video-assisted thoracic surgery "better" than thoracotomy? Ann Thorac Surg. 2007;84:225–31.
15. Cardillo G, Carleo F, Carbone L, Di Martino M, Salvadori L, Petrella L, et al. Chronic postpneumonic pleural empyema: comparative merits of thoracoscopic versus open decortication. Eur J Cardiothorac Surg. 2009;36:914–8.
16. Waller DA, Rengarajan A. Thoracoscopic decortication: a role for video-assisted surgery in chronic postpneumonic pleural empyema. Ann Thorac Surg. 2001;71:1813–6.
17. Angelillo Mackinlay TA, Lyons GA, Chimondeguy DJ, Piedras MA, Angaramo G, Emery J. VATS debridement versus thoracotomy in the treatment of loculated postpneumonia empyema. Ann Thorac Surg. 1996;61(6):1626–30.

18. Marks DJ, Fisk MD, Koo CY, Pavlou M, Peck L, Lee SF, et al. Thoracic empyema: a 12-year study from a UK tertiary cardiothoracic referral centre. PLoS One. 2012;7(1):e30074.
19. Lardinois D, Gock M, Pezzetta E, Buchli C, Furrer M, Ris HB. Delayed referral and gram-negative organisms increase the conversion thoracotomy rate in patients undergoing video-assisted thoracoscopic surgery for empyema. Ann Thorac Surg. 2005;79:1851–6.
20. Tong BC, Hanna J, Toloza EM, Onaitis MW, D'Amico TA, Harpole DH, et al. Outcomes of video-assisted thoracoscopic decortication. Ann Thorac Surg. 2010;89:220–5.
21. Drain AJ, Ferguson JI, Sayeed R, Wilkinson S, Ritchie A. Definitive management of advanced empyema by two-window video-assisted surgery. Asian Cardiovasc Thorac Ann. 2007; 15:238–9.
22. Podbielski FJ, Maniar HS, Rodriguez HE, Hernan MJ, Vigneswaran WT. Surgical strategy of complex empyema thoracis. JSLS. 2000;4(4):287–90.
23. Casali C, Storelli ES, Di Prima E, Morandi U. Long-term functional results after surgical treatment of parapneumonic thoracic empyema. Interact Cardiovasc Thorac Surg. 2009;9(1):74–8.
24. Shahin Y, Duffy J, Beggs D, Black E, Majewski A. Surgical management of primary empyema of the pleural cavity: outcome of 81 patients. Interact Cardiovasc Thorac Surg. 2010;10:565–7.
25. Solaini L, Prusciano F, Bagioni P. Video-assisted thoracic surgery in the treatment of pleural empyema. Surg Endosc. 2007;21:280–4.
26. Waller DA, Rengarajan A, Nicholson FH, Rajesh PB. Delayed referral reduces the success of video-assisted thoracoscopic debridement for post-pneumonic empyema. Respir Med. 2001;95(10):836–40.
27. Stefani A, Aramini B, Della Casa G, Ligabue G, Kaleci S, Casali C, et al. Preoperative predictors of successful surgical treatment in the management of parapneumonic empyema. Ann Thorac Surg. 2013;96:1812–9.
28. Landreneau RJ, Keenan RJ, Hazelrigg SR, Mack MJ, Naunheim KS. Thoracoscopy for empyema and hemothorax. Chest. 1996;109:18–24.
29. Luh SP, Chou MC, Wang LS, Chen JY, Tsai TP. Video-assisted thoracoscopic surgery in the treatment of complicated parapneumonic effusions or empyemas: outcome of 234 patients. Chest. 2005;127:1427–32.
30. Kim BY, Oh BS, Jang WC, Min YI, Park YK, Park JC. Video-assisted thoracoscopic decortication for management of postpneumonic pleural empyema. Am J Surg. 2004;188:321–4.
31. Lawrence DR, Ohri SK, Moxon RE, Townsend ER, Fountain SW. Thoracoscopic debridement of empyema thoracis. Ann Thorac Surg. 1997;64(5):1448–50.
32. Striffeler H, Gugger M, Im Hof V, Cerny A, Furrer M, Ris HB. Video-assisted thoracoscopic surgery for fibrinopurulent pleural empyema in 67 patients. Ann Thorac Surg. 1998;65:319–23.
33. Roberts JR. Minimally invasive surgery in the treatment of empyema: intraoperative decision making. Ann Thorac Surg. 2003;76:225–30.

Chapter 49
Optimal Management of Symptomatic Malignant Pleural Effusion

Xiao Li and Mark K. Ferguson

Abstract Malignant pleural effusion (MPE) is a common clinical problem in patients with late stage cancer. The optimal management for symptomatic MPE is still controversial. Recent findings confirmed talc to be the most effective sclerosant available for pleurodesis in MPE. Use of calibrated talc with large particle size is now firmly established in order to prevent systemic complications. Thoracoscopic talc insufflation is more favorable than beside talc slurry instillation for patients with good performance status. Tunneled pleural catheters have shown to be efficacious, cost effective, and patient friendly, and are in wide use. They have advantages over other management techniques, particularly for patients with trapped lung.

Keywords Malignant pleural effusion • Indwelling pleural catheter • Pleurodesis • Talc

Introduction

An estimated 200,000 pleural effusions due to malignancy occur each year in the United States [1]. The most common causes of malignant pleural effusions (MPE) are lung cancer in men and breast cancer in women. Together, these malignancies account for 50–65 % of all malignant effusions [2]. The majority of patients who present with a malignant pleural effusion are symptomatic. The optimal management for symptomatic MPE is controversial. Options include periodic thoracentesis, intercostal tube drainage and instillation of a sclerosant, thoracoscopy and

X. Li, MD (✉)
Department of Thoracic Surgery, Peking University People's Hospital,
No.11, Xizhimen South Avenue, Beijing 100044, China
e-mail: dr.lixiao@163.com

M.K. Ferguson, MD
Department of Surgery, The University of Chicago,
Chicago, IL, USA

M.K. Ferguson (ed.), *Difficult Decisions in Thoracic Surgery*,
Difficult Decisions in Surgery: An Evidence-Based Approach 1,
DOI 10.1007/978-1-4471-6404-3_49, © Springer-Verlag London 2014

pleurodesis, and placement of an indwelling pleural catheter. Because these effusions are often detected late in the course of disease in patients who often have limited life expectancy, selection of appropriate therapy for MPE must take into account both potential benefits and associated risks that affect duration and quality of life (QOL). We performed a literature review to examine the available evidence for the optimal management strategy for MPE. Our intent is to help inform decision making of health care practitioners and patients by weighing the risks and benefits of different management strategies for malignant pleural effusions.

Search Strategy

We performed a search in PubMed and the Cochrane database for peer-reviewed English language articles that included only human subjects for the period 2001 through September 2013. Additional articles were identified from the references in the articles identified in the search. Searches included the Medical Subject Headings (MeSH) term "malignant pleural effusion" with MeSH search terms "management/ treatment," "pleurodesis," "indwelling/tunneled pleural catheter," "talc," and "quality of life". We included randomized prospective trials when available and prospective nonrandomized studies that addressed symptoms, quality of life (QOL), and/or complications. When no prospective studies were available, large retrospective studies were included as well as meta-analyses. Review articles were used for general background information. We excluded case reports, studies involving non-malignant pleural effusions, and studies that dealt with chemotherapeutic or biologic agents.

Management Options

Thoracentesis

Thoracentesis usually is the first step in the management of MPE. It is diagnostic and, at the same time, relieves symptoms in the majority of patients. Thoracentesis also provides important information about lung expansion that helps direct subsequent therapy. However, the recurrence rate after thoracentesis for MPE is almost 100 % within 30 days. Repeated thoracentesis provides transient relief of symptoms and avoids hospitalization for patients with limited survival expectancy and poor performance status, and thus is appropriate for frail or terminally ill patients. Repeated thoracentesis without the use of sclerosing agents is associated with a high rate of infection, bleeding, pneumothorax, and the development of loculations, so repeated thoracentesis is not recommended if life expectancy is measured in more than weeks [2].

Tube Drainage and Sclerosis

Intercostal tube drainage in combination with intrapleural injection of a sclerosing agent can achieve chemical pleurodesis resulting in reduction of symptoms and improved QOL. Historically it is the most common approach to management of MPE and has a success rate of 70–80 %. However, unfavorable outcomes in some patients include infection, empyema, arrhythmias, cardiac arrest, myocardial infarction, hypotension, acute respiratory distress syndrome, and systemic inflammatory reaction secondary to sclerosing agents. This approach requires careful consideration among patients with advanced disease and limited life expectancy given the potential need for prolonged hospitalization associated with complications of the procedure.

Thoracoscopy and Pleurodesis

Thoracoscopy with administration of a sclerosing agent is a safe and well-tolerated procedure with a low perioperative mortality rate (<0.5 %). A significant benefit of thoracoscopy is the ability to obtain a diagnosis through biopsies, break down loculations to enable complete drainage of the effusion, and perform a pleurodesis during the same procedure. In patients with good performance status, thoracoscopy is appropriate for diagnosis of a suspected malignant pleural effusion and for drainage and pleurodesis of a known malignant pleural effusion.

Indwelling Pleural Catheter

Insertion of an indwelling pleural catheter (IPC) is another popular method for controlling recurrent and symptomatic malignant effusions, especially in patients with a trapped lung who are not amenable to chemical sclerosis. Several catheters have been developed for this purpose, and the published studies employing them have reported encouraging results [3–5]. Suzuki et al. reported the largest series of IPC (n=418) experience, providing evidence that IPCs are safe and effective. A recent summary of all published reports on IPC complications revealed that most complaints were minor [6]. A systematic review including 1,370 patients also has confirmed that serious complications are uncommon (<3 %) [7].

Issues

Size of the Intercostal Tube

Traditionally, tube thoracostomy and pleurodesis are performed as inpatient procedures, using a large-bore intercostal tubes (24Fr to 32Fr) because they are thought to be less prone to obstruction by fibrin plugs, but there is little published evidence to confirm this. Use of small-bore (10Fr to 14Fr) catheters for inpatient and outpatient drainage of pleural effusions has emerged as an effective

Table 49.1 Studies comparing small-bore to large bore intercostal tubes for chemical sclerosis

Author	Year	Study design	Patients	Results	Evidence quality
Clementsen et al. [10]	1998	Prospective, randomized	18 (9 small-bore, 9 large-bore)	More patients required thoracentesis in small-bore group, but were more comfortable	Moderate
Parulekar et al. [11]	2001	Retrospective, non-randomized	102 (58 small-bore, 44 large-bore)	Recurrence rates were similar, about 50 % in each group	Low
Caglayan et al. [12]	2008	Prospective, randomized	41 (21 small-bore, 20 large-bore)	Success rates similar	High

treatment for MPE and has been used more frequently in recent years. The reported experience suggests that the use of small-bore catheters is effective, safe, and well-tolerated [8, 9].

Only three studies [10–12] compared the small-bore intercostal tubes with large-bore tubes in the management of MPE. The studies using small-bore intercostal tubes with commonly used sclerosants reported similar success rates to and appeared to cause less discomfort (Table 49.1).

Sclerosant Selection

The choice of a sclerosing agent is determined by the agent's efficacy, accessibility, safety, ease of administration, number of administrations to achieve a complete response, and cost, as well as by the treating physician's personal preference [2]. A variety of sclerosing agents have been used to treat MPE, but many have proved less than optimal because of poor efficacy, a high incidence of adverse effects, difficulty in administration, or costs.

A recent Cochrane review concluded that talc is probably the optimal agent for chemical pleurodesis [13]. When comparing different sclerosants, talc was found to be the most efficacious, with overall success rate of approximately 80 %. Thoracoscopic talc pleurodesis yielded a success rate of 96 %. The relative risk (RR) of effusion non-recurrence was 1.34 (95 % confidence interval (CI) 1.16–1.55) in favor of talc compared with bleomycin, tetracycline, or tube drainage alone. This view is supported by a more recent systematic review [14], in which the authors found that talc tended to be associated with fewer recurrences when compared to bleomycin (RR, 0.64; 95 % CI 0.34–1.20) and, with less certainty, to tetracycline (RR, 0.50; 95 % CI, 0.06–4.42).

A serious complication associated with the use of talc is adult respiratory distress syndrome or acute pneumonitis leading to acute respiratory failure. There have been many reports of pneumonitis associated with talc pleurodesis, predominantly from the UK and the USA where, historically, talc of mixed particle sizes has been used. Maskell and colleagues undertook two studies to assess the association of talc particle grade and respiratory failure [15, 16]. In the first study, they concluded mixed talc worsened gas exchange and induced more systemic inflammation than talc restricted to large grade. In a subsequent cohort study of 558 patients who underwent thoracoscopic pleurodesis using large grade talc, there were no episodes of pneumonitis [16].

In the USA, bleomycin is also a more expensive sclerosant than talc, and tetracycline is no longer available for use as a sclerosant. Talc is an effective and safe sclerosant and should be the agent of choice for pleurodesis.

Talc Poudrage or Talc Slurry

Talc is administered in two ways: insufflated at thoracoscopy as dry particles using an atomizer (poudrage) or via an intercostal tube in the form of a suspension of talc particles in fluid (slurry). Four studies have directly compared talc slurry (TS) with talc poudrage (TP) [17–20].

Yim et al. [17] in 1996 designed a prospective, randomized study to compare talc slurry with thoracoscopic talc poudrage for the first time, and did not find any superiority of poudrage over slurry. One shortcoming of the study was the small sample size, and study also lacked documentation of patients' quality of life after the procedures. Data from another randomized study are available only in abstract form [18]. That study suggests superiority of poudrage over slurry, but limited data are available to validate this conclusion. More recently Stefani et al. [20] compared thoracoscopy and talc poudrage with talc slurry in a non-randomized manner. Their results suggest superiority of poudrage over slurry, but the two groups were not equivalent with respect to performance status. In the largest randomized study, Dresler et al. [19] compared talc poudrage with talc slurry. Although the study concluded that the two methods were equivalent, the subgroup of patients with primary lung or breast cancer had higher success with talc poudrage than with TS (82 % vs 67 %). Quality-of-life measurement also favored talc poudrage. Patient ratings of comfort and safety were also higher for talc poudrage (Table 49.2).

In addition to the slight superior efficacy of TS to TP, thoracoscopy also affords an opportunity to directly inspect the pleura and to address adhesions and loculations. This may be indicated for patients who have had prior ipsilateral surgery or attempted pleurodesis, or for whom there is a significant possibility of a trapped lung. TP is also perceived by patients to afford greater comfort and medical safety, as well as causing less fatigue relative to TS. These factors may importantly impact treatment preferences for patients who rank quality of life as a principal goal of care.

Table 49.2 Prospective studies comparing TP and TS for pleurodesis

Author	Year	Study design	Patients n	Results	Evidence quality
Yim et al. [17]	1996	Prospective, randomized	57 (28 TP vs. 29 TS)	Success rates similar (27/28 in TP vs. 26/29 in TS)	Moderate
Dresler et al. [19]	2005	Prospective, randomized	482 (242 TP vs. 240 TS)	Efficacy rates similar, QOL, and safety better for TP, but not significant	High
Stefani et al. [20]	2006	Prospective, non-randomized	109 (72 TP vs. 37 TS)	TP better (TP 87.5 % vs. TS 73 %)	Moderate

TP talc poudrage, *TS* talc slurry, *QOL* quality of life

Indwelling Pleural Catheter or Chest Tube and Talc Pleurodesis

Several prospective or retrospective trails have compared IPC and talc pleurodesis for the management of MPE in recent years [4, 21–27]. In a randomized controlled trail (TIME2), Davies et al. [22] compared IPC (Rocket ®) to chest tube and talc pleurodesis. They demonstrated dyspnea improvement in both groups, with no significant difference in the first 42 days. But there was a statistically significant improvement in dyspnea in the IPC group at 6 months. The duration of initial hospitalization was significantly shorter in the IPC group, with a median of 0 days compared to 4 days for the talc group. There was no significant difference in quality of life. More patients in the talc group required further pleural procedures compared with in the IPC group (22 % vs 6 %).

Another prospective randomized trial concluded that IPC (PleurX®) achieved superior palliation of unilateral MPEs than bedside talc pleurodesis, particularly in patients with trapped lungs [23].

Hunt and his colleagues also compared thoracoscopic talc to IPC. The trial included 109 patients: 59 patients had IPC placed, and 50 were treated with video-assisted thoracic surgery (VATS) and talc. Patients who underwent IPC placement had significantly fewer reinterventions for recurrent ipsilateral effusions than patients treated with VATS talc (IPC 2 % vs. talc 16 %, p=0.01), and had significantly shorter overall length of stay (LOS) (7 days vs. 8 days, p=0.006) and post procedure LOS (3 days vs. 6 days, p <0.001). Complication rates and in-hospital mortality were not significantly different. They concluded that placement of a IPC is superior to VATS talc for palliation of MPE-associated symptoms [24].

A retrospective propensity score-matched comparison of talc pleurodesis and IPC in patients undergoing diagnostic thoracoscopy also demonstrated that IPC provided palliation of patients' malignant pleural effusions and freedom from reintervention equal to that of talc pleurodesis after thoracoscopy, while resulting in a shorter mean length of hospital stay and interval to the initiation of systemic therapy. Lower rates of operative morbidity were also seen in the IPC treatment group [25].

Table 49.3 Results of studies comparing IPC and talc pleurodesis

Author	Year	Study design	Patients n	Results	Evidence quality
Putnam et al. [4]	2000	Retrospective comparison	168 (100 PleurX® vs. 68 tube + talc)	Both effective and safe, PleurX® reduced hospital stay from 7 days to 0	Low
Ohm et al. [21]	2003	Prospective, randomize	41	PleurX® efficacious in patients with trapped lung	Moderate
Davies et al. [22]	2012	Prospective, randomized	106	Relieving dyspnea equal in first 42 days, IPC better at 6 months	High
Demmy et al. [23]	2012	Prospective, randomized	57	IPC achieved superior palliation (62 % vs. 46 %)	High
Hunt et al. [24]	2012	Retrospective, chart review	109 (59 IPC vs.50 talc)	IPC with reduced LOS, fewer reinterventions	Low
Fysh et al. [26]	2012	Prospective, non-randomized	160 (only 65 in final analysis, 34 IPC vs. 31TP)	Effusion-related hospital bed days were significantly fewer with IPC (3 days vs. 10 days)	Moderate
Freeman et al. [26]	2013	Propensity-matched	60	Equal efficiency, shorter LOS for IPC	Moderate
Srour et al. [27]	2013	Retrospective, cohort	360 (100 IPC vs. 167 TP)	Better pleural effusion control and longer effusion-free survival with IPC	Moderate

IPC indwelling pleural catheter, *LOS* length of stay, *TP* talc pleurodesis

As listed in Table 49.3, an indwelling pleural catheter is therefore an effective option for controlling symptomatic malignant effusions. It is particularly useful when length of hospitalization is to be kept to a minimum, for patients who are known or are suspected to have a trapped lung, and in situations in which expertise and facilities exist for out-patient management of these catheters.

Cost-Effectiveness of Management Options

Few studies have included analysis of the cost effectiveness of different treatment options for MPE. One recent analysis by Olden et al. found treatment with talc was less costly than PleurX® with similar effectiveness. But PleurX® became more cost effective when life expectancy was 6 weeks or less. As to the small differences in cost and effectiveness, they suggested that the choice of treatment should be based on patient preferences and the clinical situation [28].

Puri et al. [29] also used decision analytic techniques to compare repeated thoracentesis (RT), tunneled pleural catheter (TPC), bedside pleurodesis (BP), and thoracoscopic pleurodesis (TP) and analyzed their cost effectiveness. Under base case analysis for 3-month survival, RT was the least expensive treatment ($4,946) and provided the fewest utilities. When under base case analysis for 12-month survival, BP was the least expensive treatment ($13,057). But when comparing the incremental cost-effectiveness ratio (ICER), TPC was both less expensive and more effective. They concluded that TPC is the preferred treatment for patients with malignant pleural effusion and limited survival; but BP is the most cost-effective treatment for patients with more prolonged expected survival.

Recommendation

The patient's symptoms, functional status, and life expectancy should be kept in mind when considering therapeutic options. Repeated therapeutic thoracentesis is a good option for patients with very limited life expectancy, with the benefit of dyspnea control despite the high rate of recurrence. The two optimal techniques for managing MPE are intercostal tubes plus pleurodesis and the use of chronic IPC. Small-bore intercostal tubes have similar success rates to large-bore tubes and appear to cause less discomfort for tube thoracostomy. The available evidence supports the need for chemical sclerosants for successful pleurodesis and the use of talc as the sclerosant of choice. Considering both efficiency and QOL, the evidence lends weight to talc poudrage rather than slurry. IPC improves symptoms for patients with MPE and is rarely associated with major complications. Based on several recent prospective randomized studies, IPC seems superior to talc pleurodesis in palliation of MPE.

As a result, we make a weak recommendation for use of small-bore catheters rather than large-bore catheters for effusion drainage and pleurodesis. Talc is the favored sclerosant because of its greater effectiveness than other agents and its low cost. When using talc for pleurodesis, thoracoscopic talc insufflation is favored. Ambulatory indwelling pleural catheter is a superior selection compared with tube and talc pleurodesis for MPE.

A Personal View of the Data

The available evidence for procedural management of MPE in patients with limited life expectancy leads us to conclude that a patient-centered approach to therapy is of paramount importance. Decision making should be tailored based on prognosis and goals of therapy.

Repeated thoracentesis provides transient relief of symptoms and avoids hospitalization for patients with limited survival expectancy and poor performance status, and thus is appropriate for terminally ill patients. Thoracoscopy has the ability to obtain a diagnosis through biopsies and break down loculations to enable complete drainage of the effusion. In patients with good performance status, thoracoscopy is appropriate for diagnosis of a suspected malignant pleural effusion and it is also can accompanied by either IPC drainage or pleurodesis according to the patient's situation.

Experience with using the IPC for MPE is becoming more widespread since its introduction in 1999. Because of its slightly higher efficacy and reduced of duration of hospital stay, we believe IPC is a better procedure for management of MPE than bedside pleurodesis and is possibly superior to VATS pleurodesis. More prospective randomized studies with larger sample size comparing the IPC to pleurodesis are needed before IPC can be definitively recommended as the best initial treatment for MPE.

Recommendations

- Both tunneled pleural catheter and talc pleurodesis provide good symptom relief for patients with symptomatic malignant pleural effusion (Evidence quality high; strong recommendation)
- Large grade talc should be used in preference to ungraded talc because of the lower rate of complications after pleurodesis. (Evidence quality high; strong recommendation)
- When using talc for pleurodesis, thoracoscopic talc insufflation is recommended for patients with good performance status. (Evidence quality moderate; weak recommendation)
- An indwelling tunneled pleural catheter is optimal for the management of malignant pleural effusions in patients who appear to have a trapped lung (Evidence quality moderate; weak recommendation)

References

1. Light RW. Pleural diseases. 5th ed. Baltimore: Lippincott, Williams & Wilkins; 2007.
2. Roberts ME, Neville E, Berrisford RG, Antunes G, Ali NJ. Management of a malignant pleural effusion: British Thoracic Society Pleural Disease Guideline 2010. Thorax. 2010;65 Suppl 2:ii32–40.
3. Qureshi RA, Collinson SL, Powell RJ, Froeschle PO, Berrisford RG. Management of malignant pleural effusion associated with trapped lung syndrome. Asian Cardiovasc Thorac Ann. 2008;16:120–3.
4. Putnam Jr JB, Walsh GL, Swisher SG, Roth JA, Suell DM, Vaporciyan AA, Smythe WR, Merriman KW, DeFord LL. Outpatient management of malignant pleural effusion by a chronic indwelling pleural catheter. Ann Thorac Surg. 2000;69:369–75.

5. Warren WH, Kalimi R, Khodadadian LM, Kim AW. Management of malignant pleural effusions using the Pleur(x) catheter. Ann Thorac Surg. 2008;85:1049–55.
6. Suzuki K, Servais EL, Rizk NP, Solomon SB, Sima CS, Park BJ, Kachala SS, Zlobinsky M, Rusch VW, Adusumilli PS. Palliation and pleurodesis in malignant pleural effusion: the role for tunneled pleural catheters. J Thorac Oncol. 2011;6:762–7.
7. Van Meter ME, McKee KY, Kohlwes RJ. Efficacy and safety of tunneled pleural catheters in adults with malignant pleural effusions: a systematic review. J Gen Intern Med. 2011;26:70–6.
8. Seaton KG, Patz Jr EF, Goodman PC. Palliative treatment of malignant pleural effusions: value of small-bore catheter thoracostomy and doxycycline sclerotherapy. AJR Am J Roentgenol. 1995;164:589–91.
9. Patz Jr EF, McAdams HP, Erasmus JJ, Goodman PC, Culhane DK, Gilkeson RC, Herndon J. Sclerotherapy for malignant pleural effusions: a prospective randomized trial of bleomycin vs doxycycline with small-bore catheter drainage. Chest. 1998;113:1305–11.
10. Clementsen P, Evald T, Grode G, Hansen M, Krag Jacobsen G, Faurschou P. Treatment of malignant pleural effusion: pleurodesis using a small percutaneous catheter. A prospective randomized study. Respir Med. 1998;92:593–6.
11. Parulekar W, Di Primio G, Matzinger F, Dennie C, Bociek G. Use of small-bore vs large-bore chest tubes for treatment of malignant pleural effusions. Chest. 2001;120:19–25.
12. Caglayan B, Torun E, Turan D, Fidan A, Gemici C, Sarac G, Salepci B, Kiral N. Efficacy of iodopovidone pleurodesis and comparison of small-bore catheter versus large-bore chest tube. Ann Surg Oncol. 2008;15:2594–9.
13. Shaw P, Agarwal R. Pleurodesis for malignant pleural effusions. Cochrane Database Syst Rev. 2004:(1):CD002916
14. Tan C, Sedrakyan A, Browne J, Swift S, Treasure T. The evidence on the effectiveness of management for malignant pleural effusion: a systematic review. Eur J Cardiothorac Surg. 2006;29:829–38.
15. Maskell NA, Lee YC, Gleeson FV, Hedley EL, Pengelly G, Davies RJ. Randomized trials describing lung inflammation after pleurodesis with talc of varying particle size. Am J Respir Crit Care Med. 2004;170:377–82.
16. Janssen JP, Collier G, Astoul P, Tassi GF, Noppen M, Rodriguez-Panadero F, Loddenkemper R, Herth FJ, Gasparini S, Marquette CH, Becke B, Froudarakis ME, Driesen P, Bolliger CT, Tschopp JM. Safety of pleurodesis with talc poudrage in malignant pleural effusion: a prospective cohort study. Lancet. 2007;369:1535–9.
17. Yim AP, Chan AT, Lee TW, Wan IY, Ho JK. Thoracoscopic talc insufflation versus talc slurry for symptomatic malignant pleural effusion. Ann Thorac Surg. 1996;62:1655–8.
18. Nuria Manes FR-P, Bravo JL, Hernandez H, Mix A. Talc pleurodesis. Prospective and randomized study clinical follow up. Chest. 2000;118:131S.
19. Dresler CM, Olak J, Herndon II JE, Richards WG, Scalzetti E, Fleishman SB, Kernstine KH, Demmy T, Jablons DM, Kohman L, Daniel TM, Haasler GB, Sugarbaker DJ. Phase III intergroup study of talc poudrage vs talc slurry sclerosis for malignant pleural effusion. Chest. 2005;127:909–15.
20. Stefani A, Natali P, Casali C, Morandi U. Talc poudrage versus talc slurry in the treatment of malignant pleural effusion. A prospective comparative study. Eur J Cardiothorac Surg. 2006;30:827–32.
21. Ohm C, Park D, Vogen M, Bendick P, Welsh R, Pursel S, Chmielewski G. Use of an indwelling pleural catheter compared with thorascopic talc pleurodesis in the management of malignant pleural effusions. Am Surg. 2003;69:198–202.
22. Davies HE, Mishra EK, Kahan BC, Wrightson JM, Stanton AE, Guhan A, Davies CW, Grayez J, Harrison R, Prasad A, Crosthwaite N, Lee YC, Davies RJ, Miller RF, Rahman NM. Effect of an indwelling pleural catheter vs chest tube and talc pleurodesis for relieving dyspnea in patients with malignant pleural effusion: the TIME2 randomized controlled trial. JAMA. 2012;307:2383–9.
23. Demmy TL, Gu L, Burkhalter JE, Toloza EM, D'Amico TA, Sutherland S, Wang X, Archer L, Veit LJ, Kohman L. Optimal management of malignant pleural effusions (results of CALGB 30102). J Natl Compr Canc Netw. 2012;10:975–82.

24. Hunt BM, Farivar AS, Vallieres E, Louie BE, Aye RW, Flores EE, Gorden JA. Thoracoscopic talc versus tunneled pleural catheters for palliation of malignant pleural effusions. Ann Thorac Surg. 2012;94:1053–7; discussion 1057–9.
25. Freeman RK, Ascioti AJ, Mahidhara RS. A propensity-matched comparison of pleurodesis or tunneled pleural catheter in patients undergoing diagnostic thoracoscopy for malignancy. Ann Thorac Surg. 2013;96:259–63; discussion 263–4.
26. Fysh ET, Waterer GW, Kendall PA, Bremner PR, Dina S, Geelhoed E, McCarney K, Morey S, Millward M, Musk AW, Lee YC. Indwelling pleural catheters reduce inpatient days over pleurodesis for malignant pleural effusion. Chest. 2012;142:394–400.
27. Srour N, Amjadi K, Forster A, Aaron S. Management of malignant pleural effusions with indwelling pleural catheters or talc pleurodesis. Can Respir J. 2013;20:106–10.
28. Olden AM, Holloway R. Treatment of malignant pleural effusion: PleuRx catheter or talc pleurodesis? A cost-effectiveness analysis. J Palliative Med. 2010;13:59–65.
29. Puri V, Pyrdeck TL, Crabtree TD, Kreisel D, Krupnick AS, Colditz GA, Patterson GA, Meyers BF. Treatment of malignant pleural effusion: a cost-effectiveness analysis. Ann Thorac Surg. 2012;94:374–9; discussion 379–80.

Chapter 50
Pleurectomy Versus Radical Pleuropneumonectomy for Malignant Pleural Mesothelioma

Shamus R. Carr and Joseph S. Friedberg

Abstract Malignant pleural mesothelioma (MPM) is a rare disease that even with therapy is almost always uniformly fatal. Modern day multimodality therapy combined with surgery has seen success with 5-year survival in a very small, select group of patients. Putting aside the controversy regarding whether surgery should be part of the treatment, there is considerable debate about which operative approach is best. These two approaches are broadly characterized as either lung-sacrificing or lung-sparing. While the available data still does not provide an absolute answer, management of MPM should take place in the setting of a multidisciplinary team with a multimodality approach, and preferably in a clinical trial setting.

Keywords Malignant pleural mesothelioma • Extrapleural pneumonectomy • Surgery • Pleurectomy • Multimodality treatment • Survival

S.R. Carr, MD
Division of Cardiothoracic Surgery, University of Utah and Huntsman Cancer Institute, Salt Lake City, UT, USA

J.S. Friedberg, MD (✉)
Division of Thoracic Surgery, Department of Surgery, University of Pennsylvania, Philadelphia, PA, USA

Department of Surgery, PENN Presbyterian Medical Center, 51 North 39th Street, 250 Wright-Saunders Building, Philadelphia, PA 19104, USA
e-mail: joseph.friedberg@uphs.upenn.edu

M.K. Ferguson (ed.), *Difficult Decisions in Thoracic Surgery*,
Difficult Decisions in Surgery: An Evidence-Based Approach 1,
DOI 10.1007/978-1-4471-6404-3_50, © Springer-Verlag London 2014

Introduction

Malignant pleural mesothelioma (MPM) is a deadly pleural-based tumor, most commonly caused by asbestos. There are approximately 3,000 cases per year in the United States and the incidence seems to have plateaued, although some have suggested that the incidence may be peaking worldwide currently [1]. MPM is still viewed as incurable, with survival typically in the 1-year range from the time of diagnosis.

At this time palliative pemetrexed-based chemotherapy is considered the standard of care for MPM [2]. The role of surgery of surgery remains controversial [3]. That said, few would contest that there appears to be a subset of patients who benefit from surgery-based multimodal treatment beyond what would be expected with chemotherapy alone [4]. Who those patients are and how to select them has not been conclusively established, but otherwise robust patients with epithelial subtype disease, minimal lymph node involvement and, sometimes, lower tumor bulk are characteristics of patients who are often included in surgical series with survivals often reported as significantly longer than what is typically reported in the nonsurgical literature. One thing is clear however: there is no role for surgery alone as a treatment for MPM, which is likely a result of the residual microscopic disease that remains after even the most aggressive operations for pleural cancers. Most experts in the field would agree that if surgery is employed in the treatment plan, the goal of surgery is to achieve a macroscopic complete resection (MCR) and other modalities must be combined with surgery in an effort to control the residual microscopic disease.

There are two approaches to achieving a MCR, lung-sacrificing and lung-sparing. The lung-sacrificing approach, extrapleural pneumonectomy (EPP), enjoys a high degree of standardization. This extends not only to the technique, but to the nomenclature as well. This operation, en bloc resection of the lung, parietal pleura, pericardium and diaphragm, with subsequent diaphragmatic/pericardial prosthetic reconstruction, is executed with a high degree of consistency among surgeons and among centers. If one surgeon tells another that an EPP was performed, it conjures a clear picture of what was done to the patient.

The lung-sparing approaches do not enjoy a fraction of this consistency. This transcends the surgical technique, which can range from a partial debulking that leaves behind gross disease to a radical resection that removes all detectable cancer and all pleural surfaces, both visceral and parietal. This variability extends to nomenclature as well. Different surgeons will employ the same term, such as "pleurectomy" to describe a multitude of procedures, while any of a number of different names may be applied to what was actually the same operation. Some of the terms that have been used to describe lung-sparing procedures include: pleurectomy, parietal pleurectomy, decortication, pleurectomy-decortication, extended pleurectomy decortication, radical pleurectomy decortication, radical pleurectomy and palliative pleurectomy.

A consensus report from the International Mesothelioma Interest Group (IMIG) has recommended more exacting definitions [5], with pleurectomy-decortication (P/D) emerging as the suggested term and extended pleurectomy decortication (EPD) for when the diaphragm and pericardium are resected. The authors find these term confusing as they include the term "decortication," which implies preservation of the visceral pleura and, in the vast majority of the cases, resection of the visceral pleura is required in order to achieve a macroscopic complete resection. The authors, therefore, will use the term "radical pleurectomy" (RP) to describe a lung-sparing operation performed with the intention of achieving a macroscopic complete resection—that is, no visible or palpable disease remaining after resection, but with preservation of the lung. Resection of both the visceral and parietal pleura is implied as well as whatever depth of diaphragm and/or pericardium are resected along with the parietal pleural surface in order to achieve a MCR. It is the authors' practice to label an operation where full thickness diaphragm is resected, for instance, as "radical pleurectomy with diaphragm resection and reconstruction". If the integrity of the diaphragm and pericardium can be preserved, while achieving a MCR, then the procedure would simply be called a "radical pleurectomy".

In addition to pemetrexed-based chemotherapy, which will be included as a component of essentially all surgery-based multimodal treatments, other modalities can be employed as well. These can be intraoperative adjuvants, such as heated chemotherapy [6], heated povidone iodine [7], and photodynamic therapy (PDT) [8] or postoperative, such as external beam hemithoracic radiation [9].

Search Strategy

A Medline search was performed in PubMed using the key words: mesothelioma, pleurectomy, pneumonectomy OR extrapleural pneumonectomy, radical pleurectomy, outcome, and prognostic factor. The search was limited to English language papers from 1999 to 2013. All titles were read by one of the authors (SRC) and were excluded if not relevant. If the decision required it, both authors read the abstract. All papers of interest were obtained from the local institutional library.

Preoperative Evaluation

A definitive diagnosis of mesothelioma must be established. If there is any question about the diagnosis, based upon a surgical biopsy, then a second opinion pathology consultation with known pathologic MPM expertise must be obtained. If there is any question about the diagnosis, as often occurs when it is based on cytology or even a core biopsy, then a surgical biopsy must be performed. This can typically be accomplished through a single 1 cm incision using a 5 mm 30° video thoracoscope and a biopsy forceps introduced through the same hole. It is best to place the incision in line with a future thoracotomy incision as MPM has a propensity to grow out of previous incision sites and if it is in the appropriate location and short in length, the biopsy incision can be easily excised at the time of thoracotomy. If there is no remaining pleural space and the lung is encased in a thick rind of cancer, then the biopsy can usually be performed with a cut down into the interspace. In either case it is important not to enter the lung as a recalcitrant air leak can result. It is also important, if palliation of a recurrent effusion is needed, not to instill talc into the chest cavity if the lung does not fully expand. If there is a trapped lung and the space gets infected in the setting of talc, a permanent foreign body, it might be impossible to clear the resulting empyema. A tunneled catheter is a safer option in the setting of a trapped lung.

The diagnosis should include the subtype. That is, it should be determined whether it is epithelial, sarcomatous or mixed. There are further subtyping categories and analyses, including the percentage of epithelial/sarcomatous in the mixed subtypes, but the distinction of pure epithelial versus non pure epithelial is important as the benefits of surgery are often much less in the subtypes that are not pure epithelial. This subtyping is critical as it allows the surgeon to be candid with the patient when the relative risks and benefits of surgery for MPM are discussed— arguably the largest and most aggressive palliative procedure in medicine. Informed consent for surgery for MPM requires that the patient understands that the role of surgery for this cancer remains investigational.

The remainder of the preoperative evaluation is directed toward making sure that the patient is a safe surgical candidate for the procedure being proposed and that the cancer is confined to one hemithorax and meets whatever other oncologic criteria determine eligibility for surgery in the surgeon's institution. As a general rule, no patient should undergo surgery for MPM without general agreement amongst the members of a multidisciplinary tumor board where the patient's case is presented. Ideally, patients undergoing surgery for MPM do so under the auspices of a clinical trial. Safety is determined using the standard testing and studies that are employed for colossal chest operations and, in the cases of EPP, likely a quantitative ventilation perfusion scan to complement the pulmonary function tests. A CT scan of the chest and upper abdomen is essential. A PET scan is helpful for staging purposes. MRI may be helpful for determining invasion, especially through the diaphragm and/or mediastinum.

Invasive staging is controversial, but likely warranted. Again, surgery for MPM is arguably the most aggressive palliative procedure in the field of medicine so it makes sense to do everything possible to assure that the disease is confined to one hemithorax and, if the institution is following a protocol where positive lymph nodes would serve as an exclusion, then invasive staging of the mediastinal lymph nodes is also warranted. Invasive staging includes laparoscopy, often with biopsy and peritoneal lavage, to rule out radiographically occult peritoneal disease. Similarly, a VATS can be performed in the opposite chest if there is any suspicion of bilateral disease. Lymph nodes can be assessed by mediastinoscopy or endobronchial ultrasound guided biopsies (EBUS).

Surgical Options

Extrapleural Pneumonectomy

Also known as pleuropneumonectomy, EPP entails en bloc resection of mediastinal/ bony hemithoracic parietal pleura, diaphragm, pericardium and lung, with subsequent prosthetic reconstruction of the diaphragm and pericardium. This approach arguably achieves the most complete resection, leaving behind the least amount of microscopic disease. It also allows for adjuvant hemithoracic radiation to treat residual microscopic disease without concern for pulmonary toxicity.

Initially operative mortality was unacceptably high, but with time EPP has been shown to be safely performed in high volume centers with operative mortality under 5 % [10–13]. Despite these improvements, post-operative morbidity remains close to 60 %, with atrial fibrillation being the most common major complication. The obvious disadvantage is that EPP leaves a patient with one lung. This can have a profound impact on quality of life and if/when there is recurrence patients, may not be able to tolerate certain treatment options which can further negatively impact their survival.

Multiple studies have identified variables that negatively impact the survival in patients who undergo EPP. These include: N2 disease, sarcomatoid subtype, advanced age, and single-modality therapy [14, 15].

Lung-Sparing Procedures (Radical Pleurectomy)

While lung-sparing procedures are not standardized, until recently even the nomenclature of the procedures were highly variable. Due to this variation, the IMIG conducted a survey of thoracic surgeons to come to a consensus on the definitions of the procedures performed for MPM [5]. The one point that has come out of lung-sparing procedures is that incomplete resection, regardless of additional adjuncts, has exceptionally poor outcomes [16].

Generally speaking the reported operative mortality for lung-sparing surgery for MPM is lower than for EPP. The foremost disadvantage of these procedures is that there seems to be higher rates of local recurrence. It seems logical to assume that this is a function of a higher burden of residual microscopic disease related to both the additional debrided surface area imposed by the remaining lung as well as the technical challenge of achieving a MCR on the entire lung surface, where the cancer can be superficially invasive into the parenchyma and with less clear margins than on some of the other "smoother" surfaces in the chest cavity. Additionally, it is currently not possible to safely deliver radiation to all surfaces after lung-sparing surgery. This eliminates radiation, likely an effective adjuvant, as a modality for a multimodal treatment protocol.

Potential advantages of lung-sparing surgery include the benefits of having two lungs. After lung-sparing surgery is has been shown that patients have significantly improved pulmonary function (FVC and FEV1) in as little as 2 months after surgery [17]. This likely translates into preservation of quality of life beyond what would be expected after pneumonectomy. At a minimum, having two lungs likely increases treatment options for the patient when the inevitable recurrence occurs. As essentially all patients recur and the vast majority will undergo treatment, it is logical to assume that patients who are candidates for more types of treatments and more aggressive treatments could see a positive impact on their overall survival, attributable to having both lungs. Some of these are the hypotheses proposed in series where lung-sparing surgery seems to have yielded a longer overall survival than EPP [8, 18].

Extrapleural Pneumonectomy vs Radical Pleurectomy

There have been multiple studies that have retrospectively reported results of lung-sparing procedures. In general, reported studies of lung-sparing procedures have median survivals that range from 10 to 30 months. There have only been a few single institution studies that have compared these operations with EPP (Table 50.1) [7, 19–21]. These are, arguably, the best current comparisons between the two procedures as the single greatest variable in surgery, the surgeon, is normalized. Still, the numbers are small and this is far from high quality evidence. There is a retrospective review of 663 patients from 3 institutions that looked at overall survival as the primary end point [11]. The two groups were relatively evenly matched, despite a statistically higher percent of patients with early stage disease in the lung-sparing group. The median survival in months was 16 and 12 for lung-sparing and EPP, respectively. This occurred with a rate of local recurrence in the ipsilateral chest being two times higher in the lung-sparing group compared to the EPP group.

At this time there is no high quality evidence that surgery is beneficial in the treatment of patients with MPM, let alone evidence to declare which operation is optimal. There are multiple issues that make it extremely difficult to study surgery for MPM. MPM is a rare cancer, an orphan disease, making the total number of patients available for study very small. Of that small number of patients with the cancer, only a small fraction, perhaps 10–20 %, undergo surgery. This makes the total denominator for patients undergoing surgery-based treatments extremely small. The very small numbers of patients having surgery are undergoing treatment at multiple centers. Consequently, it is nearly impossible for any center to conduct a trial that would carry the statistical gravitas of a trial for more common cancers like lung or breast. Further diluting the quality of comparison is the fact that mesothelioma has a tendency to behave in a more disparate manner than many other cancers. Epithelial subtype cancers often respond to treatment much differently than nonepithelial cancers. Commonly the subtypes are grouped together, arguably presenting results that are an amalgam of the treatment of two nearly different cancers.

The current staging system is not sufficiently robust to allow for valid comparisons between different centers. Missing from the current staging system are subtype, potentially the greatest prognosticator, and tumor bulk—which is emerging as

Table 50.1 Single institution studies comparing extrapleural pneumonectomy and lung-sparing surgery for malignant pleural mesothelioma

	Nakas et al. [19]	Okada et al. [20]	Lang-Lazdunski et al. [7]	Friedberg et al. [21]
# patients (lung-sparing/pneumonectomy)	165 (67/98)	87 (34/31)	76 (54/22)	28 (14/14)
Percent Stage III or IV disease (lung-sparing/pneumonectomy)	100 %/100 %	53 %/84 %	63 %/86.5 %	86 %/86 %
Percent epithelial subtypes (lung-sparing/pneumonectomy)	78 % for all patients, not listed by operation	85 %/61 %	67 %/64 %	79 %/43 %
Same surgeon for all surgery	Not specified	Not specified	Yes	Yes
Intraoperative adjuvant	None	None	Hyperthermic povidone iodine	Photodynamic therapy
Operative mortality (lung-sparing/pneumonectomy)	3 %/7 %	0 %/3.2 %	0 %/4.5 %	0 %/14 %
Median survival (lung-sparing/pneumonectomy)	13.4/14.7 months (from time of surgery)	17.0/13.0 months (from time of surgery)	23/12.8 months (from time of diagnosis)	Not reached at 25.2 months/8.4 months (from time of surgery)
Local recurrence rate (lung-sparing/pneumonectomy)	44 %/41 %	Not specified	Not specified	43 %/14 %

a possibly important staging variable. In addition, the lymph node classifications for MPM are essentially those of the lung cancer staging system and it is far from clear that this system stratifies for MPM as accurately as it does for NSCLC. Consequently, even attempting to compare different series on a stage by stage basis has potential to approach and "apples to oranges" type of comparison.

As all surgery-based treatments for MPM are multimodal, and those modalities can vary widely between institutions, it can be extremely difficult to ferret out the differences in outcomes attributable to the surgical technique employed. As essentially every patient suffers a recurrence, overall survival will be affected by the treatments for those recurrences. It is difficult, if not impossible, to standardize those post recurrent treatments for this cancer. This presents another significant barrier to assessing the role a particular operation played in a patients overall survival. Lung-sparing procedures and nomenclature is so disparate at this time that it is difficult, if not impossible, to compare results between lung-sparing series or lend true credibility to any meta-analysis type of review. There is even disparity in the time point from which overall survival is reported in surgical series. Often it is reported from the time of surgery, but sometimes it is reported from the time of diagnosis and sometimes from the initiation of a previous treatment. For a cancer where survival or incremental survival is usually reported in months, sometimes weeks, this inconsistency can be confounding and significant.

It is difficult, perhaps impossible, to achieve large enrollment in a randomized trial to definitively establish if surgery is efficacious. This cancer can often exceed a liter in volume and, at this time, there is nothing but surgery that can reliably render a patient with no evidence of disease. Patients are, understandably, reluctant to be randomized to a nonsurgical arm.

Recommendations

There remains no high quality evidence for surgery-based treatments, both with respect to lung-sparing versus lung-sacrificing or even the efficacy of surgery as a treatment. That said, most experts agree that some patients do benefit from surgery. Generally, a patient who is at low risk for surgery and has epithelial subtype disease should at least be presented at a multidisciplinary tumor board and be considered for surgery. Low tumor volume and no evidence of nodal metastases seem to make it more likely that such a patient could benefit from surgery-based treatment. There is no consensus on what operation, lung-sparing versus lung sacrificing, is best. There is general consensus that the role of surgery is to achieve a macroscopic complete resection as part of a multimodal treatment approach, regardless of which operation is performed.

The relative benefits of EPP are that it is a well characterized and standardized operation that likely leaves behind the least amount of residual microscopic disease. The downside, of course, is the effect of pneumonectomy. This not only has potential to limit pulmonary capacity, but likely quality of life and perhaps impose limitations on future treatment options.

The benefits of lung-sparing surgery are those associated with retaining both lungs. This positively impacts not only pulmonary function, but perhaps quality of life and enhancement of future treatment options as well. Most series, even those reported by the same surgeon performing both operations, usually report a lower operative mortality with lung-sparing surgery. It should also be noted that some patients who are candidates for lung-sparing surgery, and wish to pursue aggressive treatment, might not be candidates for pneumonectomy. The negatives associated with lung-sparing surgery include the fact that it almost certainly leaves behind more residual microscopic disease than EPP and that often it is more time consuming and, sometimes more technically challenging, to preserve the lung. In addition, management of postoperative air leaks after lung-sparing surgery, which can be substantial, add another level of complexity to the postoperative management.

A Personal View of the Data

Currently the data does not conclusively support one operation over the other. At this time the recommendation as to which procedure to perform, if any, hinges on institutional expertise and experience. Both procedures have their proponents and detractors and, at this time, it is not clear whether one is better all the time, in certain situations or never. Regardless, it is imperative that all patients be presented at a multidisciplinary tumor board before being offered surgery and subsequently be treated in a multidisciplinary manner. Informed consent for the patients should include recognition that surgery for MPM has not been rigorously established as the standard of care and that the disease is most likely to recur, in effect making the operation palliative. Finally, the complexity of these operations and the postoperative management is such that, if sufficient volume and expertise does not exist within an institution, it is appropriate to refer an MPM patient seeking surgery-based treatment to a center with the appropriate resources.

Surgical therapy alone does not improve survival in MPM compared to best medical therapy. We strongly recommend that treatment of MPM needs to be done by a multidisciplinary team with a multimodality approach.

Recommendations
- Patients who are at low risk for surgery and have epithelial subtype disease should be presented at a multidisciplinary tumor board and be considered for surgery. (Evidence quality low; weak recommendation)
- The current evidence is insufficient to assess whether extrapleural pneumonectomy or radical pleurectomy offers greater advantages to patients.

References

1. Hodgson JT, McElvenny DM, Darnton AJ, Price MJ, Peto J. The expected burden of mesothelioma mortality in Great Britain from 2002 to 2050. Br J Cancer. 2005;92(3):587–93.
2. van Meerbeeck JP, Scherpereel A, Surmont VF, Baas P. Malignant pleural mesothelioma: the standard of care and challenges for future management. Crit Rev Oncol Hematol. 2011;78(2):92–111.
3. Treasure T, Lang-Lazdunski L, Waller D, Bliss JM, Tan C, Entwisle J, et al. Extra-pleural pneumonectomy versus no extra-pleural pneumonectomy for patients with malignant pleural mesothelioma: clinical outcomes of the Mesothelioma and Radical Surgery (MARS) randomised feasibility study. Lancet Oncol. 2011;12(8):763–72.
4. Sugarbaker DJ, Wolf AS. Surgery for malignant pleural mesothelioma. Expert Rev Respir Med. 2010;4(3):363–72.
5. Rice D, Rusch V, Pass H, Asamura H, Nakano T, Edwards J, et al. Recommendations for uniform definitions of surgical techniques for malignant pleural mesothelioma: a consensus report of the international association for the study of lung cancer international staging committee and the international mesothelioma interest group. J Thorac Oncol. 2011;6(8):1304–12.
6. Sugarbaker DJ, Gill RR, Yeap BY, Wolf AS, DaSilva MC, Baldini EH, et al. Hyperthermic intraoperative pleural cisplatin chemotherapy extends interval to recurrence and survival among low-risk patients with malignant pleural mesothelioma undergoing surgical macroscopic complete resection. J Thorac Cardiovasc Surg. 2013;145(4):955–63.
7. Lang-Lazdunski L, Bille A, Lal R, Cane P, McLean E, Landau D, et al. Pleurectomy/decortication is superior to extrapleural pneumonectomy in the multimodality management of patients with malignant pleural mesothelioma. J Thorac Oncol. 2012;7(4):737–43.
8. Friedberg JS, Culligan MJ, Mick R, Stevenson J, Hahn SM, Sterman D, et al. Radical pleurectomy and intraoperative photodynamic therapy for malignant pleural mesothelioma. Ann Thorac Surg. 2012;93(5):1658–67.
9. Rosenzweig KE, Zauderer MG, Laser B, Krug LM, Yorke E, Sima CS, et al. Pleural intensity-modulated radiotherapy for malignant pleural mesothelioma. Int J Radiat Oncol Biol Phys. 2012;83(4):1278–83.
10. Sugarbaker DJ, Jaklitsch MT, Bueno R, Richards W, Lukanich J, Mentzer SJ, et al. Prevention, early detection, and management of complications after 328 consecutive extrapleural pneumonectomies. J Thorac Cardiovasc Surg. 2004;128(1):138–46.
11. Flores RM, Pass HI, Seshan VE, Dycoco J, Zakowski M, Carbone M, et al. Extrapleural pneumonectomy versus pleurectomy/decortication in the surgical management of malignant pleural mesothelioma: results in 663 patients. J Thorac Cardiovasc Surg. 2008;135(3):620–3.
12. Krug LM, Pass HI, Rusch VW, Kindler HL, Sugarbaker DJ, Rosenzweig KE, et al. Multicenter phase II trial of neoadjuvant pemetrexed plus cisplatin followed by extrapleural pneumonectomy and radiation for malignant pleural mesothelioma. J Clin Oncol. 2009;27(18):3007–13.
13. Weder W, Stahel RA, Bernhard J, Bodis S, Vogt P, Ballabeni P, et al. Multicenter trial of neoadjuvant chemotherapy followed by extrapleural pneumonectomy in malignant pleural mesothelioma. Ann Oncol. 2007;18(7):1196–202.
14. Balduyck B, Trousse D, Nakas A, Martin-Ucar AE, Edwards J, Waller DA. Therapeutic surgery for nonepithelioid malignant pleural mesothelioma: is it really worthwhile? Ann Thorac Surg. 2010;89(3):907–11.
15. Sugarbaker DJ, Wolf AS, Chirieac LR, Godleski JJ, Tilleman TR, Jaklitsch MT, et al. Clinical and pathological features of three-year survivors of malignant pleural mesothelioma following extrapleural pneumonectomy. Eur J Cardiothorac Surg. 2011;40(2):298–303.
16. Bölükbas S, Eberlein M, Fisseler-Eckhoff A, Schirren J. Radical pleurectomy and chemoradiation for malignant pleural mesothelioma: the outcome of incomplete resections. Lung Cancer. 2013;81(2):241–6.
17. Bölükbas S, Eberlein M, Schirren J. Prospective study on functional results after lung-sparing radical pleurectomy in the management of malignant pleural mesothelioma. J Thorac Oncol. 2012;7(5):900–5.

18. Baldini EH, Recht A, Strauss GM, DeCamp MM, Swanson SJ, Liptay MJ, et al. Patterns of failure after trimodality therapy for malignant pleural mesothelioma. Ann Thorac Surg. 1997;63(2):334–8.
19. Nakas A, von Meyenfeldt E, Lau K, Muller S, Waller D. Long-term survival after lung-sparing total pleurectomy for locally advanced (International Mesothelioma Interest Group Stage T3-T4) non-sarcomatoid malignant pleural mesothelioma. Eur J Cardiothorac Surg. 2012; 41(5):1031–6.
20. Okada M, Mimura T, Ohbayashi C, Sakuma T, Soejima T, Tsubota N. Radical surgery for malignant pleural mesothelioma: results and prognosis. Interact Cardiovasc Thorac Surg. 2008;7(1):102–6.
21. Friedberg JS, Mick R, Culligan M, Stevenson J, Fernandes A, Smith D, et al. Photodynamic therapy and the evolution of a lung-sparing surgical treatment for mesothelioma. Ann Thorac Surg. 2011;91(6):1738–45.

Chapter 51
Surgical and Medical Therapy for Malignant Pleural Mesothelioma

Christopher Cao

Abstract Malignant pleural mesothelioma is a relatively rare but aggressive form of cancer arising from pleural mesothelial cells. Current medical therapy consists of pemetrexed-based chemoradiotherapy and radiotherapy alone. Additionally, a number of novel biological and immunotherapy agents are being developed. Surgical interventions can be categorized according to technique and intent. Selected patients with adequate cardiopulmonary reserve and resectable disease may achieve long-term survival from extrapleural pneumonectomy or extended pleurectomy/decortication in the context of multi-modality therapy. The present chapter presents the current evidence on medical and surgical management of malignant pleural mesothelioma based on data from systematic reviews.

Keywords Mesothelioma • Extrapleural pneumonectomy • Pleurectomy • Trimodality therapy • Systematic review

Introduction

Malignant pleural mesothelioma (MPM) is a relatively rare but aggressive form of cancer arising from the pleural mesothelial lining with a dismal life expectancy of less than 12 months from the time of diagnosis. The peak incidence of MPM in most developed countries is projected to be between 2010 and 2020 [1, 2]. Currently,

C. Cao, MBBS, BSc (Med)
The Systematic Reviews Unit, The Collaborative Research (CORE) Group,
Macquarie University, Sydney, Australia

The Baird Institute for Applied Heart and Lung Surgical Research,
Sydney, Australia
e-mail: drchriscao@gmail.com

M.K. Ferguson (ed.), *Difficult Decisions in Thoracic Surgery*,
Difficult Decisions in Surgery: An Evidence-Based Approach 1,
DOI 10.1007/978-1-4471-6404-3_51, © Springer-Verlag London 2014

medical management in the form of chemotherapy and radiotherapy is limited in long-term efficacy but usually prescribed as adjuvant treatment in multi-modality regimens. Surgical management of patients with MPM can be broadly categorized according to therapeutic intent. For eligible candidates who are deemed to have resectable disease, surgery with a curative intent can be performed by either extrapleural pneumonectomy (EPP) or extended pleurectomy/decortication (P/D), with the aim of achieving macroscopic complete resection [3]. Less invasive procedures such as partial P/D may be performed to diagnose, prognosticate and provide symptomatic relief for patients not suitable for radical surgery. The present chapter summarizes the existing literature on medical therapy, EPP and P/D, and examines the current staging systems and important prognostic factors for patients who undergo surgery with a curative intent.

Medical Management

Chemotherapy

The standard first-line chemotherapy regimen consists of cisplatin and pemetrexed, as demonstrated by a randomized controlled trial (RCT) that reported superior survival and quality-of-life outcomes compared to cisplatin alone [4, 5]. Disappointingly, the median overall survival for this combination chemotherapy group was only 12.1 months, and an accepted second-line treatment regimen remains elusive [5]. Despite this, the prescription of neoadjuvant or adjuvant systemic chemotherapy has become the standard of care for any surgical procedure with a curative intent [6–8]. Recently, the use of intrapleural normothermic or hyperthermic chemotherapy in the setting of EPP has been reported, with the aim of eradicating microscopic disease after macroscopic complete resection [9–11]. Early results from Phase I and II studies involving hyperthermic cisplatin following extrapleural pneumonectomy have reported limited success, with a median overall survival of 12.8 months and a grade 3–4 morbidity rate of 49 % [10, 11]. However, a retrospective analysis has suggested that hyperthermic intrapleural cisplatin may prolong survival and delay disease recurrence in low-risk patients with epithelial subtype disease [12].

Radiotherapy

Postoperative radiotherapy following surgical resection has been established as an effective option for local control. Patients who undergo EPP can be treated with adjuvant radiotherapy without the risk of pulmonary toxicity to the ipsilateral lung. Compared to traditional 2-D or 3-D conformal techniques, the introduction of intensity modulated radiotherapy (IMRT) has reduced dosimetric heterogeneity and improved target volume conformality [13, 14]. Delivery techniques such as helical tomotherapy may further minimize radiation to the normal critical structures such as the heart, spinal cord, liver, kidneys and oesophagus. A number of studies on trimodality therapy involving systemic chemotherapy, EPP and IMRT have reported encouraging outcomes [15–17]. One retrospective multi-institutional study reported a median overall survival of 46.9 months for patients who underwent EPP and IMRT with a median dose of 52 Gy [18]. Another prospective study on trimodality therapy involving extended P/D, cisplatin/pemetrexed and IMRT reported a median overall survival of 30 months [19]. The emergence of IMRT and techniques such as arc therapy and helical tomotherapy are likely to replace traditional conformal methods in the treatment of MPM.

Future Directions

A number of novel treatments are being explored in Phase I and II trials, including biological and immunotherapy agents such as anti-mesothelin monoclonal antibodies [20]. The use of recombinant immunotoxins, vaccines and genetically engineered T-cells are the focus of additional studies [21]. Other targeted areas include the vascular endothelial growth factor (VEGF) and hepatocyte growth factor/c-Met pathways [5]. Combination treatment consisting of chemotherapy and the anti-VEGF antibody bevacizumab are currently underway in Phase II studies [22].

Surgical Management

Extrapleural Pneumonectomy

Extrapleural pneumonectomy involves the *en bloc* resection of the ipsilateral parietal and visceral pleurae, lung, hemidiaphragm, and pericardium. The significant morbidity and mortality associated with EPP, as well as the essential need for adjuvant therapy, was recognized by Butchart, who reported the first series of EPP in the treatment of MPM in 1976 [23]. Since then, developments in patient selection criteria, surgical technique and perioperative care have significantly improved the short- and long-term outcomes of EPP to establish this procedure as a viable option for selected patients with resectable disease. The following section presents the patient selection process, existing data on surgical outcomes and important prognostic factors for patients who undergo EPP.

Search strategy: Extrapleural Pneumonectomy

A systematic review using Ovid Medline, EMBASE, Cochrane Central Register of Controlled Trials, Cochrane Database of Systematic Reviews, and Database of Abstracts of Review of Effectiveness from January 1985 to January 2010 was performed by combining 'mesothelioma' and 'pneumonectomy' as either MeSH terms or keywords. Limitations included English language and human subjects with histologically proven MPM. After excluding irrelevant and duplicated articles, 58 studies were identified, including 3,749 patients who underwent EPP. Of these, 2,462 patients from 26 institutions were included for final analysis [24]. Studies differed in regards to adjuvant therapies, which included systemic or intrathoracic chemotherapy, radiotherapy and photodynamic therapy.

Results for EPP

Median overall survival ranged from 9.4 to 27.5 months, with the middle quartiles ranging from 12 to 20 months. Perioperative mortality ranged from 0 to 11.8 %, with the middle quartiles ranging from 3.7 to 7.6 %. Overall morbidity rates ranged from 22 to 82 %, with major morbidity being reported as 12.5–48 %. Three quality-of-life studies identified improvements in most domains at 3 months after surgery compared to baseline, but deterioration was reported after 12–24 months [25–27].

Trimodality Therapy

Search strategy: Trimodality Therapy

Currently, EPP is almost always performed as part of a multi-modality therapy. To focus on this approach, a more recent systematic review on trimodality therapy involving neoadjuvant or adjuvant chemotherapy, EPP and adjuvant radiotherapy was conducted using five databases from January 1985 to October 2012. Sixteen studies involving 744 patients who underwent EPP were identified, including eight studies on neoadjuvant chemotherapy and eight studies on adjuvant chemotherapy.

Results for Trimodality Therapy

The most robust clinical evidence can be derived from four prospective studies with a standardized neoadjuvant treatment regimen, as summarized in Table 51.1 [25, 28–30]. This series of studies reported a median overall survival of 16.8–25.5 months on intention-to-treat analysis. In contrast, a small feasibility-testing RCT comparing EPP to conservative medical management reported dismal results with a median overall survival of 14.4 months for patients who were randomized to EPP [31]. The primary objective of this RCT was to assess the feasibility of conducting a larger trial to compare EPP with medical therapy, which it concluded was not possible after recruiting only 50 patients for randomization after 3 years. However, the authors of the study retrospectively analysed their data and concluded that EPP within trimodality therapy offered no benefit and possibly harmed patients. These

Table 51.1 Summary of prospective studies on trimodality therapy involving neoadjuvant chemotherapy, extrapleural pneumonectomy and adjuvant radiotherapy for patients with malignant pleural mesothelioma

Author		Primary treatment centre	Patients undergone treatment (% ITT)			Perioperative mortality (%)	Median overall survival (months)		
			NC	EPP	Radiotherapy				
Treasure [31]	RCT	12 UK Hospitals	24 (100 %)	19 (79 %)	8 (33 %)	12.5	14.4[DR]		
van Schil [28]	OS	11 European Hospitals	58 (100 %)	42 (72 %)	38 (66 %)	6.5	ITT: 18.4[RE]	NC + EPP: NR	TMT: 33
Krug [29]	OS	Memorial Sloan-Kettering Cancer Center, NY, USA	77 (100 %)	57 (74 %)	44 (57 %)	3.7	ITT: 16.8[CC]	NC+EPP: 21.9	TMT: 29.1
Rea [30]	OS	Istituto Oncologico Veneto, Padua, Italy	21 (100 %)	17 (81 %)	15 (71 %)	0	ITT: 25.5[CC]	NC + EPP: 27.5	TMT: NR
Weder [25]	OS	University Hospital, Zurich, Switzerland	61 (100 %)	45 (74 %)	36 (59 %)	2.2	ITT: 19.8[CC]	NC + EPP: 23	TMT: NR

ITT intention-to-treat, *NC* neoadjuvant chemotherapy, *Adj* adjuvant, *NR* not reported, *TMT* trimodality therapy, *OS* observational study, *RCT* randomized controlled trial, *DR* date of randomization, *RE* date of registration, *CC* date of chemotherapy, *EPP* extrapleural pneumonectomy

claims have since been refuted by members of the surgical thoracic community who pointed out a number of protocol violations between the treatment arms and the non-standardized adjuvant therapy administered to patients [32, 33]. Indeed, with a mortality rate of 18 % for the 17 patients who underwent EPP per study protocol, the Mesothelioma and Radical Surgery (MARS) trial reported one of the highest mortality rates for EPP in the literature [8, 31].

Patient Selection and Prognostic Factors for EPP

To avoid futile aggressive surgery in inappropriate candidates, a range of preoperative investigations are performed for selected eligible patients with adequate cardiopulmonary reserve and resectable disease. High resolution computed tomography (CT) of the chest and upper abdomen remains to be the primary imaging investigation to assess the extent of locoregional disease. Magnetic resonance imaging (MRI) and positron emission tomography (PET) may provide further information on local invasion and distant metastatic disease, respectively, but are not routinely performed for all patients [6, 34]. The standardized uptake value (SUV) from PET scanning has been demonstrated to be predictive for overall survival [35]. Procedural investigations such as mediastinoscopy and laparoscopy are routinely performed in some centres to assess potential mediastinal nodal and peritoneal involvement, which may not be evident on imaging alone [36, 37]. Identification of N2 disease presents an absolute contraindication for EPP in some institutions due to its recognized poor prognosis, but it has been recognized that the pattern of nodal spread differs between MPM and NSCLC, and not all N2 disease can be identified through mediastinoscopy [38, 39]. Institutions that have performed routine mediastinoscopies, bilateral thoracoscopies and laparoscopies prior to EPP have failed to demonstrated superior survival outcomes [40]. Finally, assessment of cardiopulmonary function may include pulmonary function tests, ventilation/perfusion scanning and cardiac stress testing [6].

A number of pathological, clinical and treatment-related factors have been systematically identified as important prognostic factors for patients who undergo EPP for MPM [34]. Patients with sarcomatoid subtype and N2 nodal involvement have long been recognized to have a significantly poorer prognosis, and they are contraindicated for surgery in some institutions [16, 37, 38]. Younger age and female gender may confer some survival benefit, but this finding was not consistent in the current literature [41, 42]. For patients who undergo trimodality therapy, completeness of resection and ability to complete adjuvant therapy have been demonstrated to improve overall survival [43, 44]. Serological markers such as high haemoglobin, low white cell and low platelet counts have also been associated with improved survival outcomes [34, 45].

In conclusion, existing literature demonstrates that EPP in a multi-modality treatment setting is a viable option for selected patients deemed to have sufficient cardiopulmonary reserve and resectable disease. Prospective studies conducted in specialized centres with a standardized regimen involving neoadjuvant chemotherapy,

EPP and adjuvant radiotherapy have demonstrated median overall survival outcomes of 16.8–25.5 months on intention-to-treat analysis with an acceptable mortality rate of less than 6.5 %. However, poor outcomes for EPP within a small feasibility-testing RCT have raised doubt about this procedure within the thoracic oncology community. Due to the relative rarity of MPM and the immense logistical difficulties in conducting a multi-institutional RCT, future evidence for EPP will likely be confined to non-randomized case-series studies. Improvements in the oncological outcomes of these patients may largely be dependent on the development of more effective adjuvant therapeutic agents.

Pleurectomy/Decortication

Although pleurectomy/decortication has been described as a treatment option for patients with MPM since 1975, significant variations existed in regards to surgical technique and therapeutic intent [46]. Radical procedures with a curative intent aim to achieve macroscopic complete resection, with resection and reconstruction of the pericardium and diaphragm as required. On the other hand, less invasive procedures aim to obtain sufficient tissue to confirm diagnosis and achieve symptomatic relief from recurrent pleural effusions. Direct comparisons between these two ends of the P/D spectrum were previously impossible due to conflicting nomenclature. To unify the definition of P/D-related procedures, the International Association for the Study of Lung Cancer (IASLC) and the International Mesothelioma Interest Group (IMIG) classified P/D into partial P/D, P/D and extended P/D according to surgical technique [47]:

1. Extended P/D: parietal and visceral pleurectomy to remove all gross tumour with resection of the diaphragm and/or pericardium as required.
2. P/D: parietal and visceral pleurectomy to remove all gross tumour without resection of the diaphragm or pericardium.
3. Partial pleurectomy: partial removal of parietal and/or visceral pleura for diagnostic or palliative purposes but leaving gross tumour behind.

Based on these standardized definitions, a systematic review was carried out to classify previous studies and assess their perioperative and long-term outcomes.

Search Strategy for P/D

A systematic review was conducted using Ovid Medline, Cochrane Central Register of Controlled Trials (CCTR), Cochrane Database of Systematic Reviews (CDSR), ACP Journal Club, and Database of Abstracts of Review of Effectiveness (DARE) from January 1985 to November 2012. To maximize search sensitivity, 'pleurectomy' or 'decortication' with 'mesothelioma' we used as either keywords or MeSH terms. Limitations included English language and human patients with histologically proven MPM. This search strategy resulted in 181 potentially relevant articles.

After excluding irrelevant and duplicated reports, 34 updated studies including 1,935 patients were identified. These included 12 studies on extended P/D, 8 studies on P/D and 14 studies on partial P/D [48].

Perioperative Outcomes

From the selected studies in the systematic review, perioperative mortality ranged from 0 to 11 % for extended P/D, 0–7.1 % for P/D and 0–7.8 % for partial P/D. Overall morbidity ranged from 20 to 43 % for extended P/D, 13–48 % for P/D and 14–20 % for partial P/D. Average length of hospitalization ranged from 7 to 15 days for extended P/D, 7–14 days for P/D and 6–11 days for partial P/D. Overall, there appeared to be a trend favoring lower mortality and morbidity rates for partial P/D versus extended P/D. A summary of these findings is presented in Table 51.2 [9, 19, 49–80].

Long-Term Outcomes

Median overall survival ranged from 11.5 to 31.7 months for extended P/D, 8.3–26 months for P/D and 7.1–14 months for partial P/D. When only the middle quartiles were assessed, median overall survival ranged from 15 to 25 months, 12–18 months and 9–13 months for extended P/D, P/D and partial P/D, respectively, with a trend favoring extended P/D.

Whilst acknowledging variations in patient selection, adjuvant therapy and surgical techniques for individual patients, this systematic review demonstrated that extended P/D for patients with resectable MPM may achieve longer overall and disease-free survival outcomes compared to less invasive partial P/D procedures at the cost of higher perioperative mortality and morbidity. Overall, the vast majority of all reported P/D procedures were performed with less than 10 % perioperative mortality and 50 % morbidity.

Summary and Recommendations

Pemetrexed and cisplatin should be the first-line chemotherapy regimen for patients with MPM, but the survival benefit remains limited with medical therapy alone (evidence quality moderate; strong recommendation). For patients who undergo surgical procedures with a curative intent such as extrapleural pneumonectomy and extended pleurectomy/decortication, adjuvant therapy should be given in the form of chemotherapy and/or radiotherapy (evidence quality moderate; strong recommendation). Eligible surgical candidates with adequate cardiopulmonary reserve and resectable MPM disease benefit from trimodality therapy involving extrapleural pneumonectomy or extended pleurectomy/decortication in combination with chemotherapy and radiotherapy (evidence quality moderate; weak recommendation).

Table 51.2 Summary of perioperative and long-term outcomes for patients who underwent pleurectomy procedures in the treatment of malignant pleural mesothelioma

	Study	Perioperative mortality	Peri-operative morbidity		Length of stay (days)	Median overall survival[a]	Disease free survival[a]
			Overall	Major			
Extended pleurectomy/decortication	Lang-Lazdunski et al. [49]	0 %	27.7 %	NR	NR	23	NR
	Friedberg [50]	2.6 %	26 events	NR	NR	31.7	9.6
	Rosenzweig et al. [51]	NR	NR	NR	NR	26	NR
	Nakas et al. [52]	3 %	43 %	NR	15.3^MV	13.4	16
	Rena and Casadio [53]	0 %	NR	24 %	7	25	11
	Bolukbas et al. [19]	2.9 %	20 %	7 events	NR	30	15.8
	Flores et al. [54]	4.7 %	49 events	NR	NR	16	NR
	Okada et al. [55]	0 %	NR	15 %	NR	17	NR
	Richards et al. [56]	11 %	NR	25 %	11	13	7.2
	Lee et al. [57]	7 %	NR	4 events	9	18.1	12.2
	Rusch and Venkatraman [58]	3.4 %	NR	NR	NR	18.5	NR
	Colleoni et al. [59]	0 %	32 events	NR	NR	11.5	NR
Pleurectomy/decortication	Luckraz [60] PD only	1.1 %	18 %	NR	8	8.3	NR
	PD + ChT		15 %		9	11.9	
	PD + RT		16 %		8	10.4	
	PD + ChT + RT		13 %		8	26	
	Lucchi et al. [61]	NR	NR	NR	NR	21	NR
	Nakas et al. [62]	7.1 %	48 %	NR	14.3	14^MV	NR
	Colaut et al. [63]	NR	2 events	NR	NR	13	6
	Lampl and Jakop [64]	0 %	NR	NR	NR	14	NR
	Pass et al. [65]	NR	NR	2 events	NR	14.5	7.4
	Soysal et al. [66]	1 %	22 %	NR	NR	17	NR
	Lee et al. [67]	0 %	NR	13 %	6.5^MV	11.5	NR

(continued)

Table 51.2 (continued)

Study	Perioperative mortality	Peri-operative morbidity		Length of stay (days)	Median overall survival[a]	Disease free survival[a]
		Overall	Major			
Partial pleurectomy						
Yan et al. [68]	NR	NR	NR	NR	9	NR
Mineo et al. [69]	0 %	14 %	NR	NR	10	NR
Schipper et al. [70]	2.9 %	≥10 events	5.9 %	6.5	8.1	NR
Neragi-Miandoab et al. [71]	3.1 %	52 events	19 events	10.8^{MV}	9.4	NR
Halstead et al. [72]	2 %	NR	NR	8	13.7	NR
de Vries and Long [73]	3.8 %	NR	9 events	9	9	NR
Phillips et al. [74]	6.7 %	20 %	NR	NR	14	NR
Aziz et al. [9]	0 %	NR	2 events	NR	14	NR
Martin-Ucar et al. [75]	7.8 %	7 events	NR	7	7.1	NR
Ceresoli et al. [76]	NR	NR	NR	NR	13	NR
Hasturk et al. [77]	NR	NR	NR	NR	12	NR
Sauter et al. [78]	5 %	NR	NR	8	12	10
Allen et al. [79]	5.4 %	NR	26.8 %	NR	9	NR
Ruffie et al. [80]	NR	NR	NR	NR	9.8	NR

PD pleurectomy/decortication, *ChT* chemotherapy, *RT* radiotherapy, *MV* mean value, *NR* not reported

[a]Measured in months

A Personal View of the Data

The fact that combination therapy involving pemetrexed and cisplatin remains to be the universally accepted first-line chemotherapy over the past decade despite providing only modest improvement in overall survival summarizes the limited advances in medical therapy. However, a myriad of novel biological and immunotherapeutic agents, as well as the development of innovative radiotherapy techniques provide hope for medical management of MPM. Regarding surgery, EPP in the setting of multi-modality treatment has previously been demonstrated to be a viable option for selected patients with resectable disease. However, conflicting results from several prospective studies and a small RCT assessing trimodality therapy involving neoadjuvant chemotherapy, EPP and adjuvant radiotherapy have created significant controversy and disagreement within the thoracic oncology community. The literature does consistently provide evidence to suggest certain clinico-pathological factors such as N2 nodal disease and non-epithelial subtype have a significantly worse outcome, and these patients may not derive significant gains from radical surgery. Finally, comparative data on P/D procedures have previously been difficult to analyse due to inconsistent surgical techniques and nomenclature. Using the updated definition of P/D according to IASLC and IMIG, current evidence suggests that extended P/D in patients with resectable disease may achieve longer survival outcomes at the cost of higher perioperative morbidity and mortality compared to partial P/D. Any direct comparisons between EPP and extended P/D must acknowledge that these two surgical procedures, although sharing a curative intent, may not be interchangeable for individual patients.

Recommendations

- Pemetrexed and cisplatin should be the first-line chemotherapy regimen for patients with MPM, but the survival benefit remains limited with medical therapy alone (evidence quality moderate; strong recommendation).
- For patients who undergo surgical procedures with a curative intent such as extrapleural pneumonectomy and extended pleurectomy/decortication, adjuvant therapy should be given in the form of chemotherapy and/or radiotherapy (evidence quality moderate; strong recommendation).
- Eligible surgical candidates with adequate cardiopulmonary reserve and resectable MPM disease benefit from trimodality therapy involving extrapleural pneumonectomy or extended pleurectomy/decortication in combination with chemotherapy and radiotherapy (evidence quality moderate; weak recommendation).

References

1. Frost G. The latency period of mesothelioma among a cohort of British asbestos workers (1978–2005). Br J Cancer. 2013;109(7):1965–73. PubMed PMID: 23989951. Epub 2013/08/31. Eng.
2. Robinson BM. Malignant pleural mesothelioma: an epidemiological perspective. Ann Cardiothorac Surg. 2012;1(4):491–6. PubMed PMID: 23977542. Pubmed Central PMCID: 3741803. Epub 2013/08/27. eng.
3. Sugarbaker DJ. Macroscopic complete resection: the goal of primary surgery in multimodality therapy for pleural mesothelioma. J Thorac Oncol. 2006;1(2):175–6. PubMed PMID: 2007371537. English.
4. Vogelzang NJ, Rusthoven JJ, Symanowski J, Denham C, Kaukel E, Ruffie P, et al. Phase III study of pemetrexed in combination with cisplatin versus cisplatin alone in patients with malignant pleural mesothelioma. J Clin Oncol. 2003;21(14):2636–44. PubMed PMID: 12860938. Epub 2003/07/16. eng.
5. Nowak AK. Chemotherapy for malignant pleural mesothelioma: a review of current management and a look to the future. Ann Cardiothorac Surg. 2012;1(4):508–15.
6. Rusch VW. Extrapleural pneumonectomy and extended pleurectomy/decortication for malignant pleural mesothelioma: the Memorial Sloan-Kettering Cancer Center approach. Ann Cardiothorac Surg. 2012;1(4):523–31. PubMed PMID: 23977547. Pubmed Central PMCID: 3741802. Epub 2013/08/27. eng.
7. Sugarbaker DJ, Garcia JP. Multimodality therapy for malignant pleural mesothelioma. Chest. 1997;112(4 Suppl):272S–5S. PubMed PMID: 9337303. English.
8. Cao C, Tian D, Manganas C, Matthews P, Yan TD. Systematic review of trimodality therapy for patients with malignant pleural mesothelioma. Ann Cardiothorac Surg. 2012;1(4):428–37. PubMed PMID: 23977533. Pubmed Central PMCID: 3741794. Epub 2013/08/27. eng.
9. Aziz T, Jilaihawi A, Prakash D. The management of malignant pleural mesothelioma; single centre experience in 10 years. Eur J Cardiothorac Surg. 2002;22(2):298–305. PubMed PMID: 12142203. English.
10. Tilleman TR, Richards WG, Zellos L, Johnson BE, Jaklitsch MT, Mueller J, et al. Extrapleural pneumonectomy followed by intracavitary intraoperative hyperthermic cisplatin with pharmacologic cytoprotection for treatment of malignant pleural mesothelioma: a phase II prospective study. J Thorac Cardiovasc Surg. 2009;138(2):405–11. PubMed PMID: 2009377141. English.
11. Zellos L, Richards WG, Capalbo L, Jaklitsch MT, Chirieac LR, Johnson BE, et al. A phase I study of extrapleural pneumonectomy and intracavitary intraoperative hyperthermic cisplatin with amifostine cytoprotection for malignant pleural mesothelioma. J Thorac Cardiovasc Surg. 2009;137(2):453–8. PubMed PMID: 2009042395. English.
12. Sugarbaker DJ, Gill RR, Yeap BY, Wolf AS, DaSilva MC, Baldini EH, et al. Hyperthermic intraoperative pleural cisplatin chemotherapy extends interval to recurrence and survival among low-risk patients with malignant pleural mesothelioma undergoing surgical macroscopic complete resection. J Thorac Cardiovasc Surg. 2013;145(4):955–63. PubMed PMID: 23434448. Epub 2013/02/26. eng.
13. Chi A, Liao Z, Nguyen NP, Howe C, Gomez D, Jang SY, et al. Intensity-modulated radiotherapy after extrapleural pneumonectomy in the combined-modality treatment of malignant pleural mesothelioma. J Thorac Oncol. 2011;6(6):1132–41. PubMed PMID: 21532502.
14. Rimner A, Rosenzweig KE. Novel radiation therapy approaches in malignant pleural mesothelioma. Ann Cardiothorac Surg. 2012;1(4):457–61. PubMed PMID: 23977536. Pubmed Central PMCID: 3741784. Epub 2013/08/27. eng.
15. Buduhan G, Menon S, Aye R, Louie B, Mehta V, Vallieres E. Trimodality therapy for malignant pleural mesothelioma. Ann Thorac Surg. 2009;88(3):870–6. PubMed PMID: 2009435227. English.
16. De Perrot M, Feld R, Cho BCJ, Bezjak A, Anraku M, Burkes R, et al. Trimodality therapy with induction chemotherapy followed by extrapleural pneumonectomy and adjuvant high-dose hemithoracic radiation for malignant pleural mesothelioma. J Clin Oncol. 2009;27(9):1413–8. PubMed PMID: 2009172492. English.

17. Patel A, Anraku M, Darling GE, Shepherd FA, Pierre AF, Waddell TK, et al. Venous thrombo-embolism in patients receiving multimodality therapy for thoracic malignancies. J Thorac Cardiovasc Surg. 2009;138(4):843–8. PubMed PMID: 2009492933. English.

18. Tonoli S, Vitali P, Scotti V, Bertoni F, Spiazzi L, Ghedi B, et al. Adjuvant radiotherapy after extrapleural pneumonectomy for mesothelioma. Prospective analysis of a multi-institutional series. Radiother Oncol. 2011;101(2):311–5. PubMed PMID: 22079529.

19. Bolukbas S, Manegold C, Eberlein M, Bergmann T, Fisseler-Eckhoff A, Schirren J. Survival after trimodality therapy for malignant pleural mesothelioma: radical pleurectomy, chemo-therapy with cisplatin/pemetrexed and radiotherapy. Lung Cancer. 2011;71(1):75–81. PubMed PMID: 19765853.

20. Hassan R, Cohen SJ, Phillips M, Pastan I, Sharon E, Kelly RJ, et al. Phase I clinical trial of the chimeric anti-mesothelin monoclonal antibody MORAb-009 in patients with mesothelin-expressing cancers. Clin Cancer Res. 2010;16(24):6132–8. PubMed PMID: 21037025. Pubmed Central PMCID: 3057907. Epub 2010/11/03. eng.

21. Villena-Vargas J, Adusumilli PS. Mesothelin-targeted immunotherapies for malignant pleural mesothelioma. Ann Cardiothorac Surg. 2012;1(4):466–71. PubMed PMID: 23977538. Pubmed Central PMCID: 3741795. Epub 2013/08/27. eng.

22. Ceresoli GL, Zucali PA, Mencoboni M, Botta M, Grossi F, Cortinovis D, et al. Phase II study of pemetrexed and carboplatin plus bevacizumab as first-line therapy in malignant pleural mesothelioma. Br J Cancer. 2013;109(3):552–8. PubMed PMID: 23860535. Pubmed Central PMCID: 3738125. Epub 2013/07/19. eng.

23. Butchart EG, Ashcroft T, Barnsley WC, Holden MP. Pleuropneumonectomy in the manage-ment of diffuse malignant mesothelioma of the pleura. Experience with 29 patients. Thorax. 1976;31(1):15–24.

24. Cao CQ, Yan TD, Bannon PG, McCaughan BC. A systematic review of extrapleural pneumo-nectomy for malignant pleural mesothelioma. J Thorac Oncol. 2010;5(10):1692–703.

25. Weder W, Stahel RA, Bernhard J, Bodis S, Vogt P, Ballabeni P, et al. Multicenter trial of neo-adjuvant chemotherapy followed by extrapleural pneumonectomy in malignant pleural meso-thelioma. Ann Oncol. 2007;18(7):1196–202. PubMed PMID: 2007396867. English.

26. Ambrogi V, Mineo D, Gatti A, Pompeo E, Mineo TC. Symptomatic and quality of life changes after extrapleural pneumonectomy for malignant pleural mesothelioma. J Surg Oncol. 2009;100(3):199–204. PubMed PMID: 2009499816. English.

27. Ribi K, Bernhard J, Schuller JC, Weder W, Bodis S, Jorger M, et al. Individual versus standard quality of life assessment in a phase II clinical trial in mesothelioma patients: feasibility and responsiveness to clinical changes. Lung Cancer. 2008;61(3):398–404. PubMed PMID: 2008420128. English.

28. Van Schil PE, Baas P, Gaafar R, Maat AP, Van de Pol M, Hasan B, et al. Trimodality therapy for malignant pleural mesothelioma: results from an EORTC phase II multicentre trial. Eur Respir J. 2010;36(6):1362–9. PubMed PMID: 20525721.

29. Krug LM, Pass HI, Rusch VW, Kindler HL, Sugarbaker DJ, Rosenzweig KE, et al. Multicenter phase II trial of neoadjuvant pemetrexed plus cisplatin followed by extrapleural pneumonec-tomy and radiation for malignant pleural mesothelioma. J Clin Oncol. 2009;27(18):3007–13. PubMed PMID: 19364962.

30. Rea F, Marulli G, Bortolotti L, Breda C, Favaretto AG, Loreggian L, et al. Induction chemo-therapy, extrapleural pneumonectomy (EPP) and adjuvant hemi-thoracic radiation in malig-nant pleural mesothelioma (MPM): feasibility and results. Lung Cancer. 2007;57(1):89–95. PubMed PMID: 2007266014. English.

31. Treasure T, Lang-Lazdunski L, Waller D, Bliss JM, Tan C, Entwisle J, et al. Extra-pleural pneumonectomy versus no extra-pleural pneumonectomy for patients with malignant pleural mesothelioma: clinical outcomes of the Mesothelioma and Radical Surgery (MARS) ran-domised feasibility study. Lancet Oncol. 2011;12(8):763–72. PubMed PMID: 21723781.

32. Weder W, Stahel RA, Baas P, Dafni U, de Perrot M, McCaughan BC, et al. The MARS feasi-bility trial: conclusions not supported by data. Lancet Oncol. 2011;12(12):1093–4; author reply 4–5. PubMed PMID: 22041539.

33. Rusch VW. The Mars trial: resolution of the surgical controversies in mesothelioma? J Thorac Oncol. 2009;4(10):1189–91. PubMed PMID: 20197731.

34. Cao C, Yan TD, Bannon PG, McCaughan BC. Summary of prognostic factors and patient selection for extrapleural pneumonectomy in the treatment of malignant pleural mesothelioma. Ann Surg Oncol. 2011;18(10):2973–9. PubMed PMID: 21512863.

35. Flores RM, Akhurst T, Gonen M, Zakowski M, Dycoco J, Larson SM, et al. Positron emission tomography predicts survival in malignant pleural mesothelioma. J Thorac Cardiovasc Surg. 2006;132(4):763–8. PubMed PMID: 17000285. Epub 2006/09/27. eng.

36. Edwards JG, Stewart DJ, Martin-Ucar A, Muller S, Richards C, Waller DA. The pattern of lymph node involvement influences outcome after extrapleural pneumonectomy for malignant mesothelioma. J Thorac Cardiovasc Surg. 2006;131(5):981–7. PubMed PMID: 2006205757. English.

37. Rice DC, Steliga MA, Stewart J, Eapen G, Jimenez CA, Lee JH, et al. Endoscopic ultrasound-guided fine needle aspiration for staging of malignant pleural mesothelioma. Ann Thorac Surg. 2009;88(3):862–8. PubMed PMID: 19699913. English.

38. Edwards JG, Martin-Ucar AE, Stewart DJ, Waller DA. Right extrapleural pneumonectomy for malignant mesothelioma via median sternotomy or thoracotomy? Short- and long-term results. Eur J Cardiothorac Surg. 2007;31(5):759–64. PubMed PMID: 2007165454. English.

39. Yan TD, Boyer M, Tin MM, Sim J, Kennedy C, McLean J, et al. Prognostic features of long-term survivors after surgical management of malignant pleural mesothelioma. Ann Thorac Surg. 2009;87(5):1552–6. PubMed PMID: 2009184697. English.

40. Alvarez JM, Ha T, Musk W, Robins P, Price R, Byrne MJ. Importance of mediastinoscopy, bilateral thoracoscopy, and laparoscopy in correct staging of malignant mesothelioma before extrapleural pneumonectomy. J Thorac Cardiovasc Surg. 2005;130(3):905–6. PubMed PMID: 2005406177. English.

41. Trousse DS, Avaro JP, D'Journo XB, Doddoli C, Astoul P, Giudicelli R, et al. Is malignant pleural mesothelioma a surgical disease? A review of 83 consecutive extra-pleural pneumo-nectomies. Eur J Cardiothorac Surg. 2009;36(4):759–63. PubMed PMID: 2009472386. English.

42. Pass HI, Temeck BK, Kranda K, Steinberg SM, Feuerstein IR. Preoperative tumor volume is associated with outcome in malignant pleural mesothelioma. J Thorac Cardiovasc Surg. 1998;115(2):310–7. PubMed PMID: 9475525. English.

43. Sugarbaker DJ, Flores RM, Jaklitsch MT, Richards WG, Strauss GM, Corson JM, et al. Resection margins, extrapleural nodal status, and cell type determine postoperative long-term survival in trimodality therapy of malignant pleural mesothelioma: results in 183 patients. J Thorac Cardiovasc Surg. 1999;117(1):54–63. PubMed PMID: 9869758. English.

44. Yan TD, Boyer M, Tin MM, Wong D, Kennedy C, McLean J, et al. Extrapleural pneumonectomy for malignant pleural mesothelioma: outcomes of treatment and prognostic factors. J Thorac Cardiovasc Surg. 2009;138(3):619–24. PubMed PMID: 2009431646. English.

45. Wolf AS, Richards WG, Tilleman TR, Chirieac L, Hurwitz S, Bueno R, et al. Characteristics of malignant pleural mesothelioma in women. Ann of Thorac Surg. 2010;90(3):949–56. PubMed PMID: 2010470411. English.

46. Martini N, Bains MS, Beattie Jr EJ. Indications for pleurectomy in malignant effusion. Cancer. 1975;35(3):734–8. PubMed PMID: 1111941.

47. Rice D, Rusch V, Pass H, Asamura H, Nakano T, Edwards J, et al. Recommendations for uniform definitions of surgical techniques for malignant pleural mesothelioma: a consensus report of the international association for the study of lung cancer international staging committee and the international mesothelioma interest group. J Thorac Oncol. 2011;6(8):1304–12. PubMed PMID: 21847060.

48. Cao C, Tian DH, Pataky KA, Yan TD. Systematic review of pleurectomy in the treatment of malignant pleural mesothelioma. Lung Cancer. 2013;81(3):319–27. PubMed PMID: 23769317. Epub 2013/06/19. eng.

49. Lang-Lazdunski L, Bille A, Lal R, Cane P, McLean E, Landau D, et al. Pleurectomy/decortication is superior to extrapleural pneumonectomy in the multimodality management of patients

with malignant pleural mesothelioma. J Thorac Oncol. 2012;7(4):737–43. PubMed PMID: 22425923.

50. Friedberg JS. Radical pleurectomy and photodynamic therapy for malignant pleural mesothelioma. Ann Cardiothorac Surg. 2012;1(4):472–80. PubMed PMID: 23977539. Pubmed Central PMCID: 3741797. Epub 2013/08/27. eng.

51. Rosenzweig KE, Zauderer MG, Laser B, Krug LM, Yorke E, Sima CS, et al. Pleural intensity-modulated radiotherapy for malignant pleural mesothelioma. Int J Radiat Oncol Biol Phys. 2012;83(4):1278–83. PubMed PMID: 22607910.

52. Nakas A, von Meyenfeldt E, Lau K, Muller S, Waller D. Long-term survival after lung-sparing total pleurectomy for locally advanced (International Mesothelioma Interest Group Stage T3-T4) non-sarcomatoid malignant pleural mesothelioma. Eur J Cardiothorac Surg. 2012; 41(5):1031–6. PubMed PMID: 22219469.

53. Rena O, Casadio C. Extrapleural pneumonectomy for early stage malignant pleural mesothelioma: a harmful procedure. Lung Cancer. 2012;77(1):151–5. PubMed PMID: 22244608.

54. Flores RM, Pass HI, Seshan VE, Dycoco J, Zakowski M, Carbone M, et al. Extrapleural pneumonectomy versus pleurectomy/decortication in the surgical management of malignant pleural mesothelioma: results in 663 patients. J Thorac Cardiovasc Surg. 2008;135(3):620.e3–6. PubMed PMID: 2008112184. English.

55. Okada M, Mimura T, Ohbayashi C, Sakuma T, Soejima T, Tsubota N. Institutional report – thoracic general. Radical surgery for malignant pleural mesothelioma: results and prognosis. Interact Cardiovasc Thorac Surg. 2008;7(1):102–6. PubMed PMID: 2008079603. English.

56. Richards WG, Zellos L, Bueno R, Jaklitsch MT, Janne PA, Chirieac LR, et al. Phase I to II study of pleurectomy/decortication and intraoperative intracavitary hyperthermic cisplatin lavage for mesothelioma. J Clin Oncol. 2006;24(10):1561–7. PubMed PMID: 16575008.

57. Lee TT, Everett DL, Shu HK, Jahan TM, Roach 3rd M, Speight JL, et al. Radical pleurectomy/ decortication and intraoperative radiotherapy followed by conformal radiation with or without chemotherapy for malignant pleural mesothelioma. J Thorac Cardiovasc Surg. 2002;124(6): 1183–9. PubMed PMID: 12447185. English.

58. Rusch VW, Venkatraman ES. Important prognostic factors in patients with malignant pleural mesothelioma, managed surgically. Ann Thorac Surg. 1999;68(5):1799–804. PubMed PMID: 10585061. English.

59. Colleoni M, Sartori F, Calabro F, Nelli P, Vicario G, Sgarbossa G, et al. Surgery followed by intracavitary plus systemic chemotherapy in malignant pleural mesothelioma. Tumori. 1996;82(1):53–6. PubMed PMID: 8623505.

60. Luckraz H, Rahman M, Patel N, Szafranek A, Gibbs AR, Butchart EG. Three decades of experience in the surgical multi-modality management of pleural mesothelioma. Eur J Cardiothorac Surg. 2010;37(3):552–6. PubMed PMID: 2010103086. English.

61. Lucchi M, Picchi A, Ali G, Chella A, Guglielmi G, Cristaudo A, et al. Multimodality treatment of malignant pleural mesothelioma with or without immunotherapy: does it change anything? Interac Cardiovasc Thorac Surg. 2010;10(4):572–6. PubMed PMID: 20053697. Epub 2010/01/08. eng.

62. Nakas A, Martin Ucar AE, Edwards JG, Waller DA. The role of video assisted thoracoscopic pleurectomy/decortication in the therapeutic management of malignant pleural mesothelioma. Eur J Cardiothorac Surg. 2008;33(1):83–8. PubMed PMID: 2007614849. English.

63. Colaut F, Toniolo L, Vicario G, Scapinello A, Visentin C, Manente P, et al. Pleurectomy/decortication plus chemotherapy: outcomes of 40 cases of malignant pleural mesothelioma. Chir Ital. 2004;56(6):781–6. PubMed PMID: 15771030. English.

64. Lampl L, Jakob R. How should we treat malignant pleural mesothelioma (MPM)? Acta Chir Hung. 1999;38(1):87–90. PubMed PMID: 10439104. English.

65. Pass HI, Kranda K, Temeck BK, Feuerstein I, Steinberg SM. Surgically debulked malignant pleural mesothelioma: results and prognostic factors. Ann Surg Oncol. 1997;4(3):215–22. PubMed PMID: 9142382. English.

66. Soysal O, Karaoglanoglu N, Demiracan S, Topcu S, Tastepe I, Kaya S, et al. Pleurectomy/ decortication for palliation in malignant pleural mesothelioma: results of surgery. Eur J Cardiothorac Surg. 1997;11(2):210–3.

67. Lee JD, Perez S, Wang HJ, Figlin RA, Holmes EC. Intrapleural chemotherapy for patients with incompletely resected malignant mesothelioma: the UCLA experience. J Surg Oncol. 1995;60(4):262–7. PubMed PMID: 8551737.
68. Yan TD, Cao CQ, Boyer M, Tin MM, Kennedy C, McLean J, et al. Improving survival results after surgical management of malignant pleural mesothelioma: an Australian institution experience. Ann Thorac Cardiovasc Surg. 2011;17(3):243–9. PubMed PMID: 21697784.
69. Mineo TC, Ambrogi V, Cufari ME, Pompeo E. May cyclooxygenase-2 (COX-2), p21 and p27 expression affect prognosis and therapeutic strategy of patients with malignant pleural mesothelioma? Eur J Cardiothorac Surg. 2010;38(3):245–52. PubMed PMID: 2010460302. English.
70. Schipper PH, Nichols FC, Thomse KM, Deschamps C, Cassivi SD, Allen MS, et al. Malignant pleural mesothelioma: surgical management in 285 patients. Ann Thorac Surg. 2008;85(1):257–64. PubMed PMID: 2007610560. English.
71. Neragi-Miandoab S, Richards WG, Sugarbaker DJ. Morbidity, mortality, mean survival, and the impact of histology on survival after pleurectomy in 64 patients with malignant pleural mesothelioma. Int J Surg. 2008;6(4):293–7. PubMed PMID: 2008368393. English.
72. Halstead JC, Lim E, Venkateswaran RM, Charman SC, Goddard M, Ritchie AJ. Improved survival with VATS pleurectomy-decortication in advanced malignant mesothelioma. Eur J Surg Oncol. 2005;31(3):314–20. PubMed PMID: 15780570.
73. de Vries WJ, Long MA. Treatment of mesothelioma in Bloemfontein, South Africa. Eur J Cardio Thorac Surg. 2003;24(3):434–40. PubMed PMID: 12965317. English.
74. Phillips PG, Asimakopoulos G, Maiwand MO. Malignant pleural mesothelioma: outcome of limited surgical management. Interact Cardiovasc Thorac Surg. 2003;2(1):30–4. PubMed PMID: 17669981. Epub 2007/08/03. eng.
75. Martin-Ucar AE, Edwards JG, Rengajaran A, Muller S, Waller DA. Palliative surgical debulking in malignant mesothelioma. Predictors of survival and symptom control. Eur J Cardiothorac Surg. 2001;20(6):1117–21. PubMed PMID: 11717014.
76. Ceresoli GL, Locati LD, Ferreri AJ, Cozzarini C, Passoni P, Melloni G, et al. Therapeutic outcome according to histologic subtype in 121 patients with malignant pleural mesothelioma. Lung Cancer. 2001;34(2):279–87. PubMed PMID: 11679187.
77. Hasturk S, Tastepe I, Unlu M, Cetin G, Baris YI. Combined chemotherapy in pleurectomized malignant pleural mesothelioma patients. J Chemother. 1996;8(2):159–64. PubMed PMID: 8708749.
78. Sauter ER, Langer C, Coia LR, Goldberg M, Keller SM. Optimal management of malignant mesothelioma after subtotal pleurectomy: revisiting the role of intrapleural chemotherapy and postoperative radiation. J Surg Oncol. 1995;60(2):100–5. PubMed PMID: 7564374.
79. Allen KB, Faber LP, Warren WH. Malignant pleural mesothelioma. Extrapleural pneumonectomy and pleurectomy. Chest Surg Clin N Am. 1994;4(1):113–26. [Review] [45 refs]. PubMed PMID: 8055276. English.
80. Ruffie P, Feld R, Minkin S, Cormier Y, Boutan-Laroze A, Ginsberg R, et al. Diffuse malignant mesothelioma of the pleura in Ontario and Quebec: a retrospective study of 332 patients. J Clin Oncol. 1989;7(8):1157–68. PubMed PMID: 2666592. Epub 1989/08/01. eng.

Part VII
Mediastinum

Chapter 52
Extended Versus Standard Thymectomy for Myasthenia Gravis

Paul E. Van Schil, Rudy Mercelis, and Marco Lucchi

Abstract Myasthenia gravis is an autoimmune disorder with a highly variable clinical expression, course and prognosis. Although only moderate quality evidence is available, thymectomy is generally indicated in patients with early onset myasthenia gravis and positive acetylcholine receptor antibodies or in case of associated thymoma. Several surgical approaches to the thymus exist, the specific technique depending on the experience of the thoracic surgeon performing the procedure, also taking the preference of the patient into consideration. A multidisciplinary approach is advocated to ensure a high-quality level of preoperative, intraoperative and postoperative care. Due to the lack of large comparative or randomized trials no specific recommendations can be made regarding the best available approach to the thymus. Sternotomy remains the gold standard against which all other approaches should be evaluated and compared including thoracoscopic and robotic procedures. Despite the fact that available evidence is low, it seems that the less thymic tissue that has been left behind, the better the long-term results that are achieved.

Keywords Thymus • Myasthenia gravis • Acetylcholine receptor antibodies • Thymectomy • Diagnosis • Therapy • Surgery • Prognosis

P.E. Van Schil, MD, PhD (✉)
Department of Thoracic and Vascular Surgery, Antwerp University Hospital,
Wilrijkstraat 10, Edegem (Antwerp), B-2650, Belgium
e-mail: paul.van.schil@uza.be

R. Mercelis, MD
Department of Neurology, Antwerp University Hospital, Edegem (Antwerp), Belgium
e-mail: rudy.mercelis@uantwerpen.be

M. Lucchi, MD
Division of Thoracic Surgery, Cardiac Thoracic and Vascular Department, Azienda
Ospedaliero-Universitaria Pisana, Pisa, Italy
e-mail: m.lucchi@med.unipi.it

M.K. Ferguson (ed.), *Difficult Decisions in Thoracic Surgery*,   677
Difficult Decisions in Surgery: An Evidence-Based Approach 1,
DOI 10.1007/978-1-4471-6404-3_52, © Springer-Verlag London 2014

Introduction

The thymus is associated with highly variable disease entities often related to auto-immune disorders. Pathologically, thymic hyperplasia, cysts and different kinds of tumors may occur. Their clinical behavior ranges from benign to aggressive with symptoms due to invasion of neighboring mediastinal structures or pericardial and pleural cavities.

In this chapter patients with myasthenia gravis are considered whether or not associated with a thymoma (*patient population*). Surgical treatment consists of thy-mectomy (*intervention*) which remains a highly controversial procedure, not only regarding the specific indications but also concerning the best surgical approach in order to obtain a complete thymectomy.

In this evidence-based approach we focus on three questions: What are the current indications for thymectomy in myasthenia gravis? The neurologist gives his point of view regarding the operative indications based on recent literature data. Secondly, we discuss the different ways to reach the thymus trying to answer the question "Which is the best surgical approach to the thymus?" (*comparison*). Lastly, the specific procedure of thymectomy is highlighted with the discussion centered on the question "Is extended thymectomy better than standard thymectomy?" (*comparison*). Remission of myasthenic symptoms is considered the main *outcome* parameter.

Search Strategy

To retrieve relevant publications a PubMed search was performed with key words "myasthenia gravis" and "thymectomy", current guidelines and major thoracic surgical text books were reviewed and references of included publications were screened for additional evidence.

Current Indications for Thymectomy in Myasthenia Gravis

Myasthenia gravis is an autoimmune disorder directed against the postsynaptic part of the neuromuscular junction. A wide variation in clinical severity is found ranging from occasional ptosis or diplopia with spontaneous remission to severe generalized weakness requiring temporary artificial ventilation. In some patients the symptoms remain limited to the extraocular muscles: these patients have ocular myasthenia in contrast to generalized myasthenia gravis. Most patients have antibodies against the acetylcholine receptor (AchR) itself, while a minority have antibodies against the receptor-like muscle-specific kinase (MUSK), low-density lipoprotein receptor-related protein 4 (LRP4) or no detectable antibodies with the currently available assays [1, 2].

AchR antibody positive myasthenia gravis is subdivided in early and late onset according to the initial diagnosis before or after age 50. While there is a predominance of women in the early onset group there is an increasing incidence of late onset patients with a predominance of men. About 10 % of myasthenic patients of all ages with positive AchR antibodies have a thymoma. Thymoma patients and late onset non-thymoma patients frequently have antibodies against titin or the ryanodine receptor, while these antibodies are rare in early onset non-thymoma myasthenia gravis. In contrast, thymic follicular hyperplasia is frequent in early onset non-thymoma patients and rare in late onset patients. There is evidence that the thymus is involved in the pathogenesis of all types of AchR myasthenia, while its role is unclear in MUSK myasthenia and unknown in LRP4 and seronegative myasthenia [3].

It is generally accepted that surgery is required when a thymoma has been diagnosed. It is common practice to recommend thymectomy in early onset non-thymoma patients with generalized myasthenic symptoms. This recommendation is supported by the pathogenetic mechanism of myasthenia gravis, observational studies and non-randomized trials, although a definite controlled randomized clinical trial is still lacking.

In formulating a practice parameter for the American Academy of Neurology, Gronseth and Barohn reviewed the evidence available until 2000 [4]. They concluded that all currently published studies had serious methodological flaws that prevented definite conclusions regarding the benefit of thymectomy. These flaws included the absence of randomized allocation to thymectomy and non-thymectomy treatment, the absence of standardized, blinded outcome determinations and confounding differences in enrollment in the surgical and non-surgical groups. Because most studies showed a positive association between thymectomy and remission or improvement of myasthenic symptoms, they recommended thymectomy as an option to increase the probability of remission or improvement in non-thymomatous autoimmune myasthenia gravis. This recommendation was supported in the guidelines for the treatment of autoimmune neuromuscular transmission disorders by the European Federation of Neurological Societies in 2010 [5]. Patients with AchR antibodies and generalized disease were most likely to improve. Thymectomy was also recommended for seronegative patients but not for patients with MUSK antibodies.

The presence of conflicting data concerning the effect of thymectomy in ocular myasthenia was confirmed in a Cochrane Review in 2012 [6]. According to a survey of the Thymic Working Group of the European Association for Cardio-Thoracic Surgery (EACTS) most surgeons do not operate on myasthenic patients with exclusively ocular symptoms [7].

A recent retrospective study of 98 thymectomies in myasthenic patients over a 12-year period confirmed the generally accepted chance of one out of three of complete stable remission after the procedure with a variable degree of improvement in the other patients [8].

In 2006 a "Multicenter, single-blind, randomized study comparing thymectomy to no thymectomy in non-thymomatous myasthenia gravis patients receiving

Table 52.1 Indication for thymectomy according to myasthenia subtype

Myasthenia subtype	Thymectomy indicated	Quality of evidence	Recommendation
AchR thymoma	Yes	Moderate	Weak
AchR early onset generalized	Yes	Moderate	Weak
AchR early onset ocular	No	Low	Not recommended
AchR late onset	No	Low	Not recommended
MUSK	No	Low	Not recommended
LRP4	Unknown		
seronegative	Unknown		

AchR acetylcholine receptor, *MUSK* muscle-specific kinase, *LRP4* lipoprotein receptor-related protein 4

prednisone" was initiated under impulse of the late John Newson-Davis [9]. In this ClinicalTrials.gov NCT00294658 study patients were recruited with an age range from 18 till 65, with onset of AchR antibody positive myasthenia gravis over the last 5 years, excluding patients with only ocular symptoms. Treatment with prednisone alone is compared to the combination of prednisone and thymectomy. Extended transsternal thymectomy is the only accepted surgical procedure. The last patient was enrolled in 2012, the first results are expected in 2015. This trial will answer the question whether thymectomy and steroids are better than steroids alone. The issue whether thymectomy only is better than no treatment, and which is the best surgical approach will remain unanswered. Current indications for thymectomy in myasthenia gravis are listed in Table 52.1.

Optimal Surgical Approach to the Thymus

The thymus originates from the third and fourth pharyngeal pouches which move towards the midline and subsequently descend into the mediastinum. The thymus has a typical H-shape with two cervical poles which are less developed, and two mediastinal poles which are broadly extending along the pericardium inferiorly as far as the anterior cardiophrenic recesses. A highly variable anatomy has been described which has profound surgical implications when discussing thymectomy and the most appropriate surgical approach [10]. Precise anatomical and pathological studies have demonstrated that additional ectopic thymic tissue may be discovered in 32–98 % of patients when an extended resection has been performed [10, 11]. Non-encapsulated lobules of thymus and microscopic foci of thymus may be present in the pretracheal and anterior mediastinal fat from the level of the thyroid to the diaphragm and bilaterally from beyond each phrenic nerve. Microscopic foci of thymus have also been found in subcarinal fat and in the aortopulmonary window.

Many different approaches exist to perform a thymectomy and these can be subdivided into open procedures, minimally invasive and combined interventions (Table 52.2). The different steps of these procedures have been described in detail

Table 52.2 Surgical
approaches to the thymus

Open procedures
Partial median sternotomy
Full median sternotomy
Lateral thoracotomy
Hemi-clam shell incision
Clam shell incision
Minimally invasive techniques
Cervicotomy ± sternal retractor (increases exposure)
VATS: left, right, combined left and right
RATS: left, right
Combined procedures
Cervicotomy + VATS
Cervicotomy + RATS
Subxiphoid incision + VATS

VATS video-assisted thoracic surgery, *RATS* robotic-
assisted thoracic surgery

[12–14]. The specific indication discussed within a multidisciplinary setting, the experience of the thoracic surgeon and the patient's preference will determine the ultimate choice. In case of myasthenia a "maximal" thymectomy is advised removing as much thymic tissue as possible with surrounding mediastinal fat from the cervical region to the diaphragm extending laterally to both phrenic nerves, and also incorporating the mediastinal fat in the aortopulmonary window. In this way ectopic thymic tissue will be removed to a maximal extent.

In case of combined myasthenia and suspected or proven thymoma it is important to completely remove the thymic lesion. When present, its capsule should not be breached in order to avoid spilling of malignant cells into the mediastinum or pleural cavities.

Unfortunately, no randomized trials exist that compare the different surgical approaches to determine mortality, frequency of postoperative complications and evaluate long-term results. So, no high-quality evidence is available.

No doubt, sternotomy remains the current gold standard allowing an extended thymectomy by an anterior approach with complete removal of the thymus and surrounding fatty tissue, allowing opening of both pleural cavities, control of major mediastinal blood vessels and extensive dissection along the pericardium into the cardiophrenic recesses [14]. On the other hand, it requires a large incision necessitating an extensive osteotomy which may result in increased pain, higher morbidity, slower recovery and prolonged hospitalization time. However, a direct comparison of sternotomy with alternative incisions for similar patient groups is not available. A partial upper sternotomy provides good visualization of the upper mediastinum but evaluation of more caudal regions is not feasible [12]. Large mediastinal tumors invading major mediastinal structures may be approached by a lateral thoracotomy or combined incisions. The latter include hemi-clam shell or clam shell approaches, consisting of partial sternotomy combined with an anterolateral thoracotomy or bilateral anterior thoracotomy with transverse sternotomy, respectively. Especially for patients with myasthenia gravis and generalized complaints including respiratory problems, less invasive methods were developed to decrease morbidity in relation to the incision but still allowing an extended thymectomy.

By a cervicotomy it is possible to remove the entire thymus and surrounding fatty tissue, especially when a sternal retractor is used [13]. With the advent of video-assisted thoracic surgery (VATS), new methods became available to perform a thymectomy by small thoracoports. Recently, robotic-assisted thoracic surgery (RATS) was introduced providing optimal three-dimensional visualization facilitating dissection with the aid of highly flexible robotic arms [15–17].

Within the surgical community there is an ongoing discussion whether a right-sided, left-sided or bilateral thoracoscopic approach is indicated to perform a complete thymectomy. In some centers combined procedures are used as VATS in combination with a cervicotomy or a subxiphoid approach, in this way avoiding a scar in the cervical region [18]. The thymus may thus be approached from different angles allowing complete removal.

Regarding the incision no definite recommendations can be made due to the lack of randomized trials. Median sternotomy remains the gold standard. So, the experience of a surgeon and a specific center but also the preference of the patient after all relevant information has been provided, will determine the final approach.

Another controversial topic remains the role of a minimally invasive approach in patients with myasthenia and suspicion of thymoma. Depending on the location and size of the thymoma recent data indicate that well-encapsulated tumors without invasion into the mediastinum or large vessels can safely be removed by a thoracoscopic or especially, a robotic technique [15, 17, 18]. Invasion in large mediastinal vessels is a contra-indication for a VATS or robotic approach. The size limit is usually considered to be 4–5 cm [19]. However, as thymomas are slowly growing tumors, long-term results are still awaited for before definite conclusions will be reached regarding long-term oncological outcome.

Extended Thymectomy vs Standard Thymectomy

The role of thymectomy in the treatment of myasthenia gravis has not been elucidated yet [20]. Until recently, variable patient selection, timing and type of surgery and analytical methods rendered the conclusions of the most important retrospective studies inconsistent. Moreover, there are no controlled prospective studies and the unique randomized trial comparing thymectomy versus non-thymectomy in patients treated by steroids is still ongoing as outlined earlier [9].

Before dealing with the extent of the thymectomy to be performed for myasthenia gravis, it is crucial to emphasize that the thymus is a *functional* entity not limited to the gland itself and thymic cells may be found outside the main capsule. As outlined before, surgical and anatomical studies already showed many years ago that the thymus frequently consists of multiple lobes in the neck and mediastinum, often separately encapsulated and not necessarily contiguous [21, 22]. This results in the recommendation that as much mediastinal thymic tissue as possible should be removed for the treatment of non-thymomatous myasthenia gravis. This statement is supported by a review of published papers on the results of thymectomy [4, 20, 22–25]. Further proof comes from the presence of residual thymic tissue in most of the re-operations after previous transcervical and standard transsternal thymectomy, with improvement or remission of the myasthenic symptoms [26].

The original standard transsternal thymectomy used by Blalock was limited to removal of the thymic gland with its cervical and mediastinal lobes [27]. Unrelated to the surgical approach, the resection is currently more extensive than originally described and includes, at least, removal of all visible mediastinal thymic lobes and also part of the mediastinal and low cervical fat [4, 23–25].

The extended transsternal thymectomy also called "aggressive transsternal thymectomy" and "transsternal radical thymectomy" consists of en-bloc resection of all fat and thymic tissue in the neck and mediastinum. Dissection starts at the inferior part of the thyroid lobes proceeding caudally to the diaphragm and extending laterally from one phrenic to the contralateral one. Removing cervical tissue by a VATS or robotic procedure starting from below without a neck incision, may result in an incomplete resection which is less radical than a transcervical and transsternal thymectomy [20, 22]. However, because it is less invasive with low morbidity, this approach has been adopted by many thoracic surgeons dealing with myasthenia gravis. Retrospective studies comparing extended thymic resections with standard thymectomy, also supported the premise that the more thymic tissue is removed, the higher the remission rate will be [20].

However, we must consider that inappropriate statistical analysis has led in the past to incorrect conclusions about the relative merits of the extension of thymectomy. Unfortunately, uncorrected crude rates have been used in the most important retrospective series and this form of analysis did not include all relevant follow-up information including the median length of follow-up [4]. As a matter of fact, uncorrected crude data should not be used anymore in the comparative analysis of results of thymectomy for myasthenia gravis. Life table analysis using the Kaplan–Meier method, is currently the statistical technique of choice for the analysis of remissions following thymectomy [20].

Several other biases, such as the selection of patients for thymectomy, the different clinical classifications of myasthenia gravis, the lack of quantitative scoring systems and the different schedules of medications used in the preoperative and postoperative course make the comparative analysis based on existing published information unreliable [20].

From 2000 on, based on recommendations of the task force of the Myasthenia Gravis Foundation of America (MGFA), precise definitions of remission and life table analyses have been adopted in some but not all studies reporting the outcome of thymectomy in myasthenic patients.

Because of the lack of well-designed, controlled, prospective studies that compare thymectomy versus non-thymectomy, standard versus extended versus maximal thymectomy and finally, different surgical approaches to the thymus, we can only select and extrapolate data from well-performed observational trials.

Table 52.3 Indication for extended versus standard thymectomy according to myasthenia subtype

Myasthenia subtype	Quality of evidence	Recommendation
AchR + early onset generalized	Moderate	Weak
AchR + thymoma	Moderate	Weak
Thymoma without myasthenia gravis	Low	Weak

AchR acetylcholine receptor

Despite the fact that the available evidence is of low quality, it seems that the less thymic tissue has been left behind, the better the long-term results are achieved.

We agree with Jaretzki and Sonett statements that the transcervical-transsternal maximal thymectomy should remain the benchmark against which all other thymectomy techniques have to be evaluated and that in the absence of controlled prospective studies comparing the various thymectomy techniques, it is not possible to define a procedure of choice [20]. Alternatively, in the hands of experienced surgeons, an extended transsternal thymectomy removes most of the thymic variations in the neck with less risk of injury to the recurrent laryngeal nerves. Good results have been reported and according to a recent European Survey, it is probably the most commonly performed procedure [7].

All thoracic surgeons should be convinced of the importance of complete removal of the thymus and commit the necessary time and care to achieve this goal safely. However, because the need for complete removal of all gross and microscopic thymus has not been definitively confirmed, it may be preferable to leave behind small amounts of suspected thymus than to cause injury to the recurrent laryngeal, left vagal or phrenic nerves, which can be devastating in a patient with myasthenia gravis.

As already mentioned, clearance of the neck region is a controversial point for most of the minimally invasive techniques (thoracoscopic or robotic-assisted) and this point needs to be addressed by further studies. Up to now the minimally invasive techniques proved to be feasible and safe but we must wait for a longer follow-up time and especially, high-quality comparative studies [24, 25].

Resections less than a standard thymectomy have never been considered for the treatment of non-thymomatous myasthenia gravis. Also for patients with encapsulated thymoma, non-invasive or microinvasive lesions, corresponding to Masaoka stages I and II, complete excision including an extended thymectomy is currently considered to be the procedure of choice, even in non-myasthenic patients. Recently, Onuki et al. conducted a retrospective comparative study of 79 patients and tested the hypothesis that limited thymectomy is not inferior to total thymectomy for stage I or II thymomas in terms of surgical outcome and postoperative complications [28]. The authors concluded that there were no statistical differences in the incidence of postoperative myasthenia gravis and disease-free survival between the two groups, but this was a retrospective historical comparative study and the neurologic inclusion criteria and outcome did not meet any MGFA recommendations.

Based on the low to moderate scientific evidence derived by the literature, thoracic surgeons should perform an extended thymectomy by the least invasive operation possible (Table 52.3).

Recommendations

Thymectomy is indicated in patients with early onset, generalized myasthenia gravis and positive acetylcholine receptor antibodies or in case of associated thymoma (evidence quality moderate; weak recommendation). Sternotomy is the best approach to perform a maximal, extended thymectomy (evidence quality low; weak recommendation). In case of myasthenia gravis with positive acetylcholine receptor antibodies extended thymectomy yields better long-term results than standard thymectomy (evidence quality low; weak recommendation).

A Personal View of the Data

In patients with early onset, generalized myasthenia gravis and positive acetylcholine receptor antibodies we favor an extended thymectomy. In case of thymic hyperplasia a robotic approach is preferred as it is feasible to perform a complete thymectomy. As the bulk of thymic tissue is usually located on the left side in front of the pericardium, most cases are approached from this side. In case of myasthenia gravis associated with thymoma, sternotomy remains our standard approach. Exceptions include tumors <5 cm without invasion of major vessels or structures which are resected with the robot from the left or right side depending on their precise location. The ultimate aim is complete excision without breaching the capsule.

Recommendations

- Extended thymectomy yields better long-term results than standard thymectomy for management of myasthenia gravis. (Evidence quality low; weak recommendation)
- Sternotomy is the best approach for performing an extended thymectomy. (Evidence quality low; weak recommendation)

References

1. Meriggioli MN, Sanders DB. Autoimmune myasthenia gravis: emerging clinical and biological heterogeneity. Lancet Neurol. 2009;8(5):475–90. Epub 2009/04/21.
2. Cossins J, Belaya K, Zoltowska K, Koneczny I, Maxwell S, Jacobson L, et al. The search for new antigenic targets in myasthenia gravis. Ann N Y Acad Sci. 2012;1275:123–8. Epub 2013/01/03.
3. Marx A, Pfister F, Schalke B, Saruhan-Direskeneli G, Melms A, Strobel P. The different roles of the thymus in the pathogenesis of the various myasthenia gravis subtypes. Autoimmun Rev. 2013;12(9):875–84. Epub 2013/03/29.

4. Gronseth GS, Barohn RJ. Practice parameter: thymectomy for autoimmune myasthenia gravis (an evidence-based review): report of the Quality Standards Subcommittee of the American Academy of Neurology. Neurology. 2000;55(1):7–15. Epub 2000/07/13.
5. Skeie GO, Apostolski S, Evoli A, Gilhus NE, Illa I, Harms L, et al. Guidelines for treatment of autoimmune neuromuscular transmission disorders. Eur J Neurol. 2010;17(7):893–902. Epub 2010/04/21.
6. Benatar M, Kaminski H. Medical and surgical treatment for ocular myasthenia. Cochrane Database Syst Rev. 2012;12, CD005081. Epub 2012/12/14.
7. Lucchi M, Van Schil P, Schmid R, Rea F, Melfi F, Athanassiadi K, et al. Thymectomy for thymoma and myasthenia gravis. A survey of current surgical practice in thymic disease amongst EACTS members. Interact Cardiovasc Thorac Surg. 2012;14(6):765–70. Epub 2012/03/01.
8. Spillane J, Hayward M, Hirsch NP, Taylor C, Kullmann DM, Howard RS. Thymectomy: role in the treatment of myasthenia gravis. J Neurol. 2013;260(7):1798–801. Epub 2013/03/20.
9. Newsom-Davis J, Cutter G, Wolfe GI, Kaminski HJ, Jaretzki 3rd A, Minisman G, et al. Status of the thymectomy trial for nonthymomatous myasthenia gravis patients receiving prednisone. Ann N Y Acad Sci. 2008;1132:344–7. Epub 2008/06/24.
10. Shields T. The thymus. In: Shields T, editor. Mediastinal surgery. Philadelphia: Lea & Febiger; 1991. p. 6–13.
11. Sonett J. Thymectomy for myasthenia gravis: optimal approach. In: F MK, editor. Difficult decisions in thoracic surgery an evidence-based approach. London: Springer; 2007. p. 469–73.
12. Trastek VP PC. Standard thymectomy. In: Shields T, editor. Mediastinal surgery. Philadelphia: Lea & Febiger; 1991. p. 365–8.
13. Kirby TG RJ, et al. Transcervical thymectomy. In: Shields T, editor. Mediastinal surgery. Philadelphia: Lea & Febiger; 1991. p. 369–71.
14. Jaretzki III A. Transcervical / trans-sternal "maximal" thymectomy for myasthenia gravis. Mediastinal surgery. Philadelphia: Lea & Febiger; 1991. p. 372–6.
15. Mussi A, Fanucchi O, Davini F, Lucchi M, Picchi A, Ambrogi MC, et al. Robotic extended thymectomy for early-stage thymomas. Eur J Cardiothorac Surg. 2012;41(4):e43–6; discussion e7. Epub 2012/03/01.
16. Ruckert JC, Sobel HK, Gohring S, Einhaupl KM, Muller JM. Matched-pair comparison of three different approaches for thymectomy in myasthenia gravis. Surg Endosc. 2003;17(5):711–5. Epub 2003/03/05.
17. Ruckert JC, Swierzy M, Ismail M. Comparison of robotic and nonrobotic thoracoscopic thymectomy: a cohort study. J Thorac Cardiovasc Surg. 2011;141(3):673–7. Epub 2011/02/22.
18. Zielinski M, Czajkowski W, Gwozdz P, Nabialek T, Szlubowski A, Pankowski J. Resection of thymomas with use of the new minimally-invasive technique of extended thymectomy performed through the subxiphoid-right video-thoracoscopic approach with double elevation of the sternum. Eur J Cardiothorac Surg. 2013;44(2):e113–9. Epub 2013/06/14.
19. Kimura T, Inoue M, Kadota Y, Shiono H, Shintani Y, Nakagiri T, et al. The oncological feasibility and limitations of video-assisted thoracoscopic thymectomy for early-stage thymomas. Eur J Cardiothorac Surg. 2013;44(3):e214–8. Epub 2013/06/14.
20. Sonett JR, Jaretzki 3rd A. Thymectomy for nonthymomatous myasthenia gravis: a critical analysis. Ann N Y Acad Sci. 2008;1132:315–28. Epub 2008/06/24.
21. Masaoka A, Nagaoka Y, Kotake Y. Distribution of thymic tissue at the anterior mediastinum. Current procedures in thymectomy. J Thorac Cardiovasc Surg. 1975;70(4):747–54. Epub 1975/10/01.
22. Jaretzki 3rd A, Wolff M. "Maximal" thymectomy for myasthenia gravis. Surgical anatomy and operative technique. J Thorac Cardiovasc Surg. 1988;96(5):711–6. Epub 1988/11/01.
23. Zielinski M, Kuzdzal J, Szlubowski A, Soja J. Comparison of late results of basic transsternal and extended transsternal thymectomies in the treatment of myasthenia gravis. Ann Thorac Surg. 2004;78(1):253–8. Epub 2004/06/30.
24. Meyer DM, Herbert MA, Sobhani NC, Tavakolian P, Duncan A, Bruns M, et al. Comparative clinical outcomes of thymectomy for myasthenia gravis performed by extended transsternal

and minimally invasive approaches. Ann Thorac Surg. 2009;87(2):385–90; discussion 90-1. Epub 2009/01/24.

25. Mantegazza R, Baggi F, Bernasconi P, Antozzi C, Confalonieri P, Novellino L, et al. Video-assisted thoracoscopic extended thymectomy and extended transsternal thymectomy (T-3b) in non-thymomatous myasthenia gravis patients: remission after 6 years of follow-up. J Neurol Sci. 2003;212(1–2):31–6. Epub 2003/06/18.

26. Rosenberg M, Jauregui WO, De Vega ME, Herrera MR, Roncoroni AJ. Recurrence of thymic hyperplasia after thymectomy in myasthenia gravis. Its importance as a cause of failure of surgical treatment. Am J Med. 1983;74(1):78–82. Epub 1983/01/01.

27. Blalock A, Mason MF, Morgan HJ, Riven SS. Myasthenia gravis and tumors of the thymic region: report of a case in which the tumor was removed. Ann Surg. 1939;110(4):544–61. Epub 1939/10/01.

28. Onuki T, Ishikawa S, Iguchi K, Goto Y, Sakai M, Inagaki M, et al. Limited thymectomy for stage I or II thymomas. Lung Cancer. 2010;68(3):460–5. Epub 2009/09/01.

Chapter 53
Optimal Approach for Resection of Encapsulated Thymoma: Open Versus VATS

Joshua Sonett and Peter Downey

Abstract Thymomas make up the majority of mediastinal masses in adults and are the most common thymic neoplasm. The standard of care for the treatment of encapsulated thymoma (Masaoka stage I) has classically been total resection via an open approach, most commonly by conventional sternotomy. Minimally invasive techniques have begun to gain application in the resection of these thymomas but the optimal approach remains to be established. Recent studies have explored the technical feasibility and the oncological safety of the minimally invasive approach. This chapter will review the most current literature surrounding the topic and we will provide our assessment and current approach these patients.

Keywords Thymoma • Thymectomy • Encapsulated • Masaoka stage I • Minimally invasive • Recurrence

Introduction

Thymomas are both interesting and challenging problems. Thymomas make up the majority of mediastinal masses in adults and are the most common thymic neoplasm. They are now thought to be malignant by definition. Most patients are diagnosed between 40 and 60 years old. Men may be slightly more commonly affected than women. In 30–40 % of cases, thymomas are associated with myasthenia gravis,

J. Sonett, MD (✉)
Division of Thoracic Surgery, Columbia University Medical Center,
New York-Presbyterian Hospital, New York, NY, USA
e-mail: js2106@columbia.edu

P. Downey, MD
Department of Surgery, Columbia University Medical Center,
New York-Presbyterian Hospital, New York, NY, USA

M.K. Ferguson (ed.), *Difficult Decisions in Thoracic Surgery*,
Difficult Decisions in Surgery: An Evidence-Based Approach 1,
DOI 10.1007/978-1-4471-6404-3_53, © Springer-Verlag London 2014

or more rarely other paraneoplastic syndromes such as pure red cell aplasia or thymoma-associated multi-organ autoimmunity [1].

This chapter will be specifically focused on the surgical management of Masaoka Stage 1 thymomas. The standard of care for the treatment of encapsulated thymoma (Masaoka stage I) has classically been total resection via an open approach, most commonly by conventional sternotomy. Over the past 10–20 years, the use of minimally invasive techniques has gained wide acceptance in the treatment of many thoracic surgical diseases given the associated decrease in morbidity. Its application to encapsulated early stage thymomatous disease has also been considered but has been slow to gain full acceptance. For Masaoka Stage I encapsulated thymoma, the reported 10-year recurrence rates for standard open thymectomy range from 1 to 4 % with operative mortality ranging from 0 to 2 % [2, 3]. With such excellent oncologic results from a safe and proven technique, the primary reason surgeons are cautious to adopt thoracoscopic resection is the potentially higher rates of recurrence exposing patients to further morbidity and mortality.

This chapter will serve as an updated review of the most current literature surrounding this topic. We will again address the technical feasibility of the minimally invasive and pathologically safe thymectomy, the evidence surrounding the morbidity, mortality, and recurrence rates following minimally invasive thymoma resection, and the evidence of recurrence rates associated with the minimally invasive techniques.

Search Strategy

An English-language literature search was performed in PubMed from 1960 to present using the search terms "minimally invasive," "thymectomy," and "thymoma" resulting in 48 publications. Review was limited to case series including at least six thymomas resected by minimally invasive techniques and larger outcomes studies with survival and recurrence results.

Definitions

Staging

The Masaoka staging system is widely accepted as the gold standard for characterizing the extent of thymomatous disease at the time of operation [4]. The Masaoka staging system is a 4-tiered staging system proposed in 1981 that is based on extent of invasion and evidence of metastasis. Masaoka Stage I thymomas are defined as those that are fully encapsulated without any microscopic or macroscopic transcapsular invasion into the surrounding fatty tissue.

Minimally Invasive Thymectomy

A 2011 report from the International Thymic Malignancy Interest Group published their proposal of a broad definition of minimally invasive thymectomy [5]. Minimally invasive thymectomy is defined as "any approach as long as no sternotomy (including partial sternotomy) or thoracotomy with rib spreading is involved and in which a complete resection of the tumor is intended." Included in this definition are those procedures involving removal of the xiphoid or a rib cartilage as long as the remainder of the procedure is carried out minimally invasively as stated. Resection must include the thymoma, the entire thymus, and the surrounding fat. Incomplete resections were not considered acceptable reasons to complete a minimally invasive procedure without conversion to open.

Technical Feasibility

Minimally Invasive Versus Open Resection for Thymoma

When directly compared to open resection at the same institution, the minimally invasive approach appears to be comparable in terms of safety. In 2012, Weksler's group published their experience with open versus robotic thymectomy for stage I-III disease [6]. Fifteen patients underwent robotic resection; three patients were stage I, and seven patients were stage II. There was one post-operative complication (supraventricular arrhythmia) and no mortalities in the robotic group. There were 20 post-operative complications and 1 death in the trans-sternal group. In the robotic group, the average tumor size was 4.5 cm, which was not statistically different from that of the open group.

In 2012, Jurado et al published a larger comparison study addressing this issue [7]. This group evaluated 72 patients from 2000 to 2011 undergoing thymectomy for Masaoka Stage I, II, or III thymoma. A total of ten patients underwent thoracoscopic thymectomy (four stage I and six stage II thymomas). The median thymoma specimen size was smaller in the minimally invasive group (4.45 cm vs. 6.5 cm). Their early operative and pathological experience has shown a decreased estimated blood loss, decreased operative time, and decreased length of ICU and hospital stay without significant change in the operative time, transfusion requirements, morbidity, or mortality as compared to 57 non-matched patients undergoing open thymectomy for the same stage of disease.

Several groups have since published larger retrospective studies comparing their experience with minimally invasive thymectomy versus open thymectomy. Kimura's group evaluated 74 patients with either stage I or II disease undergoing thymectomy [8]. Forty-five underwent thoracoscopic thymectomy (41 Stage I, 4 Stage II) and 29 underwent resection via open sternotomy. There were no mortalities or immediate post-operative complications in the thoracoscopic group, but three patients (6.7 %) who underwent thoracoscopic resection suffered recurrence within 5 years. Two of these patients did have known capsule disruption at the time of resection as compared to none in the open group. The average tumor size in the thoracoscopic group was 4.8 cm, but was as high as 10 cm.

Ye's group compared their robotic thymectomy experience to their open approach for 74 Masaoka stage I or stage II patients [9]. Twenty-three patients underwent robotic-assisted thymectomy and 51 patients underwent transsternal thymectomy. In this group, there were no mortalities, no significant post-operative complications, and no recurrences at 5-year follow-up. The average tumor size in the robotic group was 3.0 cm but extended to 10.7 cm.

Operative and Perioperative Safety

As the standard of care, open resection for Masaoka stage I thymoma is associated with up to 1.6 % mortality and 6 % recurrence [2, 10]. Minimally invasive thymectomy has been cautiously adopted secondary to some theoretical concern for increased morbidity and possibly increased recurrence due to suboptimal resection margins if the operator is not skilled in the technique [11]. The current literature on minimally invasive thymectomies is summarized in Table 53.1.

Reported operative complications in early experience with minimally invasive thymectomy included vascular injury, chylothorax, phrenic nerve injury, and diaphragmatic injury. In 2007, Cheng and colleagues reviewed 44 video-assisted thoracic surgery (VATS) thymectomies, 27 of which were Masaoka stage I [13]. In their group, there were no mortalities and no reported "major" complications. This was one of the first series establishing the safety of the VATS procedure for thymoma.

In 2008, Ruckert et al. published their series of 95 consecutive robotic-assisted thymectomies for the treatment of myasthenia gravis [20]. Although not all patients had associated thymoma, their group was able to perform a technically complete thymectomy in all patients with overall zero mortality and only 2 % morbidity. Complications included one phrenic nerve injury and one bleeding episode. In 2011, their follow-up study comparing 79 VATS to 74 robotic-assisted thymectomies showed a significant improvement in complete stable remission of myasthenia gravis [21]. Although this series included patients undergoing thymectomy for various indications, their large-scale results indicate the technical safety, feasibility and possibly improved completeness of the robotic-assisted thymectomy.

In 2013, three groups published larger outcomes studies of minimally invasive thymectomy for thymoma. Odaka et al published a retrospective outcomes study of 62 thoracoscopic thymectomies for thymoma [18]. Twenty-nine patients had Masaoka stage I with tumor size ranged from 1.4 to 9.5 cm. There were no mortalities and three post-operative complications in the entire study group (4.8 %), none of which was described as a major surgical complication. Kimura's experience with 45 thoracoscopic thymectomies, 41 of which were for stage I disease, showed no mortalities, no "major" complications, and 0 recurrences at 5 years in patients with stage I disease [8]. Marulli et al. published a review of 79 patients undergoing minimally

Table 53.1 Studies of minimally invasive resection for thymoma

Studies	Year	No. of patients	Mortality (%)	Complications	Negative margins (%)	Follow-up (months)	Recurrence(s)	Quality of evidence
Agasthian and Lin [12]	2010	58, 25 stage 1	0	NR	100	58.8 (a)	2	Moderate
Cheng et al. [13]	2007	44, 27 stage 1	0	0 "major"	100	39.6 (a)	0	Moderate
He et al. [14]	2013	15, 6 stage 1	0	4	100	12–33	0	Low
Jurado et al. [7]	2012	10, 4 stage 1	0	7	100	29 (m)	0	Moderate
Kimura et al. [8]	2013	45, 41 stage 1	0	0 "major"	100	53.7 (a)	3	Moderate
Maggi et al. [15]	2008	71 thymoma	0	NR	NR	92.4 (a)	3	Moderate
Marulli et al. [16]	2013	79, 30 stage 1	0	2	100	51.7 (a)	1	Moderate
Mussi et al. [17]	2012	13, 7 stage 1	0	2	100	14.5 (m)	0	Low
Odaka et al. [18]	2013	62, 29 stage 1	0	3	100	43 (a)	3	Moderate
Pennathur et al. [19]	2011	18, 5 stage 1	0	5	NR	27 (a)	1	Low
Ruckert et al. [20]	2008	12 thymoma	0	2	100	19.8 (a)	NR	Low
Ruckert et al. [21]	2011	17 thymoma	0	4	100	42 (a)	NR	Moderate
Savitt et al. [22]	2005	14 thymoma	0	0 "surgical"	100	12 (m)	NR	Low
Takeo et al. [23]	2011	35, 15 stage 1	0	3	NR	65 (a)	1	Moderate
Ye et al. [9]	2013	23, 21 stage 1	0	1	100	1–48	0	Low
Zielinski et al. [24]	2012	24, 21 stage 1	0	1	100	29.9 (a)	0	Moderate

NR not recorded

invasive resections, 30 of whom had stage I disease [16]. They had 0 mortalities, two complications, and 0 recurrences in patients with stage 1 disease at 5 years (Table 53.1). These reports suggest at least equivalent and possibly improved perioperative safety from a technical standpoint with minimally invasive techniques.

Oncologic Efficacy

Completeness of Resection

Traditionally, general principles include complete removal of all thymic tissue at the time of resection for thymomatous disease [5]. The intended goal of complete removal of all thymic tissue is the prevention of delayed presentation of paraneoplastic diseases. For Masaoka stage I disease, enough emphasis cannot be placed on the intact removal of the thymoma, without disruption of the capsule and with clear tumor margins on pathological evaluation.

Some initial concern has been associated with various VATS or robotic approaches, specifically with respect to adequate visualization of the thymoma and surrounding structures, such as the phrenic nerve. Zielinski et al have presented a unique approach of a subxyphoid-right VATS approach with double elevation of the sternum which has specifically addressed this concern [24]. They published results of 24 patients operated on for Stage I-III thymomas. One patient required conversion to sternotomy for a large stage III tumor, but in two other patients with stage III disease, it was possible to completely resect tumor infiltrating the right lung. All other patients underwent complete resection as well. There was zero mortality, one bleeding complication and no recurrences during the follow-up period of 30 months.

In the Odaka study, of the 29 patients undergoing minimally invasive thymoma resection, only 8 had either total thymectomy or extended thymectomy [18]. The remainder had complete tumor resection, but only either a subtotal thymectomy or a left or right hemithymectomy. Their mid-term survival for stage I disease has been 100 %. In Cheng's group of 44 patients, 27 stage I, who underwent minimally invasive resection, they state that for all stage I disease, all residual thymic tissue was removed, but not necessarily at the time of tumor resection [13]. They also reported no recurrences. Other studies acknowledge the principle of complete resection, but are less explicit about the full extent of their resections. Again, long-term data is needed to fully understand the oncologic impact of thymoma resection without total thymic tissue resection, but early data has shown outcomes to be relative only to the completeness of the tumor resection.

Ability to Predict Encapsulation

The ability to reliably predict encapsulation on preoperative CT scan has been critical to appropriate patient selection for a minimally invasive approach for Masaoka stage I disease. The 5-year survival of stage II disease has previously been reported to be lower than that of stage I [25]. This would question the appropriateness of a minimally invasive approach to a potentially under-staged patient. However, a recent meta-analysis of retrospective data from 2,451 patients has shown no significant difference in overall survival or disease-free survival between stage I and stage II disease following thymectomy [26]. This raises the issue of the value of differentiating between stage I and stage II disease and ultimately may place less emphasis on the ability of pre-operative CT to predict encapsulation.

Long-Term Survival and Recurrence

Long-term survival after minimally invasive thymectomy for thymoma has been difficult to predict secondary to the overall indolent nature of thymic cancer, the relatively smaller tumor burden, and need for extended post-operative follow-up. The most important factor predicting long-term survival in the literature on open resection is the completeness of resection [5]. Encouraging mid-term survival data following minimally invasive thymoma resection is developing in the literature.

In the Odaka series mentioned above, for Masaoka stage I thymoma resection, the 5-year disease-free survival rate for Masaoka stage I was 100 % [18]. Of the 57 patients who had stage I or stage II disease, 7 underwent post-operative radiation. While encouraging, they acknowledge the need for longer-term follow-up to establish true disease free survival. Jurado et al. also showed no mortalities or recurrence of disease at 5 years for the minimally invasive group, but acknowledged a potential for lead-time bias given the median duration of follow-up was 29 months as compared to 80 months for the open group [7].

Summary and Recommendations

The level of evidence for thoracoscopic or robotic-assisted resection of encapsulated thymoma is low to moderate. There are no randomized trials comparing either technique to the open technique. The oncological outcome of any technique remains the primary concern. Recent studies in increasing volume are being published encouraging wider adaptation of minimally invasive techniques for resection of Masaoka stage I thymomas citing comparable if not improved safety and short- and mid-term recurrence rates.

The initially positive results with minimally invasive thymectomy in terms of immediate outcomes and mid-term survival are likely reflective of the improving technical skill of minimally invasive thoracic surgeons as well as careful patient selection. As minimally invasive approaches to thymectomy gain wider acceptance, we anticipate further experience will continue to show similar results. The growing body of literature in this area collectively agrees that long-term results and prospective studies will be necessary to truly establish the safety and oncologic outcome of the minimally invasive techniques.

A Personal View of the Data

In performing a minimally invasive thymectomy, we believe it is critical the operator has extensive experience with minimally invasive techniques in the treatment of benign disease of the thymus prior to an attempt at oncologic resection. We encourage a no-touch technique of the thymus itself as a means of preventing capsular disruption, and a low threshold to resect pericardium under the thymoma. While some centers have reported success with minimally invasive resection of tumors as large at 10 cm, we initially limited our thoracoscopic resections thymomas to less than 6 cm. Our present paradigm, which has evolved with experience, is to initially approach thymoma resection via VATS to assess resectability, and proceed with bilateral VATS approach with tumors that are not invading vascular structures. Any incidence of capsule disruption is considered absolutely unacceptable, as the open approach has been shown to have a negligible incidence of capsule disruption in fully encapsulated tumors. Additionally, completeness of resection by either technique is of critical importance in the management of this disease. We strongly recommend against the minimally invasive approach if there is any chance of capsule disruption or incomplete resection of the tumor.

We look forward to longer-term outcomes studies and larger case series evaluating the minimally invasive techniques for this disease. We also remain hopeful that larger trials may eventually be employed to provide sound rationale for either approach.

Recommendations

- We recommend minimally invasive thymectomy for encapsulated thymomas (Evidence quality low; weak recommendation).

References

1. Singhal SK, Kaiser LR. Surgery for myasthenia gravis. In: Pearson's thoracic and esophageal surgery. 3rd ed. Philadelphia: Churchill Livingstone/Elsevier; 2008. p. 1549–61.
2. Regnard JF, Magdeleinat P, Dromer C, Dulmet E, de Montpreville V, Levi JF, et al. Prognostic factors and long-term results after thymoma resection: a series of 307 patients. J Thorac Cardiovasc Surg. 1996;112(2):376–84. PubMed PMID: 8751506. Epub 1996/08/01. eng.
3. Blumberg D, Port JL, Weksler B, Delgado R, Rosai J, Bains MS, et al. Thymoma: a multivariate analysis of factors predicting survival. Ann Thorac Surg. 1995;60(4):908–13. PubMed PMID: 7574993; discussion 14. Epub 1995/10/01. eng.
4. Detterbeck FC, Nicholson AG, Kondo K, Van Schil P, Moran C. The Masaoka-Koga stage classification for thymic malignancies: clarification and definition of terms. J Thorac Oncol. 2011;6(7 Suppl 3):S1710–6. PubMed PMID: 21847052. Epub 2011/09/29. eng.
5. Toker A, Sonett J, Zielinski M, Rea F, Tomulescu V, Detterbeck FC. Standard terms, definitions, and policies for minimally invasive resection of thymoma. J Thorac Oncol. 2011;6(7 Suppl 3):S1739–42. PubMed PMID: 21847056. Epub 2011/09/29. eng.

6. Weksler B, Tavares J, Newhook TE, Greenleaf CE, Diehl JT. Robot-assisted thymectomy is superior to transsternal thymectomy. Surg Endosc. 2012;26(1):261–6. PubMed PMID: 21898017. Epub 2011/09/08. eng.

7. Jurado J, Javidfar J, Newmark A, Lavelle M, Bacchetta M, Gorenstein L, et al. Minimally invasive thymectomy and open thymectomy: outcome analysis of 263 patients. Ann Thorac Surg. 2012;94(3):974–81. PubMed PMID: 22748641; discussion 81–2. Epub 2012/07/04. eng.

8. Kimura T, Inoue M, Kadota Y, Shiono H, Shintani Y, Nakagiri T, et al. The oncological feasibility and limitations of video-assisted thoracoscopic thymectomy for early-stage thymomas. Eur J Cardiothorac Surg. 2013;44(3):e214–8. PubMed PMID: 23761417. Epub 2013/06/14. eng.

9. Ye B, Li W, Ge XX, Feng J, Ji CY, Cheng M, et al. Surgical treatment of early-stage thymomas: robot-assisted thoracoscopic surgery versus transsternal thymectomy. Surg Endosc. 2014;28(1):122–6. PubMed PMID: 23963682. Epub 2013/08/22. Eng.

10. Moore KH, McKenzie PR, Kennedy CW, McCaughan BC. Thymoma: trends over time. Ann Thorac Surg. 2001;72(1):203–7. PubMed PMID: 11465180. Epub 2001/07/24. eng.

11. Detterbeck FC, Zeeshan A. Thymoma: current diagnosis and treatment. Chin Med J (Engl). 2013;126(11):2186–91. PubMed PMID: 23769581. Epub 2013/06/19. eng.

12. Agasthian T, Lin SJ. Clinical outcome of video-assisted thymectomy for myasthenia gravis and thymoma. Asian Cardiovasc Thorac Ann. 2010;18(3):234–9. PubMed PMID: 20519290. Epub 2010/06/04. eng.

13. Cheng YJ, Hsu JS, Kao EL. Characteristics of thymoma successfully resected by videothoracoscopic surgery. Surg Today. 2007;37(3):192–6. PubMed PMID: 17342355. Epub 2007/03/08. eng.

14. He Z, Zhu Q, Wen W, Chen L, Xu H, Li H. Surgical approaches for stage I and II thymoma-associated myasthenia gravis: feasibility of complete video-assisted thoracoscopic surgery (VATS) thymectomy in comparison with trans-sternal resection. J Biomed Res. 2013;27(1):62–70. PubMed PMID: 23554796. Pubmed Central PMCID: PMC3596756. Epub 2013/04/05. eng.

15. Maggi L, Andreetta F, Antozzi C, Baggi F, Bernasconi P, Cavalcante P, et al. Thymoma-associated myasthenia gravis: outcome, clinical and pathological correlations in 197 patients on a 20-year experience. J Neuroimmunol. 2008;201–202:237–44. PubMed PMID: 18722676. Epub 2008/08/30. eng.

16. Marulli G, Rea F, Melfi F, Schmid TA, Ismail M, Fanucchi O, et al. Robot-aided thoracoscopic thymectomy for early-stage thymoma: a multicenter European study. J Thorac Cardiovasc Surg. 2012;144(5):1125–30. PubMed PMID: 22944082. Epub 2012/09/05. eng.

17. Mussi A, Fanucchi O, Davini F, Lucchi M, Picchi A, Ambrogi MC, et al. Robotic extended thymectomy for early-stage thymomas. Eur J Cardiothorac Surg. 2012;41(4):e43–6; discussion e7. PubMed PMID: 22368189. Epub 2012/03/01. eng.

18. Odaka M, Akiba T, Mori S, Asano H, Marushima H, Yamashita M, et al. Oncological outcomes of thoracoscopic thymectomy for the treatment of stages I-III thymomas. Interact Cardiovasc Thorac Surg. 2013;17(2):285–90. PubMed PMID: 23633558. Pubmed Central PMCID: PMC3715184. Epub 2013/05/02. eng.

19. Pennathur A, Qureshi I, Schuchert MJ, Dhupar R, Ferson PF, Gooding WE, et al. Comparison of surgical techniques for early-stage thymoma: feasibility of minimally invasive thymectomy and comparison with open resection. J Thorac Cardiovasc Surg. 2011;141(3):694–701. PubMed PMID: 21255798. Epub 2011/01/25. eng.

20. Ruckert JC, Ismail M, Swierzy M, Sobel H, Rogalla P, Meisel A, et al. Thoracoscopic thymectomy with the da Vinci robotic system for myasthenia gravis. Ann N Y Acad Sci. 2008;1132:329–35. PubMed PMID: 18567884. Epub 2008/06/24. eng.

21. Ruckert JC, Swierzy M, Ismail M. Comparison of robotic and nonrobotic thoracoscopic thymectomy: a cohort study. J Thorac Cardiovasc Surg. 2011;141(3):673–7. PubMed PMID: 21335125. Epub 2011/02/22. eng.

22. Savitt MA, Gao G, Furnary AP, Swanson J, Gately HL, Handy JR. Application of robotic-assisted techniques to the surgical evaluation and treatment of the anterior mediastinum. Ann Thorac Surg. 2005;79(2):450–5. PubMed PMID: 15680812; discussion 5. Epub 2005/02/01. eng.

23. Takeo S, Tsukamoto S, Kawano D, Katsura M. Outcome of an original video-assisted thoraco-scopic extended thymectomy for thymoma. Ann Thorac Surg. 2011;92(6):2000–5. PubMed PMID: 22115209. Epub 2011/11/26. eng.
24. Zielinski M, Czajkowski W, Gwozdz P, Nabialek T, Szlubowski A, Pankowski J. Resection of thymomas with use of the new minimally-invasive technique of extended thymectomy per-formed through the subxiphoid-right video-thoracoscopic approach with double elevation of the sternum. Eur J Cardiothorac Surg. 2013;44(2):e113–9; discussion e9. PubMed PMID: 23761413. Epub 2013/06/14. eng.
25. Davenport E, Malthaner RA. The role of surgery in the management of thymoma: a systematic review. Ann Thorac Surg. 2008;86(2):673–84. PubMed PMID: 18640366. Epub 2008/07/22. eng.
26. Gupta R, Marchevsky AM, McKenna RJ, Wick M, Moran C, Zakowski MF, et al. Evidence-based pathology and the pathologic evaluation of thymomas: transcapsular invasion is not a significant prognostic feature. Arch Pathol Lab Med. 2008;132(6):926–30. PubMed PMID: 18517274. Epub 2008/06/04. eng.

Chapter 54
Robotic Versus VATS Thymectomy for Encapsulated Thymoma

Federico Rea and Giuseppe Marulli

Abstract Minimally invasive thymectomy for early stage thymoma has been suggested in recent years and considered technically feasible; however, due to the lack of data on long term results, controversies still exist regarding the role of thoracoscopic approach for encapsulated thymoma resection. In addition, the introduction of robotic-assisted technologies in the last decade has provided a technical improvement able to overcome some limitations of conventional thoracoscopy and potentially increasing the accuracy and safety of thoracoscopic procedures. This has led many surgeons to consider robotic thymectomy for early stage thymoma as new standard of care comparable with transternal approach in terms of oncological results and less invasive in terms of surgical impact. Compared with standard thoracoscopy, the robotic approach has several advantages in this kind of procedure: safe and precise dissection around vascular and nervous structures, better manipulation of thymus and thymoma and better vision of the operative field with less risk of capsule breach or incomplete resection. Sternotomy remains the gold standard against which all other approaches should be evaluated and compared including video assisted thoracic surgery (VATS) and robotic procedures. The VATS and robotic approaches to thymectomy in stage I thymoma are technically sound and may be pursued by appropriately trained physicians. The available data from literature are inconclusive either regarding the oncologic value of thoracoscopic thymoma resection due to the lack of long term follow-up, either regarding the difference between robotic and VATS thymectomy being absent comparative studies, therefore no evidences nor strong recommendations may be done on this issue.

Keywords Thymoma • Thoracoscopy • Robotic thymectomy • Early stage thymoma • VATS thymectomy

F. Rea, MD (✉) • G. Marulli, MD, PhD
Thoracic Surgery Division, Department of Cardiac, Thoracic and Vascular Sciences,
University of Padova, Via Giustiniani, 2, 35100 Padova, Italy
e-mail: federico.rea@unipd.it

M.K. Ferguson (ed.), *Difficult Decisions in Thoracic Surgery*,
Difficult Decisions in Surgery: An Evidence-Based Approach 1,
DOI 10.1007/978-1-4471-6404-3_54, © Springer-Verlag London 2014

Introduction

Thymoma is the most common primary tumor in the anterior mediastinum in adults. In a relatively high percentage of cases thymomas are diagnosed in a early stage when still encapsulated and potentially resectable. A complete surgical resection with safety margins is the mainstay of treatment for early stage thymoma and represents the most important prognostic factor [1]. The transternal approach for thymectomy is universally considered the standard of care giving an optimal exposure of the operative field and allowing a safe and radical resection confined to the mediastinum without the need for opening the pleural cavity and then with reduced risk of contamination or intrathoracic dissemination of the tumor [2]. Video assisted thoracic surgery (VATS) was introduced in clinical practice in the early '90s and soon gained broad acceptance for diagnostic and therapeutic interventions on benign mediastinal diseases [3, 4]. The main recognized advantages of VATS compared with open approaches are the minimal operative trauma, lower morbidity, early improved pulmonary function, shorter hospital stays and better cosmetic results [3–5]. During past two decades, video-assisted thoracoscopic surgery (VATS) has been frequently performed for the treatment of mediastinal benign diseases or for thymectomy in cases of non-thymomatous myasthenia gravis [3, 4]. The VATS approach for thymoma still remains controversial and several surgeons are reluctant to use this technique: the supposed increased risk of local recurrence, due to reduced safety margins after minimally invasive resection, the possible rupture of the capsule and implantation of the tumor during endoscopic manipulations are frequent arguments against VATS approach. Furthermore, the lack of long-term data on survival and oncologic results, and the difficult learning curve for performing the operation are additional reasons to support any doubts regarding the effectiveness of the VATS resection of early stage thymomas [6].

The introduction of robotic-assisted technologies in the late 1990s provided a technical improvement able to overcome the limitations of conventional thoracoscopy: the three-dimensional vision system and the multiarticulated instruments of the da Vinci (Intuitive Surgical, Inc., Sunnyvale, CA, USA) Surgical Robotic System allow an intuitive, 'open-like' intervention but with minimally invasive access. The application of this technology has been tested in a variety of thoracic surgery procedures, however since the beginning it was clear that the robotic system provides its best advantages when operating in tiny and difficult to-reach anatomical regions such as the mediastinum. Therefore, the mediastinal diseases were electively selected by most surgeons for clinical research using the da Vinci Robot [7, 8]. The aim of this evidence-based chapter is to discuss and answer questions related to the following issues: (a) what is the evidence regarding the safety and the feasibility of thoracoscopic and robotic thymectomy (*intervention*) in patients affected by encapsulated thymoma with and without myasthenia gravis (*target population*) compared with standard transternal approach (*surgical approach*)?, (b) does the technological advantage of robotic instrumentation allow a significant gain in terms of extension and accuracy of resection over the standard VATS?, and (c) what is the difference between the two minimally invasive approaches when long-term oncologic results are compared (*comparison*)?.

Search Strategy

A search of the MEDLINE database was performed with the keywords "thymoma", "surgery", "VATS or thoracoscopic" and "robotic thymectomy", using the following limits: english language only, humans only, and published after 1992 (the year in which the first paper on thoracoscopic thymoma resection was published). The final literature search was performed on September 1st, 2013. In addition, current guidelines and major thoracic surgical text books were reviewed and references of included publications were screened for additional evidence.

The review of the literature regarding the role of VATS and robotic thymectomy for encapsulated thymoma and the comparison between the two surgical methods has evidenced the complete absence of randomized prospective trials. In addition, the published series are limited, almost all mono-institutional, retrospective and with few cases. Only one paper [9] compared the perioperative outcome of VATS versus robotic thymectomy for Masaoka stage I thymoma and few retrospective studies compared the VATS or robotic versus transternal approach [10–13]. This means that the quality of evidence is low or very low for most of the topics for which we addressed the questions.

Results

Safety and the Feasibility of Thoracoscopic and Robotic Thymectomy

At this time, the open transternal surgical approach is widely considered the gold standard for resection of thymoma assuring the best chances of a complete resection (*level of evidence moderate*) [1, 2]. In addition, the open approach allows a better control of the mediastinal vascular and nervous structures, thus potentially reducing the risk of major complications. However, the open approach is more aggressive and could lead to higher perioperative complications, most of all if the patients are also affected by myasthenia gravis, and prolonged hospital stay. Only a few authors have systematically reviewed the surgical results of thoracoscopic (conventional or robotic) thymectomy for early stage thymoma (Table 54.1) [3, 10–21]. The available data show that this approach could be considered technically sound and safe in the hands of appropriately trained surgeons with a very low percentage of open conversion (comparable between robotic and VATS approaches) and almost absent intraoperative vascular accidents (*level of evidence very low*). Ye et al [9] reported the only available comparative study on VATS versus robotic thymoma resection and found a significant difference in duration of pleural drainage and hospital stay in favor of the robotic procedure, while a significant decreased cost was associated with the VATS procedure. No significant differences were

Table 54.1 Review of the published studies on thoracoscopic and robotic thymectomy for early stage thymoma

Author	N° patients	SA	Masaoka stage I/II	TS (cm)	5-year survival (%)	FU (months)	RR (%)	OC (%)	OT (min)	POS (days)
Roviaro et al. [3]	22	uVATS	22	–	–	–	4.5	4.5	75[a]	6[a]
Cheng et al. [12]	44	uVATS	27/17	7.7[a]	100	34.6[a]	0	0	194[a]	7.6[a]
Odaka et al. [14]	22	uVATS	–	–	–	21.6[a]	0	0	194[a]	4.6[a]
Agasthian et al. [15]	50	uVATS	25/25	5[a]	100	58[a]	2	0	150[a]	5[a]
Pennathur et al. [11]	18	bVATS	5/13	3.5[a]	100	27[b]	0	0	–	2.9
Takeo et al. [16]	34	bVATS	15/19	5.2[a]	100	65[a]	2.8	0	219[a]	10.5[a]
Kimura et al. [17]	45	uVATS	41/4	4.8[a]	–	–	6.7	0	180[a]	14[a]
Liu et al. [13]	76	u/bVATS	57/19	4.6[a]	100	61.9[a]	2.6	1.3	142[a]	7.1[a]
Odaka et al. [18]	57	uVATS	29/28	4.3[a]	100	43[a]	1.7	0	225[a]	4[a]
Mussi et al. [19]	13	Robotic	7/6	3.3[a]	100	14.5[b]	0	7.7	139[a]	4[a]
Marulli et al. [20]	79	Robotic	30/49	3.7[a]	90	51.7[a]	1.3	1.3	165[a]	4.4[a]
Ye et al. [10]	23	Robotic	21/2	2.9[a]	–	16.9[a]	0	0	97[a]	3.7[a]
Schneiter et al. [21]	19	Robotic	8/11	4.0[b]	–	26[b]	11.1	0	–	5[b]

Legend: *SA* surgical access, *bVATS* bilateral video-assisted thoracic surgery, *uVATS* unilateral video-assisted thoracic surgery, *TS* tumor size, *FU* median follow-up, *RR* recurrence rate, *OC* open conversion, *OT* operative time, *POS* post-operative length of stay
[a]Mean value
[b]Median value

found in term of intraoperative safety with a single open conversion in VATS group and no conversion in robotic group, and in the duration of the surgical procedure. Both approaches were defined safe and sound.

Is There a Technological Advantage of Robotic Compared to VATS Thymectomy?

Many surgeons are still reluctant to undertake a VATS or robotic thymectomy in patients with thymoma for several reasons that stem from technical and oncologic concerns. The main technical reasons against VATS are the following: the upper mediastinum is a delicate and, for VATS, difficult-to-reach anatomical area, with vulnerable large vessels and nerves. The two-dimensional view of the operative field, the surgeon's tremor enhanced by the thoracoscopic instruments and the fact that the instruments do not articulate, make it difficult to operate in a fixed and tiny three-dimensional space such as the mediastinum. Moreover, the VATS thymectomy is considered a technically challenging operation requiring a long learning

curve [6]. The oncologic concerns are related to the possible breach of tumor capsule with risk of tumor seeding locally or in the pleural cavity and to the difficult
evaluation of resection margins with reduced oncologic accuracy and safety.

The introduction of robotic surgical systems has added a new dimension to conventional VATS providing additional advantages and overcoming some technical
and methodological limits: (1) the improved dexterity of instruments that can articulate with 7° of freedom and rotate 360°, allows complex three-dimensional movements superior to that permitted by conventional minimally invasive instruments,
enhancing the dissection safe around vessels and nerves and more comfortable in
tiny and remote areas such as the superior horns or the contralateral mediastinum;
(2) the high-resolution, three-dimensional real-time video image permits the best
possible and magnified view of the surgical field , and (3) the filtering of hand trem-
ors allows greater technical precision. To date, however, no studies demonstrated a
superiority of robotic approach for thymoma resection compared with standard
VATS (*level of evidence very low*). As reported in Table 54.1, the rate of open conversion, the operative time, the size of the tumor were comparable in VATS and
robotic studies. No papers focused on the percentage of capsule breaching, on the
rate of open conversion related to technical reasons and on the rate of complete
resection (*level of evidence very low*). In addition there is a significant difference
between series regarding the rate of Masaoka stage I and II, the extension of resection, the size of the tumor, the selection criteria for minimally invasive approach and
the surgical technique: some authors [20] adopted a "no-touch technique" with an
"en bloc" resection of thymus and perithymic fat tissue according to the International
Thymic Malignancy Interest Group criteria [22], while other authors [14, 23] preferred a partial thymectomy. In some studies [11, 19] a limit of 3 cm of diameter of
the tumor was established, in other series [13, 15, 18, 20] a limit of 5 cm was considered safe, while some authors [12, 16] accepted also greater size. These differences were independent of surgical approach (VATS or robotic).

Oncologic Outcomes

In a systematic review, Davenport et al. [24] reported an overall 5-year survival rate
for patients with Masaoka stage I and II thymoma, after complete surgical resection,
ranging from 89 % to 100 % and 71 to 95 %, respectively. Similar data were reported
by Detterbeck et al. [25] who found also a mean recurrence rate of 4 % and 14 % for
Masaoka stage I and II, respectively. These data are refer to a series of patients operated by transternal approach and represent the benchmark for any comparison.
When data on VATS or robotic thymectomy for early stage thymoma are analyzed,
there is a lack of evidence in the current literature supporting a minimally invasive
approach compared to a standard transternal approach (*level of evidence very low*).
In fact, data are inconclusive with regard to oncologic outcome and this is mainly
due to the long (10 years) lapse of time necessary in thymoma to evaluate the survival and relapse rate. As reported in Table 54.1, almost all studies had a mean

follow-up of less than 5 years, thus making unreliable the evaluation of the survival and recurrence rates. However, despite these limitations, the reported oncologic results for VATS and robotic thymectomy are good, in line with the open approach and comparable each other.

At the time of writing of this chapter, there exists insufficient data in the literature to make comments or specific recommendations regarding the appropriateness of approaches to thymectomy in encapsulated thymoma other than sternotomy, because objective assessments of outcome are lacking. The evidence on which we based our recommendations is very low quality (i.e., retrospective uncontrolled case series).

In the absence of definitive long term data, randomized studies or at least observational comparative studies should be undertaken in order to clarify the effective role of minimally invasive techniques and the superiority of one approach versus another. To reach this aim a standardization of the technique and common selection criteria are necessary in order to avoid biases in the evaluation of the outcome.

Recommendations

The transternal approach to thymectomy in encapsulated thymoma is still the standard surgical approach to which the minimally invasive techniques have to be compared. The VATS and robotic approaches to thymectomy in stage I thymoma are technically sound and may be pursued by appropriately trained physicians. The VATS and robotic approaches to thymectomy in stage II thymomas are experimental and should be evaluated in randomized trials. The oncologic value of thoracoscopic thymectomy in early stage thymoma is still unclear because long-term outcome data are lacking. Follow-up longer than 5 years is needed to safely evaluate the clinical results. VATS and robotic approaches to thymectomy should be reserved for encapsulated thymomas with a diameter ≤3 cm, any other indication should be evaluated only in controlled trials (Table 54.2).

Table 54.2 Specific indications for VATS or robotic thymectomy for early stage thymoma

Indication	VATS/robotic thymectomy indicated	Quality of evidence	Recommendation
Masaoka stage I (≤3 cm) thymoma	Yes	Very low	Weak
Masaoka stage I (>3 cm ≤5 cm) thymoma	Yes	Very low	Weak
Masaoka stage I (>5 cm) thymoma	Yes	Very low	Weak
Masaoka stage II (≤3 cm) thymoma	Yes	Very low	Weak
Masaoka stage II (>3 cm ≤5 cm) thymoma	Yes	Very low	Weak
Masaoka stage II (>5 cm) thymoma	No	Very low	Not recommended

VATS video assisted thoracic surgery

A Personal View of the Data

Our personal view is that robotic approach for early stage thymoma has an increased safety and oncologic effectiveness when compared with VATS: in fact, the superior dexterity of robotic instruments allows a lesser manipulation of the thymic and perithymic tissue required during operation; the better evaluation of healthy tissue, as a result of the high quality image, may lead to a more precise and low risk dissection, with wide safety margins and reduced possibility of an incautious tumor breaching, incomplete resection or iatrogenic injury.

Our policy is to perform a robotic thymectomy using these specific guidelines and selection criteria. The preferred radiological characteristics to make patients eligible for robotic thymectomy are: (a) the location of the tumor in the anterior mediastinum; (b) a distinct fat plane between the tumor and the surrounding structures; (c) unilateral tumor predominance and tumor encapsulation; (d) existence of residual normal appearing thymic tissue; (e) no mass compression effect; and (f) a diameter ≤5 cm. Our preferred surgical approach is from the left side with three ports; however in case of an evident right sided unilateral predominance of the mass a right sided procedure is carried out. The exclusion criteria for a robotic approach are: (a) radiological evidence of invasion of surrounding structures (e.g., pericardium, lung, nerves, or large vessels); (b) the presence of adhesions (e.g., previous thoracic surgery or pleuritis); (c) the inability to perform single lung ventilation; and (d) a body mass index >35. We use a "no touch technique" with an "en bloc" resection of the thymus and perithymic fat tissue according to the International Thymic Malignancy Interest Group criteria [22]. During resection the thymoma should never been touched, and normal thymic tissue and perithymic fat should be used for grasping and for traction, in order to avoid a direct manipulation of the tumor, a capsular damage and a potential tumor seeding.

Recommendations

- Transternal thymectomy is the standard surgical approach for encapsulated thymomas. (Evidence quality low; weak recommendation)
- VATS and robotic approaches for stage I thymoma are reasonable if performed by appropriately trained surgeons. (Evidence quality very low; weak recommendation)
- VATS and robotic approaches for stage II thymomas are experimental and should be evaluated in randomized trials. (Evidence quality very low; weak recommendation)
- The long-term oncologic outcomes of minimally invasive treatment of early stage thymoma are unknown. (Evidence quality low; no recommendation)

References

1. Regnard JF, Magdeleinat P, Dromer C, Dulmet E, de Montpreville V, Levi JF, Levasseur P. Prognostic factors and long-term results after thymoma resection: a series of 307 patients. J Thorac Cardiovasc Surg. 1996;112:376–84.
2. Masaoka A, Monden Y, Nakahara K, Tanioka T. Follow up study of thymomas with special reference to their clinical stages. Cancer. 1981;48:2485–92.
3. Roviaro G, Varoli F, Nucca O, Vergiani C, Maciocco M. Videothoracoscopic approach for primary mediastinal pathology. Chest. 2000;117:1179–83.
4. Yim AP. Video-assisted thoracoscopic resection of anterior mediastinal masses. Int Surg. 1996;81:350–3.
5. Ruekert JC, Walter M, Mueller JM. Pulmonary function after thoracoscopic thymectomy versus median sternotomy for myasthenia gravis. Ann Thorac Surg. 2000;70:1656–61.
6. Toker A, Erus S, Ozkan B, Ziyade S, Tanju S. Does a relationship exist between the number of thoracoscopic thymectomies performed and the learning curve for thoracoscopic resection of thymoma in patients with myasthenia gravis? Interact Cardiovasc Thorac Surg. 2011;12:152–5.
7. Bodner J, Wykypiel H, Greiner A, Kirchmayr W, Freund MC, Margreiter R, Schmid T. Early experience with robot-assisted surgery for mediastinal masses. Ann Thorac Surg. 2004;78:259–66.
8. Savitt MA, Gao G, Furnary AP, Swanson J, Gately HL, Handy JR. Application of robotic assisted techniques to the surgical evaluation and treatment of the anterior mediastinum. Ann Thorac Surg. 2005;79:450–5.
9. Ye B, Tantai JC, Li W, Ge XX, Feng J, Cheng M, Zhao H. Video-assisted thoracoscopic surgery versus robotic-assisted thoracoscopic surgery in the surgical treatment of Masaoka stage I thymoma. World J Surg Oncol. 2013;11:157.
10. Ye B, Li W, Ge XX, Feng J, Ji CY, Cheng M, Tantai JC, Zhao H. Surgical treatment of early-stage thymomas: robot-assisted thoracoscopic surgery versus transsternal thymectomy. Surg Endosc. 2014;28(1):122–6.
11. Pennathur A, Qureshi I, Schuchert MJ, Dhupar R, Ferson PF, Gooding WE, Christie NA, Gilbert S, Shende M, Awais O, Greenberger JS, Landreneau RJ, Luketich JD. Comparison of surgical techniques for early-stage thymoma: feasibility of minimally invasive thymectomy and comparison with open resection. J Thorac Cardiovasc Surg. 2011;141:694–701.
12. Cheng YJ, Kao EL, Chou SH. Videothoracoscopic resection of stage II thymoma: prospective comparison of the results between thoracoscopy and open methods. Chest. 2005;128:3010–2.
13. Liu TJ, Lin MW, Hsieh MS, Kao MW, Chen KC, Chang CC, Kuo SW, Huang PM, Hsu HH, Chen JS, Lai HS, Lee JM. Video-assisted thoracoscopic surgical thymectomy to treat early thymoma: a comparison with the conventional transsternal approach. Ann Surg Oncol. 2014;21(1):322–8.
14. Odaka M, Akiba T, Yabe M, Hiramatsu M, Matsudaira H, Hirano J, Morikawa T. Unilateral thoracoscopic subtotal thymectomy for the treatment of stage 1 and 2 thymoma. Eur J Cardiothorac Surg. 2010;37:824–6.
15. Agasthian T, Lin SJ. Clinical outcome of video-assisted thymectomy for myasthenia gravis and thymoma. Asian Cardiovasc Thorac Ann. 2010;18:234–9.
16. Takeo S, Tsukamoto S, Kawano D, Katsura M. Outcome of an original video-assisted thoracoscopic extended thymectomy for thymoma. Ann Thorac Surg. 2011;92:2000–5.
17. Kimura T, Inoue M, Kadota Y, Shiono H, Shintani Y, Nakagiri T, Funaki S, Sawabata N, Minami M, Okumura M. The oncological feasibility and limitations of video-assisted thoracoscopic thymectomy for early-stage thymomas. Eur J Cardiothorac Surg. 2013;44:214–8.
18. Odaka M, Akiba T, Mori S, Asano H, Marushima H, Yamashita M, Kamiya N, Morikawa T. Oncological outcomes of thoracoscopic thymectomy for the treatment of stages I-III thymomas. Interact Cardiovasc Thorac Surg. 2013;17:285–90.
19. Mussi A, Fanucchi O, Davini F, Lucchi M, Picchi A, Ambrogi MC, Melfi F. Robotic extended thymectomy for early-stage thymomas. Eur J Cardiothorac Surg. 2012;41:43–7.

20. Marulli G, Rea F, Melfi F, Schmid TA, Ismail M, Fanucchi O, Augustin F, Swierzy M, Di Chiara F, Mussi A, Rueckert JC. Robot-aided thoracoscopic thymectomy for early-stage thymoma: a multicenter European study. J Thorac Cardiovasc Surg. 2012;144:1125–30.
21. Schneiter D, Tomaszek S, Kestenholz P, Hillinger S, Opitz I, Inci I, Weder W. Minimally invasive resection of thymomas with the da Vinci® Surgical System. Eur J Cardiothorac Surg. 2013;43(2):288–92.
22. Toker A, Sonett J, Zielinski M, Rea F, Tomulescu V, Detterbeck FC. Standard terms, definitions, and policies for minimally invasive resection of thymoma. J Thorac Oncol. 2011;6:S1739–42.
23. Sakamaki Y, Kido T, Yasukawa M. Alternative choices of total and partial thymectomy in video-assisted resection of noninvasive thymomas. Surg Endosc. 2008;22:1272–7.
24. Davenport E, Malthaner RA. The role of surgery in the management of thymoma: a systematic review. Ann Thorac Surg. 2008;86:673–84.
25. Detterbeck FC, Parsons AM. Thymic tumors. Ann Thorac Surg. 2004;77:1860–9.

Chapter 55
Video Mediastinoscopy Versus Standard Mediastinoscopy

David J. McCormack and Karen Harrison-Phipps

Abstract Standard mediastinoscopy (SM) is a safe and established procedure for biopsy of masses and lymph nodes in the mediastinum. Technological advancements have led to video assisted mediastinoscopy (VAM). We evaluated the literature relating to the two techniques to determine if there is a clinical advantage to VAM over SM. Studies directly comparing VAM to SM are sparse and confined to non-randomized, retrospective cohort studies. Nonetheless, this literature suggests an advantage in number of lymph nodes biopsied, number of lymph node stations biopsied, sensitivity, specificity and diagnostic accuracy of VAM over SM. Complication rates associated with mediastinoscopy are low, and the literature does not convincingly demonstrate a safety advantage of VAM. In units where there is a teaching commitment we view VAM as a highly important tool. The enhanced perspective, increased visual field and the ability for an audience to see the operative field allows maximal utilization of training opportunities.

Keywords Mediastinoscopy • Videos assisted mediastinoscopy • Standard mediastinoscopy • Mediastinal lymphadenopathy • Non-small cell lung cancer staging

Introduction

Cervical mediastinoscopy is a well-established technique that facilities biopsy of mediastinal tissue in benign and malignant conditions. It resides within the clinician's armamentarium of tools to establish diagnosis of mediastinal lymphadenopathy and staging of lung cancer. In the context of lung cancer, its importance is in

D.J. McCormack, BSc (Hons) MRCS (✉)
Cardiothoracic Surgery Department, King's College Hospital, Denmark Hill, London, UK
e-mail: djmccormack@doctors.org.uk

K. Harrison-Phipps, FRCS (CTh)
Thoracic Surgery Department, Guy's Hospital, Great Maze Pond, London, UK

M.K. Ferguson (ed.), *Difficult Decisions in Thoracic Surgery*,
Difficult Decisions in Surgery: An Evidence-Based Approach 1,
DOI 10.1007/978-1-4471-6404-3_55, © Springer-Verlag London 2014

determining those patients likely to gain prognostic advantage from resection. When mediastinoscopy is indicated, systematic mediastinal lymph node sampling is advocated [1]. We examine whether the technological advance of video mediastinoscopy enhances a clinician's ability to sample mediastinal lymph nodes.

Search Strategy

We used the PICO formatted question: in [patients undergoing cervical mediastinoscopy] is [video assisted mediastinoscopy] superior to [standard mediastinopscopy] in achieving better [diagnostic success and lymph node yield] to frame our search. A Medline search limited to English Language and last 10 years was performed using the search terms (((("lymph node yield"[All Fields] OR "diagnostic success"[All Fields]) OR "sensitivity"[All Fields]) OR "specificity"[All Fields]) OR "positive predictive value"[All Fields]) OR (negative[All Fields] AND predictive[All Fields] AND value[All Fields])) AND (("mediastinoscopy"[All Fields] OR ("video assisted mediastinoscopy"[All Fields] AND ("standard mediastinoscopy"[All Fields] OR "conventional mediastinoscopy"[All Fields])))).

Results

Studies directly comparing standard mediastinoscopy to video assisted mediastinoscopy are sparse and confined to retrospective analysis of case cohorts. Notwithstanding this significant limitation, some guidance can be derived from review of the literature (Table 55.1) [2–4].

Direct Comparisons of Video Assisted and Standard Mediastinoscopy

Leschber and colleagues [3] described a retrospective analysis of 377 mediastinoscopies carried out over an 18 month period at a single center (Berlin, Germany). Eleven cases were excluded due to incomplete documentation. The authors examined the safety, lymph node yield and staging accuracy of video assisted versus standard mediastinoscopy. Local guidelines necessitated mediastinoscopy in all patients with proven non-small cell lung cancer being considered for resection. Furthermore, patients with mediastinal adenopathy or masses of unknown etiology underwent mediastinoscopy if other procedures failed to establish a diagnosis. VAM (n=234) and SM (n=132) were performed contemporaneously, with patients assigned to one procedure or another according to unit resource availability. No formal randomization took place. In proven cases of operable non-small cell lung cancer, systematic lymph node

Table 55.1 Direct comparisons of SM vs VAM

Author (year)	Study type	Patient cohort	Comparison	SM lymph node yield	VAM lymph node yield	P value	Quality of evidence
Anraku et al. 2010 [2]	Retrospective cohort study	645 procedures	Lung cancer staging	5.0 (+/− 2.8)	7.0 (+/− 3.2)	P<0.001	Low
	Single center 4 years	515 SM 140 VAM	Mean number of lymph nodes Number of stations sampled	2.6	3.6	P<0.01	
Leschber et al. 2007 [3]	Retrospective cohort study	366 procedures	Number of lymph nodes dissected	6.0 (range 3–11)	8.1 (range 3–25)	N/A	Low
	Single center 18 months	132 CM 234 VAM	Number of subcarinal lymph nodes biopsied	1.5 (range 0–3)	2.2 (range 0–7)	N/A	
Ho Cho et al. 2011 [4]	Retrospective cohort study	521 procedures	Number of lymph nodes dissected	7.13 (+/− 4.9)	8.53 (+/− 5.8)	P<0.005	Low
	Single center 2 years	222 CM 299 VAM	Number of stations sampled Number of remnant nodes at thoracotomy	2.98 (+/− 0.7) 7.67 (+/− 6.5)	3.06 (+/− 0.75) 5.05 (+/− 4.5)	NS P<0.001	

SM Standard mediastinoscopy, *VAM* video assisted mediastinoscopy

dissection was performed at thoracotomy. Histopathological data was compared between mediastinoscopy and resection specimens.

Complications occurred in 4.6 % of cases with minor bleeding (1.4 %) and recurrent laryngeal nerve palsy (2.5 %) being the most common. There was no statistically significant difference in complication rates between VAM and SM groups. Thoracotomy for lung cancer resection was performed following mediastinoscopy in 171 patients (VAM = 119, SM = 52). The authors assessed the number of lymph node stations sampled and the total number of nodes dissected. Comparison was made between histological staging at mediastinoscopy and subsequent thoracotomy to derive values of negative predictive value and accuracy for VAM and SM. Particular attention was afforded to station 7, as the only station accessible to all procedures (left or right thoracotomy, VAM and SM). The mean numbers of lymph nodes resected at VAM and SM respectively were 8.1 and 6 respectively. Sub analysis of station 7 lymph nodes revealed averages of 2.4 and 1.5 resected at VAM and SM respectively. No statistically significant differences could be demonstrated. The authors reported a negative predictive value of 0.82 for mediastinoscopy (VAM 0.83 vs SM 0.81). Accuracy for VAM was 87.9 % versus 83.8 for standard mediastinoscopy.

Anraku and colleagues [2] reported data on lymph node yield, diagnostic accuracy and safety from 645 consecutive mediastinoscopies (140 VAM vs 505 SM) performed in a single Canadian center. Sub analysis was performed according to the indication for mediastinoscopy (staging of lung cancer 500, diagnostic biopsy 145). In total eight patients suffered complications (three bleeding, wound infection one, recurrent laryngeal injury one, chyle leak one, pneumonia one, myocardial infarction one). The authors demonstrated a lower complication rate in SM than VAM (0.8 % vs 3.8 %, p = 0.04). No mortalities occurred.

Within the staging group there was no difference in the total of lymph nodes sampled at each station. However, the total number of lymph nodes samples in each case was significantly higher in the VAM group than the SM group (7.0 +/− 3.2 vs 5.0 +/− 2.8, p < 0.001). The total number of stations sampled was higher in the VAM group than the SM group (3.6 +/− 1.1 vs 2.6 +/− 1.1, p < 0.01). From the 500 patients undergoing mediastinoscopy for nodal staging of lung cancer, 61 % of patients underwent subsequent pulmonary resection with systematic lymph node dissection. Eleven of 303 patients with negative mediastinoscopy were found to have N2 disease at thoracotomy (false negative rate of 2.2 %). This was significantly more common in those undergoing SM than VAM (2.5 % vs 1.0 % respectively). Sensitivity, negative predictive value and accuracy were all higher in the VAM group but did not reach statistical significance.

A study of 551 consecutive mediastinoscopies performed in a single Korean center over a 2 year period was reported by Ho Cho et al. [4]. The authors focussed on staging of non-small cell lung cancer. They compared the number of lymph nodes dissected, stations biopsied and complication rates between SM and VAM. Thirty patients were excluded from analysis due to nodal involvement in stations 3, 5, 6, 8 or 9. From the remaining 521, 299 underwent VAM versus 222 SM. Within this series a longer operation time was demonstrated in the VAM group (56.6 +/− 14.9 min vs 44.3 +/− 15.1 min, p < 0.001). Complications occurred more frequently in the SM than VAM (3.6 % vs 1.6 %, p = 0.03). Recurrent laryngeal nerve palsy was the most common complication in both groups.

Analysis of lymph node yield revealed a higher mean number of total lymph nodes sampled in the VAM group (8.5 +/− 5.9 vs 7.1 +/− 4.9). Furthermore more lymph node stations were biopsied in the VAM group (3.1 +/− 0.7 vs 2.9 +/− 0.7). Twenty-two of 521 patients with negative mediastinoscopy were found to have N2 disease during lung resection (false negative rates: VAM 4.0 % vs SM 4.5 %, non-significant). The authors showed no significant difference in the negative predictive values or accuracies between the two techniques.

Reports Focusing on Video Assisted Mediastinoscopy Experience

Karfis and colleagues [5] retrospectively reported the outcomes of their 7 year, single center experience with VAM. Within this series 139 mediastinoscopies were performed on 138 patients (one patient underwent redo mediastinoscopy to facilitate drainage of pus following biopsy of suppurative lymph nodes at initial operation). Similarly to other studies, the cohort was sub analyzed according to the indication for VAM. Eighty-seven patients had suspected or proven lung cancer, the other 51 patients underwent VAM to establish a diagnosis for mediastinal lymphadenopathy. The mean operative time was 42 min.

The mean number of stations biopsied in the lung cancer group was 2.2 +/− 0.8. Within this group the sensitivity was 81 %, specificity 100 % and accuracy 85 %. The positive predictive value was 100 % with a negative predictive value of 59.3 %. Post thoracotomy lung staging agreed with VAM in 86 % of cases.

In the second diagnostic VAM group, a diagnosis of mediastinal lymphadenopathy was confirmed in 86 % of patients. The remaining patients had no lymphadenopathy demonstrable at VAM. The sensitivity of the procedure was 93.6 %, specificity was 100 % and accuracy 94.1 %. The positive predictive value was 100 % and negative predictive value was 57.1 %.

A report from Venissac et al. [6] in Nice described the outcomes of 240 consecutive VAMs. The mean number of biopsies in this series was 6.0 from a mean number of 2.3 lymph node stations sampled. Their mean operating time was 36.6 min. In those undergoing VAM for diagnosis of mediastinal lymphadenopathy (n = 46), a benign diagnosis was established in 39 patients. The diagnosis was confirmed in all patients in the basis of follow up and other investigations. The remaining patients had a malignant diagnosis that was not non-small cell lung cancer.

Seventy one patients had a known diagnosis of NSCLC and underwent VAM as a staging procedure. In a further 84 patients, there was no histological diagnosis before VAM, but biopsies revealed NSCLC. Nineteen patients underwent negative VAM, but had NSCLC confirmed at thoracotomy (with no lymphadenopathy confirmed at thoracotomy). The authors reported a sensitivity of 98.3 %, specificity of 100 % and diagnostic accuracy of 98.6 %.

No mortalities occurred but two major complications were reported (one case of pneumothorax and a single case of injury to the innominate artery).

Video Assisted Mediastinoscopy as a Training Tool

The combination of limited visibility and proximity to major vascular structures can make the process of teaching cervical mediastinoscopy challenging. VAM permits good visualization of the surgical field by an audience. Initially this may serve as a good introduction to the trainee surgeon, allowing them to appreciate their trainer's movements. Once this phase has passed, VAM allows the trainer to see what their trainee is doing in real time and give feedback throughout the procedure. Martin-Ucar and colleagues [7] described the learning curve of two trainee surgeons performing VAM. The authors demonstrated a rapid progression with VAM to complete lymph node dissection, independence from senior intervention and reduced operative time.

Recommendations

Mediastinoscopy is a safe, specific and sensitive tool for the establishment of a diagnosis related to mediastinal lymphadenopathy and in the nodal staging of lung cancer. Video assisted mediastinoscopy should be adopted as the gold-standard because: (1) it has a higher yield of total lymph nodes; (2) it facilitates biopsy of more lymph node stations; (3) it has comparable or better safety profile. In programs where there is a teaching commitment VAM is recommended.

A Personal View of the Data

VAM represents a technological advancement of an established safe and effective surgical technique. We find that the use of VAM allows excellent visualization through an enhanced visual field, magnification and improved light delivery. The ability to better appreciate the patient's anatomy and abnormalities permits more purposeful dissection. This is reflected in biopsy yield and safety. Multiple retrospective cohort studies support our experience of enhanced lymph node yield of VAM over SM. The safety profile of mediastinoscopy is excellent with a morbidity rate between 0.5 % and 5 %. However, there is conflicting evidence when comparing VAM to SM in this context. It is likely that the frequency of complications relates to the aggressiveness of the surgical operator's dissection.

Recommendations

- The process of training new surgeons is easier and more efficient with VAM. We find that both from the stand point of demonstrating technique and supervising junior operators, the enhanced visualization that VAM facilitates a smoother and less stressful learning curve. We strongly recommend the use of VAM to units with a training interest.
- Mediastinoscopy is a safe, specific and sensitive tool for the establishment of a diagnosis related to mediastinal lymphadenopathy and in the nodal staging of lung cancer (Evidence quality moderate; weak recommendation).
- Video assisted mediastinoscopy should be adopted as the standard approach because it has a higher yield of total lymph nodes, it facilitates biopsy of more lymph node stations, and it has comparable or better safety profile (Evidence quality low; weak recommendation).
- In programs where there is a teaching commitment VAM is recommended (Evidence quality very low; weak recommendation).

References

1. De Leyn P, Lardinois D, Van Schil PE, Rami-Porta R, Passlick B, Zielinski M, et al. ESTS guidelines for preoperative lymph node staging for non-small cell lung cancer. Eur J Cardiothorac Surg. 2007;32:1–8.
2. Anraku M, Miyata R, Compeau C, Shargall Y. Video-assisted mediastinoscopy compared with conventional mediastinoscopy: are we doing better? Ann Thorac Surg. 2010;89:1577–81.
3. Leschber G, Sperling D, Klemm W, Merk J. Does video-mediastinoscopy improve the results of conventional mediastinoscopy? Eur J Cardiothorac Surg. 2008;33:289–93.
4. Cho JH, Kim J, Kim K, Choi YS, Kim HK, Shim YM. A comparative analysis of video-assisted mediastinoscopy and conventional mediastinoscopy. Ann Thorac Surg. 2011;92:1007–11.
5. Karfis EA, Roustanis E, Beis J, Kakadellis J. Video-assisted cervical mediastinoscopy: our seven-year experience. Interact CardioVasc Thorac Surg. 2008;7:1015–8.
6. Venissac N, Alifano M, Mouroux J. Video-assisted mediastinoscopy: experience from 240 consecutive cases. Ann Thorac Surg. 2003;76:208–12.
7. Martin-Ucar AE, Chetty GK, Vaughan R, Waller DA. A prospective audit evaluating the role of video-assisted cervical mediastinoscopy (VAM) as a training tool. Eur J Cardiothorac Surg. 2004;26:393–5.

Chapter 56
Debulking for Extensive Thymoma

Panos Vardas and Thomas Birdas

Abstract Since 1981, when the Masaoka classification was described for thymic tumors, the literature describing tumor debulking for extensive thymomas (stage III-IV) consists only of retrospective case series. These studies confirmed that complete resection for extensive thymoma is the best prognostic factor. Most of the literature shows no benefit for tumor debulking over biopsy. Some of these studies report a higher survival rate for thymomas with maximum debulking followed by high dose radiation therapy. Further studies with randomized controlled trials are needed for definitive recommendations.

Keywords Thymoma • Debulking surgery • Biopsy • Survival

Introduction

Thymic epithelial neoplasms are the most common neoplasms arising from the thymus and include thymomas and thymic carcinomas. The most commonly used clinical classification is the Masaoka system [1, 2] (Table 56.1). Treatment of thymic neoplasms is multidisciplinary, but surgical resection has a dominant role. The ability to completely resect a thymoma or thymic carcinoma is determined by the extent of the tumor, including the degree of invasion and/or adhesion to contiguous structures. For thymomas staged III and IV, resectability is frequently not feasible at presentation, primarily due to the diffuse nature of the tumor and involvement of the great vessels or the heart.

P. Vardas, MD • T. Birdas, MD (✉)
Division of Cardiothoracic Surgery, Indiana University School of Medicine,
545 Barnhill Dr, EH 215, Indianapolis, IN 46202, USA
e-mail: tbirdas@iupui.edu

M.K. Ferguson (ed.), *Difficult Decisions in Thoracic Surgery*,
Difficult Decisions in Surgery: An Evidence-Based Approach 1,
DOI 10.1007/978-1-4471-6404-3_56, © Springer-Verlag London 2014

Table 56.1 Masaoka staging system of thymomas and thymic carcinomas [1, 2]

Stage I	Macroscopically and miscroscopically completely encapsulated
Stage IIa	Microscopically transcapsular invasion
Stage IIb	Macroscopically invasion into surrounding fatty tissue or grossly adherent to but not through the mediastinal pleura or pericardium
Stage IIIa	Macroscopic invasion into pericardium or lung without great vessel invasion
Stage IIIb	Macroscopic invasion into pericardium or lung with great vessel invasion
Stage IVa	Pleural or pericardial dissemination
Stage IVb	Lymphatic or hematogenous metastasis

A debulking procedure is defined as a partial resection of an unresectable tumor with the intent of enhancing the efficacy of additional therapies. Debulking is useful in a limited number of malignancies, primarily gynecological ones. The value of debulking for advanced thymoma, defined as Masaoka stages III and IV, remains unclear, as there is no definitive evidence in the literature of survival benefit with this approach.

Search Strategy

The PICO criteria around which the literature search was conducted included patients with regionally advanced thymoma and compared debulking to no surgery, evaluating for survival and quality of life. A search of Medline database was performed with the keywords "debulking" or "tumor debulking" and "thymoma" or "thymic tumor" or "thymic carcinoma". Studies in languages other than English were not included. Only papers that reported comparison of debulking versus non-surgical therapy – typically characterized as surgical biopsy alone – were included. All papers were published after 1981 (the year in which Masaoka staging system was established), and they classify the patient population based on this system. Using these criteria, only ten retrospective case series were identified, which provided the best evidence for this subject. The analysis of the results is presented in Table 56.2.

Outcomes of Debulking Surgery

Although very commonly performed, the role of tumor debulking is controversial and the majority (six out of the ten studies) reported no differences in survival. Cohen et al. [3] reported no benefit in survival from debulking surgery. Instead, there was benefit for local control of the disease with irradiation post-operatively. Curran et al. [4] confirmed no difference in survival between debulking and biopsy alone, but interestingly, showed that the benefit of debulking is the reduced size of

Table 56.2 Studies on debulking surgery for stage III and IV thymomas

Author, date (n = no of patients) / Study type (quality of evidence)	Stage	Outcomes	Comments
Cohen et al. [3], (1984) (n=23) / Retrospective, Evidence quality very low	23 patients with stage III and IV	Complete resection is the most important factor affecting long-term survival. No difference in survival between group who received radiation post-operatively or not when complete resection obtained. No survival benefit in debulking	No difference in survival with cell type. Strong indicator gross invasion of tumor into adjacent structures
Curran et al. [4], (1988) (n=103) / Retrospective, evidence quality very low	Complete resection (n=13) All followed by radiation, chemotherapy or nothing	5.3 years median follow-up showed 35 % survival	Irradiation may be value of local control
	Stage III (n=36) Stage IV (n=4) Debulking (n=15) Biopsy alone (n=13)	No difference between debulking and biopsy 5 year survival 21 %	Advantage of aggressive debulking is to reduce size of radiotherapy field
Urgesi et al. [9], (1990) (n=36) / Retrospective, evidence quality very low	Stage III debulking (n=21) Stage IVa debulking (n=15) Stage III biopsy alone (n=5) Stage IVa biopsy alone (n=4)	Patients with debulking surgery in stage III had better survival than biopsy alone and marginally better survival for patients in stage IVa	Total resection showed better results
Ciernik et al. [5], (1994) (n=31) / Retrospective, evidence quality very low	Stage III and IV (n=31) Debulking (n=15) Biopsy alone (n=16)	Tumor debulking did not improve survival 5-year survival: 61 % for stage III and 35 % for stage IV (no difference between stage IVa and IVb)	Radiation therapy for local tumor control is most effective treatment
Liu et al. [7], (2002) (n=38 with thymic carcinoma) / Retrospective, evidence quality very low	Stage III (n=13)	Debulking did not improve survival. Median survival: complete resec – 35	Resectability and stage were the main predictors of survival
	Stage IV (n=22) Complete resect (n=8) Debulking (n=7) Biopsy alone (n=23)	Median survival: complete resec – 35	Chemotherapy and radiation therapy had no significant impact in survival

(continued)

Table 56.2 (continued)

Author, date (n = no of patients) Study type (quality of evidence)	Stage	Outcomes	Comments
Akoum et al. [6], (2003) (n=27)	Stage III (n=14)	Better 5-year survival with complete resection (81 %), than bebulking or biopsy alone (44 %)	Resectability is the most important survival factor. Better survival in patients who present with myasthenia gravis (early diagnosis when tumor still resectable)
Retrospective, evidence quality very low	Stage IV (n=8)	10-year survival 16 % for both debulking and biopsy alone	
Kondo et al. [10], (2003) (n=1,320 patients with all stages of thymoma, thymic carcinoma and thymic carcinoid)	Thymoma Group:	Thymoma Group 5-year survival:	In thymomas complete resection is the most important factor of survival
Retrospective, evidence quality very low	Stage III (n=204) Stage IVa (n=73) Stage IVb (n=35)	Compete res – 93 % Debulking – 64.4 % Biopsy alone – 35.6 % (p=0.0028)	Study data from a questionnaire sent to 185 Japanese institutes (62 % replied). Risk for reporting bias
Lin et al. [11], (2004) (n=27 patients with thymomas and thymic carcinomas)	Stage III (n=16)	Overall for the thymoma patients the 5-year survival with debulking is 85 % vs 64 % with open biopsy (p=0.075)	Patients receiving debulking surgery and those with irradiation dosage higher than 4,400 cGy had better survival (p=0.021 and p=0.016, respectively)
Retrospective, evidence quality very low	Stage IVa (n=11) Debulking (n=11) Biopsy alone (n=16)		
Lin et al. [8], (2005) (n=20)	Stage IVa (n=14) Stage IVb (n=6)	No difference in the modalities: debulking with adj. chemoradiation, debulking with adj. chemotherapy, debulking with adj. radiation, radiation with adj. chemotherapy, chemotherapy alone	Histology of the tumor has an important prognostic factor. Chemotherapy and radiation are important for patients with advance stage or relapsed disease
Retrospective, evidence quality very low			
Liu et al. [12], (2006) (n=43)	Stage III (n=22)	Debulking survival better than biopsy alone (107 vs 57 months, p=0.03)	Survival did not differ based on tumor stage
Retrospective, evidence quality very low	Stage IVa (n=21) Debulking (n=15) Biopsy alone (n=28)	5 year survival 71 % vs 35 %	Benefit from maximal debulking resection and surgically assisted mapping and adjuvant radiotherapy

radiotherapy target, which can protect the adjacent organs from irradiation complications. Ciernik et al. [5] in a retrospective study from 1994 showed that in a series of 31 patients with stage III and IV thymomas there was no 5 or 10-year survival benefit for debulking surgery over biopsy alone. In that series, larger tumors (>10 cm) had a worse prognosis, and radiation for local control seemed to be beneficial. Their results were in accordance with other three reports. Akoum et al. [6] failed to show survival benefit of debulking over biopsy; instead, complete resection had a survival benefit (5-year survival of 81 %). Patients with myasthenia gravis had better outcome due to early diagnosis when the tumor was still amenable to complete resection. Liu et al. in 2002 [7] and Lin et al. in 2005 [8] reported no benefit in survival of debulking surgery for thymic carcinoma. Interestingly, Lin showed that the tumor histology was an important prognostic factor, with the lymphoepithelioma-like type to be the most favorable and the non-differentiated tumors being the most biologically aggressive.

On the other hand, Urgesi et al. [9] showed that debulking surgery offered a survival benefit compared to biopsy for stage III thymoma ($p < 0.01$) in a retrospective study of 36 patients. The benefit of tumor debulking for stage IV disease was marginal. Kundo et al. [10] reported the largest number of patients in a study (n = 1320) and showed a survival benefit of tumor debulking over biopsy. Unfortunately, data were extrapolated from a questionnaire which was sent to 185 institutions in Japan, and only 62 % replied. In this case, the potential for reporting bias is large and the survival results should be interpreted accordingly. Similarly, two reports in recent years [11, 12] showed a 5-year survival benefit of debulking surgery over biopsy (85 % and 71 % respectively). In both of these studies the patients underwent adjuvant radiation therapy post-operatively, and high dosage irradiation was recommended [11].

Discussion

Although advances in the treatment of thymomas have occurred in the last two decades, there is little definitive evidence to inform best clinical practice.

The treatment of thymomas includes surgery, radiation, and chemotherapy. These modalities may be combined. The determination of which combination is chosen is reflected mostly by the stage of the disease. In case of extensive thymomas, surgery alone is seldom feasible and chemotherapy and/or radiation are often used as induction or adjuvant treatments. The current literature shows that the most important factor for survival after thymoma surgery is complete resection with negative resection margins. If a complete resection cannot be establish at the time of surgery, some authors have proposed a maximum tumor debulking procedure for extensive thymomas (Masaoka stages III–IV).

Overall, in patients with stage III or IV thymoma, complete surgical resection is the main predictive factor of outcome and survival. When complete resection is not feasible, the literature does not convincingly demonstrate that debulking surgery alone increases survival. Some data support debulking with high dose irradiation for improved survival. However, there is significant variability in the use of adjuvant treatments, both within and between individual studies, and the underlying data are very methodologically weak. This makes it extremely difficult to draw solid conclusions regarding the most valid treatment.

Extensive and high dose irradiation has its own complications. Maximum debulking minimizes the target for irradiation, decreases the damage to the surrounding tissues and overall benefits the patient.

A Personal View of the Data

The authors' preference in these complex patients involves a multidisciplinary approach, frequently with induction chemotherapy before an attempted resection [13]. Typically, preoperative imaging can identify patients with likely invasion of adjacent structures that might benefit from this approach. We are fairly aggressive in trying to achieve a complete resection, and do not hesitate to resect and reconstruct the central veins, resect pulmonary parenchyma, and sacrifice one of the phrenic nerves if involved with tumor. We believe that even patients with stage IVa disease may potentially benefit from an attempt to achieve a complete resection. Patients with pleural metastases typically require en bloc extrapleural pneumonectomy along with anterior mediastinal resection. Our preferred surgical approach in these challenging cases involves a sternotomy followed by an ipsilateral thoracotomy. Obviously, careful patient selection is paramount. In cases where surgical margins are microscopically positive or even a small volume of residual gross tumor is unavoidable, we utilize postoperative radiation therapy if it can be offered without excessive risk.

> **Recommendation**
>
> • If complete resection of extensive thymoma is not possible, tumor debulking followed by targeted adjuvant radiotherapy may be considered [evidence quality low; weak recommendation]. The effect of this approach on survival is unclear.

References

1. Masaoka A, Monden Y, Nakahara K, Tanioka T. Follow-up study of thymomas with special reference to their clinical stages. Cancer. 1981;48(11):2485–92.
2. NCCN Guidelines: thymomas and thymic carcinomas http://www.nccn.org/professionals/physician_gls/pdf/thymic.pdf2013 [10/15/2013].

3. Cohen DJ, Ronnigen LD, Graeber GM, Deshong JL, Jaffin J, Burge JR, et al. Management of patients with malignant thymoma. J Thorac Cardiovasc Surg. 1984;87(2):301–7.
4. Curran Jr WJ, Kornstein MJ, Brooks JJ, Turrisi 3rd AT. Invasive thymoma: the role of mediastinal irradiation following complete or incomplete surgical resection. J Clin Oncol. 1988;6(11):1722–7.
5. Ciernik IF, Meier U, Lutolf UM. Prognostic factors and outcome of incompletely resected invasive thymoma following radiation therapy. J Clin Oncol. 1994;12(7):1484–90.
6. Akoum R, Brihi E, Chammas S, Abigerges D. Results of radiation therapy for thymoma based on a review of 27 patients. Mol Immunol. 2003;39(17–18):1115–9.
7. Liu HC, Hsu WH, Chen YJ, Chan YJ, Wu YC, Huang BS, et al. Primary thymic carcinoma. Ann Thorac Surg. 2002;73(4):1076–81.
8. Lin JT, Wei-Shu W, Yen CC, Liu JH, Chen PM, Chiou TJ. Stage IV thymic carcinoma: a study of 20 patients. Am J Med Sci. 2005;330(4):172–5.
9. Urgesi A, Monetti U, Rossi G, Ricardi U, Casadio C. Role of radiation therapy in locally advanced thymoma. Radiother Oncol. 1990;19(3):273–80.
10. Kondo K, Monden Y. Therapy for thymic epithelial tumors: a clinical study of 1,320 patients from Japan. Ann Thorac Surg. 2003;76(3):878–84; discussion 884–5.
11. Lin CS, Kuo KT, Hsu WH, Huang BS, Wu YC, Hsu HS, et al. Managements of locally advanced unresectable thymic epithelial tumors. J Chin Med Assoc. 2004;67(4):172–8.
12. Liu HC, Chen YJ, Tzen CY, Huang CJ, Chang CC, Huang WC. Debulking surgery for advanced thymoma. Eur J Surg Oncol. 2006;32(9):1000–5.
13. Okereke IC, Kesler KA, Morad MH, Mi D, Rieger KM, Birdas TJ, et al. Prognostic indicators after surgery for thymoma. Ann Thorac Surg. 2010;89(4):1071–7; discussion 1077–9.

Chapter 57
Surgery for Palmar Hyperhidrosis: Patient Selection and Extent of Surgery

Mario Santini and Alfonso Fiorelli

Abstract Video-thoracoscopic sympathectomy is an effective therapy for patients with severe primary palmar hyperhidrosis who are reaching the latter part of their teenage years. However, the best level, the extent of sympathectomy, and the optimal technique used to interrupt the sympathetic chain remain subjects of debate. Our review shows that single resection should be preferred to multiple levels of resection. In cases of isolated palmar hyperhidrosis, T3 is the level of choice, although T4 may be also reasonable. All procedures have similar outcomes, but sympathicotomy may be preferred because it is more simple and less extensive than others.

Keywords Palmar • Hyperhidrosis • Excessive sweating • Surgery • Thoracoscopy • Sympathectomy • Sympathicotomy • Sympathotomy • Clipping • Ramicotomy

Introduction

Primary palmar hyperhidrosis (PH) is an excessive eccrine sweat production that often results in serious disruption of a patient's social and occupational behavior. It is a condition of unknown origin that begins in childhood, occurs in adolescence, and without specific treatment persists throughout life. Medical management is not very effective, often leading many patients to try multiple unsuccessful treatment modalities. Advances in video-assisted thoracoscopic surgery have allowed video-thoracoscopic sympathectomy (VTS) to become a viable first-line therapy for PH, but at present significant controversy remains regarding the best operation as suggested by recent reviews [1, 2], a Cochrane protocol [3] and an Expert Consensus

M. Santini, MD (✉) • A. Fiorelli, MD, PhD
Chirurgia Toracica, Seconda Università di Napoli, Piazza Miraglia, due, I-80138 Napoli, Italy
e-mail: mario.santini@unina2.it

M.K. Ferguson (ed.), *Difficult Decisions in Thoracic Surgery*,
Difficult Decisions in Surgery: An Evidence-Based Approach 1,
DOI 10.1007/978-1-4471-6404-3_57, © Springer-Verlag London 2014

Report [4]. The best level for sympathectomy, the extent of surgery, and the optimal technique used to interrupt the sympathetic chain remain the subjects of debate in relation to the treatment efficacy and the limitation of unwanted side-effects, especially compensatory hyperhidrosis (CH), the most frequent and feared complication. The goal of the present chapter is to provide answers for such issues.

Search Strategy

In a patients with PH, what is the best level, the proper extent, and the optimal surgical technique to obtain resolution of symptoms and limit CH? To identify all scientific literature that addressed such issues, a search was done on PubMed, EMBASE and Cochrane databases using the following terms: palmar, palm, hand, hyperhidrosis, excessive sweating, surgery, thoracoscopy, sympathectomy, sympathicotomy, sympathotomy, clipping, ramicotomy, and clinical outcomes. The time frame was restricted to articles published in the last decade (from January 2003 to July 2013). Cited references of review articles on PH treatment were manually examined to find additional articles not found in the computerized databases. Additional articles were identified from reference lists of selected articles. Clinical end-points of interest were defined a priori and included both operative and longitudinal outcomes of procedural success, long-term recurrence of symptoms, patient satisfaction with the operation and perceived quality of life, and adverse events. Non-English language papers, case reports, abstracts only, letters, reviews, incomplete reports (studies that did not specify more than one outcomes of interest among sympathectomy for PH) and unpublished data were excluded. In addition, studies were excluded if (i) the population studied included patients with secondary PH in the setting of other medical conditions or (ii) if sympathectomy was performed for other reasons, such as refractory angina pectoris, Buerger's disease, and Raynaud's phenomenon. More than 350 English language abstracts were found using the search criteria above reported; of these, 62 papers were selected for the present review and divided in three groups as follows: papers reporting clinical outcomes after single or multiple levels of VTS (Table 57.1); papers comparing the results of different levels of VTS (Table 57.2); and papers evaluating the outcomes of different VTS procedures (Table 57.3).

Results

Overview

Only a small percentage of patients with PH should be considered for surgery. Careful patient selection and preoperative counseling are important to ensure a satisfactory outcome. When evaluating a candidable patient for VTS, it is important

Table 57.1 Single or multiple levels of surgery for palmar hyperhidrosis

Author	Year	N	Procedure	F/U	Success	Recurrence	CH	Severe CH	Satisfied	Grade
Neumayer et al. [5]	2003	6	T2 sympathectomy	5.2	100 %	0	n/a	n/a	100 %	Low
Schick et al. [6]	2003	61	T2 sympathectomy	3	98 %	n/a	n/a	n/a	n/a	Low
Atkinson et al. [7]	2003	10	T2 sympathicotomy	5.6	95 %	n/a	80 %	0	100 %	Low
Lladò et al. [8]	2005	27	T2 sympathectomy	17	100 %	n/a	89 %	n/a	n/a	Low
Ting et al. [9]	2005	13	T2 sympathectomy	1	100 %	0	92 %	n/a	100 %	Low
Eisenach et al. [10]	2005	10	T2 sympathotomy	n/a	100 %	0	70 %	0	100 %	Low
Miller and Force [11]	2007	15	T2 sympathectomy	15	99 %	6.6 %	40 %	1	98 %	Low
Leis et al. [12]	2010	4	T2 sympathectomy	n/a	100 %	0	100 %	50 %	n/a	Moderate
Atkinson et al. [13]	2011	155	T2 sympathectomy	40.2	96 %	3 %	68 %	1 %	n/a	Moderate
Lin and Chou [14]	2004	102	T2 block	37	100 %	0	84 %	1 %	98 %	Moderate
Yoon et al. [15]	2003	3	T3 sympathicotomy	19.7	100 %	0	0	0	100 %	Low
Doolabh et al. [16]	2004	86	T3 sympathectomy	17	100 %	2 %	76 %	2 %	94 %	Low
Dewey et al. [17]	2006	60	T3 sympathectomy	12	n/a	n/a	81 %	11 %	n/a	Low
Weksler et al. [18]	2007	96	T3 sympathicotomy	18	99 %	n/a	71 %	3 %	97 %	Low
Lima et al. [19]	2008	57	T3 sympathectomy	1	100 %	n/a	58 %	0	100 %	Low
Fiorelli et al. [20]	2010	18	T3 sympathectomy	12	100 %	94 %	11 %	0	n/a	Low
Zhu et al. [21]	2013	14	Transumbilical thoracic T3 sympathectomy	11	100 %	0	16 %	n/a	100 %	Low
Chou et al. [22]	2005	84	T4 sympathectomy	18–42	100 %	0	2.3 %	0	100 %	Moderate
Baumgartner and Toh [23]	2003	309	T2–T3 sympathectomy	0.15	98 %	0.6 %	45 %	1 %	n/a	Moderate
Loscertales et al. [24]	2004	113	T2–T3 Sympathectomy	12	100 %	0	67 %	19 %	95 %	Moderate
de Campos et al. [25]	2005	51	T2–3 sympathectomy	12.8	90 %	n/a	96 %	72 %	n/a	Low
Sihoe et al. [26]	2007	31	T2–3 sympathectomy	0.25	100 %	0	26 %	n/a	96 %	Low
Jegenathan et al. [27]	2008	66	T2–T3 Sympathicotomy	51	98 %	4.5 %	n/a	n/a	n/a	Moderate
Little [28]	2004	31	T2–3 sympathectomy	31.2	100 %	n/a	32 %	6 %	n/a	Low

(continued)

Table 57.1 (continued)

Author	Year	N	Procedure	F/U	Success	Recurrence	CH	Severe CH	Satisfied	Grade
Georghiou et al. [29]	2004	176	T2–3 sympathectomy	6	96 %	n/a	79 %	0 %	96 %	Low
Moya et al. [30]	2006	918	T2–3 sympathectomy	18	99 %	0.2 %	48 %	n/a	88 %	Moderate
Gossot et al. [31]	2003	125	T2–4 sympathicotomy	45.6	91 %	8 %	86 %	7 %	93 %	Moderate
Coveliers et al. [32]	2013	36	Robotic T2–T4 ramicotomy	24	100 %	n/a	8 %	n/a	n/a	Low
Apiliogullari et al. [33]	2012	43	Single port T3–4 sympathectomy	14	100 %	6 %	6 %	n/a	93 %	Low
Prasad et al. [34]	2010	322	T3–4 sympathectomy	24	100 %	0.9 %	63 %	4 %	80 %	Moderate

Legend: *n/a* not available, *F/U* follow-up, *CH* compensatory hyperhidrosis

Table 57.2 Comparison of different levels of surgery for palmar hyperhidrosis

Author	Year	N	Procedure	F/U	Success	Recurrence	CH	Severe CH	Satisfied	Grade
Schmidt et al. [35]	2006	117	T2-4 sympathectomy	24	93 % (all patients)	0.8 %	17 %	6 % (all patients)	92 % (all patients)	Moderate
		61	T3-5 sympathectomy			0	4 % $p<0.05$			
Sugimura et al. [36]	2007	399	T2 clipping	10.4	95 % (all patients)	0.6 % (all patients)	n/a	15 %	74 %	Moderate
		55	T2+3 clipping					24 %	62 %*	
		273	T3+4 clipping					8 %* $*p<0.01$	85 % $*p<0.05$	
Reisfeld et al. [37]	2006	618	T2-3 clipping	17.9	99 %	n/a	90 %	8 %	93 %	Moderate
		656	T3-4 clipping	8.2	99 %		95 %	2 % $p<0.001$	98 %	
Chou et al. [38]	2006	25	T4 sympathectomy	17–35	n/a	0	0	0	100 %	Moderate
		54	T2 clipping			0	42 %	16 %	83 %	
		33	T3 clipping			0	27 %	9 %	91 %	
		324	T4 clipping			0	0	0.6 %	99 %	
		28	T5 clipping			0	0	0	100 %	
Yazbek et al. [39]	2009	30	T2 sympathectomy	20	100 %	0 %	100 %	43 %	100 %	Low
		30	T3 sympathectomy		96 %	0 %	100 %	13 % $p=0.007$	100 %	
Baumghartner et al. [40]	2011	61	T2 sympathicotomy	24	95 %	1 %	75 %	7 %	100 %	Moderate
		60	T3 sympathicotomy		95 %	4 %	58 %	6 %	97 %	
Lin et al. [41]	2006	131	T3 sympathectomy	1	100 %	0	5 %	1 %	100 %	Moderate
		207	T2-4 sympathectomy		100 %	0	28 %	10 %	96 %	
		60	T3-4 sympathectomy		100 %	0	6 %	3 %	100 %	
Miller et al. [42]	2009	179	T2 sympathectomy	26	99 % (all patients)	0.3 % (all patients)	13 %	n/a	99 %	Moderate
		103	T2-4 sympathectomy				34 % $p=0.01$		96 %	

(continued)

Table 57.2 (continued)

Author	Year	N	Procedure	F/U	Success	Recurrence	CH	Severe CH	Satisfied	Grade
Lee et al. [43]	2004	64	T2 sympathicotomy	9.7	93 %	n/a	73 %	43 %	78 %	Moderate
		83	T3 ramicotomy	6.6	68 %		49 %	15 %	68 %	
							p<0.0001	p=0.01		
Chang et al. [44]	2007	86	T2 sympathectomy	47.1	n/a	25 %*	92 %	6 %	6.3 %*	Moderate
		78	T3 sympathectomy			7 %*	92 %	6 %	7.8 %	
		70	T4 sympathectomy			22 %	80 %*	3 %*	7.9 %	
						*p=0.008	*p=0.03	*p<0.001	*p<0.001	
Mahdy et al. [45]	2008	20	T2 sympathectomy	13	90 %	10 %	60 %	n/a	60 %	Low
		20	T3 sympathectomy		95 %	5 %	45 %	n/a	75 %	
		20	T4 sympathectomy		100 %	0	10 %*	n/a	100 %	
							*p=0.001			
Kim et al. [46]	2010	56	T3 sympathicotomy	22.5	94 %	1 %	82 %	3 %	85 %	Moderate
		63	T4 sympathicotomy	21.5	19 %	3 %	17 %	0	92 %	
							P<0.01			
Liu et al. [47]	2009	68	T3 sympathycotomy	17.8	100 %	n/a	77 %	n/a	24 %	Moderate
		73	T4 sympathycotomy		100 %		56 % p=0.01		58 % p<0.0001	
Ishy et al. [48]	2011	20	T3 sympathectomy	12	100 %	n/a	100 %	5 %	n/a	Low
		20	T4 sympathectomy		100 %		75 %	5 %		
							p=0.04			
Wolosker et al. [49]	2008	35	T3 sympathectomy	6	97 %	74 %	100 %	11 %	25	Low
		35	T4 sympathectomy		94 %	17 %	71 %	0	23 (quality of life)	
Yang et al. [50]	2007	78	T3 sympathicotomy	13.8	100 %	0	23 %	0	n/a	Moderate
		85	T4 sympathicotomy		100 %	0	7 %	0		
							p<0.05			
Neumayer et al. [51]	2004	91	T2-4 sympathicotomy	22.1	86 %	n/a	55 %	5 %	80 %	Moderate
		53	T4 clipping	7.5	100 %		8 %	0	100 %	
					p=0.01		(p=0.0002)			

Author	Year	N	Procedure							
Weksler et al. [52]	2009	112	T2 or T3 sympathicotomy	20.9	n/a	n/a	74.%	n/a	96 %	Low
		88	T2–4 or T3–4 sympathicotomy				84.1 %		89 %	
Yoon and Rim [53]	2003	30	T3 sympathicotomy	16.6	100 %	0	16 %	n/a	100 %	Low
		24	T2–3 sympathicotomy	17.8	100 %	0	45 %		91 %	
							p=0.02			
Yano et al. [54]	2005	41	T2 sympathectomy	24	85 %	19 %	90 %	43 %	75 %	Low
		39	T2–3 sympathectomy		100 %	3 %	100 %	76 %	71 %	
Li et al. [55]	2008	115	T2–4 sympathectomy	12	100 %	0	28 %	9 %	89 %	Moderate
		117	T3 sympathectomy		100 %	0	21 %	3 %	96 %	
								p<0.05	p<0.05	
Aoki et al. [56]	2013	25	T2 or T3 sympathectomy	20.3	n/a	n/a	100 %	n/a	n/a	Low
		27	T2–3 sympathectomy	55.3						
Katara et al. [57]	2007	14	T2–3 (right)–T2 (left) sympathectomy	23	100 %	0	80 %	0	100 %	Moderate
		11	T2–3 (left)–T2 (right) sympathectomy		100 %	0	80 %	0	100 %	
Turhan et al. [58]	2011	29	T2–T3 sympathicotomy	20.82	100 %	3 %	86 %	6 %	97 %	Low
		49	T3 sympathicotomy		95 %	2 %	79 %	6 %	96 %	

Legend: *n/a* not available, *F/U* follow-up, *CH* compensatory hyperhidrosis

Table 57.3 Comparison of different surgical procedures for palmar hyperhidrosis

Author	Year	N	Procedure	F/U	Success	Recurrence	CH	Severe CH	Satisfied	Levels
Lee et al. [43]	2004	64	T2 sympathicotomy	9.7	93 %	n/a	73 %	43 %	78 %	Moderate
		83	T3 ramicotomy	6.6	68 %		49 %	15 %	68 %	
							p<0.0001	p=0.01		
Cho et al. [59]	2003	13	T2–T4 ramicotomy	6	n/a	21 %	90 %	54 %	n/a	Low
		13	T2–4 sympathicotomy			6 %	100 %	92 %		
Hwang et al. [60]	2013	43	T3 sympathicotomy	12	82 %	n/a	80 %	8 %	91 %	Low
		43	T2–3 ramicotomy		25 %		95 %	14 %	79 %	
Chou et al. [38]	2006	25	T4 sympathectomy	17–35	n/a	0	0	0	100 %	Moderate
		54	T2 clipping			0	42 %	16 %	83 %	
		33	T3 clipping			0	27 %	9 %	91 %	
		324	T4 clipping			0	0	0.6 %	99 %	
		28	T5 clipping			0	0	0	100 %	
Neumayer et al. [51]	2004	91	T2–4 sympathicotomy	22.1	86 %	n/a	55 %	5 %	80 %	Moderate
		53	T4 clipping	7.5	100 %		8 %	0	100 %	
					p=0.01		(p=0.0002)			
Findikcioglu et al. [61]	2013	28	T3 sympathectomy	33	93 %	19 %	71 %	7 %	83 %	Low
		32	T3 clipping		100 %	6 % p=0.01	71 %	9 %	86 %	
Inan et al. [62]	2007	20	T2–4 resection	35	19	0	15 %	n/a	95 %	Low
		20	T2–4 ablation		20	0	25 %		100 %	
		20	T2–4 resection + ablation		18	0	15 %		95 %	
		20	T2–4 clipping		19	0	25 %		90 %	
Yanagihara et al. [63]	2011	84	T3 sympathectomy	12	100 %	n/a	87 %	4 %	95 %	Moderate
		68	T3 clipping		100 %				97 %	

Study	Year	n	Extent	F/U						
Scognamillo et al. [64]	2011	24	T2–4 sympathectomy	12	100 %	13 %	33 %	0	96 %	Low
		43	T2–4 sympathectomy	12	95 %	0	26 %	0	100 %	
		15	T3–4 sympathictomy or clipping	30.6	100 %	5 %	29 %	0	100 %	
Assalia et al. [65]	2007	32	T2–3 sympathectomy	48	100 %	0	73 % (all patients)	n/a	n/a	Low
		32	T2–3 sympathicotomy		100 %	3 %				
Fiorelli et al. [66]	2012	21	T2–3 sympathectomy	6	100 %	0	4 %	0	100 %	Low
		21	T2–3 sympathicotomy		100 %	0	0	0	100 %	Low

Legend: *n/a* not available, *F/U* follow-up, *CH* compensatory hyperhidrosis

to determinate through clinical history, physical examination, and appropriate laboratory tests if hyperhidrosis is primary or secondary in origin, focal or generalized, the anatomic location (single or multiple sites), the severity, and any contraindications to surgery. Detailed quality of life assessment tests and/or tests quantifying sweat produce (Iodine test, Gravimetric test, etc.) are not routinely performed in clinical practice, yet they may helpful in making the diagnosis and/or in directing surgical treatment in selected cases. Finally, patients should also be told of the success and failure rates, and long-term results.

The bulk of the randomized trials and non-randomized comparisons identified the "ideal candidates" for VTS as those who have onset of hyperhidrosis at an early age (usually before 16 years of age), are reaching the latter part of their teenage years at the time of surgery (usually >18 years old), have an appropriate body mass index (<28), report no sweating during sleep, are relatively healthy (no other significant co-morbidities), and do not have bradycardia (resting heart rate <55 beats per minute) [4].

Choice of Level

Once the decision is made for VTS, one main question is: at what level should we perform surgery? For many years, it was believed that the ideal treatment for PH would be sympathectomy at T2, because it was thought that the T2 ganglion was the only one responsible for sympathetic innervation of the upper limbs [5–14]. Subsequently, Lin and Telaranta [67] proposed that CH could be secondary to the interruption of the afferent fibers to the anterior part of the hypothalamus. Since the interruption of the interganglionic T3-T4 trunk did not abolish the sympathetic tone to the hypothalamus, and given that most of the fibers for the hand originate from T4, the best level of section to achieve good results in terms of efficiency and lower CH rate was exactly between T3-T4. Thus, various levels of the procedure from T2 to T4 were performed in recent years [15–34] and several papers showed a correlation between the severity of CH and higher resection levels.

Schmidt et al. [35] demonstrated that changing the sympathectomy level from T2-4 to T3-5 decreased CH from 19.1 to 4.9 % (p < 0.05). Dewey et al. [17] evaluated 222 patients, of whom 60 had PH. The level of sympathectomy depended upon clinical symptoms: T2 for face/scalp, T3 for palmar, and T4 for axillary hyperhidrosis, or a combination of levels for multiarea sweating. Compared with those with other levels, patients with a T2 lesion were significantly more likely to have severe CH (48.8 % versus 16.1 %; p < 0.001) and lower degree of satisfaction. Sugimura et al. [36] evaluated 727 patients with hyperhidrosis, of whom 538 suffered from PH. The level of sympathetic clipping was T2 in 399, T2-3 in 55, and T3-4 in 273 cases. When compared with T2 or T2–3 levels, clipping at the T3-4 levels was associated with a higher satisfaction rate (p < 0.01), and a lower rate of severe CH (p < 0.05). Similarly, Reisfled et al. [37] found that clamping at T3-T4 level had higher rate of success and a lower risk of severe CH compared to T2-T3 levels. Thus, if surgery is required at T2 or T3 levels, Chou et al. [38] strongly recommended the clipping method because of its potential reversibility. The main limit of these papers [17, 35–38] is that the level of sympathectomy depended upon clinical symptoms: T2 for face/scalp, T3 for palmar hyperhidrosis, and T4 for axillary hyperhidrosis, or a combination of levels for multiarea sweating. Thus, in theory the location of the primary sweating rather than the level of resection may affect the outcomes.

Other studies including patients having only PH confirmed that T2 resection resulted in a higher incidence and more degree of CH than lower levels. Yazbeck et al. [39] evaluated T2 (n=30) versus T3 (n=30) sympathectomy. The T3 group presented a lower degree of CH in the assessment 1 month (p<0.001), 6 months (p=0.033), and 20 months (p=0.007) after the operation. Baumgartner et al. [40] in T2 sympathicotomy group (n=61) found a higher incidence of CH than in T3 group (95 % versus 58 %, respectively). Similar results were reported by other authors [41–43]. Chang et al. [44] retrospectively compared the results of T2 (n=86); T3 (n=78), and T4 (n=70) sympathectomy. All three levels of sympathectomy achieved comparable improvement of PH (p=0.1). The T4 group had the lowest incidence of CS (p=0.03), presented the least severity of CS (p=0.002); and felt the least palmar over dryness (p<0.001). However, the T3 and T4 group had a similar level of satisfaction. Mahdy et al. [45] compared T2; T3; and T4 sympathectomy (20 patients in each group). Treatment success was 90 % for T2; 95 % for T3; and 100 % for T4 groups. In the T2 (60 %) and T3 (45 %) groups a higher incidence of CH was observed than in T4 (10 %; p=0.01). The CH was mild in T4 group, whereas moderate and/or severe CH was more common in the T2 and T3 groups. All patients in the T4 group were satisfied, while 40 % of T2 and 25 % of T3 were unsatisfied with their operation. Kim et al. [46] compared T3 (n=56) versus T4 (n=63) sympathectomy. Both procedures had similar success but T4 sympathectomy resulted in less CH than T3 (82.5 % versus 17.9 %; p<0.01). Liu et al. [47] evaluated T3 (n=68) versus T4 (n=73) sympathicotomy. The success was 100 % in both groups but the incidence of CH and overly dry hands were both lower in the T4 than in the T3 group (56.5 % versus 77.4 %, p=0.011 and 1.4 % versus 12.9 %, p=0.013, respectively). The "very satisfied" rate was higher in T4 than in the T3 group (p<0.0001) while the "partially satisfied" rate was similar between two groups. Ishy et al. [48] reported similar success for T3 versus T4 sympathectomy but the incidence of CH was higher in the T3 than in the T4 group (100 % versus 74 %; p=0.047). These results were also corroborated by Wolosker et al. [49] and Yang et al. [50].

Single or Multiple Levels of Resection

The need for a combined approach towards the T2 and T3 ganglia has been based on the description of the Kuntz nerve (postganglionic fibers that would go from the T2 or T3 to the brachial plexus). For this reason, in the past some authors have advocated sympathectomy including T2-T3 levels while others proposed more extensive approach going from T2 to T4. Then, several studies reported on the relationship between the extent of thoracic sympathectomy and the severity of CH with a growing consensus that limiting the extent of sympathectomy maximized patient satisfaction and minimized the risk of severe CS [31, 51–58].

Neumayer et al. [51] found that the degree of satisfaction was greater in patients treated at single level than in those treated at multiple levels (100 % versus 80 %), but especially in the first group the incidence of CH was much lower (8 % vs. 52 %). Gossot et al. [31] reported CH rates of 72.2 % in the T2-T4 group and 70.9 % in the T4 group, but severe CH able to influence normal daily activities was described in 27 % of patients in the first group and in 13 % in the second group. Weksler et al. [52] showed that patients with more than one ganglion transected demonstrated a trend toward a higher incidence of CH, a significantly higher CH score, and were more dissatisfied with VTS. Age, surgery on T2, and high CH score were independent predictors of patient's dissatisfaction. A trial comparing T2-T3 (n=24) versus T3 (n=30) sympathicotomy was reported by Yoon et al. [53] The success rate was 100 % in both group. CH was higher in the T2-T3 group than the T3 group (45 % versus 16 %; p=0.034). 86.7 % of the T3 group and 66.7 % of the T2-T3 group were satisfied with their operation (p=0.03). Yano et al. [54] compared T2-T3 (n=39) versus T2 sympathectomy. All patients experienced early relief of their symptoms. The recurrence rates at 2 years were 3 and 19 % in the T2-3 group and the T2 groups, respectively. CH was observed in 100 % (T2-3 group) and 90 % (T2 group); the incidence of severe CH was 76 and 49 % in the T2-T3 and in the T2 groups, respectively. Li et al. [55] compared T3 (n=117) versus T2-4 (n=115) sympathectomy. The incidence of severe CH was significantly lower in the T3 versus the T2-4 group (3 % versus 10 %; p<0.05). As for satisfaction rate, group T3 was superior to group T2-4 (96.6 % versus 89.6 %, p<0.05). Aoki et al. [56] confirmed that VTS at a single level compared to two levels reduced the incidence and the severity of CH. Katara et al. [57] and Turhan et al. [58] reported no difference in terms of outcome, recurrence, CH, and satisfaction between single and multiple levels, validating that preserving the T2 ganglion was safe and did not compromise the effectiveness of the procedure.

Type of Denervation

The technique of sympathetic denervation has been modified during the last decade, with a trend towards minimizing the extent of surgery from open to minimally invasive approaches, and from resection of ganglion to ablation (sympathectomy), transection (sympathicotomy), differential dissection (ramicotomy), and clipping. The rationale of ramicotomy is to achieve a selective division of the sympathetic postganglionic fibers that supply the eccrine glands of the upper extremity. Lee et al. [43] compared patients undergoing T2 sympathicotomy vs T3 ramicotomy. CH was approximately two-thirds lower in ramicotomy group but a lower rate of success was reported in ramicotomy than in sympathicotomy group (93 % versus

68 %, respectively). Cho et al. [59] found that the incidence of severe CH was lower in ramicotomy than sympathicotomy group (54 % versus 92 %, respectively) but the first group presented a higher recurrence rates (21 % versus 6 %, respectively). Recently, Hwang et al. [60] compared T3 sympathicotomy (n=43) versus T2-3 ramicotomy (n=43) showing that sympathicotomy had better outcomes than ramicotomy in terms of success (82 % versus 25 %, respectively); CH (80 % versus 95 %); and satisfaction (91 % versus 79 %, respectively).

The less than optimal results may be due to poor visualization of the anatomy of the sympathetic chain and the communicating fibers with conventional videothoracoscopy. Thus, Coveliers et al. [32] proposed the use of robotic technology to magnify visualization of the surgical field and facilitate complex maneuvers. Thirty-six patients underwent robotic T2-4 ramicotomy. The success rate was 100 %; the incidence of CH was 8.3 %. However, the main limit of robotic procedure is the high cost.

The theoretical possibility of procedural reversibility with clamping or clipping the nerve instead of other procedures in the event of severe CH has led some authors to advocate leaving the nerve in continuity. Neumayer et al. [51] found a significantly decreased incidence of CH (86 % versus 100 %) and higher rate of satisfaction (80 % versus 100 %, respectively) in clipping compared to sympathicotomy group. Lin et al. [14] reported a success of 98 % after T2 block. In two cases with severe CH a full reversibility was obtained after unclipping. Conversely, other authors did not show any advantage of clipping versus sympathectomy or sympathicotomy. Findikcioglu et al. [61] compared T3 sympathectomy (n=28) versus T3 clipping (n=32). Both clipping and cauterization were highly effective for the treatment of PH with success rates of 93 % and 100 %, respectively. The methods were comparable in terms of effectiveness and side effects despite the fact that the recurrence rate was higher in the cauterization than clipping group (19 % versus 6 %, respectively, p=0.01). Inan et al. [62] evaluated four different VTS procedures at the T2-4 level including: resection (n=20), transection (n=20), ablation (n=20), and clipping (n=20). No significant differences were seen between the four groups with regard to success or complication rates. The overall success rate of the operation was 95 %; no recurrence was observed; and more than 20 % of patients complained of CH irrespective of the surgical technique adopted. Yanagihara et al. [63] compared T3 sympathectomy versus T3 clamping. Among two groups, there were no differences in any outcome, including CH and quality of life. Similar results were reported by Scognamillo et al. [64].

Despite the initial enthusiasm, the presumption that the patient can return for "surgical reversal" by removing the clip appears dubious. Chou et al. [38] and Sugimura et al. [36] reported a resolution of CH in 76 and 47 %, respectively, of patients undergoing the reversal procedure. The clip reversal procedures are imperfect with only a limited window in which the opportunity for reversal exists. If the clip has produced cell body death or reorganization within the spinal cord, then the abnormal modulation of sympathetic output causing CH will likely not resolve. The findings of a recent animal study [68] showed that after unclipping, although the nerve appeared to recover normal morphology, and although local inflammatory cells disappear, there was a striking and almost complete absence of amyelinate fibers suggesting that there was no nerve regeneration.

Sympathicotomy intentionally does not remove or injure ganglia of the chain or axons from spinal cord neurons innervating the ganglia. Thus, some authors [13, 15, 27] supported that such procedure had a potential lower risk of CH than sympathectomy due to the less extensive areas of skin anhydrosis. However, Inan et al. [62] showed no clear differences among two procedures. Assalia et al. [65] found that sympathectomy may achieve slightly better long term results than sympathicomy. Because both techniques were used in the same patient, the differences between techniques as to the occurrence of CH could not be assessed in this study [65]. The authors [66] found no significant difference between two procedures in terms of success, recurrence and CH but sympathectomy compared to sympathicotomy resulted in a sub-clinical disturbance of bronchomotor tone and cardiac function theoretically correlated with the extent of denervation.

Recommendations

From the analysis of the literature, surgery is indicated in patients with severe primary hyperhidrosis who are reaching the latter part of their teenage years (usually >18 years old) and in whom all secondary causes of hyperhidrosis have been ruled out. CH is significantly more likely to be severe in those patient who had the T2 ganglia excised [17, 35–43]. Seven studies compared the T3 versus the T4 level [44–50]. Resolution of symptoms was favored in the T3 groups in three studies [44, 46, 49] and the T4 group in one study [45]. Three studies were similar in outcomes [47, 48, 50]. However, all seven studies [44–50] reported a reduction of CH in the T4 groups. Nine papers compared the occurrence of CH after sympathetic chain resection at a single levels versus multiple levels [31, 51–58]. All papers but two [57, 58] showed a strong correlation between the number of levels excised and the degree of CH. Eleven papers compared different techniques of sympathetic chain resection [38, 43, 51, 59–66]. In one paper [51] clipping was superior to sympathicotomy and in another [43] ramicotomy was superior to sympathicotomy. However in both studies, the procedures were attended at different anatomical level that may affected the results. Nine papers [38, 59–66] found no significant differences among the various procedures. In the light of these results, single resection is preferred to multiple levels of resection. In case of isolated PH, T3 is the level of choice although T4 interruption may be also reasonable. Sympathicotomy may be preferred to sympathectomy because it is more simple and less extensive and has similar outcomes.

A Personal View of the Data

The literature on VTS must be carefully interpreted. Most of the current evidences comes from observational studies. Some papers comparing different level of resection present a lack of uniformity in patient populations. Not all studies assess and/

or quantify the degree of CH similarly or at the same point postoperatively. Because the incidence of recurrence and/or of CH may increase with time regardless of the level resected, the differences in the follow-up period among different papers may interfere in the analysis of the outcomes. In theory, the shortest duration of follow-up may account for the lowest incidence of recurrence and/or of CH after surgery. Objective specific tests and/or questionnaires to quantify the sweating and the clinical improvement after surgery are rarely used, and most papers simply rely on subjective reporting by the patient. Some authors do not use the term sympathectomy with extreme precision; sometimes a sympathicotomy is done, leaving the ganglion intact. Thus the true level of sympathectomy/sympathicotomy is also something that should not always be presumed accurate in various reports. Especially in novices, confusion may arise as to the true ganglion or rib level, and published errors or questions of level exist. Although the differentiation may seem subtle, the clinical implications are huge and may well impact on the mishmash of conflicting conclusions regarding the level and the extent of resection.

We currently limit the extent of our resection for isolated PH to a single level, generally T3 at the top of the third rib. In the event that patient has multisite sweating (i.e. palmar associated with facial or axillar hyperhidrosis) and requires multilevel resections, we advise the patient regarding the increased risk of CH. We have not tested clip blocking in our unit, because we are unsure of its reversibility. Sympathectomy is the procedure of choice; however, in selected cases sympathicotomy may be preferred for the lower incidence of adverse effects, especially on cardio-respiratory function. We believe that in the future a standardized nomenclature (i.e. for the level of resection and/or the procedures adopted) and follow-up algorithms or surveys should be adopted in order to allow surgeons from all over the world to better communicate with one another and compare their results.

Recommendations

- Surgery is indicated in patients with severe primary palmar hyperhidrosis who are reaching the latter part of their teenage years (Evidence quality moderate; strong recommendation)
- Single resection is preferred over multiple levels of resection. (Evidence quality low; weak recommendation)
- T3 is the level of choice, althoughT4 interruption may be also reasonable. (Evidence quality moderate; weak recommendation)
- Sympathicotomy is preferred over sympathectomy because it is more simple, is less extensive, and has similar outcomes. (Evidence quality low; weak recommendation)

References

1. Deng B, Tan QY, Jiang YG, Zhao YP, Zhou JH, Ma Z, Wang RW. Optimization of sympathectomy to treat palmar hyperhidrosis: the systematic review and meta-analysis of studies published during the past decade. Surg Endosc. 2011;25(6):1893–901.
2. Moreno Balsalobre R, Moreno Mata N, Ramos Izquierdo R, Aragón Valverde FJ, Molins López-Rodo L, de Andrés Rivas JJ, García Fernández JL, Cañizares Carretero MÁ, Congregado Loscertales M, Carbajo Carbajo M, SEPAR. Guidelines on surgery of the thoracic sympathetic nervous system. Arch Bronconeumol. 2011;47(2):94–102.
3. Rzany BBR, Spinner D. Interventions for localised excessive sweating. Cochrane Database Syst Rev. 2001; (1): CD002953. doi: 10.1002/14651858.CD002953.
4. Cerfolio RJ, De Campos JR, Bryant AS, Connery CP, Miller DL, DeCamp MM, McKenna RJ, Krasna MJ. The Society of Thoracic Surgeons expert consensus for the surgical treatment of hyperhidrosis. Ann Thorac Surg. 2011;91(5):1642–8.
5. Neumayer C, Zacherl J, Holak G, Jakesz R, Bischof G. Experience with limited endoscopic thoracic sympathetic block for hyperhidrosis and facial blushing. Clin Auton Res. 2003;13 Suppl 1:I52–7.
6. Schick CH, Fronek K, Held A, Birklein F, Hohenberger W, Schmelz M. Differential effects of surgical sympathetic block on sudomotor and vasoconstrinctor function. Neurology. 2003;60(11):1770–6.
7. Atkinson JL, Fealey RD. Sympathotomy instead of sympathectomy for palmar hyperhidrosis: minimizing postoperative compensatory hyperhidrosis. Mayo Clin Proc. 2003;78:167–72.
8. Lladó A, León L, Valls-Solé J, Mena P, Callejas MA, Peri JM. Changes in the sympathetic skin response after thoracoscopic sympathectomy in patients with primary palmar hyperhidrosis. Clin Neurophysiol. 2005;116(6):1348–54.
9. Ting H, Lee SD, Chung AH, Chuang ML, Chen GD, Liao JM, Chang CL, Chiou TS, Lin TB. Effects of bilateral T2-sympathectomy on static and dynamic heart rate responses to exercise in hyperhidrosis patients. Auton Neurosci. 2005;121(1–2):74–80.
10. Eisenach JH, Pike TL, Wick DE, Dietz NM, Fealey RD, Atkinson JL, Charkoudian N. A comparison of peripheral skin blood flow and temperature during endoscopic thoracic sympathectomy. Anesth Analg. 2005;100(1):269–76.
11. Miller DL, Force SD. Outpatient microthoracoscopic sympathectomy for palmar hyperhidrosis. Ann Thorac Surg. 2007;83(5):1850–3.
12. Leis S, Meyer N, Bickel A, Schick CH, Kruger S, Schmelz M, Birklein F. Thoracoscopic sympathectomy at the T2 or T3 level facilitates bradykinin-induced protein extravasation in human forearm skin. Pain Med. 2010;11(5):774–80.
13. Atkinson JL, Fode-Thomas NC, Fealey RD, Eisenach JH, Goerss SJ. Endoscopic transthoracic limited sympathotomy for palmar-plantar hyperhidrosis: outcomes and complications during a 10-year period. Mayo Clin Proc. 2011;86(8):721–9.
14. Lin TS, Chou MC. Treatment of palmar hyperhidrosis using needlescopic T2 sympathetic block by clipping: analysis of 102 cases. Int Surg. 2004;89(4):198–201.
15. Yoon DH, Ha Y, Park YG, Chang JW. Thoracoscopic limited T-3 sympathicotomy for primary hyperhidrosis: prevention for compensatory hyperhidrosis. J Neurosurg. 2003;99(1 Suppl):39–43.
16. Doolabh N, Horswell S, Williams M, Huber L, Prince S, Meyer DM, Mack MJ. Thoracoscopic sympathectomy for hyperhidrosis: indications and results. Ann Thorac Surg. 2004;77(2):410–4.
17. Dewey TM, Herbert MA, Hill SL, Prince SL, Mack MJ. One-year follow-up after thoracoscopic sympathectomy for hyperhidrosis: outcomes and consequences. Ann Thorac Surg. 2006;81(4):1227–32.
18. Weksler B, Luketich JD, Shende MR. Endoscopic thoracic sympathectomy: at what level should you perform surgery? Thorac Surg Clin. 2008;18(2):183–91.

19. Lima AG, Marcondes GA, Teixeira AB, Toro IF, Campos JR, Jatene FB. The incidence of residual pneumothorax after video-assisted sympathectomy with and without pleural drainage and its effect on postoperative pain. J Bras Pneumol. 2008;34(3):136–42.
20. Fiorelli A, Vicidomini G, Laperuta P, Busiello L, Perrone A, Napolitano F, Messina G, Santini M. Pre-emptive local analgesia in video-assisted thoracic surgery sympathectomy. Eur J Cardiothorac Surg. 2010;37(3):588–93.
21. Zhu LH, Wang W, Yang S, Li D, Zhang Z, Chen S, Cheng X, Chen L, Chen W. Transumbilical thoracic sympathectomy with an ultrathin flexible endoscope in a series of 38 patients. Surg Endosc. 2013;27(6):2149–55.
22. Chou SH, Kao EL, Li HP, Lin CC, Huang MF. T4 sympathectomy for palmar hyperhidrosis: an effective approach that simultaneously minimizes compensatory hyperhidrosis. Kaohsiung J Med Sci. 2005;21(7):310–3.
23. Baumgartner FJ, Toh Y. Severe hyperhidrosis: clinical features and current thoracoscopic surgical management. Ann Thorac Surg. 2003;76(6):1878–83.
24. Loscertales J, Arroyo Tristán A, Congregado Loscertales M, Jiménez Merchán R, Girón Arjona JC, Arenas Linares C, Ayarra Jarné J. Thoracoscopic sympathectomy for palmar hyperhidrosis. Immediate results and postoperative quality of life. Arch Bronconeumol. 2004;40(2):67–71.
25. De Campos de Campos JR, Wolosker N, Takeda FR, Kauffman P, Kuzniec S, Jatene FB, de Oliveira SA. The body mass index and level of resection: predictive factors for compensatory sweating after sympathectomy. Clin Auton Res. 2005;15(2):116–20.
26. Sihoe AD, Manlulu AV, Lee TW, Thung KH, Yim AP. Pre-emptive local anesthesia for needle-scopic video-assisted thoracic surgery: a randomized controlled trial. Eur J Cardiothorac Surg. 2007;31(1):103–8.
27. Jeganathan R, Jordan S, Jones M, Grant S, Diamond O, McManus K, Graham A, McGuigan J. Bilateral thoracoscopic sympathectomy: results and long-term follow-up. Interact Cardiovasc Thorac Surg. 2008;7(1):67–70.
28. Little AG. Video-assisted thoracic surgery sympathectomy for hyperhidrosis. Arch Surg. 2004;139(6):586–9.
29. Georghiou GP, Berman M, Bobovnikov V, Vidne BA, Saute M. Minimally invasive thoracoscopic sympathectomy for palmar hyperhidrosis via a transaxillary single-port approach. Interact Cardiovasc Thorac Surg. 2004;3(3):437–41.
30. Moya J, Ramos R, Morera R, Villalonga R, Perna V, Macia I, Ferrer G. Thoracic sympathicolysis for primary hyperhidrosis: a review of 918 procedures. Surg Endosc. 2006;20(4):598–602.
31. Gossot D, Galetta D, Pascal A, Debrosse D, Caliandro R, Girard P, Stern JB, Grunenwald D. Long-term results of endoscopic thoracic sympathectomy for upper limb hyperhidrosis. Ann Thorac Surg. 2003;75(4):1075–9.
32. Coveliers H, Meyer M, Gharagozloo F, Wisselink W, Rauwerda J, Margolis M, Tempesta B, Strother E. Robotic selective postganglionic thoracic sympathectomy for the treatment of hyperhidrosis. Ann Thorac Surg. 2013;95(1):269–74.
33. Apiliogullari B, Esme H, Yoldas B, Duran M, Duzgun N, Calik M. Early and midterm results of single-port video-assisted thoracoscopic sympathectomy. Thorac Cardiovasc Surg. 2012;60(4):285–9.
34. Prasad A, Ali M, Kaul S. Endoscopic thoracic sympathectomy for primary palmar hyperidrosis. Surg Endosc. 2010;24(8):1952–7.
35. Schmidt J, Bechara FG, Altmeyer P, Zirngibl H. Endoscopic thoracic sympathectomy for severe hyperhidrosis: impact of restrictive denervation on compensatory sweating. Ann Thorac Surg. 2006;81(3):1048–55.
36. Sugimura H, Spratt EH, Compeau CG, Kattail D, Shargall Y. Thoracoscopic sympathetic clipping for hyperhidrosis: long-term results and reversibility. J Thorac Cardiovasc Surg. 2009;137(6):1370–6; discussion 1376–7.
37. Reisfeld R. Sympathectomy for hyperhidrosis: should we place the clamps at T2-T3 or T3-T4? Clin Auton Res. 2006;16(6):384–9.

38. Chou SH, Kao EL, Lin CC, Chang YT, Huang MF. The importance of classification in sympathetic surgery and a proposed mechanism for compensatory hyperhidrosis: experience with 464 cases. Surg Endosc. 2006;20(11):1749–53.
39. Yazbek G, Wolosker N, Kauffman P, Campos JR, Puech-Leão P, Jatene FB. Twenty months of evolution following sympathectomy on patients with palmar hyperhidrosis: sympathectomy at the T3 level is better than at the T2 level. Clinics. 2009;64(8):743–9.
40. Baumgartner FJ, Reyes M, Sarkisyan GG, Iglesias A, Reyes E. Thoracoscopic sympathicotomy for disabling palmar hyperhidrosis: a prospective randomized comparison between two levels. Ann Thorac Surg. 2011;92(6):2015–9.
41. Lin M, Tu YR, Li X, Lai FC, Chen JF, Dai ZJ. Comparison of curative effects of sympathectomy at different segments on palmar hyperhidrosis. Zhonghua Yi Xue Za Zhi. 2006;86(33):2315–7.
42. Miller DL, Bryant AS, Force SD, Miller Jr JI. Effect of sympathectomy level on the incidence of compensatory hyperhidrosis after sympathectomy for palmar hyperhidrosis. J Thorac Cardiovasc Surg. 2009;138(3):581–5.
43. Lee DY, Kim DH, Paik HC. Selective division of T3 rami communicantes (T3 ramicotomy) in the treatment of palmar hyperhidrosis. Ann Thorac Surg. 2004;78(3):1052–5.
44. Chang YT, Li HP, Lee JY, Lin PJ, Lin CC, Kao EL, Chou SH, Huang MF. Treatment of palmar hyperhidrosis: T(4) level compared with T(3) and T(2). Ann Surg. 2007;246(2):330–6.
45. Mahdy T, Youssef T, Elmonem HA, Omar W, Elateef AA. T4 sympathectomy for palmar hyperhidrosis: looking for the right operation. Surgery. 2008;143(6):784–9.
46. Kim WO, Kil HK, Yoon KB, Yoon DM, Lee JS. Influence of T3 or T4 sympathicotomy for palmar hyperhidrosis. Am J Surg. 2010;199(2):166–9.
47. Liu Y, Yang J, Liu J, Yang F, Jiang G, Li J, Huang Y, Wang J. Surgical treatment of primary palmar hyperhidrosis: a prospective randomized study comparing T3 and T4 sympathicotomy. Eur J Cardiothorac Surg. 2009;35(3):398–402.
48. Ishy A, de Campos JR, Wolosker N, Kauffman P, Tedde ML, Chiavoni CR, Jatene FB. Objective evaluation of patients with palmar hyperhidrosis submitted to two levels of sympathectomy: T3 and T4. Interact Cardiovasc Thorac Surg. 2011;12(4):545–8.
49. Wolosker N, Yazbek G, Ishy A, de Campos JR, Kauffman P, Puech-Leão P. Is sympathectomy at T4 level better than at T3 level for treating palmar hyperhidrosis? J Laparoendosc Adv Surg Tech A. 2008;18(1):102–6.
50. Yang J, Tan JJ, Ye GL, Gu WQ, Wang J, Liu YG. T3/T4 thoracic sympathictomy and compensatory sweating in treatment of palmar hyperhidrosis. Chin Med J. 2007;120(18):1574–7.
51. Neumayer C, Zacherl J, Holak G, Függer R, Jakesz R, Herbst F, Bischof G. Limited endoscopic thoracic sympathetic block for hyperhidrosis of the upper limb: reduction of compensatory sweating by clipping T4. Surg Endosc. 2004;18(1):152–6.
52. Weksler B, Blaine G, Souza ZB, Gavina R. Transection of more than one sympathetic chain ganglion for hyperhidrosis increases the severity of compensatory hyperhidrosis and decreases patient satisfaction. J Surg Res. 2009;156(1):110–5.
53. Yoon SH, Rim DC. The selective T3 sympathicotomy in patients with essential palmar hyperhidrosis. Acta Neurochir (Wien). 2003;145(6):467–71.
54. Yano M, Kiriyama M, Fukai I, Sasaki H, Kobayashi Y, Mizuno K, Haneda H, Suzuki E, Endo K, Fujii Y. Endoscopic thoracic sympathectomy for palmar hyperhidrosis: efficacy of T2 and T3 ganglion resection. Surgery. 2005;138(1):40–5.
55. Li X, Tu YR, Lin M, Lai FC, Chen JF, Dai ZJ. Endoscopic thoracic sympathectomy for palmar hyperhidrosis: a randomized control trial comparing T3 and T2-4 ablation. Ann Thorac Surg. 2008;85(5):1747–51.
56. Aoki H, Sakai T, Murata H, Sumikawa K. Extent of sympathectomy affects postoperative compensatory sweating and satisfaction in patients with palmar hyperhidrosis. J Anesth. 2014;28(2):210–3.
57. Katara AN, Domino JP, Cheah WK, So JB, Ning C, Lomanto D. Comparing T2 and T2–T3 ablation in thoracoscopic sympathectomy for palmar hyperhidrosis: a randomized control trial. Surg Endosc. 2007;21(10):1768–71.

58. Turhan K, Cakan A, Cagirici U. Preserving T2 in thoracic sympathicotomy for palmar hyper-hidrosis: less tissue trauma, same effectiveness. Thorac Cardiovasc Surg. 2011;59(6):353–6.
59. Cho HM, Chung KY, Kim DJ, Lee KJ, Kim KD. The comparison of VATS ramicotomy and VATS sympathicotomy for treating essential hyperhidrosis. Yonsei Med J. 2003;44(6):1008–13.
60. Hwang JJ, Kim do H, Hong YJ, Lee DY. A comparison between two types of limited sympa-thetic surgery for palmar hyperhidrosis. Surg Today. 2013;43(4):397–402.
61. Findikcioglu A, Kilic D, Hatipoglu A. Is clipping superior to cauterization in the treatment of palmar hyperhidrosis? Thorac Cardiovasc Surg. 2013: (in press). PubMed PMID: 23839873.
62. Inan K, Goksel OS, Uçak A, Temizkan V, Karaca K, Ugur M, Arslan G, Us M, Yilmaz AT. Thoracic endoscopic surgery for hyperhidrosis: comparison of different techniques. Thorac Cardiovasc Surg. 2008;56(4):210–3.
63. Yanagihara TK, Ibrahimiye A, Harris C, Hirsch J, Gorenstein LA. Analysis of clamping versus cutting of T3 sympathetic nerve for severe palmar hyperhidrosis. J Thorac Cardiovasc Surg. 2010;140(5):984–9.
64. Scognamillo F, Serventi F, Attene F, Torre C, Paliogiannis P, Pala C, Trignano E, Trignano M. T2-T4 sympathectomy versus T3-T4 sympathicotomy for palmar and axillary hyperhidrosis. Clin Auton Res. 2011;21(2):97–102.
65. Assalia A, Bahouth H, Ilivitzki A, Assi Z, Hashmonai M, Krausz MM. Thoracoscopic sympa-thectomy for primary palmar hyperhidrosis: resection versus transection – a prospective trial. World J Surg. 2007;31(10):1976–9.
66. Fiorelli A, D'Aponte A, Canonico R, Palladino A, Vicidomini G, Limongelli F, Santini M. T2-T3 sympathectomy versus sympathicotomy for essential palmar hyperhidrosis: comparison of effects on cardio-respiratory function. Eur J Cardiothorac Surg. 2012;42(3):454–61.
67. Lin CC, Telaranta T. Lin-Telaranta classification: the importance of different procedures for different indications in sympathetic surgery. Ann Chir Gynaecol. 2001;90(3):161–6.
68. Loscertales J, Congregado M, Jimenez-Merchan R, Gallardo G, Trivino A, Moreno S, Loscertales B, Galera-Ruiz H. Sympathetic chain clipping for hyperhidrosis is not a reversible procedure. Surg Endosc. 2012;26(5):1258–63.

Part VIII
Chest Wall

Chapter Eight

Chapter 58
Synthetic Versus Biologic Reconstruction of Bony Chest Wall Defects

Gaetano Rocco

Abstract Biologic materials are being increasingly used alone or in combination as material of choice for reconstruction of extensive defects after chest wall resection due to their facilitated incorporation in the host and their resilience to infection. Whether these materials are destined to replace time honored synthetic prostheses is not known, especially since direct comparisons of efficacy in terms of chest wall stability, reduced postoperative infection rates and need for prosthesis removal have not yet been published. Also, biologic materials have elevated costs which may suggest careful use in selected indications.

Keywords Chest wall • Prostheses • Bioengineering • Acellular collagen matrix • Cryopreserved homografts

Introduction

Thoracic surgeons are increasingly faced with the necessity of extended and repeated resections for primary or secondary tumors of the bony chest wall [1, 2]. As a consequence, large defects in the chest wall are created and subsequently reconstructed thanks to the availability of biologic materials recently introduced in the clinical practice [1, 2]. Does this mean that synthetic materials are to be abandoned? Is there substantial evidence in the literature supporting a more liberal use of biologic composites to cover chest wall defects? A major hurdle against the accumulation of reliable evidence in this field is represented by the relative rarity of both

G. Rocco, MD, FRCSEd
Division of Thoracic Surgery, Department of Thoracic Surgery and Oncology,
National Cancer Institute, Pascale Foundation, Via Semmola 81, 80131 Naples, Italy
e-mail: gaetano.rocco@btopenworld.com

M.K. Ferguson (ed.), *Difficult Decisions in Thoracic Surgery*,
Difficult Decisions in Surgery: An Evidence-Based Approach 1,
DOI 10.1007/978-1-4471-6404-3_58, © Springer-Verlag London 2014

primary and secondary chest wall tumors. Indeed, the most recent authoritative experiences are based on series counting up to around 200 patients receiving synthetic prostheses [1, 2]. In addition, the use of biologic materials is still limited to a few centers due to their cost [1, 2]. As a result, postoperative outcomes of synthetic and biological materials are usually not analyzed separately and this adds to the uncertainty in the selection of the material for each operative indication.

Search Strategy

In order to compare synthetic vs biologic materials, the search included Medline, the Cochrane controlled trials register and publications between January 1999 and August 2013 that included terms such as: chest wall resection, chest wall reconstruction, chest wall tumors, and chest wall tumors AND [biomaterials OR cryopreserved homografts OR acellular collagen matrix]. The pre-specified primary outcome was postoperative infections of prosthesis and lack of chest wall stabilization. Only publications in English were considered. Case reports and limited (<5 patients) series were excluded from this analysis, and only studies reporting on full thickness chest wall resection and reconstruction were accepted. For their intrinsic biologic features, titanium plate studies were included in the biologic/biomimetic group.

The data were entered in a NCSS version 8 spreadsheet (NCSS, LLC. Kaysville, Utah, USA, www.ncss.com) using studies on synthetic materials as control group due to the lack of clinical studies directly comparing the two reconstructive strategies. In addition, data from studies using synthetic or biologic materials were entered and matched according to decreasing numerosity. Random effect meta-analyses were run for odds ratio in order to estimate effect sizes. Consistency of the meta-analysis was assessed by the effect-equality test for heterogeneity. Heterogeneity refers to the variation across a study that is attributable to statistical heterogeneity rather than chance. As a rule, heterogeneity is established when the Q value divided by N (number of studies) −1 equals >1 and the p value is >0.05.

Results

Neither randomized trials nor comparative studies on the use of synthetic vs biologic composites for chest wall reconstruction in a clinical setting were retrieved from the literature search. Nevertheless, 14 papers [3–16] were selected that included 1,108 and 117 patients in the papers on the use of synthetic (7 studies) and biologic/biomimetic materials (7 studies), respectively. Heterogeneity was ruled out. The results of the meta-analysis showed that 98 (8.8 %) and 12 patients (11.3 %; p=0.63) developed wound infection or prosthesis instability in the synthetic and biologic/biomimetic group, respectively. In addition, although no definitive

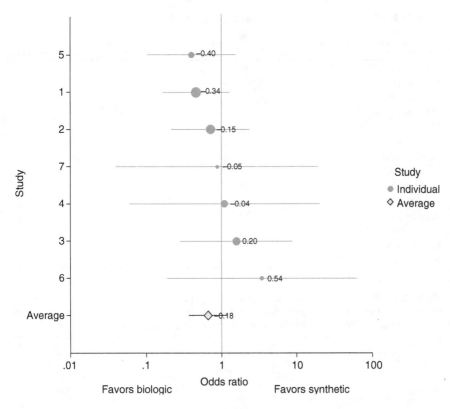

Fig. 58.1 Random effect meta-analysis of 14 papers on chest wall resection and reconstruction using biologic/biomimetic or synthetic materials

conclusions could be drawn, it appeared that the use of recently introduced biologic/biomimetic materials may be associated with a trend towards reduction of prosthetic suppurative complications compared to synthetic materials (Fig. 58.1 and Tables 58.1 and 58.2).

Biomimesis as Preservation of Structure and Function

Biomimetic reconstruction of the chest wall relies on a few fundamental principles, such as respect of the anatomy, preservation of function, selection of adequate reconstructive materials, and integration of multidisciplinary efforts [2]. For relatively limited chest wall defects, the pursuit of biomimesis is usually not a problem. Conversely, the issue of covering extensive defects while restoring osteomuscular continuity and protecting inner viscera becomes a challenging one, especially in the event of multiple reoperations and infected or previously irradiated surgical sites

Table 58.1 Dataset from 14 papers on materials used for chest wall reconstruction (7 synthetic and 7 biologic)

Studies	Total synthetic	Events synthetic	Total biologic	Events biologic
Weyant et al. [13]	262	20	32	5
Puviani et al. [3]				
Lans et al. [9]	229	22	25	3
Miller et al. [5]				
Mansour et al. [10]	200	19	24	1
Fabre et al. [15]				
Deschamps et al. [6]	197	9	11	0
Berthet et al. [12]				
Girotti et al. [14]	101	13	10	3
Ge et al. [7]				
Koppert et al. [8]	68	12	9	0
Wiegmann et al. [11]				
Kachroo et al. [16]	51	3	6	0
Barua et al. [4]				

Table 58.2 Effect-equality (heterogeneity) test for synthetic and biological materials data. The heterogeneity test is added to verify reliability of meta-analysis. Heterogeneity is established when the Q value divided by N (number of studies) −1 equals >1 and the p value is >0.05

Outcome	Cochran's Q	DF	Probability level
Odds ratio	3.4612	6	0.7491
Risk ratio	4.8987	6	0.5569
Risk difference	5.0390	6	0.5388

[2]. Ideally, appropriate reconstructive materials need to adapt to the chest wall geometry while conferring structural stability and be easily incorporated by the host [2]. Although not all defects need to be covered, it is advisable to always avoid lung herniation and scapular impingement [2].

Reconstructive Strategy

Besides the size of the chest wall defect and the condition of the area to be resected, the reconstructive options can also be dictated by its location and the contemplated use of synthetic and biologic materials alone or in combination [1, 2]. For lateral defects, titanium plates or polypropylene/polytetrafluoroethylene (PTFE) meshes are used when only one rib is removed and local anatomy mandates reconstruction; for larger defects, polytetrafluoroethylene (PTFE) patches or titanium plates can be used [12]. In the event of reoperations or in infected or heavily irradiated areas, the utilization of patches of acellular collagen matrix (ACM) may be preferred due to the characteristics of this material facilitating incorporation and resilience to infection [17]. If titanium plates are used, these need to be separated from the overlying myocutaneous layers with a rebsorbable (i.e., polyglactin) mesh to avoid friction [18]. For posterior chest wall defects, coverage may not be needed. However, patients may perceive the development of seroma as a sign of chest wall instability and an indication of an unsatisfactory postoperative outcome. This minor complication can be easily prevented by use a synthetic mesh to close the defect. For larger defects, the choice of the reconstructive material should include consideration of non-rigid, rather laminar coverage in consideration of the pressure that occurs in this region when the patient is in a recumbent position [4, 19]. A special clinical scenario is encountered when concurrent vertebral resections are required. In this context, ACM patches, due to the intrinsic biologic characteristics, confer the necessary stability and protect the exposed spine against wound infection [19].

Anterior chest wall defects mandate a reconstructive strategy primarily aimed at avoiding flail chest physiology and lung herniation. As a result, rigid materials are advocated [13, 14]. For defects resulting from the removal of one anterolateral rib segment, a non-absorbable mesh or a single titanium plate usually suffices [2]. By contrast, larger defects may require biomimetic reconstruction by restoring the intercostal space structure. To this end, the combination of titanium plates (ratio 1:2 with the removed ribs) and ACM or PTFE patches has been described, also in reoperations [12, 15, 20, 21].

When a sternal resection becomes also necessary, reconstruction with biologic materials is gaining increasing favor among surgeons [21–23]. In this setting, cryopreserved homograft material can serve as sternal replacement alone or in combination with synthetic composites [20]. In addition, titanium plates to bridge the defect and ACM or omentum to protect the mediastinum represent a reasonable alternative to PTFE or methylmethacrylate (MMM) sandwiches especially for reoperations [12, 13, 15, 23, 24].

Evidence Supporting the Use of Synthetic Materials

Synthetic materials include a wide range of time-honored composites that have been utilized for chest wall reconstruction for decades [2]. Polypropylene or polyglactin meshes and methylmethacrylate sandwich along with PTFE patches represent materials which maintain their integrity either alone or in combination with biologic prostheses [2, 10, 22, 24]. Following reconstruction with synthetic meshes, postoperative morbidity rates in terms of infection of the surgical site range between 4.6 and 23 % [1]. Local wound complications mandate removal of the reconstructive material in between 1.6 and 13 %, with an average around 7 % [1]. Lans and colleagues reported their experience with synthetic reconstruction of the chest wall yielding suppurative complications in 50 patients out of 75 developing moderate to severe complications [9]. As to residual pulmonary function, no differences between preoperative and postoperative FEV1 (forced expiratory volume at 1 s) irrespective of the associated lung resection, were noted after using MMM for reconstruction [24].

Evidence Supporting the Use of Biologic Materials

Biologic materials include mainly cryopreserved homografts and acellular collagen matrix patches [1, 2]. The main features of biologic materials include remarkable strength and user friendliness, along with easy incorporation into the host irrespective of the primary condition of the resected area (e.g., infection) [1, 2].

In spite of being synthetic, titanium plates behave as biologic composites due to the resistance to infection and the possibility to be utilized in heavily irradiated fields alone or as a support for biological or synthetic meshes [1, 2] . Cryopreserved homografts have been used by pediatric and plastic surgeons especially as sternal replacements [20]. Cadaveric sternum, iliac crest, ribs, and fascia lata have all been described to typically cover anterolateral chest wall defects [1–3, 18]. After harvesting, the bony segments undergo cryopreservation at −70 °C for at least 3 months to reduce antigenicity [18]. Implantation can be done directly or accompanied by the provision of a vascularized bed (i.e., omental flap) which revascularizes the graft, thus facilitating incorporation into the host [18]. Postoperatively, neither immunosuppressors nor steroids are used [18].

Acellular collagen matrix (ACM) patches are either human, bovine or porcine derivatives which have been implanted to cover chest wall defects originated by costovertebral, sternocostal and simple rib resections [25, 26]. These tissue patches are ready to use, do not complicate major intraoperative handling and they behave as autologous materials. A major limitation in the use of ACM patches is still represented by their cost, ranging from $ 1,750 to $ 15,000 for the largest size patches [1].

Conclusions

The intuitive concept of added usefulness of biologic compared to synthetic materials for chest wall reconstruction may be further substantiated by future studies and the availability of mature results from ongoing surgical experiences. The use of acellular collagen matrix patches alone or in combination with cryopreserved homografts and titanium plates represent today a valid theoretical alternative to time honored synthetic materials for chest wall reconstructions for previously irradiated and/or infected areas. However, refinement of indications is imperative, especially in light of the significant costs related to the use of such biologic/biomimetic composites.

Recommendations

In summary, biologic/biomimetic materials are preferred to synthetic materials due to their easy incorporation into the host and resilience to infection. Hence, these materials should be the first reconstructive choice when the resected area is infected or has been heavily irradiated.

A Personal View of the Data

Between January 2005 and May 2013, 111 procedures were done at the Division of Thoracic Surgery of the National Cancer Institute in Naples to remove chest wall tumors. In 31 % of the cases, chest wall reconstruction was accomplished through biomaterials recently introduced in the clinical practice used alone or in combination also with time-honored composites. We used titanium plates, acellular collagen matrices and cryopreserved homografts to cover extensive defects during redo operations or after heavy irradiation or localized infection. In our opinion, cost effectiveness of biomaterials is particularly advantageous for these indications to bail thoracic surgeons out of at times extremely challenging clinical scenarios.

Recommendation

- Biological materials are preferred to synthetic materials for chest wall construction, especially in patients in whom the target area is infected or has been irradiated. (Evidence quality very low; weak recommendation)

References

1. Rocco G. Chest wall resection and reconstruction according to the principles of biomimesis. Semin Thorac Cardiovasc Surg. 2011;23:307–13.
2. Rocco G. Overview on current and future materials for chest wall reconstruction. Thorac Surg Clin. 2010;20:559–62.
3. Puviani L, Fazio N, Boriani L, Ruggieri P, Fornasari PM, Briccoli A. Reconstruction with fascia lata after extensive chest wall resection: results. Eur J Cardiothorac Surg. 2013;44:125–9.
4. Barua A, Catton JA, Socci L, Raurell A, Malik M, Internullo E, et al. Initial experience with the use of biological implants for soft tissue and chest wall reconstruction in thoracic surgery. Ann Thorac Surg. 2012;94:1701–5.
5. Miller DL, Force SD, Pickens A, Fernandez FG, Luu T, Mansour KA. Chest wall reconstruction using biomaterials. Ann Thorac Surg. 2013;95:1050–6.
6. Deschamps C, Tirnaksiz BM, Darbandi R, Trastek VF, Allen MS, Miller DL, et al. Early and long-term results of prosthetic chest wall reconstruction. J Thorac Cardiovasc Surg. 1999;117:588–91.
7. Ge PS, Imai TA, Aboulian A, Van Natta TL. The use of human acellular dermal matrix for chest wall reconstruction. Ann Thorac Surg. 2010;90:1799–804.
8. Koppert LB, van Geel AN, Lans TE, van der Pol C, van Coevorden F, Wouters MW. Sternal resection for sarcoma, recurrent breast cancer, and radiation-induced necrosis. Ann Thorac Surg. 2010;90:1102–8.
9. Lans TE, van der Pol C, Wouters MW, Schmitz PI, van Geel AN. Complications in wound healing after chest wall resection in cancer patients; a multivariate analysis of 220 patients. J Thorac Oncol. 2009;4:639–43.
10. Mansour KA, Thourani VH, Losken A, Reeves JG, Miller Jr JI, Carlson GW, et al. Chest wall resections and reconstruction: a 25-year experience. Ann Thorac Surg. 2002;73:1720–5.

11. Wiegmann B, Zardo P, Dickgreber N, Länger F, Fegbeutel C, Haverich A, et al. Biological materials in chest wall reconstruction: initial experience with the Peri-Guard repair patch. Eur J Cardiothorac Surg. 2010;37:602–5.
12. Berthet JP, Canaud L, D'Annoville T, Alric P, Marty-Ane CH. Titanium plates and Dualmesh: a modern combination for reconstructing very large chest wall defects. Ann Thorac Surg. 2011;91:1709–16.
13. Weyant MJ, Bains MS, Venkatraman E, Downey RJ, Park BJ, Flores RM, et al. Results of chest wall resection and reconstruction with and without rigid prosthesis. Ann Thorac Surg. 2006;81:279–85.
14. Girotti P, Leo F, Bravi F, Tavecchio L, Spano A, Cortinovis U, et al. The "rib-like" technique for surgical treatment of sternal tumors: lessons learned from 101 consecutive cases. Ann Thorac Surg. 2011;92:1208–16.
15. Fabre D, El Batti S, Singhal S, Mercier O, Mussot S, Fadel E, et al. A paradigm shift for sternal reconstruction using a novel titanium rib bridge system following oncological resections. Eur J Cardiothorac Surg. 2012;42:965–70.
16. Kachroo P, Pak PS, Sandha HS, Lee C, Elashoff D, Nelson SD, et al. Single-institution, multi-disciplinary experience with surgical resection of primary chest wall sarcomas. J Thorac Oncol. 2012;7:552–8.
17. Rocco G, Mori S, Fazioli F, La Rocca A, Martucci N, Setola S. The use of biomaterials for chest wall reconstruction 30 years after radical surgery and radiation. Ann Thorac Surg. 2012;94:e109–10.
18. Rocco G, Fazioli F, Cerra R, Salvi R. Composite reconstruction with cryopreserved fascia lata, single mandibular titanium plate, and polyglactin mesh after redo surgery and radiation therapy for recurrent chest wall liposarcoma. J Thorac Cardiovasc Surg. 2011;141:839–40.
19. Rocco G, Serra L, Fazioli F, Mori S, Mehrabi-Kermani F, Capasso A, et al. The use of veritas collagen matrix to reconstruct the posterior chest wall after costovertebrectomy. Ann Thorac Surg. 2011;92:e17–8.
20. Rocco G, Fazioli F, Scognamiglio F, Parisi V, La Manna C, La Rocca A, et al. The combination of multiple materials in the creation of an artificial anterior chest cage after extensive demolition for recurrent chondrosarcoma. J Thorac Cardiovasc Surg. 2007;133:1112–4.
21. Rocco G, Fazioli F, La Manna C, La Rocca A, Mori S, Palaia R, et al. Omental flap and titanium plates provide structural stability and protection of the mediastinum after extensive sternocostal resection. Ann Thorac Surg. 2010;90:e14–6.
22. Chapelier AR, Missana MC, Couturaud B, Fadel E, Fabre D, Mussot S, et al. Sternal resection and reconstruction for primary malignant tumors. Ann Thorac Surg. 2004;77:1001–6.
23. Coonar AS, Qureshi N, Smith I, Wells FC, Reisberg E, Wihlm JM. A novel titanium rib bridge system for chest wall reconstruction. Ann Thorac Surg. 2009;87:e46–8.
24. Lardinois D, Müller M, Furrer M, Banic A, Gugger M, Krueger T, et al. Functional assessment of chest wall integrity after methylmethacrylate reconstruction. Ann Thorac Surg. 2000;69:919–23.
25. Cothren CC, Gallego K, Anderson ED, Schmidt D. Chest wall reconstruction with acellular dermal matrix (AlloDerm) and a latissimus muscle flap. Plast Reconstr Surg. 2004;114:1015–7.
26. Huston TL, Taback B, Rohde CH. Chest wall reconstruction with porcine acellular dermal matrix (strattice) and a latissimus myocutaneous flap. Am Surg. 2011;77:e115–6.

Chapter 59
Management of Flail Chest

Tamas F. Molnar and Szilard Rendeki

Abstract Optimal treatment of flail chest (FC), a serial and multilocular fracture of three or more adjacent ribs (+/− sternum) is challenged by changes in major trauma profiles. Pneumatic stabilization is the gold standard, while surgical interventions challenge the status quo. A review was performed of 2008–2013 Medline and PubMed data pool. The quality of evidences is moderate, the recommendations for osteosynthesis are conditional. FC patients already ventilator dependent with moderate lung contusion might be considered for surgery. Osteosynthesis is justified in FC during thoracotomy for other reason. Definitions of FC subgroups and operative details in future randomized controlled trial (RCTs) are mandatory.

Keywords Flail chest • Rib fracture • Chest trauma • Blunt thoracic injury

Introduction

Flail chest (FC) [1, 2], occasionally referred as "stove-in chest" or "crushed chest" [3], is a special scenario of serial costal fracture where at least three tandem ribs are broken in two or more places resulting in a floating segment of musculo-osteal complex [4]. A rare phenomenon is when the ribs are broken or dislodged at the costochondral junctions on both sides of the sternum, resulting in a breastplate-shaped disruption and leading to paradoxical movement of the sternum causing similar pathophysiologic consequences to lateral flail chest [5]. Four to ten percent of all hospitalized trauma patients have some sort of rib fractures [6–8]. In 30–75 % of all

The authors have no conflicts of interest to disclose

T.F. Molnar, MD, DSci (✉) • S. Rendeki, MD
Department of Operational Medicine, Faculty of Medicine, University of Pécs,
Ifjusag u 13, Pécs, Hungary
e-mail: tfmolnar@gmail.com

M.K. Ferguson (ed.), *Difficult Decisions in Thoracic Surgery*,
Difficult Decisions in Surgery: An Evidence-Based Approach 1,
DOI 10.1007/978-1-4471-6404-3_59, © Springer-Verlag London 2014

blunt trauma cases some pulmonary contusion/acute lung injury is present [6, 9]. Eighty to eighty-five percent of the severe lung contusion patients with associated extended bony chest wall injury require ventilatory support. In multiple trauma patients, the chest component greatly impacts management and the survival of these individuals. Ten to fifteen of all major blunt chest trauma causes flail chest with a mortality ranging between 8 and 20 % [6, 7, 10]. Road traffic accidents are responsible for more than three-fourths of flail chest injuries with a mortality of 5–36 % [4]. In a large reported trauma series of flail chest cases from Greece, 250 cases were seen over 12 years [10] while in another report found 262 FC among 11,966 chest injuries. Flail chest is observed in an average tertiary care/level I trauma center 10–30 times a year. Separation of a segment of the rib(sternum)-intercostal tissue unit from the rest of the thoracic musculo-osteal complex cage challenges different therapeutic concepts and provides grounds for discussing different theoretical approaches [11–13].

Flail chest is a combined injury of the osteomuscular complex of the chest wall and the underlying lung parenchyma. Basically there are two different therapeutic approaches: conservative treatment (non-operative) and aggressive intervention (surgical solution) [14–17]. At the present time, internal pneumatic stabilization (ventilation) is the gold standard, while a new wave of surgical intervention challenges the status quo [18]. While the surgical restoration of osteal continuity seems to be a fair aim, the supposed benefit to the ventilatory dynamics and the consecutive gas exchange is less convincing [19]. Orthopedic and trauma surgeons focus on the bony chest cage where dislodged rib edges should be fused, while intensive therapists see the injured bone as the roof above the main problem: injured lung parenchyma. Thoracic surgeons see chest wall as an interwoven structure where bones and muscles maintain integrity and support each other. The question is whether proper gas exchange within the pulmonary parenchyma does require restoration of chest cage integrity or not? There are excellent reviews on the road leading to where we are today [20–22]. Past publications on different therapeutic modalities applied to this pathology show a pendulum pattern between the two divergent concepts of ventilation and surgical reconstruction.

Search Strategy

A computerized search was performed using the Medline and PubMed databases focusing on English language literature for the period 2008–2013. The reference list was expanded where it seemed appropriate. PICO formatting information assisted in defining the addressed question: what are the available data for treatment outcomes for flail chest? "P" for patient/population was identified by keywords: "chest/thoracic injured/chest/thoracic trauma patient, flail chest". Additional PICO terms used apart from flail chest were: "pulmonary contusion", "rib fracture". Search for "I" for interventions was divided into "rib/chest wall osteosynthesis/fixation" vs. "ventilation/pneumatic stabilization/conservative treatment". Search for "C" for

Comparison was performed according to the same dichotomy. Finally, as "O" for outcome: "survival, death, complications, hospital stay, days on ventilator" terms were used. Hub term: "flail chest" yielded 620 items in PubMed. The following extensions were applied to the key terms: "surgery/ stabilization/ management/ treatment." Special attention was paid to the two extremes of the publication horizon: meta-analysis and technical papers/case reports. Four review/meta-analysis articles (R/MA), one randomized controlled trial RCT, four cohort studies (CS) and three case-control studies (CCS) and three extremely relevant observational series (OS) were harvested. Case studies, technical descriptions (n=37), all of them detailed in the individual reference lists of our primary sources (R/MA,RCT,CS. CCS,OS), were included as relevant but a priori biased sources, totalling up to 52 items of the source pool.

Results

The amount of published data on flail chest which should define or at least have a weighty impact on clinical decision making of the daily clinical routine is surprisingly small and their quality is far from satisfactory. There is only one randomized clinical trial (RCT) published in the last 5 years [18]; therefore two further studies published earlier had to be implemented in order to create a minimally acceptable data pool [1, 23] (Table 59.1). Marasco et al. presented their RCT on flail chest involving 23 patients in each arm in 2013 [18]. They enrolled multitrauma patients already ventilator dependent without hope of weaning within the following 48 h. The patients of the surgical arm had a superior outcome to the ventilatory group in length of ICU stay (285 h vs 319 h) but not in the duration of invasive mechanical ventilation. Surgical approach included fixing one fracture per rib, thus converting the flail segment to simple fracture, using resorbable plates with bicortical screws. Noninvasive ventilation after extubation was definitely shorter in the surgical arm (3 vs 50 h). Follow up lung function and quality of life did not differ in the two groups. Secondary endpoints included pneumonia, pneumothorax, drainage, readmission to ICU, and hospital stay, without significant differences between the two groups. Tracheostomy was required more frequently in the nonoperative group (70 % vs 39 %) However there was an average cost saving of 14,443 USD per patient who was operatively treated in Australia. Equally important advantage was an extra 5 day ICU bed availability per operated patient. The two other randomized studies coming from Japan [23] and Egypt/Germany [1] published in 2002 and 2005 respectively had altogether 77 cases in both arms and had provided moderate evidence according to the GRADE approach [24]. Both papers suffer from serious selection bias. The comparator conservative group of FC in the paper of Granetzny et al. received strapping and elastoplast packing, a heavily outdated method even in 2005 [1]. Reduced times on ventilator and related ICU stay, less frequency of pneumonia and superior postoperative lung functions favored the surgical solution in these two limited value RCT series.

Table 59.1 Main evidence for/against surgery in flail chest

Study/year/type	Patients ventilation vs. surgery	Outcome classification	Advantage of surgery	Authors' notes	Quality of evidence
Marasco et al. [18] (2013/RCT)	23/23	DV, DICU, DHS, RC, Tr'y M, failed extubation, cost	DICU, RC(P) Tr'y, cost	(+) Patient selection, absorbable plates	High
Granetzny et al. [1] (2005/RCT)	20/20	DV, DICU, DHS, RC, M CWD, LF	DV, DICU, DHS LF	(−) Outdated conservative treatment, 7/20 vs 9/20 pts ventilated	Moderate
Tanaka et al. [23] (2002/RCT)	18/19	DV, DICU, RC, Try' M	DV, DICU RC(P), Tr'y	(−) No invasive pain control/ obligatory ventilation	Moderate
Leinicke et al. [25] (2013/R/MA)	319/219	DV, DICU, DHS, RC, Tr'y, M	DV, DICU, DHS, RC(P), Try', M	(−) Mixed database on RCT, CS, CCS	Moderate
Slobogean et al. [26] (2013/R/MA)	Total of 753	DV, DICU, DHS, RC, Tr'y, M, CWD, pain	DV, DICU, DHS, RC(P), Tr'y, M CWD	(−) Wide range of techniques, study period span: 1972–2008	Low
Bhatnagar et al. [27] (2012/R/MA)	Unknown see (US) National Trauma Data Bank v.5.0	DV, DHS RC(P), Tr'y M sepsis, cost intubation	DV, DHS, cost	(−) Missing source data	Low
deMoya et al. [29] 2011/CC	32/16	DV, DICU, DHS, RC, M Pain	Pain (need of narcotics/ relief)	(+) Measure/match of lung contusion	Moderate
Althausen et al. [30] 2011/CC	28/22	DV, DICU, DHS, RC Tr'y	DV, DHS RC(P)	Short admission/op interval	Moderate
Balci et al. [38] (2004/CS)	37/27	DV,DHS, Tr'y, M, pain	DV,DHS, Tr'y, M, pain	Short admission/op interval	Moderate
Nirula et al. [39] (2006/CC)	30/30	DV, DICU, DHS	DV, DICU, DHS	(+) Prospective surgical arm	Moderate
Demirhan et al. [40] (2009/OS)	72/0	M	Mortality for FC: 11.1 %	One armed observation on a significant number of cases	Low
Cannon et al. [22] (2012/OS)	162/2	Ma	Mortality for FC 9.1 %	Significant number of cases (+) Measure of lung contusion	Low
Athanassiadi et al. [10] 2010/OS	244/6	DV, DHS	Mortality for FC 8.8 %	Significant number of cases (+) Measure of lung contusion and inclusion of ISS	Low

Abbreviations: *CCS* Case control study, *CS* Cohort study, *CWD* Chest Wall deformity, *DV* Duration of artificial ventilation, *DICU* Duration of days in Intensive care unit/ICU bed occupancy, *DHS* Duration of hospital stay, *ISS* Injury Severity Score, *FC* Flail Chest, *LF* Lung function compromise, *M* mortality, *OS* Observational series, *pts* patients, *RC* Respiratory complications, *RC(P)* respiratory complication: pneumonia, *RCT* randomized controlled trial, *R/MA* review/ meta-analysis articles (R/MA), *Tr'y* tracheostomy

Considering the scarcity of good quality primary source data there is a surprisingly vast amount of review papers and meta-analysis on flail chest. There are four important review-like papers on the topic [16, 25–27]. The most comprehensive of all is of the practice management guideline for flail chest of the Eastern Association for Surgery of the Trauma published in 2012 [16]. The literature research process yielded 37 studies published between 2005 and 2011. It replaces the previous guideline, which provided evidences for the practice 7 years ago, based on 92 studies published between 1966 and 2005 [28]. The new answer to the old question, is there a role for surgical fixation of flail chest injuries, has remained the same: yes, in certain cases. The conditional recommendations according to the GRADE approach [28] are that surgical fixation may be considered in cases of severe FC failing to wean from the ventilator. Prophylactic fracture fixation was discouraged as no benefit has been identified so far. "On the way out" osteosynthesis was included in the Recommendations [16].

A systemic review and meta-analysis of Leinicke et al. published in 2013 on 9 studies (2 RCT, 4 CS, 3 CCS) have evaluated the outcome of 538 cases [25]. There was a benefit of surgery vs pneumatic stabilization in duration of mechanical ventilation (4.52 days) and intensive care bed occupancy (3.4 days) evident in the pooled database. Relative risk (RR) for tracheostomy was 0.25 in the operative group. Statistical differences support a surgical approach for decreased mortality (RR:0.44) and pneumonia (RR:0.45), but vast heterogeneity and patient allocation in the sources cast a shadow on the validity of the observations. The paper had strong and adequate statistical power but the pre-selection bias dominating the patient pool (n: 459) seriously limited the clinical applicability of the message.

Another meta-analysis by Slobogean et al. in 2013 harvested nearly the same database [26]. The authors omitted the article of de Moya et al. from 2011 [29] focusing on pain in FC and of Althausen et al.[30] on locked plate fixation, two case-control studies considered in Leinecke's analysis. In comparison with Leinecke's work, Slobeogean et al. created a pool of 753 cases of which only 100 participated in publication in the new millennium having added the series of Borelly (n=176) [31], Kim (n=63) [32] Ohreser (n=14) [33] and Teng (n=60) [34]. One third of the cases was treated more than 30 years ago. The paper reports an advantage for surgical fixation in ventilator days (8 day difference) and pneumonia (odds ratio: 0.2). A decrease in intensive care bed occupancy (5 days) mortality (odds ratio: 0.31) septicemia (odds ratio: 0.36) and tracheostomy (odds ratio: 0.06) were also calculated. The extremely long time span and the heterogeneity of the pooled data counterweight the advantages of the analysis.

Bhatnagar et al. promising in their 2012 paper a focused look at the FC problem utilizing sophisticated statistical methods [27]. The message of their Markov model driven paper is clearly in favor of rib fracture fixation, however their utilized database is actually not visible to the average reader. Coding bias influencing their calculation based on US National Trauma Data Bank and shortcomings of primary reports detailed above make the paper unsuitable for bedside problem solving. Open reduction and internal fixation of ribs for flail chest in a clinically blind budget oriented analysis represents the most cost effective strategy by $8,400 USD. The main benefit of this paper is the letter to the editor of Paydar et al. [35] who are calling for a proper chest wall injury classification to be able to identify the very subset of patients who really might benefit from surgical approach.

There are two further papers to be mentioned here as they contribute to the present debate in a significant amount and manner. Nirula and Mayberry summarize the ruling opinions on potential indications for selective operative rib fracture in their paper with 116 references [36]. Open chest defects and pulmonary hernia are supported by case series. Decision for surgery in FC in cases of non-healing ribs and "thoracotomy on the way out" is supported by case series but the expert opinion is divided. Reduction of acute pain and disability are no go areas: unproven and controversial. Lafferty et al. in their 2011 current concepts review on chest wall injuries [37] concludes that there are occasional scenarios where osteosynthesis of broken ribs should be considered. The reference list is 103 items long. The operative indications in their interpretation are always relative. The individualized decision should be optimized to the pattern of rib fracture, the patient's overall status (age, comorbidities etc.).

There are five non-randomized observational studies [29, 30, 34, 38, 39] in the last decade suggesting that hazily defined subset of patients might benefit from surgery in terms of pneumonia and other ventilation related complications. These advanced audit like retrospective studies are bravely arguing for osteosynthesis without contextualizing their own results with respect to non-surgical alternatives i.e. pneumatic stabilization by different ventilatory strategies (invasive and non-invasive methods). On the other hand Athanassiadi and colleagues [10] in their well balanced and sober analysis of 250 flail chest injuries published in 2010 identified the high Injury Severity Score (ISS) value as the most significant prognostic factor. One hundred and five of their patients (42 %) had isolated flail chest, none of them was operated on. In addition, the resort to mechanical ventilation was not found to be necessary to achieve positive outcome [10]. The authors performed six operative stabilization "on the way out" of the 11/250 patients, who required thoracotomy for other reason. It worth to mention, that this paper of vast case number is missing from all the meta-analyses discussed above. Similar conservative attitude is reported in another observational study from Turkey in 2009, where 4205 chest trauma cases were analyzed [40]. None of their 72 flail chest patients (1.7 %) seen over 10 years of experience was operated on. Similarly, only 1.3 % of 154 flail chest patients required surgical stabilization in the series of Cannon et al. between 2001 and 2010 [22]. Their highly conservative approach resulted in a 9.1 % FC-related mortality.

Further papers highlight the importance of lung contusion/acute lung injury in outcome. As early as in 1997 the milestone study of Voggenreter et al. [41] emphasized the importance of the lung contusion in the outcome of flail chest. It is worth mentioning that two recent overviews of the question also emphasize [4, 42] the definitive role of lung injury in the optimal treatment of chest wall injury, flail chest included. In spite of this warning neither the three RCTs nor the relevant cohort studies implemented this important cofactor into their analyses. This is one of the main reasons why their results and conclusions are received with some sort of doubt. Lung injury combined with rib fracture predicts respiratory failure where CT diagnosis has a definitive role [43]. In a series of 408 multiple rib fractures lung contusion was about ten times more frequent than flail chest (22 % vs 2.3 %) which latter required artificial ventilation but no surgery in eight cases out of the ten [44]. Pulmonary contusion and flail chest were recently identified as strong predictors of development of ARDS in trauma patients [45]. It is proven, that as lung contusion and resulting injury exceeds 20 % of total pulmonary parenchyma, the probability of the onset of ARDS sharply increases [46]. Chest CT in combination with the dynamic changes of blood gases are proper tailoring tools for measuring the 20–25 % threshold which excludes surgical fixation [47].

Conclusions

In conclusion, the quality of the primary data serving as basis for evidences is suboptimal. At least three major works [10, 22, 40], which provide a vast number of cases (476 in all) a strong evidence for the more conservative approach are missing from recent meta-analyses. The quality of evidences for surgical fixation of flail chest is moderate or low according to the GRADE system [24, 28]. The recommendations in treating flail chest surgically are conditional. Few reliable data are available, and some argue for a more extensive usage of osteosynthesis in this serious clinical picture without evidence-based justification. What is clear from the reviewed papers, and no further studies are required is that in case of flail chest aggressive physiotherapy, invasive pain control and as a minimum requirement high intensity observation are needed.

Recommendations

Flail chest patients who are already ventilator dependent with up to moderate lung contusion (<25 % of surface) without expected weaning in 48 h, might be considered for rib osteosynthesis using absorbable implants. Rib fixation is justified in flail chest where thoracotomy is performed for other reason.

A Personal View of the Data

The authors' personal view is based on their perception of the development of present status of the treatment of FC/lung contusion and on the technical details of the surgical solutions. Therefore a short review of both questions is unavoidable before the definitive opinion is presented. Till the 1970s paradoxical chest wall movement was thought to be responsible for the respiratory insufficiency observed in patients with flail chest [20]. The advent of artificial ventilation brought the importance of lung contusion into the focus [48]. Internal or pneumatic stabilization with continuously evolving artificial ventilation strategies [49], optimization of intravascular fluid, pain relief, and aggressive physiotherapy became the ruling concept [5, 12].

As for the technicalities concerned, there are four concepts for osteosynthesis of broken ribs [36, 37, 42]:

(a) Cerclage using wiring/approximating stitches, which provides semi rigid apposition of the injured part or using mesh in a carpet-like fashion. Vertical bridging belongs to this group, as the implants bridge the floating segment with the intact part of the thoracic cage. Abrams rod, Nuss plates and derivatives, methyl-methacrylate prosthesis, rib grafts are also reported.
(b) Pericostal plates: Judet and U plates and their variations are struts provided with tongs to grasp the bone. Plates made of metal have alternatives of absorbable materials [50]. Dynamic compression osteosynthesis with plates and bicortical screws has been considered gold standard.
(c) Intraosseal methods: intramedullary nailing, usage of pins.
(d) Combined methods applying plates with cerclage or bicortical (locking) screws.

The dynamic concept (a) stemming from chest surgery favors anchoring the floating segments is opposed by bone-axis driven osteosynthesis-centric orthopedic ones (b, c, d) that promote tight compression and rigid fixation. Both styles have strong theoretical arguments and the literature proves that both solutions are workable in their own context. The normal breathing with a frequency of 12–18/min is a strong argument against stable fixation such as intramedullary device, screws or plate application. Wire breakage, screw dislodgement and plate fracture/dislocation are not rare. Osteomyelitis and metal piece migration are warnings that foreign bodies even made of high tech materials cannot be left in situ indefinitely just to spare costs.

It is obvious, that a properly planned RCT is required to convince the rather reluctant surgical and intensivist communities in the USA and Europe that there is opportunity to investigate operative fixation in flail chest [19]. The very first task is to create a clear and simple definition of subgroups of flail chest, an adjusted application of the principles of the TNM-like system already established in cancer surgery. Inclusion of extent and severity of lung injury is mandatory [35, 51]. Homogenization of techniques is only part of the question, as the principles are more important [52]. How many of the broken ribs should be unified? All of them, every second rib, or only the uppermost and the lowermost rib need fixation? Another question is if both ends of the ribs are to be osteosynthetized, or it is enough if the rolling door-like segment is anchored to the rest of the cage. Till we get answers to these questions, surgical reconstruction of flail chest cannot be considered as a potential solution for the problem, but as the problem itself.

Future clinical studies should focus also on implanted foreign bodies. It should be noted, that differently from other osteosynthesis indications, in the case of flail chest one needs only 1 or 2 weeks, till the integrity of the chest cage is regained, but the prosthesis stays there for long if not for good. Removal of metal plates is an independent event of hospital stay, risk and expenditure. A common methodological mistake is that ventilator time is compared in the two groups without referring to the simple fact, that this is the treatment itself in one arm. One has to calculate with the time/discomfort, narcosis and quality of life issues for a second surgery when and if the nonabsorbable plates/screws are to be removed. Definition of optimal timing of surgery also needs to agree upon. The injury-surgery time window varies between 2 and 10 days. The longer the waiting time is, the better the outcome with surgery is. While the worrying signs of respiratory insufficiency are well identified, there is little to help in selecting those patients who can be weaned within a short time, and even less to help in identifying those who are likely to develop ventilator related complications.

At the present time, we have a hazy picture of the optimal treatment of flail chest. Major trauma profiles are changing both in the civilian and the military environments [53]. Road traffic accidents, terror attacks on civilians and novel explosive techniques in modern asymmetric warfare are the main factors responsible for an ever increasing proportion of complex chest wall and lung injuries [54]. There are acceptable indications for osteosynthesis in order to restore chest wall stability [4]. Apart from fixation "on the way out" when thoracotomy is performed for another reason, chest wall stabilization might be justified for anterior flail chest using the minimally invasive Nuss method and similar techniques [55].

Clinical experience and the data presented support a cautious attitude, where surgical fixation is indicated in strictly limited circumstances, as detailed above. There is no reason to turn down the current standard of care for most of the flail chest cases, which favors upfront invasive pain control, aggressive physiotherapy and artificial ventilation if required. Other topics to be investigated are the appropriate principles for fluid management for patients with pulmonary contusions, details of sophisticated ventilatory support and non-invasive ventilatory strategies. Extracorporal lung support devices such as ECMO [extracorporeal membrane oxygenator] and pumpless lung assist systems represent new methods to consider when pro and con arguments for surgical stabilization of flail chest are at stake. Extensive underlying parenchymal derangements require PiCCO (pulse induced continuous cardiac output) monitoring [56]. Lung contusion and ISS remain the main prognostic factor and decisive elements when surgical stabilization is considered. Severe, radiologically identified injury exceeding 20–25 % of the lung surface contradicts operative intervention [4, 42]. These decisions definitely need a multidisciplinary approach where the intensivist and the thoracic surgeon are equal partners.

Whatever method adjusted to the actual situation and patient will be proven to be superior by RCTs, the innovative soul and bravery of the surgeon cannot be replaced by cold blooded protocols. Le Roux's short paper on a bygone case using fish hooks in a desperate case of FC is a herald coming from the past to teach the present [57].

Recommendations

- Flail chest patients who are ventilator dependent, with up to moderate lung contusion, and without the expectation of weaning in 48 h, might be considered for rib osteosynthesis using absorbable implants. (Evidence quality moderate; weak recommendation).
- Rib fixation is justified in flail chest where thoracotomy is performed for other reasons. (Evidence quality low; weak recommendation).

Acknowledgments Ms Veronika Martos – International Loan Services/University of Pécs Medical Library without whose generous help and unselfish contribution this manuscript would not have been realized.

Ms Andrea Varga for her generous contributions in the language editing.

References

1. Granetzny A, Abd El-Aal M, Emam E, Shalaby A, Boseila A. Surgical versus conservative treatment of flail chest evaluation of pulmonary status. J Thorac Cardiovasc Surg. 2005;4:583–7.
2. Freedland M, Wilson RF, Bender JS, Levison MA. The management of flail chest injury: factors affecting outcome. J Trauma. 1990;30(12):1460–8.
3. Bloomer R, Willett K, Pallister I. The stove-in chest: a complex flail chest injury. Injury. 2004;35(5):490–3.
4. Molnar TF. Surgical management of chest wall. Trauma Thorac Surg Clin. 2010;20(4):475–85.
5. Pettiford BL, Luketich JD, Landreneau RJ. The management of flail chest. Thorac Surg Clin. 2007;17(1):25–33.
6. Demirhan R, Onan B, Oz K, Halezeroglu S. Comprehensive analysis of 4205 patients with chest trauma: a 10-year experience. Interact Cardiovasc Thorac Surg. 2009;9:450–3.
7. Keel M, Meier C. Chest injuries – what is new? Curr Opin Crit Care. 2007;13:674–9.
8. Sirmali M, Türüt H, Topçu S, Gulhan E, Yazici U, Kaya S. A comprehensive analysis of traumatic rib fractures: morbidity, mortality and management. Eur J Cardiothorac Surg. 2003;24(1):133–8.
9. Engel C, Krieg JC, Madey SM, Long WB, Bottlang M. Operative chest wall fixation with osteosynthesis plates. J Trauma. 2005;58:181–6.
10. Athanassiadi K, Theakos N, Kalantzi N, Gerazounis M. Prognostic factors in flail-chest patients. Eur J Cardiothorac Surg. 2010;38(4):466–71.
11. O'Connor JV, Adamski J. The diagnosis and treatment of non-cardiac thoracic trauma. J R Army Med Corps. 2010;156(1):5–14.
12. Karmy-Jones R, Jurkovich GJ. Blunt chest trauma. Curr Probl Surg. 2004;41(3):211–380.
13. Hildebrand F, Giannoudis PV, van Griensven M, Zelle B, Ulmer B, Krettek C, et al. Management of polytraumatized patients with associated blunt chest trauma: a comparison of two European countries injury. Injury. 2005;36:293–302.
14. McGillicuddy D, Rosen P. Diagnostic dilemmas and current controversies in blunt chest trauma. Emerg Med Clin North Am. 2007;25(3):695–711.
15. Meredith JW, Hoth JJ. Thoracic trauma: when and how to intervene. Surg Clin N Am. 2007;87:95–118.
16. Simon B, Ebert J, Bokhari F, Capella J, Emhoff T, Hayward 3rd T, Eastern Association for the Surgery of Trauma, et al. Management of pulmonary contusion and flail chest: an Eastern Association for the surgery of trauma practice management guideline. J Trauma Acute Care Surg. 2012;73(5 Suppl 4):S351–61.
17. Slobogean GP, MacPherson CA, Sun T, Pelletier ME, Hameed SM. Surgical fixation vs nonoperative management of flail chest: a meta-analysis. J Am Coll Surg. 2013;216(2):302–11. e1.
18. Marasco SF, Davies AR, Cooper J, Varma D, Bennett V, Nevill R, Lee G, Bailey M, Fitzgerald M. Prospective randomized controlled trial of operative rib fixation in traumatic flail chest. J Am Coll Surg. 2013;216(5):924–32.
19. Mayberry JC, Ham LB, Schipper PH, Ellis TJ, Mullins RJ. Surveyed opinion of American trauma, orthopedic, and thoracic surgeons on rib and sternal fracture repair. J Trauma. 2009;66:875–9.
20. Bemelman M, Poeze M, Blokhuis TJ, Leenen LP. Historic overview of treatment techniques for rib fractures and flail chest. Eur J Trauma Emerg Surg. 2010;36(5):407–15.

21. Fitzpatrick DC, Denard PJ, Phelan D, Long WB, Madey SM, Bottlang M. Operative stabilization of flail chest injuries: review of literature and fixation options. Eur J Trauma Emerg Surg. 2010;36(5):427–33.
22. Cannon RM, Smith JW, Franklin GA, Harbrecht BG, Miller FB, Richardson JD. Flail chest injury: are we making any progress? Am Surg. 2012;78(4):398–402.
23. Tanaka H, Yukioka T, Yamaguti Y, Shimizu S, Goto H, Matsuda H, et al. Surgical stabilization or internal pneumatic stabilization? A prospective randomized study of management of severe flail chest patients. J Trauma. 2002;52:727–32; discussion: 732.
24. Brozek JL, Akl EA, Alonso-Coello P, Lang D, Jaeschke R, William JW, et al. Grading quality of evidence and strength of recommendations in clinical practice guidelines. An overview of the GRADE approach and grading quality of evidence about interventions. Allergy. 2009;64:669–77.
25. Leinecke JA, Elmore L, Freeman BD, Colditz GA. Operative management of rib fractures in the setting of flail chest a systematic review and meta-analysis. Ann Surg. 2013. doi:10.1097/SLA.0b013e3182895bb0. September Epub ahead of print.
26. Slobogan EA, MacPherson CA, Sun T, Pelletier ME, Hameed SM. Surgical fixation vs nonoperative management of flail chest: a meta-analysis. J Am Coll Surg. 2013;216:302–11.
27. Bhatnagar A, Mayberry J, Nirula R. Rib fracture fixation for flail chest: what is the benefit? J Am Coll Surg. 2012;215(2):201–5.
28. Brozek JL, Akl EA, Compalati E, Kreis J, Terracciano L, Fiocchi A, et al. Grading quality of evidence and strength of recommendations in clinical practice guidelines. The GRADE approach to developing recommendations. Allergy. 2011;66:588–95.
29. de Moya M, Bramos T, Agarwal S, Fikry K, Janjua S, King DR, et al. Pain as an indication for rib fixation: a bi-institutional pilot study. J Trauma. 2011;71(6):1750–4.
30. Althausen PL, Shannon S, Watts C, Thomas K, Bain MA, Coll D, et al. Early surgical stabilization of flail chest with locked plate fixation. J Orthop Trauma. 2011;25(11):641–7.
31. Borelly J, Aazami MH. New insights into the pathophysiology of flail segment: the implications of anterior serratus muscle in parietal failure. Eur J Cardiothorac Surg. 2005;28:742–9.
32. Kim M, Brutus P, Christides C, Dany F, Paris H, Gastinne H, et al. Résultats comparés du traitement des volets thoraciques: stabilisation pneumatique interne classique, nouvelle modalité de la ventilation artificielle, agrafage. J Chir. 1981;118(8–9):499–503.
33. Ohresser PH, Amoros JF, Leonardelli M, Sainty JM, Vanuxem P, Autran P, et al. Les sequelles functionelles de traumatismes fermes du thorax. Poumon Coeur. 1972;28(3):145–50.
34. Teng JP, Cheng YG, Ni D, Pan RH, Cheng YS, Zhu JZ. Outcomes of traumatic flail chest treated by operative fixation versus conservative approach. J Shanghai Jiaotong Univ (Med Sci). 2009;29:1495–8.
35. Paydar S, Mousavi SM, Niakan H, Abbasi HR, Bolandparvaz S. Appropriate management of flail chest needs proper injury classification. J Am Coll Surg. 2012;215(5):743–4.
36. Nirula R, Mayberry JC. Rib fracture fixation: controversies and technical challenges. Am Surg. 2010;76(8):793–802.
37. Lafferty PM, Anavian J, Will RE, Cole PA. Operative treatment of chest wall injuries: indications, technique, and outcomes. J Bone Joint Surg Am. 2011;93(1):97–110.
38. Balci AE, Eren S, Cakir O, Eren MN. Open fixation in flail chest: review of 64 patients. Asian Cardiovasc Thorac Ann. 2004;12:11–5.
39. Nirula R, Allen B, Layman R, Falimirski ME, Somberg LB. Rib fracture stabilization in patients sustaining blunt chest injury. Am Surg. 2006;72:307–9.
40. Demirhan R, Onan B, Halezeroglu S. Comprehensive analysis of 4205 patients with chest trauma: a ten-year experience. Interact Cardiovas Thorac Surg. 2009;9:450–3.
41. Voggenreiter G, Neudeck F, Aufinkolk M, Obertacke U, Schmit-Neuerburg K. Operative chest wall stabilization in flail chest-outcomes of patients with or without pulmonary contusion. J Am Coll Surg. 1998;187(2):130–8.
42. Bastos R, Calhoon JH, Baisden CE. Flail chest and pulmonary contusion. Semin Thorac Cardiovasc Surg. 2008;20:39–45.
43. Livingston DH, Shogan B, John P, Lavery RF. CT diagnosis of rib fracture and the prediction of acute respiratory failure. J Trauma. 2008;64(4):905–11.

44. Byun JH, Kim HY. factors affecting pneumonia occurring to patients with multiple rib fractures. Korean J Thorac Cardiovasc Surg. 2013;46:130–4.
45. Watkins TR, Nathens AB, Cooke CR, Psaty BM, Maier RV, Cuschieri J, et al. Acute respiratory distress syndrome after trauma: development and validation of a predictive model. Crit Care Med. 2012;40(8):2295–303.
46. Bakowitz M, Bruns B, McCunn M. Acute lung injury and the acute respiratory distress syndrome in the injured patient. Scand J Trauma Resusc Emerg Med. 2012;20:54.
47. de Moya MA, Manolakaki D, Chang Y, Amygdalos I, Gao F, Alam HB, et al. Blunt pulmonary contusion: admission computed tomography scan predicts mechanical ventilation. J Trauma. 2011;71(6):1543–7.
48. Trinkle JK, Richardson JD, Franz JL, Grover FL, Arom KV, Holmstrom FM. Management of flail chest without mechanical ventilation. Ann Thorac Surg. 1975;19(4):355–63.
49. Avery EE, Morch ET, Benson DW. Critically crushed chests: new methods of treatment with continuous mechanical hyperventilation to produce alkalotic apnea and internal pneumatic stabilization. J Thorac Surg. 1956;32:291–311.
50. Mayberry JC, Terhes JT, Ellis TJ, Wanek S, Mullins RJ. Absorbable plates for rib fracture repair: preliminary experience. J Trauma. 2003;55:835–9.
51. Kilic D, Findikcioglu A, Akin S, Akay TH, Kupeli E, Aribogan A, et al. Factors affecting morbidity and mortality in flail chest: comparison of anterior and lateral location. Thorac Cardiovasc Surg. 2011;59(1):45–8.
52. Paydar S, Mousavi SM, Akerdi AT. Flail chest: are common definition and management protocols still useful? Eur J Cardiothorac Surg. 2012;42(1):192.
53. Keneally R, Szpisjak D. Thoracic trauma in Iraq and Afghanistan. J Trauma Acute Care Surg. 2013;74(5):1292–7.
54. Propper BW, Gifford SM, Calhoon JH, McNeil JD. Wartime thoracic injury: perspectives in modern warfare. Ann Thorac Surg. 2010;89(4):1032–5; discussion 1035–6.
55. Pacheco PE, Orem AR, Vegunta RK, Anderson RC, Pearl RH. The novel use of Nuss bars for reconstruction of a massive flail chest. J Thorac Cardiovasc Surg. 2009;138(5):1239–40.
56. Oren-Grinberg A. The PiCCO monitor. Rev Int Anesthesiol Clin. 2010;48(1):57–85.
57. le Roex R. So many years ago. S Afr Med J. 2013;103(3):153.

Chapter 60
Management of Pectus Deformities in Adults

Marco Anile, Daniele Diso, Erino Angelo Rendina, and Federico Venuta

Abstract Management of chest wall deformities in adults is still controversial. Cosmetic and psychological problems along with cardiopulmonary derangement represent the main indications for surgical correction. Two surgical approaches are currently considered as viable options: open and minimally invasive repair. Both techniques have been modified during the years and show advantages and potential disadvantages with comparable results. The choice of the type of approach should be decided on the base of the morphology of deformity, functional aspects and surgeon's experience.

Keywords Pectus excavatum • Pectus carinatum • Chest wall deformities • Open approach • Minimally invasive repair • Recurrence

M. Anile, MD, PhD • D. Diso, MD, PhD
Department of Thoracic Surgery, University of Rome Sapienza,
Policlinico Umberto I Viale del Policlinico 155, 00161 Rome, Italy
e-mail: marco.anile@uniroma1.it; daniele.diso@uniroma1.it

E.A. Rendina, MD
Department of Thoracic Surgery, Sant'Andrea Hospital, University of Rome Sapienza,
Via di Grottarossa 1035, 00189 Rome, Italy

Eleonora Lorillard Spencer Cenci Foundation
e-mail: erinoangelo.rendina@uniroma1.it

F. Venuta, MD (✉)
Department of Thoracic Surgery, University of Rome Sapienza,
Policlinico Umberto I Viale del Policlinico 155, 00161 Rome, Italy

Eleonora Lorillard Spencer Cenci Foundation
e-mail: federico.venuta@uniroma1.it

M.K. Ferguson (ed.), *Difficult Decisions in Thoracic Surgery*,
Difficult Decisions in Surgery: An Evidence-Based Approach 1,
DOI 10.1007/978-1-4471-6404-3_60, © Springer-Verlag London 2014

Introduction

Pectus deformities (PD) include a wide spectrum of congenital chest wall malformations: they include pectus excavatum (PE), pectus carinatum (PC), Poland syndrome, pouter pigeon breast and sternal cleft. Based on the severity of the deformity, patients may present with different degrees of cardiopulmonary and vascular symptoms; however, usually these malformations are asymptomatic and have primarily esthetic implications. The most frequent malformations are PE and PC with a ratio of occurrence near to 12:1 and a threefold higher incidence in males [1].

The pathogenetic mechanism of both deformities is related to overgrowth of the costal cartilages; when it displaces the sternum posteriorly PE will be visible; in case of an anterior sternal dislocation PC will occur. Pectus carinatum is often recognized at adolescence while PE is almost always evident during the first years of life becoming progressively more severe during the growth. This different pattern of presentation allowed, in case of PE, the development of several theories regarding the best timing for surgical intervention; furthermore, the modifications of already consolidated treatments and the newly developed surgical techniques encouraged correction also in the pediatric population.

Historically, adolescence has been considered the more correct time for surgery [2]. In fact, a very early surgical correction (before the 4th year of life) has been advocated as the cause of the occurrence of the acquired restrictive thoracic dystrophy (acquired Jeune's disease); however, Robicsek [1] suggested that this adverse event is related due to inappropriate surgical technique; on the other hand primary PE correction in adults has often been taken into consideration only when associated with surgical treatment of a simultaneous cardiac disease. In adult patients, two new aspects have contributed to modify the surgical approach to this malformation: the increasing importance of cosmetic aspects and psychological implications (this often happens in subjects with minimal and totally asymptomatic deformities) and the development and worldwide acceptance of minimally invasive techniques; particularly, the latter contributed to reduce surgical trauma and postoperative discomfort with a shorter postoperative course and satisfactory esthetic results. In addition, in adults functional aspects are also crucial since in this subgroup of patients chest wall deformities might be associated with cardiopulmonary impairment.

Search Strategy

A Medline and Pubmed search was conducted with search terms [pectus deformities], [pectus excavatum], [pectus carinatum] AND [adults] AND [surgical repair] AND [recurrence]. English language articles published during the last 20 years (1993–2013) were included; a total of 406 papers were identified and 20 of them were selected and included as references. All papers were original articles or reviews; no case reports were considered.

Overview

Patient Assessment

Patients with PD require an accurate preoperative evaluation. Cardiac assessment is crucial because of the frequent association with the Marfan syndrome; systolic murmurs and mitral valve prolapse are often present [3]. Standard electrocardiogram shows the potential presence of arrhythmias and signs of ischemia. Echocardiography helps to evaluate the degree of sternum compression on the heart with quantification of the diastolic filling; it also evaluates valves anatomy and function (particularly the mitral and aortic valve). Because cardiac anatomy might be difficult to assess by routine transthoracic echocardiography, transesophageal echocardiography could be performed either preoperatively or during surgery [4]. Furthermore, in these patients a careful evaluation of global cardiac performance is mandatory to rule out coronary artery disease [5].

Pulmonary function tests should also be performed. A restrictive disorder due to a chest wall stiffness and decreased lung volumes relative to sternal compression are often present in case of PE; an obstructive disease may rarely occur in patients with PC because of chest wall enlargement and consequent lung parenchyma over-expansion [6].

Cardiopulmonary exercise test with the quantification of oxygen uptake (VO_2 max) under effort has gained importance. In this group of patients there is often an impairment of exercise tolerance with reduced aerobic capacity due to cardiovascular abnormalities and less frequently to pulmonary dysfunction [7]. However, differently from pulmonary surgery in which a low VO_2 max may contraindicate surgery, in these patients it may be a useful indicator for surgical repair and postoperative improvement is an excellent index to assess the objective benefit.

Radiological assessment is mandatory before surgery, in order to program the type of operation and to predict outcome. Currently, chest computed tomography (CT) is considered the gold standard to quantify the severity of chest wall deformity and the dislocation and compression of the heart and lungs. For both PE and PC there is a CT index (Haller index) [8] measured as the ratio between the antero-posterior and lateral chest diameters that quantify the degree of sternal depression or anterior displacement. For PE a CT index more than 3.2 identifies a severe degree of deformity; for PC there is not a widely accepted cutoff value, but in the majority of series the mean value of their patients was 1.9 [9, 10]. In a recent study, it has been evaluated whether the Haller index measured at chest x-ray correlated with CT before and after minimally invasive PE repair [11]; the authors showed that there was a strong correlation between these two techniques also during follow up and concluded that routine CT could not be required in this setting.

Indications

In the pediatric age the most frequent indication for surgical repair is esthetic impairment; in the adult population more importance is given to the severity of the deformity and the presence of symptoms; however, in a subgroup of patients with minor degree deformities, cosmetic concern remains a priority. As we have already reported, the severity of PE and PC calculated at CT is the most important morphological parameter to consider surgical correction [9]. This condition may be associated with paradoxical chest wall movement and chest pain potentially exacerbated by physical activity. Cardiopulmonary symptoms due to displacement or compression of the heart and lungs, such as palpitation, arrhythmia, dyspnea, low cardiopulmonary performance, are mainly related to the degree of PD and may be present at rest and/or during exertion. In patients affected by Marfan syndrome with mitral valve prolapse or patent foramen ovale or other cardiac abnormalities, the correction of PD is performed simultaneously with cardiac surgery. One challenging indication is the correction of recurrent PD, in particular PE. This event is reported with an incidence between 2 and 37 % and the majority of patients were treated by an open approach in the pediatric age [12, 13]. Liu et al. reported their experience in 18 patients undergoing resection by a minimally invasive approach with encouraging results [14].

Technical Aspects

The technical details of PD surgical correction underwent several modifications in the recent past. The subpericondrial resection of costal cartilages with sternal osteotomy proposed by Ravitch in 1949 for both deformities has been continuously modified [9, 10, 15, 16]. The skin incision, the extent of cartilage resection, the need of bar placement to support the sternum have been changed. Actually the open approach consists of a skin incision over the sternum (more often a transverse incision), mobilization of pectoralis major and rectus abdominis with resection of the xiphoid process, a subpericondrial resection of the involved costal cartilages, a transverse wedge osteotomy of the sternum and suture of the xiphoid process to the pericondrium of last two sternal ribs. In case of PC this is sufficient to warrant correction. In case of PE sternal elevation and healing may be obtained with different methods:

1. after osteotomy and section of the xiphoid process two sutures are carried through both sides of the xiphoid and around the right and left portions of the second rib. This maneuver allows relocation of the xiphoid process and rectus muscles under the sternum, keeping it elevated.
2. one or two thin stainless-steel bars are placed below the sternum after the osteotomy and sutured to the ribs on both sides.
3. after osteotomy and section of the xiphoid process the sternum is freed and bent upward; Marlex mesh is placed below the sternum and sutured to the resected costal cartilages; the xiphoid process is sutured to the mesh [1].

Open Approaches

The open approach has been recommended for patients with complex defects (often PE and PC are associated) or asymmetric deformities. The way to stabilize the sternum in the correct position is usually a surgeon's personal choice according to his experience and preference. However, the crucial principle of this technique is represented by the subpericondrial resection of the involved costal cartilages with careful and meticulous preservation of pericondrium; this allows an intact pericondrial bed to guide cartilaginous regeneration.

Minimally Invasive Approach

In 1998 Nuss proposed a new minimally invasive approach to repair PE in children [17]; this technique has rapidly gained acceptance and several studies reported a growing experience in adults. The Nuss procedure is performed by inserting behind the sternum a molded U-curved bar that subsequently is rotated with inversion of the U shape. The bar edges are fixed to the ribs with stitches or dedicated anchorage systems. This technique underwent several modifications to make it safer. In fact, the retrosternal passage of the bar was originally blindly performed after mediastinal dissection with a custom made dissector. For these reasons, the videothoracoscopic approach has been introduced with enormous advantages in terms of safety and decrease in operative time. In the adult population placement of two bars is often required to obtain a satisfactory correction and it is mandatory to fix them with stabilizers to avoid displacement [18]. The advantages reported with this technique are clearly cosmetic (skin incision), reduction of operative time and blood loss, absence of cartilage resection and osteotomy with reduced postoperative pain and risk of infection. Symmetrical deformities are the best indications for this technique, even if it has been proposed also to treat recurrent PE and also in association with cardiac surgery. After 2 years the bar(s) is usually removed.

Outcomes

Results

The international literature reports satisfactory results with PD surgical repair. In the case of PE, outcomes with the open approach and the minimally invasive technique are comparable in terms of cosmetic and functional results. In fact, a limited transverse skin incision with the open approach (usually in the submammary sulcus) allows an acceptable esthetic result similar to the lateral mid-axillary incisions required by the Nuss procedure. Correction of the deformity is achieved in the majority of patients with both techniques as reported in Table 60.1. Placement of two bars with the minimally invasive approach allows better distribution of the

Table 60.1 Surgical outcomes for pectus deformities repair

Author	Year	N°	Age	Approach	PD	PR (%)	Compl. (%)	Recur.	FUP (ms)
Mansour et al. [5]	2003	77	22	Open	PE+PC	91	14.3	1	12
Fonkalsrud et al. [9]	2002	116	30	Open	PE+PC	96.5	22	2	51.6
Wurtz et al. [10]	2012	205	25	Open	PE+PC	97.5	8.3	1	24
Fonkalsrud and Mendoza [15]	2006	275	19.8	Open[a]	PE+PC	98.1	2.9	2	17
Jaroszewski and Fonkalsrud [21]	2007	320	27	Open	PE+PC	98	4.6	6	26
Hebra [20]	2006	30	23	MIRPE	PE	86	29	n/a	n/a
Park et al. [19]	2011	102	19	MIRPE	PE	n/a	20	n/a	n/a
Liu et al. [14]	2012	18	21	MIRPE	Rec.PE	100	50	0	19

Legend: *PD* pectus deformity, *PR* positive results, *Compl.* complications, *Recur.* recurrence, *FUP(ms)* follow-up in months, *PE* pectus excavatum, *PC* pectus carinatum, *Rec.PE* recurrent pectus excavatum
[a]minimally open approach

remodeling forces with minor probability of bar displacement. From the functional point of view, symptom relief and improvement in performance status is reported in all series. Recently, a prospective study showed that in 70 patients with a mean age of 27 years cardiopulmonary exercise tests clearly improved at 6 and 12 months after surgery for PE with a modified Ravitch procedure. This report pointed out for the first time that improvement was not related to changes in lung function but in aerobic capacity with increased cardiovascular adaptation at maximal workload [7].

Complications

A number of complications are reported equally with both techniques: pneumothorax, pleural effusions, pericarditis, bleeding, seroma, skin infection, and persistent chest pain. Bar displacement is a dreadful complication almost exclusive to the minimally invasive approach; its incidence has changed during the years because of the routine use of stabilizers with a reduction from 9.5 to 2.5 % [18, 19]. The incidence of recurrence is different with the minimally invasive and the open approaches: with the former the incidence is low, ranging between 2 and 5 % [18–20]; with the open approach it is higher with a large variability (1.3–37 %) [5, 9, 21] probably due to an imprecise subpericondrial resection.

Conclusions

Surgical treatment of PD in adults is a challenge for thoracic surgeons. The two most widely used surgical techniques result in satisfactory functional and cosmetic results when the correct indications are followed; the morbidity rate is low. Although data reported in the literature are limited and no large comparative studies are present, we can recommend these two approaches for symptomatic patients with a high chance to obtain relief of symptoms and improvement of cardiopulmonary performance.

A Personal View of the Data

Management of PD in adults is still a controversial issue and indications are mainly related to patient discomfort. For complex deformities in symptomatic adults the modified open approach allows us to obtain encouraging cosmetic and functional results. For PE elevation it is generally necessary to use bars; in young patients with symmetric deformities the minimally invasive approach may be a viable option even if no long term follow up data are reported yet. Use of stabilizers is mandatory to avoid bar displacement.

Recommendation

- We recommend either open or minimally invasive approaches for correction of pectus deformities in symptomatic patients; both have a high chance of providing relief of symptoms and improvement of cardiopulmonary performance. (Evidence quality low; weak recommendation)

References

1. Robicsek F, Watts LT, Fokin AA. Surgical repair of pectus excavatum and carinatum. Semin Thorac Cardiovasc Surg. 2009;21:64–75.
2. Frantz FW. Indications and guidelines for pectus excavatum repair. Curr Opin Paediatry. 2011;23:486–91.
3. Kelly Jr RE. Pectus excavatum: historical background, clinical picture, preoperative evaluation and criteria for operation. Semin Pediatr Surg. 2008;17:181–93.
4. Krueger T, Chassot P, Chritodoulou M, Cheng C, Ris HB, Magnusson L. Cardiac function assessed by transesophageal echocardiography during pectus excavatum repair. Ann Thorac Surg. 2010;89:232–9.
5. Mansour KA, Thourani VH, Odessey EA, Durham MM, Miller JI, Miller DL. Thirty-year experience with repair of pectus deformities in adults. Ann Thorac Surg. 2003;76:391–5.
6. Malek MH, Fonkalsrud EW, Cooper CB. Ventilatory and cardiovascular response to exercise in patients with pectus excavatum. Chest. 2003;124:870–82.
7. Neviere R, Montaigne D, Benhamed L, Catto M, Edme JL, Matran R, et al. Cardiopulmonary response following surgical repair of pectus excavatum in adult patients. Eur J Cardiothorac Surg. 2011;40:e77–82.
8. Haller JA, Kramer SS, Lietman SA. Use of CT scans in selection of patients for pectus excavatum surgery: a preliminary report. J Pediatr Surg. 1987;22:904–6.
9. Fonkalsrud EW, DeUgarte D, Choi E. Repair of pectus excavatum and carinatum deformities in 116 adults. Ann Surg. 2002;236:304–14.

774   M. Anile et al.

10. Wurtz A, Rousse N, Benhamned L, Conti M, Hysi I, Pinçon C, et al. Simplified open repair for anterior chest wall deformities. Analysis of results in 205 patients. Orthop Traumatol Surg Res. 2012;98:319–26.
11. Wu T, Huang T, Hsu HH, Lee SC, Tzao C, Chang H, et al. Usefulness of chest images for the assessment of pectus excavatum before and after a Nuss repair in adults. Eur J Cardiothorac Surg. 2013;43:283–7.
12. Yüksel M, Bostanci K, Evman S. Minimally invasive repair after inefficient open surgery for pectus excavatum. Eur J Cardiothorac Surg. 2011;40:625–9.
13. Antonoff MB, Saltzman DA, Hess DJ, Acton RD. Retrospective review of reoperative pectus excavatum repairs. J Pediatr Surg. 2010;45:200–5.
14. Liu J, Zhu S, Xu B. Early results of 18 adults following a modified Nuss operation for recurrent pectus excavatum. Eur J Cardiothorac Surg. 2013;43:279–82.
15. Fonkalsrud EW, Mendoza J. Open repair of pectus excavatum and carinatum deformities with minimal cartilage resection. Am J Surg. 2006;191:779–84.
16. Masaoka A, Kondo S, Sasaki S, Hara F, Mizuno T, Yamakawa Y, et al. Thirty years experience of open repair surgery for pectus excavatum: development of a metal-free procedure. Eur J Cardiothorac Surg. 2012;41:329–34.
17. Nuss D, Kelly Jr RE, Croitoru DP, Katz ME. A 10-year review of a minimally invasive technique for the correction of pectus excavatum. J Pediatr Surg. 1998;33:545–52.
18. Hebra A. Minimally invasive repair of pectus excavatum. Semin Thorac Cardiovasc Surg. 2009;21:76–84.
19. Park HJ, Jeong JY, Kim KT, Choi YH. Hinge reinforcement plate for adult pectus excavatum repair: a novel tool for the prevention of intercostal muscle strip. Interact Cardiovasc Thorac Surg. 2011;12:687–91.
20. Hebra A, Jacobs JP, Feliz A, Arenas J, Moore CB, Larson S. Minimally invasive repair of pectus excavatum in adult patients. Am Surg. 2006;72:837–42.
21. Jaroszewski DE, Fonkalsrud EW. Repair of pectus chest deformities in 320 adult patients: 21 year experience. Ann Thorac Surg. 2007;84:429–33.

Index

CPSIA information can be obtained
at www.ICGtesting.com
Printed in the USA
LVHW06*2354020718
582513LV00001B/79/P

9 781447 164036